Mental Health Nursing

D1147944

For Churchill Livingstone:

Commissioning Editor: Jacqueline Curthoys
Project Manager: Gail Murray
Project Development Manager: Dinah Thom

Mental Health Nursing
An Evidence-based Approach

Edited by

Robert Newell BSc PhD RGN RMN RNT ENB650
Senior Lecturer, School of Healthcare Studies, Research Support Team, University of Leeds, UK

Kevin Gournay CBE MPhil PhD CPsychol AFBPsS FRCN RN
Professor of Psychiatric Nursing, Institute of Psychiatry, London, UK

Foreword by

Sir David Goldberg DM FRCP
Professor of Psychiatry, Institute of Psychiatry, London, UK

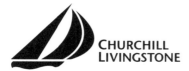
CHURCHILL
LIVINGSTONE

EDINBURGH LONDON NEW YORK PHILADELPHIA ST LOUIS SYDNEY TORONTO 2000

01152037

CHURCHILL LIVINGSTONE
An imprint of Harcourt Publishers Limited

© Harcourt Publishers Limited 2000

is a registered trademark of Harcourt Publishers Limited

The right of Robert Newell and Kevin Goumay to be
identified as authors of this work has been asserted by them
in accordance with the Copyright, Designs and Patents Act
1988

All rights reserved. No part of this publication may be
reproduced, stored in a retrieval system, or transmitted in
any form or by any means, electronic, mechanical,
photocopying, recording or otherwise, without either the
prior permission of the publishers (Harcourt Publishers
Limited, Robert Stevenson House, 1–3 Baxter's Place,
Leith Walk, Edinburgh EH1 3AF), or a licence permitting
restricted copying in the United Kingdom issued by the
Copyright Licensing Agency, 90 Tottenham Court Road,
London W1P 0LP.

First published 2000
  Reprinted 2000

ISBN 0 443 05873 3

British Library Cataloguing in Publication Data
A catalogue record for this book is available from the British
Library

Library of Congress Cataloging in Publication Data
A catalog record for this book is available from the Library of
Congress

Note
Medical knowledge is constantly changing. As new
information becomes available, changes in treatment,
procedures, equipment and the use of drugs become
necessary. The editors, contributors and the publishers have,
as far as it is possible, taken care to ensure that the
information given in this text is accurate and up to date.
However, readers are strongly advised to confirm that the
information, especially with regard to drug usage, complies
with the latest legislation and standards of practice.

19 JAN 2001

The
publisher's
policy is to use
**paper manufactured
from sustainable forests**

Printed in China

Contents

Contributors **vii**

Foreword **ix**

Preface **xi**

Abbreviations **xiii**

1. Introduction **1**
   Robert Newell, Kevin Gournay

SECTION 1   Orienting material: the
background to care **9**

2. The consumer of mental health care **11**
   Peter Campbell

3. History of mental health nursing and
   psychiatry **27**
   Peter Nolan

4. Legal aspects of mental health nursing **49**
   Damian Mohan, David Carson, Pamela J. Taylor

5. Government policy and the organisation of
   mental health care **73**
   Kevin Gournay, Malcolm Rae

6. General consultation skills **79**
   Robert Newell

7. Principles of assessment **103**
   *Wendy Maphosa, Mike Slade, Graham
   Thornicroft*

8. Evaluation in mental health nursing **121**
   Derek Milne

SECTION 2   Mental health care: approaches to
client problems **145**

9. Schizophrenia **147**
   Kevin Gournay

10. Disorders of mood: depression and mania
    165
    Robert Gareth Hill, Geoff Shepherd

11. Suicide and self-harm **187**
    Sarah Kelly

12. Phobias and rituals **207**
    Kevin Gournay, Lindsey Denford

13. Somatisation and inappropriate illness
    behaviour **225**
    Trudie Chalder

14. Eating disorders **243**
    Janet Treasure, Gill Todd, Ulrike Schmidt

15. Anger and impulse control **265**
    Tracey Swaffer, Clive R. Hollin

16. Post-traumatic disorders **291**
    Karina Lovell, Sheena Liness

17. Children's and adolescents' difficulties **313**
    Richard Soppitt, Panos Vostanis

18. Mental disorders of older people **341**
    Peter Ashton, John Keady

SECTION 3   Mental health initiatives: new directions in mental health care **371**

19. Advocacy   **373**
    Bob Gates

20. Self-help initiatives   **391**
    Bhavna Tanna, Kevin Gournay

21. Alternatives to traditional mental health treatments   **405**
    Peter Huxley

Index   421

Contributors

Peter Ashton BA MSc RMN DipCBT CPNCert BPsychCert CertEd RNT
Senior Lecturer in Nursing, School of Nursing, University of Wales Bangor, Bangor, UK

Peter Campbell BA(Hons)
Freelance Writer and Trainer

David Carson LLB
Reader in Law and Behavioural Sciences, Faculty of Law, University of Southampton, Southampton, UK

Trudie Chalder MSc PhD ENB650 RMN SRN
Lecturer, Academic Department of Psychological Medicine, Institute of Psychiatry, London, UK

Lindsey Denford BEd(Hons) RMN RNT DipCBT HND ENB650 ENB620
Senior Tutor, Institute of Psychiatry, London, UK

Bob Gates MSc BEd(Hons) DipNurs(Lond) RNMH RMN CertEd RNT
Director, East Yorkshire Learning Disability Institute, University of Hull, Hull, UK

Kevin Gournay CBE MPhil PhD CPsychol AFBPsS FRCN RN
Professor of Psychiatric Nursing, Institute of Psychiatry, London, UK

Robert Gareth Hill BSc MSc MA PhD
Previously a Research Associate, The Sainsbury Centre for Mental Health, London. Completing a Doctorate in Clinical Psychology, University of Surrey, UK

Clive R. Hollin BSc PhD
Professor of Criminological Psychology, Centre for Applied Psychology, University of Leicester, Leicester, UK

Peter Huxley BA(Hons) MSc PhD CQSW
Professor of Psychiatric Social Work and Head of the School of Psychiatry and Behavioural Sciences, University of Manchester, Manchester, UK

John Keady RMN DipPP CertHEd RNT
Senior Lecturer in Nursing, School of Nursing, University of Wales Bangor, Bangor, UK

Sarah J. Kelly BA(Hons) RMN
Assistant Research and Development Coordinator, Dales, Hull, UK

Sheena Liness BA(Hons) RMN ENB650
Nurse Tutor, Behavioural Psychotherapy, Institute of Psychiatry, London, UK

Karina Lovell BA(Hons) MSc PhD RMN ENB650 PGDC(Ed)
Lecturer in Nursing, University of Manchester, UK

Wendy Maphosa BSc RMN Thom Dip
Nurse Specialist, PRSM, Institute of Psychiatry, London, UK

Derek Milne BSc MSc PhD DipClinPsych FBPsS
Centre for Applied Psychology, Newcastle University, Newcastle upon Tyne, UK

Damian Mohan MRCPsych
Lecturer in Forensic Psychiatry, University of Southampton, Southampton; Professorial Unit, Broadmoor Hospital, Crowthorne, UK

Rob Newell BSc PhD RGN RMN RNT ENB650
Senior Lecturer, School of Healthcare Studies, Research Support Team, University of Leeds, UK

Peter W. Nolan BA(Hons) MEd PhD RMN RGN DN RNT
Professor of Mental Health Nursing, School of Health Sciences, The Medical School, University of Birmingham, Birmingham, UK

Malcolm Rae OBE SRN RMN
Nursing Officer, Department of Health, London, UK

Ulrike Schmidt MPhil PhD MRCPsych
Consultant Psychiatrist, Eating Disorder Unit, Institute of Psychiatry, London, UK

Geoffrey Shepherd MPhil PhD
Previously Head of Service Planning, The Sainsbury Centre for Mental Health; Joint Chief Executive, The Health Advisory Service (HAS 2000); Chair in Psychiatric Rehabilitation, St Thomas's and Guy's Medical School, London, UK

Mike Slade BA BSc PsychD RMN CPsychol
Lecturer in Clinical Psychology, PRSM, Institute of Psychiatry, London, UK

Richard Soppitt MB ChB MRCPsych MMedSci
Consultant Child and Adolescent Psychiatrist, Northbrook Child and Family Centre, Solihull, UK

Tracey Swaffer BSc(Hons) PhD
Senior Lecturer in Psychology, School of Health and Social Sciences, University of Coventry, Coventry, UK

Bhavna Tanna PhD
Clinical Psychologist, Three Bridges Forensic Service, West London NHS Healthcare Trust, Ealing Hospital, London, UK

Pamela J. Taylor MB.BS MRCP FRCPsych
Professor of Special Hospital Psychiatry, Institute of Psychiatry, London; Honorary Consultant Forensic Psychiatrist, Broadmoor Hospital, Crowthorne; South London and Maudsley NHS Trust, UK

Graham Thornicroft BA(Hons) BS MB MA MSc PhD MRCPsych
Professor of Community Psychiatry and Director, PRSM, Institute of Psychiatry, London, UK

Gill Todd BH(Hons) RMN
Clinical Nurse Leader, The Gerald Russell Unit, Eating Disorders Unit, Bethlem Royal Hospital, Beckenham, UK

Janet Treasure PhD FRCPsych FRCP
Consultant Psychiatrist, Eating Disorder Unit, Institute of Psychiatry, London, UK

Panos Vostanis MB MD MRCPsych
Senior Lecturer in Child and Adolescent Psychiatry, University of Birmingham, Birmingham, UK

Foreword

Evidence-based medicine (EBM) has come to stay. Where previously doctors often relied upon precedent and received opinion, they are now expected to know whether a particular intervention is supported by evidence or not. In some ways, the practitioner of EBM is like Molière's 'Bourgeois Gentilhomme', who discovers that he has been speaking prose all his life without realising it. It is mistaken to believe that before EBM we ignored evidence, and it is certainly not the case that we have good evidence for everything that we still find ourselves having to do.

What is probably new is that the number of treatment trials have increased exponentially in recent years, and no one can be expected to have read all the papers published – even in a specialised field. The techniques of 'meta-analysis' have therefore been used to combine the results of a series of trials of a particular treatment, weighting each reported trial by the size of the population included in the trial, and excluding trials that do not reach specified scientific standards. Even here though, we can reach misleading conclusions, since trials reporting negative results are much less likely to be published than those reporting positive results. The editors of this book are aware of these shortcomings and discuss them in their opening chapter.

Nevertheless, well conducted meta-analyses are probably the best that we have at present,

and are certainly greatly preferable to the rules of thumb of eminent practitioners, however distinguished they may be. As you read through the chapters of this book, it will become apparent that although the era of EBM may have come, available facts still lag far behind what we would wish to have. In too many fields, the assertions are still based on received wisdom or on studies consisting of rather small numbers of patients. The great strength of EBM, however, is that it encourages students to be aware of the evidence base that exists for a particular assertion, so that they have a clear idea of which of their opinions are probably sound and which may well be revised in the course of their professional work.

In practice, we are often called upon to make decisions, or to embark on one line of management rather than another, in the absence of the sort of evidence that we all would like to have. EBM deals with groups of patients, but each reader of this volume will find themselves having to care for individual patients, who may well have characteristics that demand special attention. Evidence-based medicine may be the ultimate goal, but we may need to ask ourselves what the *patient-based evidence* is for a particular line of treatment, and to reconcile ourselves to the fact that we sometimes have no alternative but to rely on 'established wisdom'.

The arrival of nurse therapists has been one of

the most important advances that have occurred in my lifetime, in that it has transformed the role of the psychiatric nurse from mainly custodial and supportive to being the purveyor of active – and often highly effective – interventions. The cognitive–behavioural approach is referred to repeatedly and it is likely to set mental nursing on a new course in the next century.

This approach is still not taught to many of those who qualify as community psychiatric nurses (CPNs), and is still not practised by many established CPNs. Too many of the roles that a CPN is expected to perform involve the nurse in risk-taking and in pressurising reluctant patients to take medication: the low morale and high burn-out seen in inner-city community mental health services are the price we are paying for not having trained the workforce in a full range of skills, so allowing them to practise a much more satisfying profession. It is to be hoped that this book will assist tomorrow's nurses to become aware of the full potential of the profession that they are about to enter.

David Goldberg

Preface

We believe this first edition of *Mental Health Nursing: An Evidence-based Approach* represents an important departure from the usual way in which education and training in mental health nursing are resourced. We have avoided, where possible, the kind of evidence which used to be the staple of our clinical practice and which is still, unfortunately, present in much pre-registration training of mental health nurses, nurses in general and other health care professionals, including doctors: unsubstantiated opinion. This form of writing very often led to textbooks which relied on endless exhortations to the reader about apparent forms of best practice, which in fact had very little in the way of evidence behind them. Indeed, much of the problem arose simply from the *lack* of good available evidence and the requirement to address the needs of distressed people even in the absence of such evidence. This lack of evidence still remains throughout nursing, and mental health nursing is certainly no exception, although it must be noted that mental health nurses have, in the past, often been at the forefront of criticising care based on inadequate evidence, often to the detriment of their own careers.

The rise of the evidence-based care and clinical effectiveness movements is important to us as a profession, provided we are able to respond appropriately, because it will enable us to question inappropriate practice from a stronger knowledge base than ever before. In a clinical world in which nurses still have a level of therapeutic and administrative power that is considerably less than that of other clinicians, notably doctors, this knowledge base will form an extremely important part of our voice in fighting for more appropriate patient care. As nurses, we have wished, in recent years, increasingly to work alongside patients in their desire to have a say in the way in which their care is organised and delivered. The use of the best available evidence will help us to do so, and it is to be hoped that we will, as a profession, use this evidence to empower patients to insist on care which is based upon such evidence, rather than upon custom and practice.

This book is organised into three sections. In the first, we offer general *Orienting Material* that we expect will be a valuable general setting for some of the material which follows in the subsequent sections. The second section, *Mental Health Care*, is largely specific to particular client difficulties, and is the most extensive section of the book. It also contains material where a considerable amount of the evidence we seek in order to guide our care is available. In mental health, nurses and other practitioners have increasingly worked, both with each other and with clients, to introduce new approaches to care, and the final section, *Mental Health Initiatives*, addresses three key areas.

The book is intended principally for nurses, both at pre- and post-registration levels, and is aimed at colleagues with a wide range of academic backgrounds and qualifications. Since mental health care has been at the forefront of multidisciplinary working for many years, we expect there will be much here to interest non-nursing colleagues also. Contributing authors have organised their chapters so that general issues, including clinical features, interventions and evidence appear first, and are of common interest to all disciplines. The implications for nursing care are described later in the chapters, but will also be of interest to non-nurses, since the boundaries of care are becoming increasingly flexible.

Evidence-based care and clinical effectiveness are young initiatives in health care, and, quite correctly in the case of new initiatives, have begun to be subjected to criticism. For example, some medical practitioners have seen these approaches to care as threats to their clinical judgement, presumably because their existence might be expected to lead to a prescriptive attitude to care. Similarly in nursing, some commentators have suggested that evidence-based care is not client-centred, since it supposedly applies proven interventions to suitable client *groups*. As nurse behaviour therapists, we well remember these criticisms being levelled at ourselves and colleagues during the development of nurse therapy as a discipline, often by practitioners whose own therapeutic approaches had received little or no empirical support. We strongly refute both these suggestions; evidence-based care is a framework which is designed to support individual clinicians' decision-making in response to the unique profile offered by each client with whom we interact. Evidence-based care and clinical effectiveness provide the best possible evidence to enhance our decision-making, rather than supersede it. Since good information about efficacy reduces our reliance on custom, precedent and so-called expert opinion, it increases client-centredness, rather than reducing it.

Perhaps if we were to identify a single aim for this book, it would be the reduction of such reliance. In mental health care, our history is littered with ineffective treatments, many of which have done untold harm to clients. The role of nursing within mental health care has increased tremendously in recent years. With this greater role goes an increase in responsibility for our actions with clients. The practice of evidence-based care is at least as much about avoiding harm through inaction or inappropriate action as it is about appropriate intervention. In our experience, the single greatest concern of clients is whether the interventions which are being offered to them will be effective in addressing their life problems and, if so, when. As a profession, we must all be concerned with intervention outcome, because we owe it to clients to be able to answer this question with honesty and accuracy.

R. N.
K. G.

Leeds and London 2000

Abbreviations

AA	Alcoholics Anonymous
ACT	assertive community treatment
AD	Alzheimer's disease
ASW	approved social worker
BDI	Beck Depression Inventory
CAPO	Campaign Against Psychiatric Oppression
CBT	cognitive-behaviour therapy
CFS	chronic fatigue syndrome
CICB	Criminal Injuries Compensation Board
CMHT	community mental health team
CPA	Care Programme Approach
CPN	community psychiatric nurse
CPS	Crown Prosecution Service
CPT	cognitive processing therapy
DSH	deliberate self-harm
DSM	Diagnostic and Statistical Manual
EBP	evidence-based practice
ECT	electroconvulsive therapy
EE	expressed emotion
EMDR	eye movement desensitisation and reprocessing
GAD	generalised anxiety disorder
HBRS	Helper Behaviour Rating Scale
ICD	International Statistical Classification of Diseases and Related Health Problems
IED	intermittent explosive disorder
IMMEL	Index for Managing Memory Loss
MDF	Manic Depressive Fellowship
MHAC	Mental Health Act Commission
MHRT	Mental Health Review Tribunal
MIND	National Association for Mental Health
MMPI	Minnesota Multiphasic Personality Inventory
NAS	Novaco Anger Scale
NIMH	National Institute of Mental Health (USA)
PE	prolonged exposure
PTSD	post-traumatic stress disorder
RCT	randomised controlled trial
RMO	responsible medical officer
SANE	Schizophrenia A National Emergency
SDO	Supervised Discharge Order
SIT	stress inoculation training
SOAD	second opinion appointed doctor
SPSSB	Scale for Predicting Subsequent Suicidal Behaviour
STAXI	State-Trait Anger Expression Inventory
SUDS	subjective units of discomfort
VOC	validity of cognition

CHAPTER CONTENTS

Key points   1

The aim of this book   2

The nature of evidence-based practice and clinical effectiveness   3

The need for evidence-based care   5

Challenges to evidence-based care   5

About this book   6

Exercise   7

Key texts for further reading   7

References   7

1

Introduction

Robert Newell   Kevin Gournay

KEY POINTS

- This book addresses the need for evidence upon which to base mental health nursing practice.

- There should be no innovation without evaluation.

- Evidence-based care involves: production of evidence, making evidence available and using evidence.

- There are five generally accepted levels of evidence: systematic reviews, randomised controlled trials, non-randomised experimental studies, well-designed non-experimental studies and expert opinion.

- Evidence-based care aims to keep care up to date and thus optimise good practice.

- Adequate practice of evidence-based care requires good evidence and good appraisal skills.

- This book is aimed at students and practitioners at all levels of educational attainment and clinical experience.

THE AIM OF THIS BOOK

Mental Health Nursing: An Evidence-based Approach has the simple aim of responding to a pressing need within mental health nursing – the need for appropriate evidence upon which to base our clinical practice as nurses. This need is itself related to two further needs. Mental health nurses need to be in a position to participate fully within research and practice development initiatives in the multidisciplinary teams of which they form part. We also need to have a coherent, authoritative voice within the discipline of mental health care, contributing to the organisation and development of the discipline through participation in the National Health Service's (NHS) evidence-based practice, clinical efffectiveness and clinical governance agendas. Both contributing to research and practice development and developing a voice within the discipline require, from the outset, a grasp of the evidence which relates to our practice.

Taking the examples of research and practice development, it is immediately clear from an examination of proposals for funding that the interesting questions are invariably asked by those researchers, clinicians and managers who have a keen grasp of the relevant literature and how it relates to practice. This grasp gives relevance and clarity to the questions they pose. The same is true of reviews of services.

In terms of contributing to the direction of mental health services, it should be noted that nurses are, as in all elements of the NHS, the most numerous group. Moreover, we have the most frequent contact with patients and clients. Despite this, ours has not, in the past, been a strong voice within mental health care provision, and nurses are entirely familiar with the different levels of power possessed by different professions within the NHS. The evidence-based practice, clinical effectiveness and clinical governance

agendas offer an opportunity to change, because of the notion within these initiatives that care provision should be based on an allocation of resources according to effectiveness of the proposed care provided and adequacy of the systems for monitoring that care, rather than vested professional interests (Department of Health 1996, 1997; National Health Service Executive 1996). It is, however, unlikely that these initiatives will cause existing power structures to whither away. On the contrary, nurses may find the need for evidence particularly acute. Since ours is traditionally a less powerful profession, with a less developed research base, we may find that we, in particular, are judged by our grasp of the evidence. Moreover, that grasp may constitute our most important source of professional power (Newell 1997).

Since evidence is regarded as crucial to good mental health care, this book has attempted to assemble accounts of current good practice which are based on the best available evidence. As we shall see in Section 1, evidence comes at different levels of authoritativeness, at the very lowest of which is unsubstantiated opinion. In consequence, this book contains very little information of that lowest kind. Sometimes this has led to gaps in the content we have presented. For example, counselling in general practice for minor psychological disorders, relationship difficulties and other life crises appears to take up a considerable amount of mental health nursing time, yet a recent review found no definitive evidence for the effectiveness of counselling of this general sort (Centre for Dissemination and Reviews 1997). Similarly, some mental health nurses have introduced what are usually referred to as 'complementary' approaches, such as aromatherapy and massage, into their care. While this kind of expansion of the therapeutic armamentarium to be employed by nurses in their interactions with clients is potentially of considerable value, these initiatives are, alas, often introduced without adequate attempts to evaluate their effectiveness. We regard it as a useful general principle in clncal practice that there should be no innovation without evaluation, and have used this principle in deciding what areas should be included. As a rule, therefore, no subject areas are included where evidence for effectiveness is totally lacking, either because such studies that have been undertaken are negative in their findings, or because insufficient adequate studies have been undertaken. As a result, we can make no claims to comprehensiveness in the subject matter this book covers.

We have not, however, attempted to restrict the content of this book to work derived from randomised controlled trials (RCTs) – the supposed 'gold standard' of evidence-based practice. For one thing, an exclusive reliance on this form of evidence would considerably reduce the evidence base upon which much of mental health care currently relies. Moreover, the inclusion of RCTs alone would itself present a biased picture of the range of clinical practice for which research-based evidence is available. Finally, there are some areas of practice which are potentially so important that we have relied on comparatively modest evidence in order to indicate the direction in which research and practice are going. The chapters on advocacy and self-help are good examples of this. In all such areas, however, chapter authors have taken a critical approach to what is currently available.

Finally, we recognise that there are some areas where the definition of evidence is somewhat different from clinical practice. Much of the information in Section 1 – Orienting Material – is of this form. Thus, chapters which examine such issues as policy, law and consumer views draw on evidence which is different in form from much clinical evidence – evidence such as historical discussion, precedent and personal testimony.

However, as in the clinical chapters, the authors have examined their topics in a critical way. It is, perhaps, this attempt to present arguments in a way which is as transparent to the reader, and as considered and analytical as possible, which most accurately defines both the evidence-based practice movement and the intent of this book.

THE NATURE OF EVIDENCE-BASED PRACTICE AND CLINICAL EFFECTIVENESS

Evidence-based practice and clinical effectiveness are broadly similar terms, since both emphasise the importance of clinical practice which, when delivered to patients and clients, is effective in achieving health gain for them. However, evidence-based practice is the broader term, and includes not only clinical effectiveness (care which achieves health gain) but also cost-effectiveness (care which achieves this gain economically), dissemination (making effective care available to health care workers and to patients) and development of clinical guidelines (effective routine implementation of care which is known to be effective).

Muir Gray (1997) identifies three broad stages in the practice of evidence-based health care:

- production of evidence
- making evidence available
- using evidence (getting research into practice).

While producing evidence is predominantly the responsibility of researchers, making this evidence available is also a critical part of the researchers' role, and the importance of an appropriate dissemination strategy is emphasised by most grant-awarding bodies, since such strategies determine the eventual impact of the research undertaken. Indeed, in the case of secondary research, such as systematic reviews, the dissemination strategy is at least as important as other elements of the research. Moreover, the importance of dissemination in the practice of evidence-based care is now so widely recognised that there is considerable primary research activity aimed at evaluating the most effective methods of dissemination and implementation.

The third element – using research – is, of course, predominantly the responsibility of clinicians, in their daily contact with clients, and of managers, via the health policies they develop and implement. Clinicians and managers themselves need support, both through the provision of evidence-based information itself and through the provision of educational opportunities which empower them to appraise and use this information effectively. Accordingly, a number of initiatives, most notably the Cochrane Collaboration and the Centre for Reviews and Dissemination have attempted to collect, appraise and synthesise evidence related to key clinical topics, and to make these available to clinicians in a way which is readily understandable to them either without additional research training or with minimal additional educational input.

The evidence-based care movement is itself seen as an educational initiative and is described as a 'process of life-long, self-directed learning' (Sackett et al 1997). Clinicians are seen as responding to the clinical problems posed by patients and clients in a structured way which emphasises the search for and examination of the best available, relevant evidence. The process, shown in Box 1.1, is described as consisting of five phases through which clinicians address their information needs.

Readers will readily recognise this cycle as a problem-solving process similar to the nursing process. While we are concentrating here on evidence derived from research, it should be noted that clinical evidence derived from observation and diagnositic tests is also included in the appraisal process.

Box 1.1 The process of evidence-based care (adapted from Sackett et al 1997)

1. Converting information needs to answerable questions
2. Tracking down (with maximum efficiency) the best available evidence
3. Critically appraising that evidence for its validity and applicability
4. Applying the results of this appraisal in clinical practice
5. Evaluating performance

Evidence is regarded as being hierarchically organised in terms of its strength. Thus, the most reliable, valid evidence is thought to be that derived from systematic reviews of randomised controlled clinical trials, while the least useful is thought to be that derived from expert opinion (see Box 1.2).

Box 1.2 Levels of evidence (adapted from Muir Gray, 1997)

1. Strong evidence from at least one systematic review
2. Strong evidence from at least one randomised controlled trial of appropriate size
3. Evidence from well-designed non-randomised trials
4. Evidence from well-designed non-experimental studies from more than one research group or centre
5. Expert authority opinion or reports of expert committees

To the five levels in Box 1.2, we might easily add a further, still less reliable level: the opinion of other clinicians with whom we are in contact, who may or may not be experts in the field. Our own, personal, clinical opinions form even a further level of evidence, but it is difficult to place this level of evidence within the hierarchy. If the opinions are solely the product of clinical observations from within our own caseload, they may be very unreliable indeed, but many clinicians base their opinions on a complex synthesis of the six levels of evidence identified here. Indeed, the process of judging the applicability of research to our own clinical needs requires just such a complex synthesis. Nevertheless, clinicians often place considerable reliance on clinical experience alone. It is one of the tasks of practising evidence-based care to move away from this reliance.

THE NEED FOR EVIDENCE-BASED CARE

It might be argued that clinicians have always sought to practise the best possible care for their patients and clients. If this is so, we might wonder why there is any need for a new 'initiative' to bring this best practice into being. Nevertheless, Sackett et al (1997) suggest a number of compelling reasons for a formal approach to enhancing the ability of clinicians to deliver such effective care. First, new evidence and new forms of evidence are continually accruing. In particular, the rise in popularity of the RCT as the litmus test of treatment efficacy has the potential to exert considerable influence upon practice. However, there is a commensurate increase in the amount of time and effort required of clinicians who wish to keep up to date with this increase in available information. Second, this new information is not usually effectively disseminated into clinical practice. Third, as a result of the first two factors, the level of a clinician's up-to-date knowledge deteriorates over time. Since appropriate knowledge is thought to be associated with the provision of good care, the effectiveness of the clinician in practice will also deteriorate. Fourth, previous attempts to address this decline in currency of knowledge have not been effective. Finally, the three strategies of learning to practise evidence-based care, seeking and applying summaries of evidence-based care and accepting evidence-based clinical guidelines

have been shown, at least in the field of medicine, to keep clinical practice up to date.

CHALLENGES TO EVIDENCE-BASED CARE

Lest it be thought that the use of evidence in the pursuit of effective care is unproblematic, there are a number of difficulties in the practice of evidence-based care. First, there are practical problems of access to appropriate evidence. Consider the case of the nurse working in a primary care setting. In order to benefit adequately from the evidence-based care movement, the nurse must be able to have ready access to a library or other facility which contains appropriately compiled reviews of relevant research (such as those provided by the Centre for Reviews and Dissemination at York University). If the nurse works in an area (such as mental health) where few such reviews exist, the nurse must be able to access the original papers (which requires time and resources) and be able to appraise them appropriately (which requires training and experience). Finally, there may be insufficient original papers to appraise, particularly if a nursing perspective is sought. In mental health nursing, this is a particularly pressing need. Indeed, we have, in putting together this book, become aware of areas where the knowledge base is extremely thin.

Second, even if these practical problems of access could be overcome, work in evidence-based care is currently overwhelmingly biased towards RCTs, and, in many cases, meta-analyses of these RCTs. While such approaches are clearly powerful tools in the investigation of clinical practice, there is a danger that their distillation and dissemination to clinicians will result in an uncritical acceptance of their findings. This would be particularly unfortunate in mental health care, since we have the example of the

Smith & Glass (1977) meta-analysis, a review of the effects of psychotherapy which has been repeatedly cited both in the clinical effectiveness and evidence-based care literature and in the field of mental health care. The conclusion of this review (that all psychotherapies are roughly equal in effectiveness) has rarely been challenged, and has itself been repeatedly cited by advocates of all schools of psychotherapy. However, the critique of this review by Rachman & Wilson (1980) highlights numerous errors and biases in the original paper which have largely been ignored by later commentators, particularly those from a psychodynamic background. There is, therefore, no reason to suppose that the meta-analysis is in any way less susceptible to bias than any other form of review.

Since the existence of short, readable synopses of published research is not a guarantee of the excellence of the original research upon which they are based, such synopses may not be the shortcut to effective care which they appear to be. Readers of such synopses need the same ability to critically appraise what they read as do the researchers compiling such reviews, particularly in the field of mental health, where outcome research is often at an early stage, with a consequent reliance on the evidence of 'expert' clinicians. As we suggested earlier, nurses, who have only recently begun to be perceived as experts, need to be particularly vigilant in their examination of both primary research and reviews of such research. This vigilance itself requires access to training in appraisal skills.

ABOUT THIS BOOK

As we noted at the beginning of this chapter, this book is aimed at answering a need for appropriate evidence upon which to base practice. The need for evidence is the responsibility of all clinicians working in mental health care. In nursing,

we face serious challenges to our ability to provide high-quality, research-based care. Not least of these is the current position of research within the profession. It has been noted (Department of Health 1992) that there are deficits in the research capacity of nursing at every level – from pre-registration training to doctoral preparation and beyond. There is also a shortage of clinical researchers within nursing, and within the fields of primary care and mental health (Department of Health 1996). Moreover, despite the large clinical impact of nursing, most of the effort towards introducing evidence-based care has, so far, been directed towards medicine. We believe that textbooks for nursing in general, and for mental health nursing in particular, should break away from the traditional approaches of, on the one hand, prescribing a range of activities which nurses 'should' do, or, on the other, exploring countless elements of the nursing role, all without any noticeable appeal to evidence other than precedent and opinion.

Since there are deficits in research-based knowledge at all levels in nursing, this book is not aimed at any particular 'level' of practitioner. We have gone to some lengths to encourage contributors to write in a way which is accessible to *all* practitioners, regardless of their educational level or background, and we expect that students and clinical practitioners will all be able to gain from the contributions. At the same time, we have not imposed a particular 'house style' on contributors. People write differently, and we expect that readers will benefit from the change of pace from one chapter to another. Certainly, some contributors write in what would would generally be regarded as a more 'academic' or 'popular' style, and some chapters are more demanding of the reader than others. Once again, we have chosen to retain this diversity, and hope readers will find it both challenging and rewarding.

As far as possible, we have tried to offer evidence, rather than supplying assertion, and contributors have consciously avoided a prescriptive approach to what nurses 'should' do in clinical practice. Nevertheless, wherever possible, the implications for nursing practice are drawn by contributors. In keeping with the skills-based focus of this book, and the emphasis on evidence, we have included both practical exercises and key texts for further reading at the end of each chapter. There is a good deal to be gained simply from reading this material, and indeed, many of the authors are leaders in their fields. However, we hope that readers will also engage with the exercises as fully as possible. Most of the exercises have an experiential flavour which will help readers to get the most from the material and to apply it in their clinical practice. Similarly, the best way to practise evidence-based care is to become as confident and competent as possible in accessing, appraising and applying the evidence in clinical practice. We hope this book will contribute to your desire and ability to do so.

Exercise

In this chapter, a number of challenges to the practice of evidence-based care were identified. Which of these affect you most? Draw up an action plan which will help you to address these issues. Be sure to include your current strengths as well as needs. Ensure that your plan is truly practical. What will you do tomorrow to improve your ability to deliver evidence-based care?

KEY TEXTS FOR FURTHER READING

Muir Gray, J A 1997 Evidence-based healthcare: How to make health policy and management decisions. Churchill Livingstone, New York. *An excellent general introduction to the practice of evidence-based health care. Well written and accessible to the interested non-specialist reader.*

Sackett D L, Richardson W S, Rosenberg W, Haynes R B 1997 Evidence-based Medicine: How to Practice and Teach EBM. Churchill Livingstone, New York. *An excellent alternative to Muir Gray, with more of a focus on day-to-day clinical practice, but, as the title suggests, an almost exclusive concentration on medical care.*

Rachman S J, Wilson G T 1980 The effects of psychological therapy. Pergamon, Oxford. *An extended review of the effectiveness (or otherwise!) of a range of psychotherapeutic approaches. Particularly important for the rigour the authors bring to the examination of published research findings, and their comments about the process of psychotherapy research.*

Fonagy A, Roth P 1996 What works for whom. Guilford Press, New York. *A fairly comprehensive, recent review of effectiveness in psychotherapeutic approaches. This book is important because it is so comprehensive, but requires critical reading, since it is sometimes over-accepting of the claims of some therapeutic approaches.*

REFERENCES

Centre for Dissemination and Reviews 1997 Mental health promotion in high risk groups. Effective Health Care 3(3):1–10

Department of Health 1992 Report of the taskforce on the strategy for research in nursing, midwifery and health visiting. HMSO, London

Department of Health 1996 Research capacity strategy for the Department of Health and the NHS. A first statement. HMSO, London

Department of Health 1997 The new NHS. HMSO, London

Muir Gray J A 1997 Evidence-based healthcare: How to make health policy and management decisions. Churchill Livingstone, New York

National Health Service Executive 1996 Promoting clinical effectiveness: a framework for action in and through the NHS. NHS Executive, Leeds

Newell R J 1997 Editorial: Towards clinical effectiveness in nursing. Clinical Effectiveness in Nursing 1(1):1–2

Rachman S J, Wilson G T 1980 The effects of psychological therapy. Pergamon, Oxford

Sackett D L, Richardson W S, Rosenberg W, Haynes R B 1997 Evidence-based medicine: How to practice and teach EBM. Churchill Livingstone, New York

Smith M L, Glass G V 1977 Meta-analysis of psychotherapy outcome studies. American Psychologist 32:752–760

Orienting material: the background to care

SECTION CONTENTS

2. The consumer of mental health care 11

3. History of mental health nursing and psychiatry   27

4. Legal aspects of mental health nursing 49

5. Government policy and the organisation of mental health care   73

6. General consultation skills   79

7. Principles of assessment   103

8. Evaluation in mental health nursing 121

CHAPTER CONTENTS

Key points   11

Introduction   12

Recent changes in the status of mental patients
    within mental health services   13

Reasons for recent changes in the status of
    mental patients   15

Mental patients as individual consumers of
    mental health care   16

Limitations in the view of mental patients as
    consumers of mental health care   17

Beyond a view of mental patients as consumers
    of mental health care   19

Mental patients as providers of mental health care
    20

Mental patients as experts on madness   22

Mental patients as citizens   23

Implications for mental health nurses in the
    changing status of mental patients   24

Conclusion   25

Exercise   25

Key texts for further reading   26

References   26

2

The consumer of mental health care

Peter Campbell

KEY POINTS

- Questions about the status of mental patients have become vitally important as community care develops.

- Balance between care and custody will be central both to the future lives of community mental patients and the future work of mental health nurses.

- Mental patients are now in a position to influence rather than control services.

- Mental patients now have a presence as legitimate stakeholders in the process of shaping mental health service provision.

- Information, advocacy and the Care Programme Approach give opportunities to mental patients to become active consumers.

- The essential relationship of mental patient to services is not that of a conventional consumer.

- The compulsory element in care and lack of power to choose obstructs consumer status.

- Mental patients in society are more concerned with their status as citizens than as service users.

KEY POINTS (*contd*)

KEY POINTS (*contd*)

- After 10 years of consumer involvement, many service-user organisations would describe efforts to involve as tokenistic.

- Representation is a key issue clouding consultation.

- The idea of mental patients as providers of care remains controversial.

- Nurses who experience mental distress face problems in their profession.

- New understandings of mental illness are as important as new services.

- The majority of mental patients want to live an ordinary life in the community.

- It is possible that enthusiasm for the rights of mental patients has already passed its peak.

- The challenge for nurses and service-user organisations is to convert official rhetoric into concrete benefits for people using services.

INTRODUCTION

In the eyes of contemporary British society, the consumer of mental health care remains, first and foremost, a mental patient and mentally ill. Whatever designations we would rather choose, either as people with a mental illness diagnosis or as professionals trained in the care and treatment of people with such diagnoses, the reality is that the terms mental patient and mentally ill would be easily recognised, understood and accepted throughout our society in a way that the description 'consumer of mental health care' would never be.

The position of those diagnosed as mentally ill, both as recipients of mental health services and as participants in the wider community, is changeable and has changed substantially over the last 200 years. The pace of such change may now be accelerating. A century ago, as the asylum building programme continued and ever larger institutions overflowed with inmates for whom there were no cures and precious few treatments, the asylum dweller was widely seen as a degenerate element undermining the fabric and future of civilised society. Less than 60 years ago, the concept of 'life unworthy of life', advocated by the psychiatrist Alfred Hoche in 1920, justified the murder of hundreds of thousands of mental patients in Nazi Germany. Only within the last 30 years has the right of mental patients to consent to treatment become an issue for serious debate. Only within the last 15 years has the possibility of mental patients as agents of change within services been entertained. Although becoming a consumer of mental health care may still not imply an enviable status, it could be argued that we have come a long distance fairly quickly.

It could also be argued that a primary function of mental health nurses, indeed of all mental health professionals, is to secure further improvements in the status of the diagnosed mentally ill as a social group. But even if such a view is currently unfashionable and one believes that the crux of a nurse's work lies in the individual caring relationship with particular clients, the actual and potential status of those individuals within services and society is of vital importance. The destinies of the powerless are not just bound up in the progress of illnesses but are intimately constrained by who the majority deem them to be and by who they will allow them to become.

As we approach the end of the 20th century, questions about the status of mental patients may have reached a particularly sensitive point.

Some of the old certainties about their status and potential role have been dissolved by changing understandings and ideologies and by the existence of many people with a mental illness diagnosis in the community alongside the bulk of citizens. But, while there may be new possibilities opening up, it is by no means certain what destination these people will eventually achieve. Is the status of 'consumer of mental health care' a desirable and appropriate end-point of progress? Is it merely a staging post, perhaps on the way to better prospects, perhaps on a return journey to an inferior but more realistic position?

These are not idle questions. Community care will prove to be a failure unless it leads to the greater social participation of mental patients. But the terms on which such participation is to be established remain debatable. At a time when the Mental Health Act 1983 is criticised by prominent establishment spokespersons for swinging the pendulum too far in the direction of individual rights yet is resolutely defended by the majority of consumer organisations and when there is an obvious disjunction between official promotion of the diagnosed mentally ill as key agents in the development of community services and public perception of community mental patients as dangerous, destructive and unpredictable elements on the streets, we cannot afford to be complacent about the direction in which we are travelling. The balance between care and custody will be central both to the future lives of community mental patients and the future work of community mental health nurses.

RECENT CHANGES IN THE STATUS OF MENTAL PATIENTS WITHIN MENTAL HEALTH SERVICES

If the Mental Health Act 1983 can be viewed as a triumph for the idea of the mental patient as an individual possessing definable rights, the idea of a collective of mental patients as an essential creative agent in developing mental health services has been the product of subsequent years. There were few service-user organisations at the time when the Mental Health Act was being developed and it was little influenced by direct contributions from mental patients. The current recognition of mental health service users as legitimate stakeholders in service development was only just emerging. The 1985 House of Commons Social Services Select Committee Report on Community Care illustrates the transitional situation at that time, complaining on the one hand about the difficulty 'of hearing the authentic voice of the ultimate consumers of community care' and recommending that 'all agencies responsible ensure that plans for services are devised with as well as for mentally disabled people and their families' but at other points clearly focusing on the individual and on individual rights to be involved. Yet in 1986, the Disabled Persons (Services, Consultation and Representation) Act secured the involvement of disabled people in certain consultations and by the time of the NHS and Community Care Act 1990, the connection between involving service users collectively in local community care planning and the creation of appropriate services had been clearly established.

Mental patients now have the opportunity to take a much more active role within mental health services. Although the types of care and treatment available over the last 30 years may have changed comparatively little, the possibility for individuals to be involved in their own care has certainly improved in the last decade. In 1993, there was little or no independent advocacy available to enable mental patients to express their concerns more effectively. Now, partly as a result of the Mental Health Act 1983 itself, the provision of individual advocacy is extensive.

There is still no legal right to advocacy for informal patients. But the desirability of advocacy is now seldom challenged openly (Mental Health Task Force User Group 1994). At the same time, the introduction of the Care Programme Approach (CPA) from 1991 has increased the occasions on which mental patients can discuss their wants and needs. Although care planning and advocacy increase influence rather than secure control, in certain respects it may now be more appropriate to think of the individual mental patient as an active consumer of care rather than a passive recipient.

Involvement of mental patients in the general development of new and existing services is still restricted to a minority. Nevertheless, changes in this area of activity have been dramatic. Mechanisms for consulting consumers and consumer groups exist in almost every area and region of the country. Major mental health voluntary organisations like MIND (National Association for Mental Health) have established clear procedures to enable their campaigns to be directly influenced by the contributions of consumers. Individual mental patients and consumer organisations are employed by service providers as trainers and consultants. Few important conferences or seminars will omit a presentation of the consumer perspective on the topic under discussion and there is now a substantial literature by mental patients on community mental health issues. Although the capacity of mental patients to change the nature of mental health provision through collective action is open to question, their presence as legitimate and proactive stakeholders in the process can no longer be doubted (Barker & Peck 1996).

Between 1992 and 1994, the Mental Health Task Force, set up by the Department of Health as a small group to encourage the closure of large psychiatric institutions and to hasten their replacement with local community services, worked extensively with consumer groups in England. At the end of the initiative, a number of publications were produced by the Task Force User Group: Advocacy – A Code of Practice; Building on Experience. A training pack for mental health service users working as trainers, speakers and workshop facilitators; Guidelines for a Local Charter for Users of Mental Health Services.

In the mental health nursing sphere, the 1994 Report of the Mental Health Nursing Review Team 'Working in Partnership. A Collaborative Approach to Care' talks of the work of mental health nurses as 'starting and finishing' in the relationship with people who use services and includes, among its recommendations, the following:

> we recommend the representation and participation of people who use services and their carers on service planning, education and research groups

and

> we recommend that people who use services and their carers should participate in teaching and curriculum development.

The latter recommendation led the English National Board in 1996 to produce 'Learning from each other. The involvement of people who use services and their carers in education and training'. This practical document not only fulfils the work of the Mental Health Nursing Review but sees itself as meeting the NHS medium-term priorities for 1996 to 1997 'to give greater voice and influence to users of NHS services and their carers in their own care'. Alongside the two earlier examples of the collaborative approach, 'Learning from each other' shows not only that there has been a move beyond official rhetoric towards practical results but, in its close connection of consumer input into training with increasing influence over individual care, confirms that both in an ideological and a practical sense we have moved significantly beyond the 1985 House of Commons Social Services Select Committee Report.

REASONS FOR RECENT CHANGES IN THE STATUS OF MENTAL PATIENTS

The emergence of mental patients as consumers of mental health care with a right to greater involvement in shaping mental health services is the result of a complex interweaving of factors, some of which have been touched upon above. The emphasis on consumer and civil rights in the USA during the 1970s, extending to mental patients' rights and advocacy, contributed to the work surrounding development of the Mental Health Act 1983 and the emphasis on individual rights it secured. It could also be argued that a fundamental underlying factor has been the major change in lifestyle for mental patients since the 1950s as a result of the introduction of open door policies in psychiatric hospitals and the extensive development and use of psychiatric medications that assisted people with long-term problems to spend more time in the community and less in institutions (Barham 1992). The growth of action by independent consumer organisations in the 1980s may be related to the fact that by then there were substantial numbers of long-term mental patients who had spent most of their patient careers predominantly in the community, who were thus both keenly aware of their inferior status and able to do something about it and who, after 20 years or more of living with a mental illness diagnosis, had too little left to lose not to make the attempt.

Other important factors include:

The emphasis on consumer-led and consumer–orientated services. This is partly the result of dissatisfaction with the post-war welfare state that was intensified following the election of a Conservative government in 1979 with its continuing concern about the capacity of the welfare state to create dependency and its preference for mechanisms of the market. At the same time, concern about the quality and paternalism of services and increasing complaints from organisations of people in receipt of those services reinforced the need for different approaches and the realisation that only by consulting consumers could efficient and effective services be created.

The break-up of asylum-based systems of mental health care. This made the development of new approaches and services more likely. It also challenged the dominance of psychiatry within mental health care and encouraged the idea that people with other expertise (including even mental patients) might have a contribution to make. At the same time, certain groups of mental health professionals were becoming more organised and more assertive in challenging psychiatrists' hegemony. These groups were more open to new alliances. A number of independent consumer organisations were helped through their early stages of development by radical mental health workers including psychologists (Barker & Peck 1987).

Scepticism about professional expertise and the rise of self-help. Public awareness of the power and danger of medical technology has been accompanied by higher levels in understanding of and interest about psychological issues. While professional expertise has continued to be incapable of producing cures or often even clear-cut, positive outcomes for people with diagnosed mental illnesses, self-help initiatives have blossomed (not only in respect of mental health). This has been significant not only because there is a crossover between self-help and consumer action principles but because it has created the possibility for the direct experience of mental patients to be more positively valued in professional and public arenas.

Emergence of concern about equal opportunities. Action by women, black people and other minority groups to challenge discrimination has been reflected within services where the failure to provide equal access, equal treatment and appropriate services has been very clear.

The growth in action by disabled people, creating their own organisations and seeking to establish alternative services controlled by disabled people. This work is informed by a new social model of disability, emphasising the importance of social factors like discrimination, exclusion and oppression rather than individual impairments in producing disability.

The development, particularly since 1985, of organisations controlled by mental patients. Although partly the product of broader changes, these organisations have influenced the pace and direction of changes in the status of mental patients (Campbell 1996).

MENTAL PATIENTS AS INDIVIDUAL CONSUMERS OF MENTAL HEALTH CARE

A number of the general changes that have moved patients towards a more powerful position within mental health services have already been described. But any assessment of the true position and the extent to which it approaches the ideal of the consumer in other markets demands a more detailed examination of the day-to-day life of mental patients in the light of some of the major principles within consumerism: information, access, choice, redress and representation.

The quality and availability of information for mental patients whose first language is English have improved markedly in the last 15 years. It is now unusual for detained patients not to receive information about their rights and restrictions under the Mental Health Act. Written information about treatments, including electroconvulsive therapy (ECT) will usually be available and is often displayed in admission wards and other locations. As discharge approaches, patients may now receive individualised packs of information about services and opportunities in the local community. An increasing proportion of information is now produced in direct consultation with those who will be using it or by consumer organisations themselves. Although there continue to be difficulties around the balance of information to include in leaflets about psychiatric treatments – how full does full information about the negative effects of medication need to be? – there have been examples of successful and imaginative initiatives (Leader 1995). Mental patients do not have absolute rights to their records and in some services it may not be easy to gain access to them. Nevertheless, the introduction of client-held records (Stafford & Hannigan 1997) and the possibility of drug contracts (Mosher & Burti 1994) reveal the extent to which services are moving towards greater openness.

The increased power of mental patients is also visible in the provision of independent advocacy. Although the idea of advocacy is not novel to mental health professionals, it is only in the last decade that mental health services have moved away from an understanding of advocacy as something provided by nurses and social workers as part and parcel of their work to an acceptance of the need for advocacy undertaken by discrete agents and agencies that are independent of service provision. There is currently no coherent system of mental health advocacy covering the UK and services may vary significantly from area to area, both in terms of availability and in the quality and character of what is offered.

Comprehensive training programmes for advocates are still comparatively rare. Despite this, there can be little doubt that increasing numbers of mental patients have access to skilled support in their most important transactions within the health and social welfare system, whether these be with psychiatrist, social worker, benefits officer or nurse. In addition, there is evidence that greater emphasis on the principle of self-advocacy, whereby the advocate prioritises support for individuals to act for themselves and intervenes on their behalf only as a last resort, combined with commitment to promote the wishes of mental patients rather than their best interests, can produce a type of advocacy that more effectively gives the individual power as a consumer (Brandon 1995).

The mental patient's position as a consumer is currently grounded in the CPA introduced from 1991. This offers each individual important tools for exercising a meaningful influence within the care process: planning meetings with relevant professionals, a written and agreed care plan that is regularly monitored and an identified key-worker. In theory, such a mechanism could realise much of the desire for a consumer-led service. In practice, there must be significant reservations. Implementation of the CPA has been extremely slow and it is not yet a comprehensive system. Moreover, there is initial evidence that the process, which is anyway a means of targeting services and assessing needs rather than creating a greater range of services, does not itself give power to the consumer. An audit of care plans in one locality identifies a series of shortcomings, including divergence between the contents of care plans and assessments performed and a poor reflection of clients' own views within care plans (Perkins & Fisher 1996). Although the CPA promises greater sensitivity to consumers, attitude changes that could make such sensitivity a reality still seem to be absent.

LIMITATIONS IN THE VIEW OF MENTAL PATIENTS AS CONSUMERS OF MENTAL HEALTH CARE

Any presentation of the proposal that mental patients can be validly seen as consumers of care immediately encounters serious difficulties. In the first place, mental patients in the UK appear quite reluctant to describe themselves as consumers. This is particularly true of those involved in organisations controlled by people who use services where the term is seldom chosen, but is evident even among the wider constituency. When describing themselves in relationship to the services they use or to problems in their lives, people with a mental illness diagnosis are more likely to use their own diagnosis term or speak of themselves as service users, members, recipients or psychiatric system survivors. While self-description may not always have great significance and may be dictated by fashion, mental patients often have specific and coherent reasons for rejecting the status of consumer.

These objections tend to focus around two issues: the inappropriateness of the consumer model in capturing mental patients' essential relationship to services and the limitations inevitably imposed on any understanding of the lives of people diagnosed as mentally ill by the assumption that the most important aspects of their existence are bound up with consumption of care and treatment.

A member of the Campaign Against Psychiatric Oppression, a prominent survivor group in the early 1980s, once remarked that 'Survivors of the mental health system are no more consumers of mental health services than cockroaches are consumers of Rentokil' (Barker & Peck 1987). We should not overlook the unfortunate reality that the majority of people consuming mental health care are doing so out of necessity rather than choice and that they would reckon the opportunity to cease such consumption to be a most desirable goal. Nor can we ignore the significant and growing minority who are being legally compelled to consume various elements on the mental health care menu. The Mental Health Act 1983 allows mental patients to be detained for the purposes of treatment over substantial periods. Under certain circumstances, the Act permits people to be forced to receive exactly those treatments they have said they do not want. So-called consumers of mental health care can be locked alone in seclusion rooms and can be forcibly injected. Such interventions are regulated and there are opportunities for appeal and redress. But they hardly imply the freedoms and privileges normally attached to consumer status.

The compulsory element in mental health care has direct implications for the relationship between mental health nurses and mental patients and calls into question the usefulness of the consumer model in describing the status of service recipients whether they are detained in hospital under the Mental Health Act or not. The Mental Health (Patients in the Community) Act 1995 gives supervision order supervisors (who will often be community psychiatric nurses) power to convey their supervisees against their will to a defined place for treatment purposes. Section 5.4 of the Mental Health Act 1983 allows designated nurses to prevent informal mental patients from leaving hospital in order that an assessment for detention under the Act can be undertaken. While powers of this kind exist, it is perhaps understandable that so many mental patients question the reality of informal status. Even with the improvements outlined in the previous section, the power of individual mental patients is very limited. More and better quality information, independent advocacy and the CPA have not secured mental patients the power to choose. Unlike consumers in other markets, they

do not have the right to choose or withhold choice, to enter or exit the market. Focusing on the lives of people with a mental illness diagnosis as if they were pre-eminently consumers of care carries a real danger of totally missing the essential nature of their experience. A journey through a shopping mall and a journey through mental health services are simply worlds apart.

Whatever the power to choose may be, it is only meaningful to the extent that there are alternatives to choose between. Absence of choice has been a long-standing feature of mental health services which the movement towards consumer-led services and the development of internal markets in health were intended to address. While there is certainly greater awareness that certain parts of the service system offer a poor or even a reduced range of choices and that some important groups of consumers are receiving services that are demonstrably inappropriate to their real needs, progress to create new services has not been rapid and there is still a marked variation from area to area. Thus, although the need for 24-hour crisis services has moved from rhetoric to a firm place on most plans for comprehensive local services in the course of the last 10 years, many areas still are not providing them. In the last 15 years, the needs of black and ethnic minority groups have been increasingly highlighted and specialised services are beginning to be created for them (Huka 1996). But mainstream services remain insensitive to their needs and their passage through mental health services is often still significantly rougher and tougher than it is for the majority of mental patients. The particular needs of women are also now more directly addressed by services. Yet, in-patient facilities are often unsafe for women and the Patients' Charter Mental Health Services (1997) assures single sex accommodation and the choice of a health professional of your own gender as an expectation rather than a right.

Accompanying these major concerns about the choices currently available, must be a recognition of the frequent divergence between what mental health professionals think mental patients most need and what mental patients themselves think. Mental health care is a field of controversial treatments whose outcomes are rarely clear cut. In these circumstances, there is the possibility for genuine disagreements that cannot simply be attributed to the recipient's lack of insight. Yet even when research confirms differences in perceptions between groups of mental patients and groups of mental health nurses about the value of specific interventions, there is a tendency to attribute this to a lack of true understanding in the former rather than the erroneous priorities of the latter (Sharma, Carson & Berry 1992). One of the important shortcomings of a simple model of consumerism is that it overlooks that what is being discussed is not what the consumer wants but what the mental patient needs. The balance of power is completely different. Unlike the traditional consumer, the mental patient's capacity even to know what he or she wants is by definition fatally compromised. It is a final irony that the classic position of mental patients as consumers of care is to be always in the wrong rather than always right.

BEYOND A VIEW OF MENTAL PATIENTS AS CONSUMERS OF MENTAL HEALTH CARE

The relationship between mental patients and mental health services is evidently complicated and may not be easily captured in one concept. Although in a neutral sense mental patients can be seen as service users, their predicament while using services can perhaps be described as somewhere between that of recipients and that of consumers and moving slowly towards the latter status. That an increasing number of mental patients might now acknowledge their status as psychiatric system survivors merely underlines the powerful and complicated dynamics of a relationship where people can feel themselves to be consumed rather than consuming.

Yet a major part of the criticism of a consumer model relates not to its failure to accurately describe a relationship but to its focus on a limited and limiting aspect of mental patients' lives. Although service-user organisations have devoted much of their energies to changing mental health services and continue to define themselves in relation to such systems, they have also campaigned for a recognition of their potential role within society. Ultimately, their concern is with their status as citizens not as service users. In pursuit of these goals, service users have exploited alliances not only with mental health professionals but with oppressed groups in society and have worked both within and around the spirit of government initiatives to develop consumer-led services and, increasingly, in fields where more radical and challenging ideologies prevail.

Collective involvement of mental patients in shaping mental health services has, as we saw earlier, become an integral part of governmental efforts to develop community care. In a sense, such consultation has its roots in popular ideas of consumerism. But it also moves significantly beyond these ideas towards offering a proactive role in the management, planning and monitoring of services that would not usually be implied in other markets. Buying baked beans is unlikely to entitle you to a position in the Heinz boardroom.

The range of mechanism being used to consult with mental patients is extremely wide, from consumer surveys and questionnaires to the employment of groups as advisers to purchasers both in establishing contract specifications and monitoring their performance. In some services, particularly those run by voluntary organisations, mental patients will be involved on the management committee. In others, they may be involved in the selection process for new staff. In rare instances, mental patients have even been appointed to the boards of Mental Health Trusts. At the heart of these consultative initiatives are a variety of planning groups and committees where mental patients are recognised as legitimate stakeholders and provide representatives.

In many respects, these developments do indicate a remarkable shift in the focus of mental health service planning and mark the genuine arrival of a new partner in the consultative process. Nevertheless and perhaps inevitably at this relatively early stage, there are still significant gaps between ideals and reality. Many of the problems are not particularly related to the new partners being mental patients but revolve around practical difficulties in involving experts and non-experts that are common in all joint working of this kind. But there can be little doubt that the experiences and lives of mental patients do require a sensitive and flexible response from planning mechanisms and may require an investment of time, energy and money that service providers, planners and purchasers are not currently prepared to give. After 10 years of 'user involvement', many service-user organisations still characterise their participation as essentially tokenistic and this seems to relate to the degree of involvement on consultative groups (not enough representatives, decisions taken outside meetings), the amount of support for involvement (not enough time or information to prepare for meetings, no resources to help contact with own constituents) as well as to the results of involvement.

Representation is a key issue clouding all such consultation and is not openly addressed (Beresford & Campbell 1994). While there may be a divergence between two types of involvement (representation and direct participation), it is clear that much of the difficulty is caused by the rules for involvement being left unclear and the criteria for representativeness changing from area to area and from occasion to occasion in a manner that is frustrating and destructive to continuing partnerships. A recent review of involvement by mental health service users with social services departments following the NHS and Community Care Act indicates little evidence of power sharing with service users, limited commitment of resources to make further participation possible and, most significantly, confusion about the meaning and purpose of user involvement (Bowl 1996). Although government commitments to consumer-led services clearly imply the collective involvement of mental patients in planning and monitoring and the mechanisms to facilitate it are substantially in place, evidence of substantial shifts in attitude is disappointing.

MENTAL PATIENTS AS PROVIDERS OF MENTAL HEALTH CARE

No-one who has spent time on a psychiatric ward or who has listened to recently discharged acquaintances talking about how they received more help from fellow-patients than from nurses can remain unaware of mental patients' capacity to provide as well as consume mental health care. Recognition and promotion of self-help – the capacity of people with similar life experiences and problems to help each other and themselves – have been a major feature of health provision in the UK since the foundation of the NHS. In the late 1990s, it would be hard to find many psychiatric categories for which there was not a network of self-help groups. As a society we seem to have accepted, indeed to have endorsed with some enthusiasm, the possibility that direct personal experience can be a valuable therapeutic tool. Even so, the recognition that mental patients can make a contribution as paid mental health workers or can organise and run their own mental health services is a very recent development that remains highly controversial.

Although some people with a mental illness diagnosis have always been attracted to work within mental health services and have managed to do so, until recently this has been predominantly a secret activity. Only since the mid-1980s have mental health organisations – initially in the voluntary sector – placed advertisements that encouraged applications from current or former mental patients and positively valued such life experiences. At the same time, an increasing number of newly formed, independent, service-user organisations began to employ workers and to become involved in service provision, particularly in mental health advocacy where many paid workers now have direct experience of services. The direction in which we are travelling can be seen in the announcement in 1997 by the Pathfinder Trust in South London that it will actively seek to recruit people who have experienced mental health problems and that having had such problems will be seen as a desirable attribute in selection criteria. The Trust's target is to ensure that 10% of its 521-strong nursing workforce has experienced a mental health problem.

It can be convincingly argued that the role of mental patients in providing mental health services is comparatively small. The new purchasing arrangements that have been inadequate in expanding choice have so far failed particularly in respect of the most innovative projects. In the USA, some of the potential has been more fully realised. Not only are more services organised by mental patients themselves but schemes, like the Case Management Aides project in Denver, Colorado, enable mental patients to work as employees in mainstream services. Mental patients have provided their own drop-in and day-care services in the UK and there are plans for user-controlled crisis provision. But, at present, much of what mental patients are providing is not a real alternative to existing services or is on the periphery of mental health care – mental health advocacy, training and education.

The predicament of people with a mental illness diagnosis who are employed in mental health services remains unenviable and appears to be increasingly problematic the closer their direct involvement in providing care becomes. To succumb to mental illness still seems to be a fate worse than death, even for those professionals most intimately involved in the lives of those with such difficulties. Mental health nurses are by no means immune from this prejudice. In the wake of the Beverley Allitt case and the Clothier Inquiry Report recommendations, nursing journals like the *Nursing Times* have regularly featured letters and articles charting the discrimination encountered by nurses whose mental distress becomes public. It seems likely that most mental health professionals who experience mental distress do not feel able to be open about it at work and will take steps to conceal their problems. Such circumstances are tragic in themselves but they also raise fundamental questions: Is the status of the mental patient as a provider of care anything more than a comforting illusion? If the experience of mental illness is such a negative attribute among the nursing profession, on what basis do mental health nurses set out to care for those with a mental illness diagnosis?

Once again, the emergence of people with a mental illness diagnosis from the restraint of traditional mental patient status has produced a situation of confusion and contradictions where there is potential for progress but no clear sense of direction. The Clothier Inquiry Report (1994) recommendations included:

- No-one with evidence of a major personality disorder should be employed in the nursing profession.
- Further consideration should be given to proposals that any nursing applicant with excessive absence through sickness, excessive use of counselling or medical facilities or self-harming behaviour such as attempted suicide, self-laceration or eating disorder, should not be accepted for training until they have shown the ability to live without professional support and have been in stable employment for at least 2 years.

The English National Board for Nursing, Midwifery and Health Visiting in 'Learning from each other' (1996) states:

> People who use health care services and carers have a valuable contribution to make to the development of health services: they can work in partnership with health care professionals to ensure that health services are truly responsive to their needs. Equally people who use services and carers have an important contribution to make to pre- and post-registration, education and training…

These two quotations are not directly contradictory. But they certainly reveal very different assessments of the contribution that anyone with a mental illness diagnosis might hope to make. It might not be going too far to suggest that in their potential capacity to deliver care mental patients will always remain outsiders in the judgement of mental health professionals

MENTAL PATIENTS AS EXPERTS ON MADNESS

Whatever the preferred agenda of mental health professionals, the work of independent, service-user organisations in the UK has always focused as much on the experience of living with a mental illness diagnosis as on the consumption of care. Their starting point has often been profound dissatisfaction with medical explanations of madness and opposition to professional approaches that discount personal experiences of madness or relegate it to a very debased position in the hierarchy of acceptable evidence. For them, new understandings have been as important as new services.

The history of psychiatry has been filled with individual protests by madpersons challenging their treatment and setting out personal interpretations of their experiences (Porter 1987). These have increased in recent years (for reasons already outlined) and have been accompanied by collective initiatives to promote alternative, non-medical understandings. The National Self-Harm Network, growing out of conferences and publications by service-user organisations in the UK over the last 10 years, has promoted self-help and analysis based on direct experience (Pembroke 1995). The National Hearing Voices Network, based on work begun in the Netherlands, is now well established in this country and assists people to understand and live with hearing voices. As Baker (1995) describes:

> To date, very little has been written about this experience and its meaning, usually it is regarded as a symptom of mental illness and is not talked about because it is a socially stigmatising experience. The information in this booklet is based on research and practical work carried out in the Netherlands and the United Kingdom over the last ten years, which for the first time comes directly from the experts, the voice hearers themselves.

Such initiatives and the huge growth in literature devoted to the mental patient perspective worldwide are encouraging signs of diversity in debates about the nature and meaning of madness. But their significance should not be overstated. The content of an individual's psychotic episodes is still likely to be ignored or valued negatively. Many mental health nurses are trained not to 'collude' with a mental patient's delusions and some appear to believe that talking too much about these phenomena carries a risk of infection. While a minority of well-organised mental patients are winning an audience for their understandings among a minority of professionals, the majority who confront the service system in their isolation and distress must still fit their experiences into professionally sanctioned frameworks in order to gain credibility.

The assumption that the professional knows best dominates the delivery of mental health care. It is supported by the concept of insight which can be described with only a little unfairness as being the capacity of mental patients to agree with mental health professionals that not only is there something wrong but on the nature of what is wrong and the necessary treatment. Disagreement on any of these can be taken as lack of insight which in turn may not only be sufficient justification for discounting opposition but even ultimately for compulsory treatment. These are attitudes that place very significant obstacles in the way of anything but a narrow interpretation of consumer expertise and appear often to be structural rather than superficial.

It is important to make a clear distinction between the reception mental patients are likely to receive when they present their experience in using mental health services and when they present their understandings of their difficulties, particularly if these include new views of psychosis or other devalued experiences and behaviours. Mental health professionals may have been forced to make room for mental patients as partners in designing services, but they have scarcely begun to recognise the contribution of those with a mental illness diagnosis to debates on what mental illness really is.

MENTAL PATIENTS AS CITIZENS

In previous sections, we have been concentrating on the potential roles of mental patients in relation to services, whether as consumers or providers of care. This should not lead us to overlook the likelihood that it will always be a minority who are interested in the details of their relations with service systems or involvement in managing and running services. What primarily concerns the majority is the opportunity to live an ordinary life in the community. As moves towards comprehensive community care accelerate and increasingly allow a higher proportion of mental patients, even those with a diagnosis of long-term and enduring mental illness, to live most of their lives outside hospital locations, issues of social integration and equal citizenship are becoming central.

In their detailed study on the marginalisation of a group of long-term mental patients in the community, Barham & Hayward (1995) capture the uncertainty of society in the face of their new neighbours:

> mental patients may be more of a mystery today, living among us, than they were when hidden away in the asylum. We do not know them, because they are neither outside society in the world of exclusion, nor are they full citizens – individuals who are like the rest of us. Being neither self nor other, they are a new kind of social construction.

The terms on which mental patients are to be offered new participation in society are by no means decided but there are already indications that, in the absence of any coherent promotion of their case by government or professional organisations, the community mental patient may receive a disadvantageous settlement. Since the NHS and Community Care Act, the national media have featured a series of dramatic cases which have chronicled the supposed failure of community care for this group and promoted an awareness of its threat to fellow citizens, for example, Ben Silcock, who walked into the lions' den and Christopher Clunis, who killed a total stranger on an Underground station platform;

these are among the most notorious on a long list. Although a tiny proportion of mental patients are violent, it is perhaps not surprising that a recent study (Rose 1996) found that two-thirds of community mental patients interviewed believed the general public were definitely afraid of people with a mental health problem and a further 21% thought they sometimes were. Such perceptions are a recipe for isolation not integration.

The type of citizenship available to mental patients depends not only on the degree of shelter, support and occupational opportunity provided by community care services but on the attitudes that inspire those facilities and inform public opinion. It is possible that enthusiasm for the rights and the contribution of mental patients has already passed its peak. As Muijen (1996) writes:

> Whether one likes this or not, the priority in mental health care has fast become the safety of the public rather than the quality of life of 'victims of psychiatric oppression' less than a decade ago. The opinions of people clamouring for yet more places in secure units and yet more restrictive care in the community, as reflected by the Mental Health Act, can be seen and heard everywhere.

The introduction of the Disability Discrimination Act 1995 and continuing campaigns in support of full civil rights for disabled people can be seen as encouraging signs to set against the concerns expressed above. But the Act has particular shortcomings for people with mental health problems and it is certainly arguable that the special connection of incompetence and violence to people with a mental illness diagnosis may ultimately lead to a separation of this group from disabled people in general – in the public mind if not in legislation. As it is, mental patients now stand in a doubtful position, confronted by a society that cannot easily come to terms with the discovery that madness is not a permanent condition and that has not yet concluded whether community mental patients are essentially capable or incapable of making decisions like other citizens. In the meantime, advertising slogans like those of the prominent mental health charity SANE – 'You don't have to be mentally ill to suffer from mental illness' – are a reminder of the negative contribution mental patients are deemed to be making to society.

IMPLICATIONS FOR MENTAL HEALTH NURSES IN THE CHANGING STATUS OF MENTAL PATIENTS

The uncertain journey of those diagnosed as mentally ill away from a simple mental patient status has been accompanied and to some extent prompted by another journey from institution to community. It was perhaps inevitable that the initial reaction to the increased visibility of mental patients would create difficulties and that the cold welcome we are currently witnessing is a temporary phenomenon. Even so, it is hard to see how community care is ever going to become more than another barren dumping ground unless mental health nurses do more to challenge social attitudes and practices. A recent article (Hopton 1997) suggests:

> The most appropriate socialist–humanist response to a person's mental distress is to encourage and facilitate direct action against those social and political forces which have precipitated that distress. This will lead to a restoration and enhancement of creative potential, whereas traditional approaches promote a resigned acceptance of the status quo as being 'good enough if not ideal'.

Although this approach may have the practical support of a minority of nurses and goes some way beyond the boundaries of mental health consumerism, it is closely linked to many of the propositions of service-user organisations and at least acknowledges the long-term goals that some mental patients are now contemplating.

Even if wider change is considered to be outside the remit of mental health nurses, the transition from mental patient to consumer presents challenges to nursing practice. Mental health nurses must now be effective information-providers, prepared to work with independent advocates and even, on occasion, to consult with service-user representatives. It is likely that they will be increasingly asked to open their practice up to consumer scrutiny and to participate in consumer-led debates around awkward issues ranging from 'Why do nurses spend so much time in the nursing office?' to 'What makes a good mental health nurse?' Although mental health nurses still retain great power in the caring relationship with service users, the changes described in this chapter certainly imply a recognition that collaboration and mutual exchange should be the essence of this relationship rather than an expert–subordinate transaction. The experience of recent years suggests that open acknowledgement of the mental patient's expertise on madness as opposed to expertise on consuming services may be a long way off. On the other hand, the belief that we are involved in a dialogue rather than a monologue now seems quite secure.

CONCLUSION

People with a mental illness diagnosis are a low status group. None of the developments described in this chapter has altered the predominantly negative way in which society views mental patients. Social stigma is a commonplace of nurse training courses. It is no less real for all

that. At the same time, it is important to be cautious when assessing the increasing power of mental patients within services. While certain advances towards consumer status have been made with improved choice, information, access and redress, the consumer model remains inadequate in its failure to describe the essential powerlessness of mental patients in the face both of compulsory powers of the Mental Health Act and the system's enduring slowness to provide real choices either in services or understandings. What has changed is that service users (mental patients are no longer part of official language) have been recognised as essential partners in the planning and provision of community mental health services. The creation of consultative mechanisms and the enthusiastic response of small but significant numbers of service users, not just to consultation but to involvement in areas of training, education and research, do indicate a potential shift in the balance of power. The challenge for mental health nurses and service-user organisations is how to transform the good intentions and rhetoric of official documents into concrete benefits for people using services.

Exercise

How much do you know about service-user involvement in your local mental health services? Discover as much as you can about service-user action in your area. Identify your local service-user group, make contact with it and discover the nature and range of its activities. Are mental health nurses involved in working with service-user activists? Is there an advocacy service in your area? If so, make contact with it and find out what it does; if not, find out why.

KEY TEXTS FOR FURTHER READING

Chamberlin J 1988 On our own: patient-controlled alternatives to the mental health system. MIND, London

Romme M, Escher S 1993 Accepting voices. MIND, London

Rogers A, Pilgrim D, Lacey R 1993 Experiencing psychiatry: users' views of services. Macmillan/MIND, London

Barham P 1997 Closing the asylum: the mental patient in modern society, 2nd edn. Penguin, Harmondsworth

Read J, Reynolds J (eds) 1996 Speaking our minds: an anthology. Macmillan/Open University, London

REFERENCES

Baker P 1995 The voice inside. Hearing Voices Network, Manchester

Barham P 1992 Closing the asylum: The mental patient in modern society. Penguin, Harmondsworth

Barham P, Hayward R 1995 Relocating madness: From the mental patient to the person. Free Association Books, London

Barker I, Peck E 1987 Power in strange places: User empowerment in mental health services. Good Practices in Mental Health, London

Barker I, Peck E 1996 User empowerment – a decade of experience. Mental Health Review 1(4):5–13

Beresford P, Campbell J 1994 Disabled people, service users, user involvement and representation. Disability and Society 9(3):315–325

Bowl R 1996 Involving service users in mental health services: social services departments and the NHS and Community Care Act 1990. Journal of Mental Health 5(3):287–303

Brandon D 1995 Advocacy: Power to people with disabilities. Venture Press, Birmingham

Campbell P 1996 The history of the user movement in the United Kingdom. In: Heller T, Reynolds J, Gomm R, Muston R, Pattison S Mental health matters. Macmillan and Open University, London, ch 26, p 218

Clothier Inquiry Report 1994 aka The Allitt Inquiry: Report of the independent inquiry relating to the deaths and injuries on the children's ward at Grantham and Kesteven General Hospital during the period February to April 1991. HMSO, London

English National Board 1996 Learning from each other. The involvement of people who use services and their carers in education and training. English National Board for Nursing, Midwifery and Health Visiting, London

Hopton J 1997 Towards a critical theory of mental health nursing. Journal of Advanced Nursing 25: 492–500

Huka G 1996 The Sanctuary project. In: Tomlinson D, Carrier J (eds) Asylum in the community. Routledge, London, ch 10, p 207

Leader A 1995 Direct power: A resource pack for people who want to develop their own care plans and support networks. Brixton Community Sanctuary, Pavilion Publishing and MIND, London

Mental Health Task Force User Group 1994 Advocacy – A code of practice. Department of Health, London

Mosher L, Burti L 1994 Community mental health: A practical guide. W W Norton, New York

Muijen M 1996 Splendid isolation or dirty power? Breakthrough 2(4):3

Pembroke L 1995 Self harm: Perspectives from personal experience. Survivors Speak Out

Perkins R, Fisher N 1996 Beyond mere existence: the auditing of care plans. Journal of Mental Health 5(3):275–286

Porter R 1987 A social history of madness. Weidenfeld and Nicholson, London

Rose D 1996 Living in the community. Sainsbury Centre for Mental Health, London

Sharma T, Carson J, Berry C 1992 Patients' voices. Health Service Journal 102(5285):20–21

Stafford A, Hannigan B 1997 Client-held records in community mental health. Nursing Times 93(7):50–51

CHAPTER CONTENTS

Key points   27

Introduction   28

Early forms of mental health care   29

Asylums   32

Reflections from within   35

The romance of military psychiatry   37

Legacy of war-time psychiatry   39

The 1960s and the decline of the old order   41

Walking backwards into the future   44

Conclusions   46

Exercise   46

Key texts for further reading   46

References   47

3

History of mental health nursing and psychiatry

Peter Nolan

KEY POINTS

- The history of mental health care enables mental health workers to appreciate the origins and development of service provision, treatment methods and therapeutic interventions.

- A knowledge of the history of mental health care can provide valuable insights into the current state of mental health services.

- History helps us hear the 'user's voice' through the centuries so that we appreciate the continuity of need over time.

- A considerable contribution to the growth of mental health services has been made by voluntary and church organisations, particularly the Quakers.

- A mental health service that is not well grounded on sound therapeutic knowledge is likely to be at the whim of economic and political agendas.

INTRODUCTION

Interest in the history of mental health care has been enjoying a revival not only in the UK but also in the Western world more generally during the past three decades. According to Berrios (1996), the inspiration behind the revival was the Symposium on the History of Psychiatry which was held at Yale University in 1967. Participants were enabled to appreciate how an understanding of the history of one's profession could enable practice with keen insights and enable it to be proactive. They were reminded that the great 19th century alienists – Mercier, Bucknill, Tuke, Pinel, Connolly and Griesinger – were all accomplished historians as well as medical practitioners. These individuals certainly did not consider the study of history an exercise in antiquarianism; on the contrary, it was a means of enriching their understanding of how best to care for mentally ill people. The lessons of the past could inform and improve services for patients in the future. Although people who have come into mental health care as nurses or doctors have traditionally been offered little formal teaching about the history of psychiatry or of mental health nursing, most psychiatric hospitals, while they existed, cherished their own history and new staff found themselves surrounded by photographs of former medical superintendents, chief male nurses, matrons, many generations of hospital football and cricket teams and pictures of other significant events in the lives of staff and patients. Most hospitals boasted one or two ardent amateur historians amongst their staff, people who kept safe the archives of the hospital, and could recite names and dates from the time when the hospital was founded until the present day.

The writings of the founders of modern psychiatry provide valuable insights into the nature of mental illness, and also demonstrate their atti-

tude towards the past. Pinel adopted a 'presentistic' approach in his work; he was very much of the opinion that the history of psychiatry was a museum of failed endeavours and that only what was happening now had clinical, scientific or philosophical merit. This same assumption permeated the work of Bucknill & Tuke (1858), but their aim was to show that psychiatry had developed so far as to be able to embrace both medical and other broader perspectives. Their book, *A Manual of Psychological Medicine*, included such chapters as 'Lay descriptions of insanity', 'Opinion of medical writers', 'The concept of insanity' and 'A critique of treatment and classification'. Nonetheless, until the 1960s, historiography focused almost exclusively on the work of members of the medical profession, but has more recently broadened its outlook to include accounts and analyses of the work of other groups involved in mental health care and of the patients and clients who received it. Berrios (1996) and Porter (1987) have written persuasively about the need for historians of mental health care to look far beyond what it was that doctors were doing and to examine a much wider variety of primary source materials. In recent years, Andrews (1991) has shed new light on the work of the attendants and nurses who worked at the Bethlem Hospital, and Arton (1981), Carpenter (1988), Nolan (1993) and Clarke (1994), among others, have further added to the growing body of literature on the history of mental health nursing.

Hunter (1956) insisted that mental health care professionals needed to revisit and reconstruct their past. He sought to challenge the stereotype of psychiatry as a discipline outside the scientific arena, lacking in direction, and engaged in by people of limited intellectual and clinical abilities. What he felt was needed was well-conducted research into and analysis of the achievements of psychiatry, and accurate accounts of the work and inspiration of the people who have contributed to the care of the mentally ill. Walk (1961), an ardent advocate for the need to include history in all mental health care training curricula, was firmly of the opinion that professionals who have no understanding of the past can have only a partial understanding of the present.

The rationale behind including a chapter on history in a book which is concerned with the practical application of theories of mental health care is to emphasise that today's mental health nursing is the end-point of a long tradition of helping people suffering from mental illness in a variety of contexts. This chapter will show that our predecessors diligently sought ways of managing and treating mental illness – in some instances with considerable success – and where they had no success, continued their search for more effective ways of caring. It must be impressed on the reader that an overview such as this chapter provides is certainly not exhaustive; instead what follows is highly selective and provides only limited insights into the care of mentally ill people in the past. It is intended as a spur to prompt readers to get involved in a branch of research that is stimulating and under-developed. The art and science of caring can be studied from many different perspectives such as political, economic, sociological and literary, and each of these provides additional dimensions to our understanding.

EARLY FORMS OF MENTAL HEALTH CARE

It is necessary to reach far back into history to set the stage upon which the drama of the history of mental health care has been played out. One of the earliest institutional forms of care for people suffering from mental illness was provided by the monks whose monasteries thrived from the 4th to the mid-16th centuries in the UK.

Monasteries were at the forefront of Europe's scholarship and the spearhead of civilisation in the early Middle Ages. Scholar-monks passed their lives reading and writing books and also doing good works which included caring for people with physical and 'spiritual diseases'. Monks known as 'soul friends' befriended the melancholic in order to 'steer them back into social harmony with kith and kin' (Nolan 1993). The monastic environment was one of peace and orderliness and was deemed therapeutic for those whose minds were disturbed. Mentally ill people might spend some time living in an isolated monastic community on an island or in a hamlet so as to escape the world and be helped to recover (Nolan 1993). The kind of care and spiritual sustenance offered by the monks to the mentally ill was the same as that described many centuries before by the great Roman orator Cicero, who considered that those who suffered in the mind needed carers who could show empathy and protect them from fear, anger and guilt. He considered that appropriate carers were those who could foster civilised behaviour in the sick person through inspiring conversation, reading aloud, playing music and pointing out the beauties of nature (Clarke 1975).

In April 1536, during the reign of King Henry VIII, there were scattered throughout England and Wales more than 800 monasteries, nunneries and friaries and within them lived 10 000 monks, canons, nuns and friars, many of whom were engaged in tending the sick. By April 1540, all of them had ceased functioning and many of them were destroyed. Following the dissolution of the monasteries, the structure of health care which had been developed by the religious communities fell apart. From the late 16th to the mid-18th centuries, it is difficult to chronicle the provision of care for mentally ill people. Private madhouses sprang up to replace the care provided by the religious houses and access to the very varied services they provided was dependent on having the means to pay for them. The quality of care on offer was extremely uneven; some madhouses were run according to the Christian virtues which the monastic communities had espoused, while others were driven primarily by profit and were characterised by overcrowding, under-staffing and an ethos of containing people rather than healing them. The many sufferers who could not afford private care wandered aimlessly from village to village or were incarcerated in prisons and workhouses.

Private entrepreneurs had, in the main, no philosophical, religious or therapeutic ideas upon which to base the care they provided. It was not until the late 18th century that new ideas about caring emerged and the mentally ill again found champions who had the courage and com-passion to consider what was in their best inter-ests and to speak out on their behalf.

One such innovative carer was Nathaniel Cotton who owned and ran a private madhouse near St Albans which was founded in the mid-18th century. Cotton provided a pleasant physi-cal environment at his madhouse and was equally concerned that there should be a healing emotional atmosphere. With this in view, he employed 'servants' who were endowed with patience and good humour and could inspire patients with hope and determination. Cotton's most famous client was the poet William Cowper who spent 18 months in his care. Cowper confided to his diary that his recovery (sadly, not permanent) owed much to Cotton:

> a man well known for his humanity and sweetness of temper and who daily engaged me in the most delightful themes from the Bible.
>
> Cowper 1816

However, Cowper reserved his highest praise for Sam Roberts, the personal servant allocated to him by Cotton. It is apparent that Roberts combined qualities of gentleness, watchfulness and an ability to be happy which had a highly therapeutic effect on those for whom he cared. There is certainly much to interest students of mental health today in the 'healing relationship' that existed between Cowper and Roberts who finally left Cotton's employ to care for Cowper until the end of his days.

Elsewhere, however, the practices employed to contain and restrain the mentally ill in the pri-vate asylums were harsh in the extreme. 'Muffling' was common; that is, tying a towel round the mouth of a noisy patient. The circling swing, described as a 'mechanical exercise', was regarded as a safe and satisfactory remedy for mania. The patient was strapped into a kind of swivel chair and revolved up to 110 times per minute with the direction being changed every 6 minutes, which had the effect of stimulating the victim to empty his or her stomach, bowels and bladder – the desired effect.

> With the patient in the erect position, care was required to prevent the hanging over of the head, otherwise the suffusion of the countenance was found to leave ecchymosis. If no evacuation occurred, the patient became in any case so subservient to his physician's wishes as willingly to take any medicine prescribed. The full effect of the swing was calculated to produce a remarkable prostration of strength to the relief of all concerned, except perhaps the patient.
>
> Rosie 1948

The madness of King George III was highly fortuitous in turning the tide of neglect, cruelty and exploitation against the mentally ill and gov-ernment finally stepped in to enact legislation to improve the situation for this highly vulnerable section of the population. Private asylums were henceforth required to be licensed; they had to submit to regular inspections and could not admit patients without a doctor's order. Inspections were carried out in London by two

Commissioners, and in the provinces by two Justices of the Peace and a doctor. Reports of the provincial inspections were sent to London through the Clerk of the Peace.

Far more significant than the legislation coming out of London was the opening in 1794 of what was to become the most famous private madhouse not only in the UK but the world. This was The Retreat at York, founded by a devout Quaker, William Tuke, and run on Christian humanitarian principles. Tuke had a personal interest in the care of the mentally ill because of a local scandal in 1792 involving the death at the York Asylum of Hannah Mills, a Quaker patient. Hannah was admitted to the asylum suffering from melancholia on 15 June, 1790, and died there 6 weeks later. On investigation it was found that during her stay, she had not been permitted any visitors and that she had died alone in great mental anguish. Hannah's story had a profound impact on Tuke and the local Quaker community, so much so that he resolved to devote some of his vast wealth to building an asylum for 'Friends deprived of their reason' (Scull 1982). Tuke's philanthropy was coupled with an ability to select first-rate staff, which led him to employ as his first Superintendent, George Jepson, a man as devout and committed to caring as Tuke was himself, and immensely skilled in managing and treating the mentally ill (Digby 1985).

Jepson set about building a community at The Retreat, a community of patients cared for by staff with proven religious principles and dedicated to the alleviation of suffering. Every morning, he brought together residents and carers to discuss the management of the community and the progress each resident was making. Civility was a ground rule at The Retreat and physical restraint of residents was forbidden. In his effort to create an environment in which residents could enjoy warmth and security, Jepson invited Catherine Allen, a nurse at another Quaker

Institution, Brislington House near Bristol, to work with him at The Retreat. They later married and, as a husband and wife team, were able to provide the family-like atmosphere which both thought so beneficial to residents.

The Tuke family will always be credited with the founding and development of The Retreat. However, as Scull (1982) has argued, Tuke was not the only philanthropist concerned with the fate of the mentally ill during the second half of the 18th century. Men like John Ferriar at the Manchester Lunatic Asylum and Edward Fox who ran a madhouse for aristocrats in Bristol were convinced that:

> The first salutary operation in the mind of a lunatic (lies) in creating a habit of self-restraint, which could be achieved by the management of hope and apprehension, the dispensation of small favours and inspiring confidence, rather than coercion.
>
> Ferriar 1795

They appreciated that physical coercion would only bring about outward conformity and did not help the patient to internalise moral values and civilised standards. Only by treating the patients as rational beings and building up self-esteem, they thought, was it possible to re-educate them to discipline themselves and regain the power of reason (Ferriar 1795). These ideals were fundamental to what became known as the 'moral treatment' movement and they found their most powerful expression in The Retreat. 'Moral treatment' represented:

> A disavowal of physical therapies including bleeding and the administration of drugs, in favour of a psychological approach. Ideally, the stricken patient was quickly removed from his or her home to the calm of a small, isolated institution staffed by numerous empathetic but firm attendants. Under their watchful and reasoned guidance, the lunatic was given distracting work, a sound diet, gentle amusements and religious instruction. The

exciting cause was removed and the physical lesion in the brain slowly healed.

Ewing 1977

This was not kindness for kindness' sake, but rather designed to encourage the individual's own efforts to rediscover his powers of self-control (Ewing 1975). While undoubtedly more humane than previous approaches, the rhetoric of moral treatment concealed a desire to replace external restraint with internalised values of work, prayer and appropriate recreation as defined by those running the institutions. The pay-off for madhouse keepers was that moral treatment was ultimately less demanding than constant physical coercion; it also allowed carers to experience the satisfaction of feeling that they stood on the moral high-ground which those in their charge were struggling to reach (Short 1986).

Some critics of the moral treatment movement argue that the establishment of The Retreat was both courageous and arrogant in that Tuke had no evidence that the kind of care he wanted to offer at The Retreat would benefit the patients for whom he assumed responsibility (Belkin 1996). Rothman (1971) considered that Tuke's hidden agenda and personal need was to impose order, defend social control and sustain certain models of behaviour in an age of disruptive industrialisation and religious dislocation. Furthermore, The Retreat satisfied Tuke's desire to assert the superiority of the Quaker religion over other religions in its capacity to transform the mentally disordered person into a well-adjusted, law-abiding and productive citizen.

Despite such criticisms, it is nonetheless remarkable that no patient was re-admitted to The Retreat during its first 15 years (Tuke 1813) – a record which any contemporary psychiatric institution would be proud of! The great 19th century reformer Lord Shaftesbury was highly influenced in his campaign for a national mental health care strategy by what he saw at The Retreat. He and Dr John Connolly, also an advocate of humane care and opponent of physical restraint, aimed to reform public attitudes towards the insane. To their combined endeavours can be attributed the passing of the Lunatics Act 1845 which, for the first time, committed local authorities to providing specialist facilities for the mentally disordered. Within the next 50 years 100 institutions were built across the country providing from a few hundred to nearly a thousand beds.

ASYLUMS

Asylums were required to produce an annual report detailing what had transpired during the previous year and highlighting problems that were obstacles to the smooth running of the system. The annual reports of the Lincoln Lunatic Asylum provide information about the work that was undertaken there. They attempted to define the type of care patients required but soon spoke of good care as a 'mysterious process' and unique in the way that it was provided by each carer and received by each patient. A member of the Lincoln Board of Governors, writing in 1833, stated that:

> The mental condition of lunacy is rather a matter of metaphysical curiosity than medical value. It seems to consist in an impaired control of the will over the current of ideas. This defective control varies in degree from moral insanity, passing ultimately to that condition in which an educated lunatic describes his ideas as flitting involuntarily before his mind like a rack of clouds.
>
> Proceedings of the Lincoln Lunatic Asylum 1847

In its report of 1843, the new humanitarianism inspired by Shaftesbury and The Retreat is very apparent:

1. This Board is more and more confirmed in its reprovision of instrumental restraint and the

use of instruments and other violent processes and to avoid seclusion as a means of coercion.

2. That the introduction into this house of the Whirling Chair, the Bath of Surprise, the Douche and other such violent and abrupt practices towards the patients is hereby interdicted.

3. That no system of warming this house by which patients may breathe a heated atmosphere is hereby interdicted.

4. That the practice of shaving the heads of lunatics, blood-letting, the cold bath, baths above blood heat, the process of subduing violence by the use of tartarised Antimony or of Narcotics, the practice of enforcing sleep by Opiates, and the courses of Drastic Medicines are hereby interdicted.

Proceedings of the Lincoln Lunatic Asylum 1847

The Board was at pains to emphasise the importance of kind and caring relationships which would enable the mentally disordered to regain control over themselves and their lives. Wholesome food, regular exercise and civilised behaviour were the main ingredients of the new regime. Attendants had the responsibility of ensuring that the highest standards of care were maintained at all times and that all patients were treated with the respect that they deserved.

On 11 August, 1852, the Worcester Pauper Lunatic Asylum was opened to accommodate 200 patients who were admitted from various workhouses within the county, from private establishments, and from their own homes. By the end of 2 months, 152 people were in residence. The earliest treatment regimes at the asylum consisted of alternating cold and tepid sponging, opiate enemata, tonics, stimulants and counter-irritants modified to suit the particular symptoms of individual patients. Cod-liver oil was considered to be beneficial in improving the prognosis for a number of seemingly hopeless cases of dementia. Potassium iodide was used in cases of general paralysis of the insane but was not found to be as effective as the various mercu-

rial preparations available (Hassal & Warburton 1964).

It is not easy to find accounts written by patients of what it was like to be an inmate of a 19th century asylum. In this respect, the memoirs of Christian Watt, who was born in Fraserburgh in 1833 and who died 90 years later having spent almost half her life in Aberdeen Cornhill Asylum for the Insane, are remarkable. Christian entered domestic service at the age of 8 and worked as a laundry-maid, fish-gutter and house-maid to the aristocracy, eventually marrying a fishmonger. Her account of her life, her poverty, the deaths of her husband and some of her children, and of leaving other young children behind her on entering the asylum are poignant. In 1878, life was hard:

> My elder son was at sea, but I still had seven bairns to feed and clad. I wore myself out with hard work. In buying fish at the Broch market, I could not compete with the Fish merchants, so got little to barter for food in the country. I was sick with worry, neither eating nor sleeping, for I had no money except my son's allowance of 4/-. I know now I should have gone to the Parish for help, but I was far too proud. It may be wrong but that was how we were brought up; and selling your possessions is a degrading game.
>
> Fraser 1983: 106

She was admitted to the Aberdeen Royal Mental Asylum leaving her cousin, Mary, to look after the children, the eldest of whom, Isabella, was only 10. On the morning of her departure for the Asylum, 'the saddest day of my life', Mary and daughters Annie and Isabella saw her onto the train. Christian entered the asylum through a small gate set in a high granite dyke. She was taken through endless corridors and as she passed through each section of the asylum, she noticed that doors were firmly locked behind her. The next morning, at breakfast, she observed her fellow patients 'gulping and stomaching their porridge in such a slovenly and distasteful manner' and was comforted by a nurse who promised her, 'If you take a job in the kitchen, you can eat there.' Later that morning she spent an hour with the Medical Superintendent Dr Jamieson and insisted that under no circumstances was any of her children to be allowed to visit her. As an expert needlewoman, Christian was allocated the job of teaching her skills to other women patients. She also worked in the hospital laundry which serviced the big hotels and boarding houses in Aberdeen, thus providing income to keep the asylum financially secure. Despite her reluctance to go into the asylum, Christian found it a haven of peace and she had special words of praise for the nursing staff:

> Nurses are to medicine what glasses are to a person with failing sight.
>
> Fraser 1983: 111

The critical importance of nursing in mental hospitals was highlighted by the Scots doctor W.A.F. Browne, who was appointed to the post of Medical Superintendent at the Royal Edinburgh Asylum in 1838. He described what he considered an ideal hospital to be:

> A spacious building resembling the place of a peer surrounded by extensive grounds and gardens, the interior fitted with workshops and music rooms, the sun and air allowed to enter unobstructed by shutters and bars. The inmates are actuated by the common impulse of enjoyment. All are busy and delighted by being so. The house and all around it appear a hive of industry.
>
> MacNiven 1960

Browne recognised that the chief obstacle to creating what he considered to be an appropriate atmosphere in the asylums for the care and treatment of the mentally ill was the lack of suitable staff. It was ironic in Browne's opinion that the people who were closest to the patients, who spent most of their time with them, and who managed them when they become distressed, were nurses and attendants who were largely untrained. In an attempt to improve this situation, Browne inaugurated a course of lectures for nurses in 1854 at the Royal Edinburgh Asylum, 6 years before Florence Nightingale founded her Training School at St Thomas's Hospital. In his report of 1855, he records:

> A course of thirty lectures was commenced in October 1854 and continued weekly until May, in which mental disease was viewed in various aspects; in which the relations of the insane to the community, to their friends, and to their custodians, were described; in which treatment, so far as it depends on external impressions, the influence of sound minds, of love, and fear and imitation, were discussed. The descriptions were powerfully aided by portraits of patients familiar to the auditors, and graphically executed by a patient who had lost and regained his genius as an artist. The classes consisted of the officers, male and female attendants, some of the patients who belonged to the medical profession and occasionally a visitor. The attendance, though perfectly voluntary, was numerous, attentive and grateful.
>
> Williams 1989

These lectures were a landmark in the history of mental health nursing. Browne's insistence that nursing staff played an influential part in the recovery of mental patients echoed Esquirol's plea:

> First, cure your attendant and when you have succeeded you may proceed to treat the patient.
>
> Esquirol 1820

The need to attract better quality staff into nursing and to retain them was a constant theme of the annual reports of state asylums. Some felt that to make the work more attractive by offering better pay and conditions would assist in recruitment while others felt that money should be spent on training whoever came forward to ensure that they were brought up to standard. However, even training for doctors working in mental health remained sketchy until 1885 when a national training scheme leading to the Diploma in Psychological Medicine was introduced. In the same year, the first manual for attendants/nurses working in mental hospitals was published. The *Handbook for the Instruction of the Attendants on the Insane* contained 64 pages, was bound in red hardboard and included an appendix listing all the public and private asylums in the UK and the names of their superintendents. The 'Red' Handbook was unequivocal that the first duty of the attendant was to exercise personal discipline and to impose discipline on patients by setting an example of industry, order, cleanliness and obedience. For the first time, the knowledge and skills expected of attendants were written down, boosting both their status and their morale. Indeed, so popular did the manual prove that by 1902, 15 000 copies had been sold (Rollin 1986).

At its Annual General Meeting of 1889, the Medico-Psychological Association (MPA) (the association founded in 1841 by asylum superintendents) resolved to introduce on a nationwide basis, a course for attendants and nurses working with the mentally ill. Training began almost immediately and the first students took their examination in May, 1891. The content of training was based on the 'Red' Handbook and included basic anatomy and physiology, general principles of nursing, the mind and its disorders, care of the insane and the general duties of the attendant/nurse.

REFLECTIONS FROM WITHIN

Two books that had a profound impact on mental health care provision at the beginning of the 20th century were Clifford Beers' *A Mind That Found Itself*, published in 1937, and Montagu Lomax's *Confessions of an Asylum Doctor*, which appeared in 1922. Both authors sought to change the system by speaking out about their own experiences.

Beers was a highly intelligent and articulate American university student who suffered a serious breakdown during the course of his studies. He observed in minute detail the deterioration in his ability to think logically, to engage in conversation with others and to manage his own life. His experience of professional care was that it was grossly inadequate; staff appeared to him to be lacking in empathy, interest and skill. *A Mind That Found Itself* is a gripping account of a mentally ill person's attempt to understand what is happening to him and to assist in his own recovery. After his recovery, Beers founded the National Committee for Mental Hygiene, membership of which was revolutionary in that it included both physicians and lay people. Branches were soon established in many countries including the UK, and aimed to:

1. promote the early diagnosis and treatment of mental illness
2. develop appropriate practices for hospitalised patients
3. stimulate research activities
4. secure public understanding of and support for psychiatric and mental hygiene activities
5. provide individuals and groups with the appropriate skills to implement mental hygiene principles
6. co-operate with governmental and private agencies whose work touches the field of mental hygiene.

Beers argued that mental hygiene should be a concern not just of those who were ill, but equally importantly, of those who were still well:

> Mental health today means not merely freedom from mental disease but the ability to build up and maintain satisfactory relationships. It takes

in personal and social adjustment of all sorts. It stands for the development of wholesome, balanced, integrated personalities, able to cope with difficult life situations.

Beers 1908: 325

The Mental Hygiene Movement in the UK sought to promote mental health on a national scale and campaigned for improved services for women during pregnancy and the puerperium, for the establishment of child guidance clinics and for a better awareness of mental health issues in schools and the work place. One of the Movement's principal strategies for accomplishing its aims was to bring about improvements in the education of health professionals regarding mental health and illness.

Lomax's book, *Confessions of an Asylum Doctor*, complemented Beers' in that it explored the care of the mentally ill from the standpoint of a medical professional. Lomax described how at the Prestwick Asylum where he had worked, epileptic and tubercular patients were housed together, patients were constantly drugged and purged, clothed in rags and accommodated in miserable wards. He was outraged that assistant medical officers in state asylums were appointed at a salary of £150 per year on a contract that included a dismissal clause if they married. His book aroused such a storm of controversy that a Royal Commission was set up to investigate its allegations. The Commission's Report entitled 'Administration of Public Mental Hospitals' did not accept all that Lomax had said, but did recommend that in future mental hospitals should be limited to 1000 patients in order to avoid overcrowding with its consequent reduction in the quality of inmates' living and staff's working conditions. Further recommendations included that:

— all Medical Superintendents of asylums should hold the Diploma in Psychological Medicine

— mental and general nursing should be brought closer together
— every asylum should have at least one qualified general nurse on its staff.

Lomax's book doubtless acted as a spur to the first National Review of Mental Nursing which reported in 1924 (Ministry of Health 1924). Although none of the recommendations made in its report, 'Nursing in County and Borough Mental Hospitals', was ever implemented, nevertheless the report provides fascinating insights into the state of mental nursing at that time. It records that the total number of mental nurses in England and Wales in 1923 was 16 949, comprising 7418 male nurses and 9531 female. There was one male nurse to every nine male patients and one female nurse to every 10 female patients; at night, the ratio was one nurse to 55 patients. While the mental hospitals had clearly become a major source of employment for both men and especially women, the Report accused many hospitals of not enquiring sufficiently closely into the suitability of people applying for nursing posts. It felt that asylum work could be made more attractive to a better quality of applicant if hours were reduced and holiday entitlement and wages increased so that the wages of mental nurses were 10% higher than that paid to general nurses and male nurses received 20% more than female nurses. The report recommended that nurses' accommodation and recreational facilities should be improved. It also suggested that mental nurses would benefit from training alongside general nurses and that general nurse tutors and nurses should be appointed to mental hospitals as a means of improving care and raising the status of mental nursing.

The 1924 report commended the fact that the management of the mental hospitals had been removed from the Home Office to the Ministry of

Health in 1919. It felt that this would be helpful in reducing the stigma of mental illness *and* improving the status of psychiatry. It suggested that every County Borough Council should have a Health Committee to manage local mental hospitals. The poor state of the economy during the 1920s meant that none of these recommendations was seriously addressed.

THE ROMANCE OF MILITARY PSYCHIATRY

War has had a considerable influence on the history of psychiatry and the types of services provided for patients. The first reference to caring for servicemen with mental health problems dates from 1711 when the Royal Hospital at Kilmainham was enlarged in order to accommodate men quartered in Ireland who were suffering from mental illness. The accommodation was extended in 1730 and again in 1807; the hospital finally closed in 1849 when all mental patients were removed to the military asylum in England (Rosie 1948). In 1819, following revelations concerning inhumane treatment endured by patients in civilian mental hospitals, the army decided to establish its own hospital for the treatment of insane soldiers. This was Fort Clarence, situated near Chatham. Staff Surgeon Murray provides an insight into the management of the Military Hospital in his report of 1821:

> The minutest attention to the moral management of the patients continues to form the principal feature in the practice of the asylum. The patients are required to rise early, make their beds, wash and clean themselves and then play ball, marbles, or be exercised at the dumb-bell. Three times a day, the majority are regularly marched to the extremity of the grounds to the sound of the clarinet. The officer patients amuse themselves with quoits, ninepins, cards or backgammon and are

supplied with a daily newspaper which is afterwards passed on to the men.

> Rosie 1948

Dr Scott, Surgeon to the Forces, writes in his annual report for 1833:

> The attendants are enjoined to treat the inmates with consideration and kindness. They must be treated like children, with gentleness and constant watching.

> Rosie 1948

The role of the attendants was clearly to encourage patients to work, although the regime was less strict for officers who could choose the type of work they undertook. Further insights into the life of the attendants are provided in the annual report for 1840:

> The married attendant is commonly necessitous and must have much firmness of principle to resist such opportunities as are afforded in the asylum to appropriate to the use of his family articles of food. Moreover, the single men are more easily kept at their posts. They ask for less leave, and are satisfied with more confinement. I apprehend it might be an advisable rule to establish as part of the Standing Orders that no married soldier should be taken on as an orderly.

> Rosie 1948

In 1846, on the advice of Her Majesty's Commission in Lunacy, Fort Clarence was closed because of overcrowding and the damp dreariness of its accommodation for staff and patients. The patients were removed to the Royal Naval Hospital at Great Yarmouth which had been purpose-built. By 1854, all use of instruments of restraint had ceased, except for the strait-jacket. In 1870, another new military asylum was opened at Netley and appears to have been run along progressive and humane lines. In the mid-1950s Netley became the main mental hospital for all three services, army, navy and air-force, until 1978, when the last soldiers to be treated there had served in Northern Ireland. Shortly after it ceased as a mental hospital for services personnel, the site was converted to a Training Headquarters by the Hampshire Constabulary. One of the first reports of the Commissioners in Lunacy concerned itself with the most minute details of patient care:

> We observe that they have to drink their porter out of quart basins and we beg to recommend that pint mugs be substituted.
>
> Rosie 1948

The forces, therefore, had an excellent track-record in providing top quality psychiatric care for their men long before the First World War produced enormous numbers of shell-shock victims requiring nursing. Nurses working in the forces during the two world wars inherited a tradition of humane and progressive care which enabled them to be pioneers in care. The memoirs of John Greene (personal communication 1995) provide an excellent record of the work that was done by mental nurses during the Second World War and of how they were able to influence mental health provision after demobilisation.

Early in 1940, Greene read an advert placed by the Admiralty in the *Nursing Mirror* for applications from mental nurses to work with psychiatrists in establishing a psychiatric nursing service for the Royal Navy. Greene was one of 24 men recruited and after initial training, was sent with five other mental nurses to the Royal Naval Hospital at Chatham where he assisted two recently recruited psychiatrists, Dr G. V. Stephenson from the Priory Hospital at Roehampton and Dr K. Cameron from The Maudsley, in setting up a neurosis ward and a psychosis ward. The nursing staff had the help of sick bay attendants who had been given a minimal training in nursing by the navy and a number of ordinary sailors who were referred to as

'mental guards'. The job of the mental guards was to control the patients which they did by confining them to their beds all day. These men had been selected far more for their physical bulk than for any aptitude for tending the sick and the newly arrived mental nurses quickly requested that they be removed from the wards. They also asked for all use of restraints to be forbidden, including the padded cells.

During their first days at Chatham, the Battle of Britain was at its height and clearly visible in the skies at night. The incessant bombing of army, navy and air-force positions soon took its toll and military patients began to arrive on the wards in various stages of fatigue and distress, many in psychotic states. The most common form of treatment for patients with fear and exhaustion was continuous narcosis, prolonged in some cases for up to 3 weeks. The most common form of fear and fatigue manifested itself in what was referred as to as 'the 2000 year stare', where patients stared vacantly into space and were oblivious to everything around them. The nurses' job was to record the temperature, pulse and respiration of these patients every quarter of an hour and to wake them at frequent intervals for food. Having to cope with such a volume of patients set the nurses on a steep learning curve; they were quickly in demand on medical and surgical wards to help with patients in altered states of consciousness. So successful was the experiment of recruiting mental nurses that others were called up after the Battle of Britain.

Greene was allocated to join the hospital ship Vita and spent the war sailing the Indian Ocean, treating war casualties in Aden, the Seychelles, Mombasa, Karachi, Bombay, Colombo, the Maldives and Mauritius. The ship was fully equipped with medical, surgical and psychiatric wards and an operating theatre. During the Burma Campaign, the Vita was the base hospital ship at Trincomalee Harbour in Ceylon. Nurses were expected to conduct physical and psychiatric assessments and initiate treatment, often without medical support. The number of casualties treated by mental nurses far exceeded what had been anticipated and the efficiency with which they worked impressed not only their senior officers, but the nurses themselves. Their experience gave them confidence and skills to work independently and demonstrated what could be achieved by nurses in the absence of institutional bureaucracy.

Psychiatrists and mental nurses who had served in the war together had a special working relationship that overcame professional allegiances and enabled them to inaugurate many improvements in mental health care after their demobilisation. Many ex-military nurses joined the Society of Registered Male Nurses since full membership of the Royal College of Nursing remained closed to them until 1960 when the College's Charter was amended (Nolan 1993). The Society was an energetic forum for progressive mental nurses who sought to improve the status and practice of nursing. Greene took a post at Herrison Hospital in Dorset where he played an important role in establishing the nurse training school, and in developing therapies such as electroconvulsive therapy (ECT), deep insulin therapy and prefrontal leucotomies. The routine of the civilian psychiatric hospital was very mundane to those returning from war service and gross overcrowding of the wards made nursing difficult and unsatisfying.

LEGACY OF WAR-TIME PSYCHIATRY

Although nurses and doctors who had seen active service during the war had developed many skills which made them able to be innovative practitioners in civilian life, their experiences had by no means been comprehensive. It was noted that doctors and nurses returning to work in psychiatric hospitals had no understanding of or skills in managing chronic conditions and tended to treat all patients as if they were neurotic (Trethowan, personal communication 1996).

The post-war period saw the rise and fall of a variety of treatments in mental health care. Hydrotherapy, which had been in widespread use since the turn of the century, was just beginning to fall into disrepute. This involved patients being laid on canvas stretchers and submerged for hours just below water level in baths kept slightly above body temperature. Hydrotherapy was a non-specific treatment prescribed for patients suffering from a variety of conditions and although no evidence was ever established to show that it had any effect, patients frequently stated that they felt better afterwards. It may be that the continuous attention of a nurse which the therapy required was in itself therapeutic, denoting that it was more a placebo effect than anything inherent in the procedure itself.

As hydrotherapy fell out of favour during the late 1940s, continuous narcosis therapy was in the ascendancy. This treatment was prescribed only for refractory patients and large doses of barbiturates were administered either orally or intramuscularly, which resulted in patients sleeping for up to 20 hours a day. The regime was continued for up to 3 weeks. Reflecting on his own ideas at this time, Sir Aubrey Lewis commented:

> Continuous narcosis was very much to my taste. I could understand its logic and it seemed likely to me to succeed. I was very keen on such simple practical measures as the allaying of anxiety by continuous baths. I became quite adept at regulating continuous baths; the attendant risks were completely out of court and the advantages were maximised.
>
> Shepherd 1993

Continuous narcosis was another therapy that demanded close nursing attention, especially when epileptiform seizures occurred as happened not infrequently. Patients also tended to develop chronic urinary and chest infections and by the end of the 1950s, continuous narcosis was being replaced by insulin therapy and ECT (Trethowan, personal communication 1996). Insulin units flourished all round the country in the late 1950s and early 1960s. Every patient was allocated a nurse for the duration of his or her treatment and having been fasted overnight, insulin was administered intravenously. Patients remained in a coma for approximately 7 minutes after which time, glucose was administered to bring the patient round. In some instances, patients suffered from irreversible coma and died. Once awake, patients sweated profusely and were ravenously hungry and ready to eat a hearty breakfast which was also part of the treatment because many were so grossly underweight. This treatment was mainly managed by nurses and Trethowan (personal communication 1996) recalls that the remark 'If you want to increase nurses' morale, start an insulin unit!' was frequently used by doctors who were concerned about the well-being of nurses.

Among the many nurses and doctors who had served in the war and who strove to introduce into civilian practice ideas they had developed during their military careers was John Barry who worked at St Francis Hospital in Haywards Heath. Barry was an active member of the Society of Mental Nurses and became chairman of the Chief Male Nurses' Association. His aim was to raise mental nursing to the same status that it had enjoyed in the services. Another was Peter Dawson who was employed at St Ebba's Hospital in Epsom and became recognised for his campaign to encourage mental nurses to gain a qualification in general nursing as well as mental nursing. He believed that the training mental nurses received was inadequate for the types of conditions they encountered and

consequently many patients were inappropriately cared for. Dawson held the view that many Medical Superintendents sought to curtail the ambitions of nurses and felt threatened by nurses with wartime experience who had developed considerable leadership skills. This was not true of all Superintendents; some, such as Francis Pilkington who became Medical Superintendent at Moorhaven Hospital in 1949 and later President of the Royal College of Psychiatrists, believed that the future of psychiatry lay in building alliances between nurses and doctors.

Within a short time of his arrival at Moorhaven, Pilkington had transformed it into one of the finest psychiatric hospitals in the country. He invited students studying in a variety of paramedical disciplines to come on placement at the hospital, increased the number of social workers and occupational therapists employed and introduced industrial therapy. He invited lecturers from nearby Dartington Hall to talk to staff and patients about art and attempted to broaden the range of creative activities available to the patients. Pilkington was fortunate in having the services of John Greene as his Chief Male Nurse. In many respects, the relationship between Greene and Pilkington might be considered to resemble the famous 18th century working partnership between Tuke and Jepson. It is little wonder that Moorhaven Hospital was at the forefront of developing community services in the early 1960s.

When the NHS was founded on the 5 July, 1948, there were 480 000 beds available in 2690 hospitals; 270 000 beds were for mentally ill patients and those with learning difficulties (Webster 1985). As during the 1920s, the majority of in-patients in psychiatric hospitals were working class people; the middle classes were more likely to be found in the out-patient sector. Increasingly, however, hospitals started to introduce open-door policies, (Warlingham Park 1942, Belmont 1944, Mapperly 1945, Dingleton 1947, Crichton Royal 1950) enabling patients to take week-end leave rather than being removed completely from their families during the period of their hospital stay. Slowly a new spirit of liberalism was beginning to replace the oppressive post-war atmosphere that prevailed in mental hospitals throughout the country.

As the 1950s progressed, a number of factors, amongst the most important of which were severe overcrowding in the mental hospitals, staff shortages, new medications and growing anxiety about the massive costs in providing a national health service, provided an impetus for non-hospitalised forms of care to be developed. The open-door policy demonstrated that it was not necessary to confine every patient with mental health problems within a hospital, but that many patients recovered more quickly and were better able to return to their everyday lives if they spent time in their own communities during the period of their treatment.

THE 1960s AND THE DECLINE OF THE OLD ORDER

The great mental hospitals, however, continued to flourish well into the 1960s and provided an invaluable service to people who could not obtain help from any other sector of the health service. The medical and nursing staff who worked in them remained devoted to their particular hospital although this was less true of members of the more recently established professions, such as psychology, social work and occupational therapy, who were increasingly employed to work with mental health clients. The treatment provided for hospitalised patients was largely drug-based, supported by ECT and occupational and industrial therapy. In some institutions, the principles of the 'therapeutic community' as defined by Maxwell Jones, a prominent psychiatrist whose ideas stemmed from his war-time experiences, were adopted. Hospital staff enjoyed first-rate sporting and recreational facilities, good accommodation, and active staff social clubs. These facilities served both to create an esprit de corps and to suppress the dissent which might easily have been the result of the frustration of working with people largely rejected by society. In the 1960s, psychiatry still seemed to those working within it to be firmly established within an institutional context.

The reality was different, however; the apparent calm of the day-to-day running of the mental hospitals concealed a morass of problems which it was increasingly difficult to contain. Where the great humanitarian reformers such as Tuke, Shaftesbury and Connolly had conceived the mental asylums as a system of caring for vulnerable people, the system had in essence become a means of warehousing large numbers of people for whom society chose this convenient method of administering welfare. Overcrowding with its attendant dehumanisation and lack of privacy and choice for patients had become accepted as a matter of course by medical and nursing staff. The mental hospitals were still finding it extremely difficult to recruit 'progressive' staff even when those in authority wanted such innovators. Staff working in the hospital system tended to react to situations rather than being able to take a proactive stance. Nurse training only served to reinforce this as it involved apprenticing students to the system and assessing them in terms of their ability to conform to the system. Little attempt was made to define good nursing practice and there was immense variation in the way that different hospitals cared for and treated their inmates (Nolan 1993).

It was inevitable that the apathy which characterised the mental hospitals should find itself challenged by the highly charged individualism of the 1960s. Nor was it possible for the mental hospitals to withstand the economic realities of the health service and its ever escalating costs. Enoch Powell was the first Minister of Health to declare that:

> Mental hospitals are doomed institutions, part of a bygone age and must disappear.
>
> Powell 1961

A year later, Powell published his Hospital Plan (1962) which, in conjunction with the Mental Health Act 1959, was to have a significant influence on the future of mental health services. The Plan anticipated that the number of hospital beds available to mental health patients would be halved by the mid-1970s and replaced by beds on general hospital wards and services in the community. The not-so-hidden agenda aimed to guarantee the demise of the old psychiatric hospitals by withholding maintenance expenses (Rogers & Pilgrim 1996). Later in his life, Powell reflected that by the 1960s, mental hospitals had become unmanageable and impervious to outside influences, so entrenched were they in their own bureaucracies (Powell 1988). There was no satisfactory way of monitoring costs or staffing levels as lines of accountability were either blurred or non-existent. Nurses spent most of their time on trivial, domestic chores and were therefore overtrained. Powell's aim as Minister of Health was to curtail the rising costs of the health service and as mental health care was clearly both inadequate and expensive, it seemed to him an obvious place to start making cutbacks. He invited professional and public bodies to scrutinise psychiatry and targeted it as a key area for reform.

Psychiatry thus found itself under attack from external bodies. It was also under attack from within. A small but highly influential group of psychiatrists voiced their opinion that psychiatry could not justify its claim to be a branch of medicine as it was neither 'scientific' nor 'benign' in its attempts to improve the lot of suffering humanity. The term 'anti-psychiatry' which had first been used by Beyer in 1912 was revived by Cooper (1967) to describe the views of those who considered psychiatry to be a 'game' played by bourgeois psychiatrists on their 'victims' (patients) in order to reduce them 'to nothing more than the wretched forsaken condition into which the psychiatrists themselves had fallen' (Tantam 1991). Barton, Laing and Esterson in the UK, Szasz and Goffman in the USA and Basaglia in Italy exposed the imprecision of the term 'schizophrenia', the non-reciprocity between doctor and patient in situations of mental health care, the undue reliance on neuroleptic drugs which they described as 'abortifacients of the spirit', and the tendency of psychiatry 'to close experience down rather than open it up' (Tantam 1991: 333). Ignatieff summed up the environment of the average psychiatric hospital thus:

> The vast grey space of state confinement: on the wards of psychiatric hospitals, the attendants shovel gruel into the mouths of vacant, unwilling patients; in the dispensaries the drugs are prepared ... needs are met, but souls are dishonoured. Natural man – the 'poor, bare forked animal' is maintained; the social man wastes away.
>
> Ignatieff 1984

During the 1960s it became quite clear that the old mental hospitals could not and would not accommodate new approaches to care although new wards were still being opened and the autocratic rule of the Medical Superintendents continued. Gradually, the bureaucratic infrastructure of the mental hospital system began to be dismantled. In 1963, the post of Medical Superintendent was abolished and the management of the mental institutions fell to Hospital Groups. Services formerly available in mental hospitals such as radiography, pathology and surgery were relocated in general hospitals; malarial treatment for patients with general paralysis of the insane was replaced by sulphonamides; new drugs obviated the need for tuberculosis and epilepsy wards; leucotomies and insulin therapy were abandoned and ECT became the preferred treatment. With the establishing of 'psychiatric wards' and 'psychiatric units' in general hospitals in the mid-1960s, psychiatry was dealt another severe blow. The better psychiatric staff, doctors and nurses were selected to work in these new settings, thus leaving the less able to manage as best they could in the psychiatric hospitals. The majority of these staff, as later events were to demonstrate, were unable to rebut the increasing criticism of the psychiatric system or reverse the gradual erosion of humane practices within the system. The inevitable public inquiries into psychiatric hospitals during the 1960s and 1970s further served to weaken and fragment psychiatric nursing. These inquiries were largely instrumental in generating in nurses a sense of low self-esteem and powerlessness.

What was overlooked by those who sought, for the best reasons, to reform the mental health care system was that the psychiatric hospitals were refuges for many disadvantaged people who saw them as their homes. Such insensitivity seems, at least in retrospect, very uncaring. The abolitionists, however, won the day and whereas in 1960, there were 130 mental hospitals, many with more than 1000 beds, by 1993, 38 of these had closed and a further 21 were earmarked for closure. Of the hospitals remaining, only 14 were sure to survive until the end of the century. The number of hospital beds for mentally ill people fell by 44% from 1979 to 1992; that is, from 89 000 beds to 50 000 (Eaton 1994).

The state of uncertainty and transition in psychiatry did not ease its recruitment problems. While hospital training schools published brochures describing psychiatric nursing as 'one of the most satisfying jobs that young people could contemplate entering' (Tonks & Smout 1982), there was a persistent lack of response from indigenous applicants and many hospitals were forced to employ nurses from overseas, even some who did not speak English. The Salmon Report (Department of Health and Social Security 1966) attempted to strengthen the management structure of nursing and to encourage staff not to look upon the hospital at which they had trained as the place where they would work until retirement. Instead, they were invited to seek promotion at other hospitals. Seconding general nurse students to psychiatric hospitals was a further attempt to break down the insularity of the institutions although the stated reason was that the students would have the chance to 'develop the skills of establishing relationships with patients' (Nolan 1993). 'Psychiatric Nursing Today and Tomorrow' (Ministry of Health 1968) was rightly sceptical of this argument; it was equally sceptical about the way in which psychiatric nurses were being trained and about the scope of training to alter nursing practice within the institutions. The last few nails were put in the coffin of institutional psychiatry when a series of enquiries into alleged maltreatment of patients took place at the end of the 1960s (Martin 1984). Poor professional practice, chronic overcrowding, bad management, seriously inadequate nursing care and lack of accountability were all brought to public attention.

It was therefore inevitable that during the next two decades there would be a very marked shift towards providing care for mentally ill people in the community. Barham (1992) described the return of mental health patients to the community as the return of a people from exile. Szasz (1985) commented that the dismantling of the institutions revealed that psychiatry had never been anything more than a system of providing homes for the homeless and that the community care intended to replace it would simply be a form of outdoor relief. The translocation of services to the community meant that nurses and doctors had to engage in a radical reassessment of their working practices and learn to collaborate with professional and non-professional groups in a way they had never had to before.

There was a steep increase in the number of training courses for community-based staff and Project 2000 attempted to bring mental health and general nurse students closer together during their training, a development which had been considered desirable at the end of the 19th century and recommended in reports during the 1920s. The ethos of mental health nursing changed beyond recognition and mental health nurses were forced to redefine their role and justify their practice as they had never had to before. Instead of working in teams, community psychiatric nurses (CPNs) began to take responsibility for their own caseloads. Many found themselves isolated, having to manage their own time and seek support and advice on an ad hoc basis. As the hospital base of psychiatry was increasingly undermined, the hospital-based Schools of Nursing also began to disappear and to be reconstituted firstly as Colleges of Nursing, and, very soon afterwards, as Departments of Nursing in further and higher education.

Among the first psychiatric nurses to move out into the community were those keen to escape the restrictive atmosphere of the institutions and to establish themselves as professionals on an equal footing with other medical and paramedical health carers. Community-based work offered better job prospects than hospital nursing where career opportunities were declining. Unfortunately, the optimism with which some nurses greeted the advent of community care was short-lived. Throughout the 1970s and especially the 1980s and 1990s, the resources made

available for community care did not match the speed at which hospital beds were being closed. Carson et al (1996) and Nolan et al (1995) have identified a variety of factors that cause particular distress to nurses in the community; for example, unpropitious working conditions, inadequate resources, lack of support from colleagues and other professionals and self-doubt regarding their ability to care for very ill people in a non-clinical environment. Gournay & Brooking (1996) observed that CPNs were being used in widely differing ways across the country, regardless of their skills. The issues of educational training and support were addressed by White (1996) who found that the content of Project 2000 courses was not adapted to meet the needs of mental health nurses and despite much endeavour to provide appropriate educational support in the community, it remained inadequate. The rapid rate of service development in a new context of care means that education and training will necessarily lag behind practice for some time. Collaboration between practice areas and educational institutions so that teaching and research are shared is perhaps the best model with which to proceed.

WALKING BACKWARDS INTO THE FUTURE

The immense changes which have taken place in mental health nursing over the last 20 years have not reduced the concern felt by many about the quality and availability of mental health care. Pope (1997) reports that the strain placed on mental health services in big cities is becoming intolerable and that approximately 5000 severely mentally ill people are not receiving appropriate care and treatment. Levels of stress amongst staff working in the community are known to be extremely high (Carson et al 1995, Cushway et al 1996). Although today's health services aim to be evidence-based, the 'scientific' basis of mental health care is weak compared with that of other branches of health care and research undertaken by mental health nurses, although increasing, is still in its infancy. As a result, mental health clients are subjected to fashions in care in the absence of hard evidence as to how they might best be helped. There is still a readiness on the part of mental health professionals to adopt any new model of care regardless of whether it has been validated or not. Nursing in general and mental health nursing in particular are still not sufficiently secure to be able to debate, analyse and test approaches to care before implementing them on a large scale.

The number of nursing students entering mental health care has been falling gradually since the introduction of Project 2000, although it was hoped that strengthening the educational base of nursing would improve the status of all branches of nursing. The gap between educational institutions and the service arena has widened both physically and philosophically, thus making it ever harder for nurses to integrate theory and practice. Project-based approaches to innovation are funded but cannot be properly carried through because there is a shortage of appropriately skilled nurses. This is a very real problem in the short term, although soon a new generation of highly educated, critical and research-skilled nurses will emerge from higher education to set nursing on a firmer footing. It is hoped that these nurses will be able to resist pressures from government and professional bodies to pursue politically driven agendas in health care which are not in the best interests of clients and their carers.

Today's mental health clients face many difficulties in addition to their mental health problems. These include unemployment, substandard housing, poor education, stigmatisation and fragile or non-existent social networks. It is now apparent that reforming the health services will not be effective unless housing, education and employment issues are also addressed. The mental health nurses of the future will need to do more than merely assist in managing the symptoms of patients; they will have to work closely with people to help them manage various aspects of their lives as well as agitating for better conditions than people with mental health problems have had hitherto.

A dilemma that must be confronted by mental health nurses in the very near future is whether to align themselves with primary care teams and forge new relationships with general practitioners, practice nurses, health visitors and community midwives, or whether to remain with the mental health services. Both options are attractive and challenging. Attachment to the primary health care team could provide ideal opportunities for mental health nurses to identify and address mental health problems at an early stage of their development, to assume responsibility for mental health promotion programmes and to act as a resource for other health professionals. On the other hand, nurses, because of their traditional caring role, have a considerable contribution to make to the care provided by mental health teams who tend to work with people who have severe and enduring mental health problems.

Among the many lessons that can be learned from studying the history of mental health nursing is that a clear account of what one is expected to do boosts both personal and professional confidence. Nurses will need to re-invent themselves if they are to survive within the new health service and meet the far-ranging health and social needs of their clients. In order to define, clarify, raise and protect their status and in order to safeguard nursing care for mental health clients, nurses need intellectual skills, confidence and enthusiasm to identify, analyse and disseminate good working practices.

The work currently being undertaken by mental health nurses is not clearly defined (Tilley 1997) nor has it a coherent and rigorous scientific or philosophical basis (Morrall 1997). Multidisciplinary training and working is currently very much to the fore; however, its success depends on people feeling secure in their professional roles. Mental health nursing is vulnerable at a time when professional boundaries are being negotiated, the ownership of skills contested and roles redefined.

CONCLUSIONS

This brief overview has tried to explore how mental health nursing has reflected and engaged with social, intellectual and political developments over the last three centuries. It can be seen how the past permeates the present in a critical and challenging way. While certain charismatic individuals exert a significant influence on their profession, the thousands of ordinary carers who have made nursing what it is today must not be forgotten. Research should be carried out into the work and philosophies of such pioneers of mental health care as George Jepson, Catherine Allen and Clifford Beers *and* into the work and attitudes of ordinary carers such as Sam Roberts. Whole periods remain to be explored as far as nursing is concerned – the years immediately after the First and Second World Wars have, for example, hardly been considered in the literature. This research needs urgently to be done so

that mental health nurses can understand, define and defend the unique essence of nursing. Indeed, unless nurses move quickly to demonstrate that what they have to offer contributes to the mental well-being of their clients and their clients' families, then they will enter the 21st century in a weaker position than they entered the 20th.

Acknowledgement

I would like to acknowledge my debt to the Wellcome Institute for the History of Medicine for financial assistance in undertaking part of this work.

Exercise

Select a service or therapeutic intervention with which you are familiar. Ask yourself why this type of service or intervention is needed at this time. Now ask yourself 'How were the people who are currently receiving this service cared for in the past?' Look up your hospital records; go to the libraries and ascertain what kind of provision there was for these clients 100 years ago. Try to locate official documents and old photographs; find out who were the key secular and religious figures involved in providing care. Who exactly were the people receiving care? What type of work did they do? Did they reside in one place or did they move around a lot? If they were described as poor, what did that mean at the time? What sorts of help did they receive? How useful was it?

Compare the service provided a century ago with the service you currently provide. Is the service for these clients better today, and if so, in what ways? Is it worse? Try to be as detailed as you can in comparing the conditions and services of the two periods.

KEY TEXTS FOR FURTHER READING

Belkin G 1996 Moral insanity, science and religion in nineteenth century America: the Gray-ray debate. History of Psychiatry vii:591–613

Berrios G E 1996 The history of mental symptoms. Cambridge University Press, Cambridge

Conrad L I, Neve M, Nutton V, Porter R 1995 The Western medical tradition 800 BC to AD 1800. Cambridge University Press, Cambridge

Freeman H, Berrios G E (eds) 1996 150 years of British psychiatry, vol 11: the aftermath. Athlone Press, London

Mulhall A 1995 Nursing research: what difference does it make? Journal of Advanced Nursing 21:576–583

Rafferty A M 1996 The politics of nursing knowledge. Routledge, London

Rothman D J 1971 The discovery of the asylum. Little Brown, Boston

REFERENCES

Andrews J 1991 Bedlam revisited: A history of Bethlem Hospital 1634–1770. PhD thesis, University of London

Arton M 1981 The development of psychiatric nurse education in England and Wales. Nursing Times 3:124–127

Barham P 1992 Closing the asylum. Penguin, Harmondsworth

Beers C W 1937 A mind that found itself. Doubleday, Doran, New York

Berrios G E 1996 The history of mental symptoms. Cambridge University Press, Cambridge

Bucknill J, Tuke D H 1858 A manual of psychological medicine. John Churchill, London

Carpenter M 1988 Working for health – The history of the Confederation of Health Service Employees. Lawrence and Wishart, London

Carson J, Fagin L, Ritter S 1995 Stress and coping in mental health nursing. Chapman and Hall, London

Clarke B 1975 Mental disorder in earlier Britain. University of Wales Press, Cardiff

Clarke L 1994 The opening of doors in British mental hospitals in the 1950s. History of Psychiatry iv:527–551

Cooper D 1967 Psychiatry and anti-psychiatry. Tavistock, London

Cowper W 1816 Memoirs of the early life of William Cowper Esq. R Edwards, London

Cushway D, Tyler P, Nolan P 1996 Development of a stress scale for mental health professionals. British Journal of Clinical Psychology 35:279–295

Department of Health and Social Security 1966 The Salmon Report – The report of the Committee on Senior Nurse Staffing Structure. HMSO, London

Digby A 1985 Madness, morality and medicine – A study of the York Retreat. Cambridge University Press, Cambridge

Eaton L 1994 Why is community care failing the mentally ill? Community Care (Supplement on the mentally ill: the facts) 12:5

Esquirol E 1820 Melancolie. In: Dictionnaire des sciences medicales. Panckouke, Paris

Ewing M 1975 Jonathan Hutchinson FRCS. Annals of the Royal College of Surgeons of England 57:301

Ewing M 1977 Sir William Ferguson (1808–1877). Journal of the Royal College of Surgeons of Edinburgh 22:127–135

Ferriar J 1795 Medical histories and reflections. London 111–112

Fraser D 1983 (ed.) The Christian Watt papers. Paul Harris Publishing, Edinburgh

Gournay K, Brooking J 1996 The community psychiatric nurse in primary care: An economic analysis. In: Brooker C, White E (eds) Community psychiatric nursing, vol 3. Chapman and Hall, London

Hassal C, Warburton J 1964 The new look in mental health – 1852. Medical Care 4:14–16

Hunter R 1956 The rise and fall of mental nursing. Lancet i:98–99

Ignatieff M 1984 The needs of strangers. Chatto and Windus, London

Lomax M 1922 Confessions of an asylum doctor. George Allen and Unwin, London

MacNiven A 1960 The first commissioners: reform in Scotland in the mid nineteenth century. The Journal of Mental Science 106:451–457

Martin J P 1984 Hospitals in trouble. Basil Blackwell, London

Ministry of Health 1924 Nursing in county and borough mental hospitals. HMSO, London

Ministry of Health 1968 Psychiatric nursing today and tomorrow. HMSO, London

Morrall P A 1997 Lacking rigour: a case-study of the professional practice of psychiatric nurses in four community mental health teams. Journal of Mental Health 6:173–179

Nolan P 1993 A history of mental health nursing. Chapman and Hall, London

Nolan P, Cushway D, Tyler P 1995 A measurement tool for assessing stress among mental health nurses. Nursing Standard 9:36–39

Pope N 1997 Danger mental patients evade care. The Sunday Times 20 April: 28

Porter R 1987 Mind-forg'd manacles. Athlone Press, London

Powell J E 1961 Speech by the Minister of Health, the Rt Hon Enoch Powell. Report of the Annual Conference of the National Association for Mental Health, London

Powell J E 1988 My years as Health Minister. The Spectator 20 February: 8–10

Proceedings of the Lincoln Lunatic Asylum and Communications with Her Majesty's Commissioners in Lunacy 1847 Longman, London

Rogers A, Pilgrim D 1996 Mental health policy in Britain. Macmillan, London

Rollin H R 1986 The red handbook: an historic centenary. Bulletin of the Royal College of Psychiatrists 10:279

Rosie R 1948 The early days of army psychiatry. Journal of the Royal Army Medical Corps XC:93–100

Scull A 1982 Museums of madness. Penguin, Harmondsworth, p 67

Shepherd M 1993 Interview with Sir Aubrey Lewis by Professor Michael Shepherd. Psychiatric Bulletin 17:738–747

Short S E D 1986 Victorian Lunacy. Cambridge University Press, Cambridge

Szasz T 1985 A home for the homeless: the half-forgotten heart of mental health services. In: Terrington R (ed) Towards a whole society. Richmond Fellowship Press, London

Tantam D 1991 The anti-psychiatry movement. In: Berrios G E, Freeman H (eds) 150 years of British psychiatry 1841–1991. Gaskell and Royal College of Psychiatrists, London, Ch 22

Tilley S 1997 Introduction. In: Tilley S (ed) The mental health nurse. Blackwell Science, Oxford

Tonks P, Smout L 1982 Rubery Hill Hospital – a short history. Published privately

Tuke W 1813 Descriptions of the Retreat, York

Walk A 1961 The history of mental nursing. Journal of Mental Science 107:1–17

Webster C 1985 Nursing and the early crisis of the National Health Service. The history of nursing group at the RCN. Bulletin 7:12–24

White E 1996 Project 2000: the early experience of mental health nurses. In: Brooker C, White E (ed) Community psychiatric nursing, vol 3. Chapman and Hall, London

Williams M 1989 History of Crichton Royal Hospital. Dumfries and Galloway Health Board, Dumfries

CHAPTER CONTENTS

Key points   49

Introduction   50

Law and mental health   50
  Principles and types of law affecting work in mental
    health services   50
  Enforcing the law   52

Status and rights of patients   52
  Individualism and capacity   52
  Standards   54

Mental health law   55
  Mental Health Act 1983   56
  After-care and legal responsibilities   61

Patients in the criminal justice system   63
  Arrest and prosecution   63
  Court   63

**Nursing detained patients: creating a safe
    environment   66**
  Searching a room   66
  Restricting visitors' access   66
  Mail censorship   67
  Retaking an absconded patient   67
  Use of force   67
  Seclusion   67
  Assault against a nurse   68

Civil law and the patient   68
  Compensation   68
  Managing financial affairs   69
  Making a will   69

**Preparing a report for courts and other statutory
    bodies   69**

Conclusion   70

Cases cited   70

Glossary   71

Key texts for further reading   71

References   71

4

Legal aspects of mental health nursing

Damian Mohan   David Carson
Pamela J. Taylor

KEY POINTS

- The law recognises diminished capacity and responsibility.

- Legislation and case law are the two sources of law in common law countries.

- Nurses are subject to general law, the requirements of their professional body and their contracts of employment.

- Nurses have special protections against litigation by patients.

- Adult patients with capacity can decide for themselves.

- Good practice statements can help deter litigation by being explicit about standards.

- Mental Health Review Tribunal orders release from a detention order not discharge from hospital.

- A supervised discharge order does not authorise a discharged patient to be medicated against the patient's will.

INTRODUCTION

All health care practice is bound by ethical principles and law. Each person who presents to health services for help is presumed to have rights over determining what happens to his or her own body, to have a capacity to be able to do so and to have certain responsibilities for the nature of his or her own behaviour. If someone develops a mental disorder, then more often than not such capacities and responsibilities are unremarkable compared to a mentally healthy peer. For an important minority of people with a mental disorder, however, capacity for decision-making and/or responsibility for behaviour is impaired. In most developed and many developing countries the law takes account of this. The effect is intended, as far as possible, to safeguard patient rights in such circumstances, but also to protect health care staff in the delivery of appropriate care and treatment even in the absence of real consent when the health or safety of the patient or the safety of others might otherwise be at risk. Nurses have a key role in ensuring that patients' civil liberties and other rights are respected.

For an even smaller group of people with a mental disorder, antisocial or dangerous behaviour may emerge, and the law recognises diminished capacity and responsibility and it allows for the possibility that the individual cannot be held fully responsible for such acts and/or should be dealt with primarily as presenting health care problems rather than in the criminal justice system.

This chapter seeks to explore the main principles embodied in mental health and related law and practice. Reference is almost exclusively to England and Wales, since this is where our experience lies. Details of legislation and practice vary between jurisdictions, even within the UK.

Nevertheless, the principles which we will be illustrating from practice in England and Wales are remarkably similar between common law countries. Countries formally under the influence of Napoleon have very different legal systems, but still the core concepts of autonomy, capacity and responsibility underpin their legislation (for a summary and example of international differences see Harding 1993).

LAW AND MENTAL HEALTH

Principles and types of law affecting work in mental health services

In essence, in common law countries, like England and Wales, there are two sources of the law concerned with mental health: legislation and case-law precedents. Legislation for England and Wales includes Acts (such as the Mental Health Act (MHA) 1983) and delegated legislation such as the Mental Health (Hospital Guardianship and Consent to Treatment) Regulations 1983 (SI 1983 No. 893). An excellent text which covers this legislation and relevant case law is Hoggett (1996). As Scotland and Northern Ireland have their own court systems and legislation, the Mental Health (Scotland) Act 1984 and the Mental Health (Northern Ireland) Order 1986 follow similar principles, but differ in important respects. Government circulars do not have the authority of legislation unless (which is rare) they are declarations issued under the National Health Service Act 1977 or Local Authority Social Services Act 1970 (both as subsequently amended); nevertheless, they are influential. Codes are not legislation and they are not binding, unless the Act, which requires them to be drafted, stipulates that they are to be taken into account by courts and tribunals. The MHA 1983 required that a Code be prepared. It was firstly with the 1993 Code of Practice (Department of Health and Welsh Office 1993), and more latterly a new Code of Practice has been issued (Department of Health and Welsh Office 1999). The Act does not stipulate enforcement. All staff working in the field ought, however, to be aware of its guidance and, if deviating in practice, to be prepared to justify that explicitly. Breaches of the Code might leave practitioners liable to civil action. International declarations (e.g. the United Nations Declaration on the Rights of Mentally Retarded Persons 1971) and similar ethical cases are not part of UK law unless and until they are adopted by legislation. If that happened to the European Declaration of Human Rights, as the current government has promised, then its provisions could be enforced in English courts. Already it is possible for patients to seek support for their position through the European Court in Strasbourg when national options have been exhausted.

While many areas of the law affecting people with mental disorders are covered by statute, many others are not. The law concerning negligent treatment, or duties of confidentiality, for example, is not dealt with by any Act of Parliament. These are among the issues which are covered by 'case law'. This means that the courts have established the legal principles, over years, on a case-by-case basis. To discover the law on a particular issue it is necessary to examine the precedents. This requires a search for a similar case that has been before the courts. If the judges agree that the *relevant* legal facts of your case are the same as in a previous case decided by a superior court, then they are bound to apply the same law as in that precedent case. The same happens with the interpretation of legislation. If the court interprets a word or phrase in a particular way, then subsequent courts should follow that interpretation, unless they can find a way of distinguishing the two cases or a higher court has overturned the earlier decision.

Aside from specific mental health legislation, three 'types' of law apply to nurses working in the mental health field. First, there is law in the widest sense, which applies to everyone. That is the most extensive and important kind of law. Second, nurses, like some other professions, are also regulated by special legislation. The Nurses, Midwives and Health Visitors Act 1997 retains the United Kingdom Central Council for Nursing, Midwifery and Health Visiting (UKCC) and National Boards The UKCC's principal functions are 'to establish and improve standards of training and professional conduct for nurses, midwives and health visitors.' The Council registers nurses. It also maintains a Code of Practice on professional standards. Nurses found to have acted unprofessionally, which will involve breaching the Code, can lose their registration. Without registration a person cannot, lawfully, be employed as a registered nurse.

The third 'type' of law is employers' law. When people make a contract, the courts will, if it is necessary (and lawful), enforce it. So, for example, if a nurse is bound, by her or his contract of employment to 'blow the whistle' on any colleague who abuses patients then she or he must do so, or if not, the employer will be entitled to treat it as misconduct. Action may be taken by employers and/or the professional organisations, even though no other law has been broken. In employment, as in other aspects of civil law, the standards of proof rest on the balance of probabilities (although the seriousness of the allegations is taken into account), whereas the criminal law requirement is for evidence 'beyond reasonable doubt'. Thus, a nurse could be sacked under employment law for hitting a patient, even though there was insufficient evidence for a criminal prosecution of assault.

Enforcing the law

An important consideration when reading law books is the emphasis these place on legal points rather than factual disputes. Most cases involving nurses will primarily be about what happened. The nurse says this happened; the patient says that occurred. What the relevant law is will depend upon what the facts were. This is a very important point for practice. It will not matter that a nurse knew and followed the law if a court decides that what actually happened was different from what the nurse claims. Lawyers will always consider the chances of proving that the facts were as their client claims. Thus, nurses should take care with records and think about how they can prove their version of events. How could you convince a court or tribunal that what you say is what you advised the patient, that what you recorded as given on the prescription card is what you injected? Documentation is very important not just to ensure quality communication with others but also to prove what was done should there be a dispute.

Those who bring cases to the courts must prove them (and fund them if they are not eligible for legal aid). In the criminal court the prosecution must find the defendant guilty beyond reasonable doubt. This is a high standard of proof to satisfy. A rare exception allows the defence of insanity (here with its special legal meaning) to be proved on the balance of probabilities, but the onus is on the defendant to prove. In civil cases the standard is the balance of probabilities. If, for example, a patient is suing a nurse for breach of confidence, the patient (the plaintiff) will have to prove his or her case is more likely to be true than the defendant nurse's (i.e. the balance of probabilities favours the plaintiff). However, the courts increasingly state that the level of proof required is linked to the seriousness of the allegations.

Section 139 of the MHA 1983 provides nurses, and others acting or claiming to act under the authority of that act, with special protections. They cannot be sued for such actions without the permission of the High Court, or prosecuted without the consent of the Director of Public Prosecutions, and they will not be liable unless it is also proved that they acted in 'bad faith or without reasonable care'. Case law is unclear about the limits of these extra protections; for example, whether they apply to patients who have not been detained. Section 139 does not apply to patients while challenging their detention, such as by seeking a writ of *habeas corpus*, or with respect to a challenge over the provision or non-provision of services. A patient might seek a declaration from the court that treatment is not to be imposed (see *Re C* below).

The court has powers to review the actions of national and local government, including health authorities and hospitals. The court is, however, anxious not to trespass too far into the political arena, such as by requiring hospitals to provide services for which they do not have the funds. Basically, the court will only intervene when a minister, public official or authority takes a decision which 'no responsible, properly informed, official would take'.

STATUS AND RIGHTS OF PATIENTS

Individualism and capacity

Mental disorder or learning disability is, on its own, legally irrelevant. No English law authorises different treatment of people just because they have a mental disorder or learning disability. For special treatment, more must be demonstrated. The MHA is principally concerned with the detention and involuntary treatment of a small proportion of in-patients and with the management of property under the Court of Protection (see further below).

Other areas of health care and treatment or problem management are not covered by statute. The matter of consent to treatment for disorders other than mental disorders is among the most important. Such areas are covered by case law. The Law Commission (1995), which is an official body set up to review the law, has proposed major changes. The government could implement the Commission's proposals using the draft Act of Parliament that they have provided. Until there is new legislation, however, the court must make decisions based upon the existing precedents.

Re C provides one such example. This concerned a man diagnosed as having paranoid schizophrenia who was detained in a secure hospital. He developed gangrene in a leg and was told, by physicians, that he would die unless it was amputated. He refused and asked a court to declare that, if the doctors amputated his leg without his permission, they would be breaking the law. The judge acknowledged the patient's mental illness but also noted that, during lucid periods, he was able to – and did – understand the issues involved and make a free decision for himself. So the judge gave him the declaration he sought. The judge did not assume incapacity either from the patient's illness or from his detention. He undertook an individualistic assessment.

The patient favoured death over amputation; it was not for the court to judge the patient's value system – the judge and the doctors might have thoroughly disapproved of it for themselves; the court's role was merely to rule on the patient's capacity to make that judgement. It is important to re-emphasise that the treatment (the amputation) was not for a mental disorder. If it had been – for example, if he had a confusional state secondary to toxicity from the gangrene – treatment of the confusional state might have been authorised under the MHA 1983, although still not necessarily the amputation. If the mental disorder had been more pervasive, the court might have taken a different view with respect to the man's wishes had they only been expressed during a disordered state. The position is very different for children.

The Law Commission has recommended that a person should be treated as lacking capacity to make a legal decision (e.g. to make a will or consent to treatment) if he or she is unable, because of mental disability, to make the decision for himself or herself, or cannot communicate the decision. The test of incapacity proposed is:

a. he is unable to understand or retain the information relevant to the decision, including information about the reasonably foreseeable consequences of deciding one way or another or of failing to make the decision; or
b. he is unable to make a decision based on that information

Clause 2(2)

Since this is not, and may never become, statute law why mention it? Because in *Re C* the judge based his decision on such a definition and thus, by precedent, in effect this is English law already.

A great deal of support has been expressed for the Law Commission's proposals, but the incapacity test is more demanding than the Commission appears to have intended! All of us, with or without a mental disability, have difficulties coping with lots of pieces of information at the same time. Think of what happens – or should happen – when patients are asked to consent to a treatment. They must be as fully informed as possible about the nature of the problem in general terms (although the law does not require so much information be given), from which they are suffering, and then of any variation they may encounter because of their individual make-up; individuals then need to know about the positive effects of the treatment – including the chances of its achieving cure, symptom reduction, limitation, prevention – and, then a grasp of any short- and longer-term adverse effects, and perhaps, too, how the proposed treatment may interact with others. That, as minimum, is a lot of information to be able to take in, and then to organise in order to make a decision. Nurses have a vital role to play in assisting patients with decisions, providing they are themselves well informed. Repetition of information is often necessary and a good indicator of some understanding is that the patient asks pertinent questions for more. Good decision-making often takes more than a few minutes and the more continuous contact with nursing staff than other disciplines is helpful.

If patients have capacity, and have not been detained under the MHA 1983, then they are entitled to make their own decisions, and may vary them. They may, for example, withdraw consent to being touched. If you did touch without consent, then it could be a trespass for which you could be sued or even prosecuted. In practice, this is most unlikely to occur, providing the act was done in good faith and genuinely in the interests of the patient, or it was a reasonable step in self-protection. Forcible restraint or injection would be a different matter. (A patient was found not guilty of assaulting a police officer when he tried to escape from a doctor, who wished to sedate him, but who had not first detained him under the MHA.) Detaining someone without authority, such as given by the MHA 1983, or the individual's consent, is false imprisonment.

Standards

While the law of trespass is very important for determining basic principles concerning the rights and dignity of patients, it is rarely relied upon. If a complaint arises, particularly about standards of care, it is more likely to be associated with the concepts surrounding the law of negligence. Nurses, like all other health care professionals, can be sued for negligence. Similar, but not identical, issues and considerations will apply if an employer or professional body were to take action against a nurse. The professional code, issued by the UKCC, closely reflects the requirements of the law of negligence.

The law of negligence involves five key elements. First, the person injured must have been owed a duty of care by the person being sued. Basically, we owe duties to those people we can reasonably foresee would be injured by our actions or inaction. For nurses, that includes patients, clients they are assessing for a service, colleagues with whom they are working, and it should include those members of the public with whom nurses place patients. It does not, however, include everyone. Judges decide who owes whom a duty of care.

The second point is that the injury or loss must have involved a breach of the duty of care. In practice, this is the most important issue in negligence claims. The question is whether the nurse's actions, for example in not seeking the admission of a patient threatening suicide, would be supported by a responsible body of professional opinion (Bolam test). Expert witnesses will be called to say whether they think any or many professionals doing that work would have so acted. The judge determines, from this evidence, what the standard is for the purpose of the hearing and whether the actions under scrutiny met it or not. Minority practices can meet this test. It does not depend on what the best or most nurses would have done. If professional protocols, describing current standards, are developed, they can help prevent litigation because everyone will have a clearer idea of what the contemporary standards are.

Third, in the law of negligence, the breach of the duty of care must have *caused* the losses. If they would have occurred anyway, then they were not due to the breach. Employers and professional bodies, however, are entitled to discipline nurses who behave badly (i.e. breach the duty of care) even though no harm results.

The fourth and fifth requirements in negligence are that the harm suffered must be of a kind that the law recognises (there has been, for example, a dispute in recent years about compensation for post-traumatic stress disorder arising from events experienced indirectly). The harm must also have been reasonably foreseeable.

Only if all five requirements of the law of negligence are proved, on a balance of probabilities, will a nurse be liable. If the nurse was working within the broad remit of his or her employment, then the employers will be responsible for meeting the compensation claim. This is called vicarious liability. Negligence can also be committed directly by managers, for example by allocating untrained or insufficient staff to a particular task.

The law of negligence is also relevant to questions surrounding consent to treatment. Presuming that the patient is capable of consenting (as discussed above), and has not been detained so that treatment may be imposed (see below), the issues are whether the patient actually consented, and about the nature and quality of that consent. If consent has been based on insufficient accurate and relevant information in terms appropriate for the patient, then it will be invalid and any contact will be a trespass. How is the question of sufficient information answered? By using the same sort of test as for the standard of care in the law of negligence. The legal question is whether a responsible body of professionals of the same discipline would have provided that amount of information.

MENTAL HEALTH LAW

Patterns of mental health care and treatment have evolved rapidly since the 1950s, when voluntary admission to hospital became the norm. For England and Wales, Department of Health (1995) figures show that 91% of patients admitted between 1987 and 1993 were admitted voluntarily, in precisely the same way as a patient with any other health problem needing hospital admission.

The decision by the Court of Appeal in the case *R. v. Bournewood Community and Mental Health NHS Trust* may substantially change the position with regard to compulsory detention. At the hearing in December 1997, the Court of Appeal upheld the decision that a hospital could informally admit a person for treatment for a mental disorder under Section 131 of the MHA only with the person's consent. It is clear from this decision that inability to consent makes detention illegal. Mr L, the appellant, was autistic. His needs were described as complex; he had no ability to communicate dissent or consent to treatment, or consent or dissent to detention. He had been resident in Bournewood Hospital for 30 years and in March 1994 he went to live with carers in their own home. Mr L had been living successfully in the community and his carers treated him as one of the family. He did, from time to time, develop tantrums and on one occasion in July 1994, while attending the local day centre, he developed a tantrum. He was given a sedative and taken to Accident and Emergency from where he was referred to Bournewood Hospital to allow for a full reassessment. Mr L made no objection and was compliant to this. His RMO said that she would place him on a Section, should he decide to leave. A request by his carers to bring him home resulted in legal proceedings being instituted on his behalf, challenging the nature of the admission (not the need for it) on the grounds that he did not have the capacity to make a decision about admission, and so the absence of refusal, resistance or distress that attended it could not be taken as consent. In effect, for the admission to have been legal, he should have been compulsorily detained under the provisions of the MHA 1983. This decision was upheld by the Court of Appeal. The court took the view that the critical issue was whether the staff had the ability to, and would, prevent the patient leaving the ward if he decided to do so. However, the House of Lords reversed the decision of the Court of Appeal in June 1998. This outcome leaves a number of important questions unanswered. Protection of the rights of people who lack capacity remains a deficiency in the current MHA 1983 and will clearly need to be addressed in the proposed reform of the MHA 1983.

Community options for treatment have grown, further increasing numbers of people in voluntary treatment. What follows in this chapter is in the same spirit. It will and must only apply to a minority of patients, but discussion of the legal provision for compulsory detention is important because of their potential for unfamiliarity.

The MHA 1959 repealed previous mental health legislation, under which compulsory admission was the rule, and emphasised, under Section 5, that its own subsequent emphasis on compulsory detention should not be taken as preventive of informal admission wherever possible. The MHA 1983 makes the same point (Section 131).

In order to detain a patient against his or her wishes in hospital, a recommendation is required by a health care professional and a social worker. Except in an emergency, the former means two independent doctors, one of whom must have special experience in psychiatry (S12(2)); the social worker must have received special training and be 'approved'. The social work position

should follow consultation with the nearest relative, assessment of family views and suitable accommodation. When the application package is complete, managers of the hospital where the patient is to be detained must formally accept the papers or the detention is not valid or legal.

Mental Health Act 1983

The MHA 1983 has 10 parts. Part I deals with the definition of mental disorder; Part II deals with the civil procedures for compulsory admission to hospital for assessment and treatment, and guardianship; Part III is concerned with patients in criminal proceedings or under sentence; Part IV covers the law in relation to consent to treatment and Part V deals with the independent review of the legality of continued detention, the Mental Health Review Tribunal (MHRT). The remaining five parts of the Act deal with such matters as the removal and return of patients within the UK, management of property and affairs of patients, the functions of local authorities and the Secretary of State for Health, offences against the Act and miscellaneous provisions ranging from duties to inform patients' relatives, or correspondence of patients, to bringing the mentally disordered to a place of safety for assessment. Among the functions of the Secretary of State is the maintenance of the Special Health Authority, the Mental Health Act Commission (MHAC), members of which may see patients and scrutinise the records of all detained patients with the goal of protecting their rights and interests.

Formal admission procedures

Table 4.1 summarises the principal routes to compulsory admission to hospital or community health services on the grounds of mental disorder.

Table 4.1 Summary of provisions available under the Mental Health Act 1983

Objective	The order	Section	Duration/effect
Emergency assessment	1. The patient is already in hospital:		
	a. nurse's holding power	5(4)	Until arrival of doctor (maximum 6 hours)
	b. doctor's holding power	5(2)	Up to 72 hours from making the order
	2. Emergency admission	4(2)	Up to 72 hours from time hospital managers receive papers
	3. Place of Safety Order	136	Up to 72 hours from arrival (not necessarily hospital)
Extended assessment	1. Assessment Order (civil)	2	28 days maximum (application to MHRT must be within first 14 days of detention)
	2. In criminal proceedings:		
	a. For report to a court	35	Up to 28 days – renewable to a maximum of 12 weeks
	b. Interim hospital order	38	Initial period of 12 weeks – with further periods of 28 days up to 1 year* maximum. Comes to an end when sentenced
	(Assessment of 'treatability' prior to sentencing but post conviction)		
Treatment	1. Treatment Order (civil)	3	6 months maximum (renewable for 6 months then annually) can appeal to MHRT once in each period of detention; must be referred if no appeal in 3 years
	2. Hospital Order (criminal court)	37	Initial period of 6 months, first renewal period 6 months, subsequent renewal periods 1 year (MHRT appeal not permitted in first 6 months)
	Restriction discharge	41	Usually indefinite
	3. Remand for treatment while under criminal proceedings:		
	a. Remand Order	38	Crown Court only. 28 days renewable up to 12 weeks
	b. Prison Transfer Order	48	Terminates on return to prison or change of sections by court
	4. Transfer of sentenced prisoners	47	Maximum duration is up to earliest release date; or may be terminated by Home Secretary; may be extended under S37 (i.e. notional 37)
		49	Restriction order
	Hybrid order	45A/B	May serve entire sentence in hospital or transfer to prison
Community provisions	1. Guardianship	7	6 months renewable
	2. Guardianship Order	37	Usually indefinite
	3. Court mandated restrictions allowing conditions (usually) supervision on discharge for the duration	41	Usually indefinite
	4. Supervised discharge order**	25a	6 months renewable or can appeal to MHRT

*Increased to 1 year by Crime (Sentences) Act 1997.
**The Mental Health (Patients in the Community) Act 1995.

Emergency assessment. *1a Compulsory retention in hospital.* If a patient is already voluntarily in hospital, but decides to leave and cannot be persuaded otherwise, there are two provisions in the MHA 1983 to safeguard the patient's health or safety, or the safety of others if as a result of the mental disorder the patient would be compromised by the departure. Section 5(2) allows the patient's retention for up to 72 hours from the signature of the doctor responsible for the patient (the RMO), or the RMO's designated deputy, to allow completion of assessment.

If a doctor is not immediately available, a registered mental health (or learning disabilities) nurse may similarly (S5(4)) prevent departure, but for a shorter period (see Table 4.1). The doctor may extend the period up to the full 72 hours permissible if necessary. A nurse invoking this provision is entitled to 'use the minimum force necessary to prevent the patient from leaving the hospital' (Code of Practice, para 9.6). The nurse must provide a written record to an authorised person as soon as is possible. When the power has lapsed, the nurse must complete a Form 16. It is the responsibility of the senior nurse on duty to inform the patient why it has been necessary to detain the patient under Section 5(4) and what may happen next.

Under the holding powers, the MHA does not provide for treatment without the patient's consent; however, in a bona fide emergency, the general rules under common law apply, and treatment prescribed by a doctor which may be life saving or prevent serious injury or harm may be given regardless of the patient's immediate wishes.

1b Emergency admission. In any case of urgent necessity, an application for admission for assessment can be made under Section 4(2) of the MHA 1983. This 'emergency application' is made either by an approved social worker or by the nearest relative of the patient *and* any one doctor. For up to 72 hours, the patient can then be more thoroughly assessed as an in-patient. Guidance from the Code of Practice is that this approach to detention should only be used in truly exceptional circumstances, because of concern that the rights of the patient may be more vulnerable to inappropriate detention. Reasons for the concern

include the minimal criteria for admission and the absence of any appeal process. In practice, the use of 28-day detention has risen as the use of this 3-day order has fallen (Webster et al 1987) so the balance of protections for the patient is not entirely clear.

Admission for extended assessment. Section 2 allows for compulsory admission and detention for up to 28 days for assessment or assessment followed by treatment for mental disorder. This should be when the diagnosis or role of treatment is unclear, but it is in the interests of the patient's health *or* safety *or* the protection of others for the patient to be so detained. The period of detention is not renewable and, if continued detention is required, then an application for a treatment order (Section 3) must be made. Under both assessment (S2) and treatment (S3) orders, application must be by an approved social worker (ASW) *and* two doctors as described on page 56.

It is often a nursing responsibility to make the initial checks on behalf of the hospital management that the forms are correct, and to receive them formally on behalf of the managers.

The patient may be discharged from the order by completion of the 28 days without further order, by the RMO discontinuing the order, or by an MHRT (see below).

In relation to patients involved in criminal proceedings, the remand for assessment provisions

Table 4.2 Other legislation

Criminal Procedure (Insanity and Unfitness to Plead) Act 1991	A plea used by defendant when because of mental disorder she/he is not responsible for actions which offend against the criminal law	Disposal is at discretion of court which hears psychiatric evidence: ranges from NHS hospital to Special Hospital
Crime (Sentences) Act 1997	Hospital Direction Order (Hybrid Order)	At discretion of court
Other provisions which may have conditions of treatment attached	Bind over, Suspended prison sentence with supervision, Life licence, Probation order, Parole	At discretion of court

were introduced to provide important safe-guards, particularly for nursing staff. Under regular bail arrangements, even if a condition of residence is attached, there are no legal powers to prevent a patient leaving hospital if the patient chooses to go. A nurse or other hospital staff member can only inform the police and the court. Under MHA remand provisions, the day-to-day powers are similar to those for holding any detained patient.

The treatment order. Section 3 provides for the compulsory admission of a patient to hospital for treatment, which can last for an initial period of up to 6 months, and is renewable (see Table 4.1). For this section, the nature of the mental disorder must be sufficiently well understood for the legal classification to be specified.

The categories of mental disorder allowed by the MHA are mental illness (not further defined), severe mental impairment, mental impairment and psychopathic disorder. Sexual problems and alcohol or other drug dependency as sole mental health problems are explicitly excluded. The MHA 1983 introduced the concept of varying degrees of mental impairment for the first time. It is defined as the combination of (severe) impairment of intelligence *and* social functioning *and* abnormally aggressive or seriously irresponsible conduct. In other words, none of the following:

- impairment of intelligence alone
- impairment of intelligence in combination only with impairment in social functioning even if susceptible to treatment and in the interests of the patient's health are sufficient to allow legal detention of a patient.

Only England and Wales retains the term 'psychopathic disorder'. While the terminology is outdated and in itself can require work with patients to reassure them and explain its technical meaning, retention of a separate category to cover personality disorder seems to us to be use-ful. It will undoubtedly, however, be one of the issues under scrutiny when mental health legislation again comes under review.

Consent to treatment

Concepts of consent to treatment have already been introduced. Capacity to make a decision is part of common law. Generally, the patient's autonomy and right to decide about treatments is paramount. Informal patients are empowered to withhold consent should they decide to do so. Part IV of the MHA applies to any patient liable to be detained under the Act except for those liable to be detained by virtue of an emergency application (Sections (4) or 5(2) or 5(4) or 35 see below).

In the UK and most common law countries, there is recognition that mental capacity need not be impaired in relation to all tasks, and the MHA 1983 reflects this. People may not be able to take an appropriate decision about where they are treated, but still they may be competent to decide about specific treatments. They may be content, and/or sufficiently competent to decide to live in a psychiatric hospital or nursing home, but not competent to manage complex financial affairs.

With respect to treatment, every engagement with the patient must be with the patient's consent and co-operation. Even when consent to specific treatment has to be overruled, or even when it may be necessary to restrain a patient physically to deliver that treatment, every effort should be made to continue to explain to the patient what is happening and why. The law, however, has important protective value for nurses and other clinicians in seeking to deliver effective treatment to an uncomprehending or protesting patient. The MHA 1983 referring to patients detained for more than 72 hours recognises consent to treatment as follows:

1. *Treatments described as 'not requiring consent' (S63).* This means consent only in the strict legal sense of the Act. These treatments include any treatment otherwise unspecified in the Act or regulations, but given under medical direction for the treatment of mental disorder. Nursing care has been clarified as belonging to this group. Psychological treatments, including psychotherapy, would also be included.

2. *Treatments requiring consent* or *a second opinion are treatments 'specified by regulations made by the Secretary of State' under Section 58.* At present, the list includes ECT and any psychotrophic medication once prescription has gone on for longer than 3 months in any period of continuous detention. In other words, there is an expectation that for many, probably most patients, recovery on specific medication is likely to be sufficient within 3 months to allow them to take their own decision about continuing, but in any event to provide both patient and staff with the safeguard of formal review. At this point, either the patient's consultant (RMO) must sign a form to confirm that the patient is competent to make a decision about this treatment and is consenting *or* must apply to the MHAC for their second opinion appointed doctor (SOAD) to attend as an independent person to review the treatment plan.

The nurse has an important role to play in the consultation process undertaken by the SOAD. Before providing a signature certifying that either the patient is incapable of consenting or not consenting, but that treatment may be given, the SOAD must be given a full treatment plan by the RMO and 'consult two other persons who have been professionally concerned with the patient's medical treatment'. It is explicit in the MHA that one of them 'shall be a nurse' (and one neither a doctor nor a nurse).

A difficulty with this provision is that the appointed doctor's certification has only the force of advice, albeit legally sanctioned advice, and may not be expert. Fortunately, conflicts of interest for patients or staff arise very rarely, but the responsibility for the treatment decision remains firmly with the patient's RMO. The appointed doctor is not held liable for his/her advice. If, however, the RMO acquiesces to bad advice, say a refusal to certificate neuroleptic treatment for psychosis, that RMO may be held liable if the patient suffers harm as a result and it was argued that the RMO's actions were not acceptable by a responsible body of opinion. Nurses should only attempt to give prescribed specific treatments to a patient if they have verified for themselves that the appropriate consent forms have been completed and remain valid. It is good practice for long-stay patients for forms to be reviewed annually by the whole clinical team; it is essential that changes of psychiatric medication are as well represented on the consent form as on the prescription card. It is vital to remember that a patient's capacity for consent may change over time and this too must be reflected. In any rare instances where there may be deviance from usual clinical practice or Code of Practice Guidance in this regard, this should have been discussed widely in the clinical team and clearly documented.

3. *'Urgent treatment'.* Section 62 allows for 'urgent treatment', which means that any treatment that is 'immediately necessary to save the patient's life' may be given pending compliance with this formal consent process, providing it has no unfavourable irreversible physical or psychological consequences. Immediate prevention of suffering or harm to self or others includes also the caveat that the treatment should not entail 'significant physical hazard'. In practice, this section provides recognition that on rare occasions ECT may be life-saving and a course may be started without delay were an SOAD not to be almost immediately available.

4. *Treatments requiring consent* and *a second opin-*

ion *(S57) are very rarely given.* They are treatments with a high, if not certain, likelihood of permanent change to the individual. At present only psychosurgery, and hormones *implanted* (i.e. a pellet of slow-release hormones surgically inserted into the body) for control of sexual drive are listed.

Anxiety about these treatments is such that no-one may be trusted to consent to them without independent assessment. Whether a patient is detained or not, in hospital or not, in all other respects obviously competent or not, first the patient's specific competence to consent to such a treatment must be checked by an MHAC-appointed team of three, possibly including a nurse. If the competence is in doubt, then the treatment cannot proceed. If it is not, then an appointed doctor must review and consult as under Section 58, and certify that the treatment should be given.

Right of appeal against detention

Most detained patients are entitled to appeal against detention to an MHRT. The exceptions are emergency detentions, and there are also certain times within periods of detention when applications cannot be made, for example the second 14 days of the assessment order (S2) or the first 6 months of a hospital order (S37). An MHRT consists of a panel of three: an independent doctor, a person with a legal training (who for restricted cases must have had judicial experience) and a lay person. An MHRT is fully independent of the detaining hospital. It may order the release from detention of a patient or that the patient continue to be detained. Any other decision, for example to support a transfer recommendation of a restricted patient, has only the force of a recommendation. It is useful to be clear about two points : the MHRT orders *release* from a *detention order*, **not** discharge from hospital.

Some patients may leave as soon as the order is lifted; some may choose to stay. In a very exceptional case, a patient may lawfully be redetained almost immediately (*South Western Hospital Managers*). It is important to have a reasonable grasp of these limitations as the task of explaining detained patients' rights to them is very commonly the task of nursing staff.

Increasingly, nurses are expected to give evidence to an MHRT, or indeed wish to. This is to be welcomed, as it is the nurse who has most day-to-day contact with the patient and is therefore familiar with the daily activities, mental state and associated behaviour of the patient who is appealing against detention.

The patient may, and often does, stay voluntarily for some period after being discharged from a detention order. In the case of transferred prisoners with unspent sentences, discharge from the order (S47 ± 49) has only the effect of returning the patient to prison.

After-care and legal responsibilities

Most people with a mental disorder will live most of their time in the community. Many will need care, specific treatments and even supervision in the community. In response to concerns that such people receive insufficient care in the community, the government has proposed various initiatives, the most important this decade being the Care Programme Approach (CPA) (Department of Health 1990). This provides a structure which sets standards for the after-care of every such person in the community. People who have been detained patients have special rights under Section 117 of the MHA 1983.

Care Programme Approach

The CPA was implemented in April 1993. It applies to all people referred to and accepted by specialist mental health services, and all psychiatric patients considered for discharge from hospital. The objective of the CPA is to ensure that all individuals are properly assessed, and that no-one who is vulnerable can slip through the safety net of care. Its key elements are: the systematic assessment of health and social care needs, an agreed care plan, the allocation of a key-worker, often a nurse, and regular review and monitoring of progress. The patient must be involved in all aspects of the care planning process.

Supervision Register

Discharged patients who need to be more closely supervised, because of the risk that they are judged to pose to themselves or others, may have their names placed on the Supervision Register. They must be told that this has happened. This is to help ensure that they get the follow-up and services that they require. Like CPA, the Supervision Register is part of Department of Health guidance, with the same force.

Section 117

Section 117 places a legal duty on health and local (social services) authorities to provide after-care for detained patients from the point of discharge until they 'are satisfied that the person is no longer in need of such services'.

The Mental Health (Patients in the Community) Act 1995 and MHA 1983 Guardianship

On 1 April 1996, The Mental Health (Patients in the Community) Act 1995, which provides for the Supervised Discharge Order (SDO), came into effect. It was a government response to the high profile case of Christopher Clunis, a man with a mental disorder who killed a stranger in a public place. The ensuing public inquiry (Ritchie et al 1994) recommended such an order. It allows for patients who have previously been detained under Sections 3, 37, 47 or 48 without restrictions, or patients who are on Section 17 leave of absence, who present a 'substantial risk of serious harm' to the health and safety of themselves or others, to be supervised while living in the community. The application with specific requirements, such as place of residence, is made by the RMO to the patient's catchment area health authority. Consultation must take place with the patient, informal carers and the nearest relative. This Act does not permit discharged patients to be medicated against their will. Nor does it authorise entry into the patient's home without his or her consent. If the patient refuses access, then a warrant under Section 135 of the MHA must be obtained from a magistrate.

Guidance in the Code of Practice states that the supervisor is permitted to authorise any responsible adult to convey the patient, and this includes the police. Nurses remain unsure of how much force that they are legally entitled to use when conveying a patient. The Code of Practice again states that 'unreasonable force must never be used when conveying a patient neither should the power (or threat of using it) be used to coerce a patient into accepting medication or treatment'. There are no guidelines available to differentiate between what might be considered to be 'reasonable' force and 'unreasonable' force, however common sense dictates that nurses operating singly or even in pairs should seek co-operation, not confrontation. Concerns about treatment refusal or deterioration of health or behaviour will generally be taken back and a review will be undertaken by the team resulting in an appropriate plan of care being formulated. It is possible that this might include compulsory admission to hospital if the situation is serious or likely to become so.

The Mental Health (Patients in the Community)

1995 Act was introduced amid much criticism, principally, that it simply restated current policy on community care, that it lacked any powers not already allowed under guardianship and that it was not followed by any additional funding.

Guardianship (S7, MHA 1983) requires commitment from social services, but the designated guardian need not be a social worker. It confers powers to require residence at a specified place, attendance at places for the purpose of medical treatment, occupation, education or training and, unlike the new power does confer powers of access to the patient for any registered doctor, approved social worker or specified person (who could be the community psychiatric nurse (CPN)).

PATIENTS IN THE CRIMINAL JUSTICE SYSTEM

Arrest and prosecution

People with some mental disorders are more prone than their healthy peers to come into conflict with the law. Having a mental illness or learning disability does not provide any automatic defence to criminal liability. At every stage of the criminal justice process, however, the law makes provision for the possibility that a mental disorder may impair ability: when making a statement to the police, surviving remand on criminal charges, pleading in court, in relation to guilt and in relation to sentencing in the event of a conviction. Expert reports from the mental health professionals to the courts or other relevant authorities may be required and increasingly nurses are expected to contribute to this process.

Police and Criminal Evidence Act 1984

When a mentally disordered person is interviewed by the police there is a risk of miscommunication, possibly leading to false evidence or false confessions. In England, the Police and Criminal Evidence Act (PACE) 1984 requires the presence of an 'appropriate adult' during police interviews. An 'appropriate adult' may be a relative or guardian of the detainee, or any professional person with experience of dealing with mental health problems with a task 'to advise the person being questioned about the purpose of the interview, to observe whether or not the interview is being conducted properly and fairly, and to facilitate communication with the person being interviewed' (Home Office 1991). A comprehensive account of PACE and 'Fitness for interview' during police detention is provided by Gudjonsson (1995).

Crown Prosecution Service

Should the police consider there is sufficient evidence to pursue charges they must put this to the Crown Prosecution Service (CPS), a national agency of prosecuting lawyers created by the Prosecution of Offences Act 1985. The CPS will make the decision on whether or not to proceed with a particular case on two principal factors: whether the evidence is likely to lead to a conviction and whether proceeding is in 'the public interest'. In the latter context, the CPS is directed by its Code of Practice to pay attention to mental disorder.

Court

After being charged, the defendant must be brought before a magistrates' court. The case may then be remanded for trial. The remand can be on bail or in custody. Lesser offences are likely to remain in the magistrates' court, while the more serious are referred to the Crown Court. At the extremes, the person charged has no say in the type of trial he or she may have. An offence like 'drunk and disorderly' may only be heard at summary trial, a murder charge only before a jury. Some offences in the middle ground may be dealt with 'either way' and the charged person may choose. If the defendant has a mental disorder, then the courts may take this into account at almost any stage of the hearing.

Court diversion

In 1990, a Home Office circular (66/90) (Home Office 1990) reaffirmed government policy that offenders with a mental disorder should be diverted to the health and social services, rather than be detained in the criminal justice system. Court diversion schemes were established to make rapid psychiatric assessments available to magistrates' courts. Where these do not exist, then comparable schemes, such as Bail Information Service, might, in a not dissimilar way, provide verified information at an early hearing in the magistrates' court to assist in decisions about the public interest and possible discontinuance of proceedings, or about best placement of the accused pending trial. The mental health schemes vary in different parts of the UK and internationally in the lead profession. The service in Auckland, New Zealand, for example, was one of the early ones to be CPN-led (Chaplow et al, 1993).

Fitness to plead

Before standing for trial, the defendant must be fit to plead. The legal meaning of 'fitness to plead' requires that the defendant has the mental capacities to understand the nature of the charges against him or her, the meaning of the pleas available to him or her, to know that a juror can be challenged, be able to instruct legal advisers as to his or her defence and to follow evidence. Very few people (less than 40 annually) are found unfit to plead.

Insanity and diminished responsibility

For there to be criminal responsibility, the prosecution must prove, invariably beyond reasonable doubt, that the defendant caused the prohibited act (*actus reus*) with the proscribed mental state (*mens rea*) and that there was no applicable defence. As a few crimes such as murder require intention, the defendant will not be guilty if incapable of intending.

A psychiatric opinion may be sought about what the state of mind of the accused was at the time of the offence in order to help the court with the question of *mens rea*. It is for the defence to consider raising the question of insanity (although others may also raise it), which may apply to any offence, but the criteria for this legal concept are tough, and the defence is hardly used in England and Wales. The Homicide Act 1957 introduced a defence of diminished responsibility for murder cases. An important problem is that a murder conviction carries a mandatory sentence of life imprisonment, but if the person convicted has a mental disorder, the person may be more safely treated as a patient. Under Section 2 of the Homicide Act 1957 a person who kills 'shall not be convicted of murder if he was suffering from such abnormality of mind (whether arising from a condition of arrested or retarded development of mind or any inherent causes or induced by disease or injury), as substantially impaired his mental responsibility for his acts and omissions in doing or being a party to the killing'. Abnormality of mind here is interpreted in a very broad sense: it 'means a state of mind so different from that of ordinary human beings that the reasonable man would term it abnormal'. That is what must happen in practice. It is not a matter of clinical opinion but entirely a matter for the jury in court. If the defence is accepted, then a conviction for manslaughter follows and any sentence is possible. The judge may consider a life sentence appropriate, but his options include a hospital order or a community penalty.

Sentencing

If the sentencing stage is reached, this is the most likely point in a trial that medical recommendations may influence outcome. Evidence of mental disorder may be taken as mitigation and could lessen a sentence. Coupled with a recommendation for treatment of some kind, it is likely to influence subsequent placement.

For patients convicted of an offence which could attract a sentence of imprisonment, sentence may be set aside and a Hospital Order (S37) with or without restrictions (S41) made (see also Table 4.1). The latter can only be imposed in a Crown Court if a psychiatrist gives evidence in person and the court considers the public may be at special risk from the person.

For a good many people, the case for psychiatric treatment may be unclear or unrecognised. In the former case, most usually in relation to the legal category of psychopathic disorder, a recommendation may be made to the court for an interim hospital order. This allows for the patient to be tested in treatment for up to 1 year before the court makes a definitive decision on sentencing.

For those who slip through the net and receive a sentence of imprisonment notwithstanding a mental disorder, or who develop mental disorder in prison, then the MHA 1983 provides for their transfer from prison to hospital, and back again if they recover sufficiently and this otherwise seems appropriate and safe.

A development which came into effect on 1 October 1997 is the Crime (Sentences) Act 1997. This Act amends the MHA 1983 with the introduction of a Hospital Direction Order (SS 45A & 45B, MHA 1983). This amendment permits the Crown Court to attach a Hospital Direction when imposing a sentence of imprisonment on a mentally disordered offender (see Table 4.2). It enables the courts in cases where they are going to pass a prison sentence to send the offender to hospital and therefore gives the courts greater flexibility to deal with somebody who *might* respond to treatment. It was conceived amid anxieties about hospital treatment for 'psychopathic disorder'. The Hospital Direction Order is being introduced in phases; in the first phase it only applies to the legal category of 'psychopathic disorder'. The provision remains for its extension to other categories should that be seen to be appropriate. It is available in respect of all prison sentences, except those fixed by law, that is life sentence for murder. Admission takes place within 28 days of sentencing; the management of the order is similar to that for any transferred, sentenced prisoner (S47). A Limitation Direction can be added by the court, the equivalent restriction on discharge. The prisoner may serve the entire sentence in hospital or can be transferred back to prison if treatment is not thought to be making any difference. It is hard to see what this adds to existing MHA 1983 provisions, but perhaps time will tell.

There is not space here to consider the range of possibilities for liaison through sentencing between mental health and criminal justice services. It is useful to be aware, however, that the court may make 'orders' of various kinds, such as a probation order with a condition of treatment or a bind over. The condition of the order will generally request the offender to attend a probation officer and a mental health worker, almost invariably a psychiatrist. These orders are 'voluntary' in the sense that the offender agrees to abide by them in court, but in the event of not complying with the conditions, the offender may be returned to court in breach of the order and possibly re-sentenced.

It is particularly important if there is a question of admission of a person to mental health services – whether in hospital or in the community – that nursing staff are directly involved in the assessment for placement if they are to be involved in care. While there is no rigid divide between disciplines in the tasks appropriate to a comprehensive assessment, broadly the psychiatrist's task is to assess the personal characteristics of the patient, using family/personal informants as well as the patient as far as possible, and to provide an overall integrative framework for the assessment. The social work tasks are principally around family and social network assessment and evaluation of the community options for placement. Psychologists offer evaluation for specific deficits or, generally, task-orientated treatment packages. Nurses are particularly well qualified to assess environmental aspects of risk, and indeed are principally responsible for environmental safety within a hospital setting. The tasks range from consideration of the physical structure and context of a placement to observation of interpersonal abilities, or lack of them, and implementation of care programmes and treatment.

NURSING DETAINED PATIENTS: CREATING A SAFE ENVIRONMENT

Nursing detained patients gives rise to special clinical issues which require specialist skills. The creation of a secure environment means stable deployment of experienced staff, clear leadership and predictable, clearly structured roles and events (Friis & Helldin 1994). Skills in observation, assessment, prevention and diffusion of violence are all important. From a legal perspective most of the work is uncontentious, but appropriate observations may mean carrying out a room search or monitoring a patient's visitors and mail. Testing patient progress often means taking the patient out of the building; the patient may

abscond and need retaking. All such tasks have ethical and legal implications as well as carrying higher than average risks for personal physical safety and being tasks which most staff find distasteful and emotionally draining. The focus of the following sections is because of the possible legal implications rather than in proportion to their role in maintaining safety.

Searching a room

The MHA does not provide specific authorisation for the searching of patients and their personal belongings. The position depends on the general law. The Code of Practice, however, gives some guidance on procedures that should be followed. It advises that each authority should have an operational policy on the searching of patients and their belongings, which has been checked with legal advisers. Routine searches are not advised outside hospitals or units providing special security and, in the absence of lawful justification, the personal search of a patient or his possessions without his consent would constitute a trespass to the person. In any setting (including security) if there are grounds for a search, the patient's consent should be sought. In the absence of a patient's consent, staff should consult the unit general manager or deputy. Such a search should be carried out by a staff member of the same sex, preferably two nurses rather than one, and the patient's co-operation and involvement maintained as far as possible. An unwitnessed search leaves the nurse more vulnerable to accusations of improper conduct. If items are removed, the patient should be informed where these are being kept.

Restricting visitors' access

Communication with others is cherished by most people and it is important that it is maintained as far as possible for detained patients. Reasons for detention, however, may include risk to others and this may have to lead to some limits on communication by letter, telephone or visits. A visitor may also be excluded because the visitor threatens health or security. Grounds might include: incitement to abscond, smuggling of illicit drugs or alcohol into the hospital, transfer of potential weapons or unacceptable aggression or unauthorised media access. If it is considered necessary by the nurse to exclude a visitor, a full discussion should take place as soon as is practically possible with the patient's multidisciplinary team. The decision should be clearly documented and, where appropriate, the person concerned should be informed. In practice, the limiting of visitors rarely arises as a problem.

Mail censorship

Occasions for interfering with the correspondence of patients are rare and no mail addressed to Members of Parliament, legal or medical advisors, and a court or a statutory body may be intercepted or searched. The MHA 1983 provides for withholding other mail from or to a detained patient only when that is in the interests of the patient or for the protection of others.

Retaking an absconded patient

Most patients, even when hospitalised, are free to come and go as they wish, even those under legal orders including bail remand. Staff may make reasonable efforts to dissuade patients from leaving inappropriately, but for patients detained under the MHA 1983 they have powers in law to bar departure or to retake absconding patients if it is safe to do so, and to escort them back to the hospital. Safety is paramount; the law does not protect from injury, so, while a nurse may have a legal right to restrain a departing patient, if to do

so would result in certain injury to one or both of them, alternative strategies such as simply alerting others may be better in the first instance. Documentation of actions and reasons for them is again vital. The police should be informed at once of the escape or absence without leave of a patient who is considered dangerous. The Code of Practice advises that whenever the police are asked for help in retaking a patient they must be given guidance on a timescale of risks. It is good practice to be able to supply an accurate description and, preferably, a photograph of the patient in such circumstances.

Use of force

The Criminal Law Act 1967 allows 'a person to use such force as is reasonable in the prevention of crime,' and the Code of Practice advises use of 'the minimum necessary (restraint) to deal with the harm that needs to be prevented'. Physical restraint is generally for the last resort, and, when it is used, care must be taken to document the antecedent behaviour in the build-up to the incident as well as the incident itself. Attempts must be made to maintain verbal contact with and reassurance of the patient during any restraint. A specialist technique of restraint known as 'control and restraint' or C & R became popular because staff trained in its use can use minimum force to immobilise a patient, and indeed fewer staff are needed to achieve this. Maintenance of training is essential both for safeguarding patients and indemnifying staff who use the procedures correctly. A comprehensive account on the 'Use and abuse of control and restraint' is provided by Tarbuck (1992).

Seclusion

The Code of Practice defines seclusion as 'the supervised confinement of a patient alone in a room which may be locked for the protection of others from significant harm'. The guidance in the Code is generally unremarkable and sensible. Seclusion should be used as infrequently and briefly as possible. Hospitals should have clear, written guidelines on the use of seclusion, the roles and responsibilities of each member of staff, and the procedures for recording, monitoring and reviewing the seclusion. The decision to place a patient in seclusion can be made by any qualified doctor or nurse. In the absence of a doctor, arrangements must be made for a doctor to attend immediately. A nurse should be readily available within sight and sound of the seclusion room at all times and present at all times with a patient who has been sedated. It is the responsibility of the nurse to document a report every 15 minutes. A review should be carried out every 2 hours by two nurses in the seclusion room and every 4 hours by a doctor. If it is necessary to continue seclusion beyond 8 consecutive hours, or for more than 12 hours intermittently, then an independent review must take place by a senior doctor and a team of nurses who were not directly involved in the care of the patient at the time of the incident. Any use of seclusion should be accompanied by detailed records in the patient's case notes and cross-referenced to a special seclusion book which should contain a step-by-step account of the seclusion procedure. The principal entry should be made by the nurse in charge of the ward and the record should be countersigned by a doctor and a unit nurse manager. The details of observation, supervision, security and recording are to safeguard both the staff involved in the decision to seclude and maintain the seclusion *and* the patient. Patients who require seclusion are generally particularly ill and vulnerable.

Assault against a nurse

Each employing NHS Trust has a duty of care to the patient *and* the staff member. Health and Safety regulations set minimum standards to ensure that employees are operating in a safe environment. Nonetheless, nursing staff are from time to time at the receiving end of an assault, occasionally a serious one. Staff are then faced with the question of whether to involve the police or not and, if so, how far to press an often reluctant police force to pursue the matter with the CPS. In general, it is a useful guide from the clinical perspective that if the process were to have a reasonable chance of influencing patient management for the better, it is worth encouraging proceedings. It may be, for example, that proceedings could lead to a hospital order and a different basis for treatment. It may be that patients who have difficulty in doing other than shifting all responsibility for their actions on to their mental disorder may be enabled to reappraise their responsibility.

CIVIL LAW AND THE PATIENT

Matters in civil law where the patient may be in conflict with the nurse over negligence, trespass or false imprisonment have already been dealt with. The patient, however, may need recourse to law in other civil matters and look to clinicians for help.

Compensation

Recovery of losses and/or compensation after injury or trauma is one principal area that may come to civil law. In criminal cases, the criminal courts may make a compensation order, or the patient may take matters to the Criminal Injuries Compensation Board. Levels of compensation through these routes are generally low, and other possible sources of redress include specially appointed tribunals or a civil action in the High

Court. All such actions tend to be stressful and call for greater levels of support.

Managing financial affairs

Most psychiatric patients can manage their affairs most of the time, but some, for example those with dementia, become unable to do so. As far as possible in such conditions it is helpful to anticipate problems and discuss with patients whether they might be in a position to confer power of attorney to someone of their choice in the event of becoming incapacitated. If, however, incapacitation happens before arrangements of choice can be made, then the Court of Protection may have to be involved. It is very expensive for the patient. It is an office of the Supreme Court, which is administered as part of the Lord Chancellor's department and dealt with in detail under Part VII of the MHA 1983. In practice, the Court of Protection usually exercises its jurisdiction by appointing a receiver whom it grants specified powers. Anyone (usually a relative) can apply for Court of Protection on behalf of the patient. The government has issued a green paper on this topic, so important legislative changes are likely in the next few years.

Making a will

Testamentary capacity essentially refers to the ability to make a will. The testator has to be 'of sound disposing mind' and fulfil the following criteria:

1. understand the nature and implications of making a will
2. appreciate the extent of his/her property
3. know the persons who are the objects of his/her will
4. appreciate which persons reasonably expect to benefit, and the manner of distributing his/her property between them.

It is unusual for wills to be challenged on grounds of impaired capacity, and when they are it can be difficult to assist the court with pertinent clinical advice, since it is post-mortem assessment of the mental state at the time of the making of a will that is likely to be at issue.

PREPARING REPORTS FOR COURTS AND OTHER STATUTORY BODIES

It is not uncommon for a nurse to be asked to prepare a report for legal purposes. This request might be from a court, an MHRT, an inquiry panel or indeed any statutory body. There are principles in preparing reports that apply to any health service practitioner.

The most notable differences, which have ethical implications, between a clinical interview and an interview for the purpose of preparing a report lie in the purpose and subsequent distribution of the information. In ordinary clinical practice, there are reasonable expectations of confidentiality of information given and that the patient's best interests will be paramount. Once a report passes out of the clinical service into another sort of service neither the patient nor the writer can be assured of control of its distribution. The report may, in effect, become a public document. Further, even when a report has been prepared explicitly on behalf of a patient, the use to which it is put may not necessarily prove to be to the patient's advantage. All these things need to be aired clearly with the patient before the process of report writing starts.

Clause 9 of the second edition of the UKCC's 'Code of Professional Conduct for the Nurse Midwife and Health Visitor' gives guidance to nurses on matters of confidentiality (UKCC 1987). It recommends that each nurse shall 'respect confidential information obtained in the course of professional practice and refrain from disclosing such information without the consent of the patient/client, or a person entitled to act on his or her behalf, except where disclosure is required by law or by the order of a court or is necessary in the public interest.' When a nurse interviews a person, whether or not already a patient, primarily for the purpose of preparing a report which will go outside the clinical setting, it must be done with the valid consent of that person.

The essentials then of the preparation and history of the report are to clarify the issues to be addressed, to make the sources of information clear, to verify information as far as possible, to avoid gratuitous information giving and restrict it to that pertinent to the questions at issue, to write in plain English (or at least non-technical language), to distinguish between information and opinion and to confine opinion to what is relevant for the court or body and consonant with expertise. More detailed guidance may be found elsewhere (e.g. Grounds et al 1985)

CONCLUSION

Some of the legal issues that may directly affect the nurse–patient contact in mental health services have been considered. Some aspects of law inescapably affect all practice. Traditionally, doctors and social workers have been most directly involved with using the law in treatment settings but nurses are increasingly involved in a number of ways, particularly in informing detained patients about their rights. They can only do that from a position of knowledge. A special detaining power has been given to nurses, but of more importance in numerical terms is their potential role in review of, or appeals against, continuing detention. Statute law, such as in the Mental Health Act 1983, is relatively easy to follow because it is the most visible. As more recognition is accorded to the rights and competencies of people who have mental disorders, nurses will be not only be expected, but duty bound, as a responsible body of professionals, to ensure that they are aware of the more subtle issues that arise in day-to-day management and over consent to assessments and treatments. As the law is continually undergoing change, refresher training is an important adjunct to experience. The law affecting mental health nursing is an area of practice, that either directly or indirectly, has an impact on every patient's care. A clear knowledge of mental health law should not promote an adversarial relationship between nurses and their patients; on the contrary, nurses have begun to realise that an understanding of the legal issues involved in patient care enhances and reinforces what is their most important goal: a good professional working relationship with the patients that they care for and seek to treat.

Acknowledgement

The authors wish to express their appreciation to Graham Allison, Care Services Manager at Broadmoor Hospital Authority, Berkshire, UK for his advice in drafting the outline of this chapter; and to Christine Tonks for preparing the manuscript.

CASES CITED

Re C (Adult: Refusal of Treatment) ([1994] WLR 290)
South Western Hospital Managers R v. *South Western Hospital Managers and another*, ex parte M [1992] QB; All ER (1994) 161–163

R v. *Bournewood Community and Mental Health NHS Trust.* ex parte L [1998] 1 ALL ER 634

GLOSSARY

All ER   All England Law Reports
QB   Queen's Bench Division.

KEY TEXTS FOR FURTHER READING

Gunn J, Taylor PJ (eds) 1993 Forensic psychiatry: Clinical, legal and ethical issues. Butterworth-Heinemann, Oxford

Hoggett B 1996 Mental health law, 4th edn. Sweet and Maxwell, London

REFERENCES

Chaplow D, Chaplow R, Maniapota W 1993 Addressing cultural differences in institutions: changing health practices in New Zealand. Criminal Behaviour and Mental Health 3:307–321

Department of Health 1990 Joint Health/Social Services 1990. The care programme approach for people with a mental illness referred to specialist psychiatric services. Circular No. HC(90) 23, LASSL (90) 11

• Department of Health and Welsh Office 1983 Code of Practice on the Mental Health Act 1983, 2nd edn. HMSO, London

Department of Health and Welsh Office 1993 Mental Health Act 1983: Code of Practice, laid before Parliament pursuant to Section 118(4) of the Mental Health Act 1983, revised. HMSO, London

• Department of Health and Welsh Office 1999 Mental Health Act 1999: Code of Practice. Stationery Office, London

Department of Health 1995 Inpatients formally detained under the Mental Health Act and other legislation, England 1987–88 to 1992–93. Department of Health Statistical Bulletin 1995/4, London

Friis S, Helldin L 1994 The contribution made by the clinical setting to violence among psychiatric patients. Criminal Behaviour and Mental Health 4:341–352

Grounds A T 1985 The psychiatrist in court. British Journal of Hospital Medicine 33:55–58

Gudjonsson G H 1995 'Fitness for interview' during police detention: a conceptual framework for forensic assessment. Journal of Forensic Psychiatry 6:185–197

Harding T 1993 A comparative survey of medico-legal systems. In Gunn J, Taylor P J (eds) Forensic Psychiatry: Clinical, legal and ethical issues. Butterworth-Heinemann, Oxford p. 118–166

Hoggett B 1996 Mental health law, 4th edn. Sweet and Maxwell, London

Home Office 1990 Provision for mentally disordered offenders. Circular 66/90. HMSO, London

Home Office 1991 Police and Criminal Evidence Act (S66) Codes of Practice (revised). HMSO, London

Homicide Act 1957. HMSO, London

Law Commission 1995 Mental Incapacity Law Commission No. 221. HMSO, London

Mental Health Act 1983. HMSO, London

Police and Criminal Evidence Act 1984. HMSO, London

Ritchie J H, Dick D, Lingham R 1994 Report of the inquiry into the care and treatment of Christopher Clunis. HMSO, London

Tarbuck P 1992 Use and abuse of control and restraint. Nursing Standard 6(52):30–32

United Kingdom Central Council for Nursing, Midwifery and Health Visiting (UKCC) Advisory Paper 1987 'Confidentiality; An elaboration of Clause 9 of the second edition of the UKCC's Code of Professional Conduct for the Nurse Midwife and Health Visitor'. UKCC, London

Webster L, Dean C, Kessel N 1987 Effect of the 1983 Mental Health Act on the management of psychiatric patients. British Medical Journal 295:1529–1532

CHAPTER CONTENTS

Summary of the strategy for modernising mental health services 75
   Failures of the past 75
   Modernising mental health and social care 75
   Investment for reform 76

References 78

5

Government policy and the organisation of mental health care

Kevin Gournay   Malcolm Rae

At the time of writing, at the end of 1998, the new government has been in power for just over 18 months. There have already been some welcome developments which have been underpinned by extra money for mental health services. One of the first actions concerning mental health was the setting up of an Independent Reference Group (IRG), which comprised individuals from a number of different stakeholder perspectives. This group had the task of examining hospital closure and was also used to inform policy development. In the summer of 1998, the government announced the first two national service frameworks (NSFs) and mental health and coronary heart disease have been chosen as the first priority areas. The NSFs will set national standards and link these standards with new initiatives on effectiveness led by the National Institute for Clinical Excellence (NICE) and health improvement led by the Commission for Health Improvement (CHIMP). The NSF is being informed by an External Reference Group (ERG), which, like the IRG comprises a range of different perspectives including users, carers, health professionals and policy makers. The ERG is working to tight deadlines and the framework for mental health is due to be published in July 1999. In the wider context, the government has also set up initiatives to reduce social exclusion – a topic which is obviously of great importance for those with long-term mental illness who are often one of the most marginalised groups in society. As a corollary of these initiatives, the Chief Nursing Officer, Mrs Yvonne Moores, is leading the development of a new strategy for Nursing, Midwifery and Health Visiting, which will be published in late 1999. We are also awaiting the outcome of a review which may see changes in the structure and function of the UKCC and the National Boards.

To understand the current policy position regarding mental health, and to appreciate the context, one needs to examine some of the recent developments in both mental health nursing and the mental health services more generally. 1994 saw the publication of *Working in Partnership* (Department of Health 1994) which was a result of a 2-year-long review of mental health nursing. One of the clear messages from this review, which was in accord with other developing mental health policy, was that there should be a focus on people with serious and enduring mental illness. Subsequently, the Clinical Standards Advisory Group (CSAG) on Schizophrenia (Department of Health 1995a) set out a range of standards for working with people with schizophrenia, both in hospital and in the community. This was the first time that government had attempted to set national standards for the care and treatment of any mental health group, and this initiative has preceded more recent attempts to underpin practice with evidence. CSAG has now started work on depression, and within 18 months or so, practitioners, service planners, and managers will be given clear standards for the care and treatment of people with depression, a condition which affects one in five of us. It is also very pleasing to note that the CSAG Depression Committee contains four nurses in its membership, thus ensuring that the nursing perspective in this work will be robust. It is of course entirely logical that standards of care are led by

evidence; however, the evidence of efficacy of treatments for mental health problems is sometimes difficult to find. Indeed, recently Lewis et al (1997) in a consideration of the issues of evidence-based medicine in psychiatry, suggested that the task of reviewing evidence in mental health care was 'truly Herculean'.

Another major guiding principle for those working in mental health services is of course the Care Programme Approach (CPA) (Department of Health 1990). This set out the principle of key-working and emphasised the requirement for systematic assessments of health and social care and the regular review of an established care plan. Subsequently, *Building Bridges* (Department of Health 1995b) described how the care plan could be tiered so as to prioritise services for those with the most severe problems. More recent developments of the CPA have included a focus on risk assessment and management, with Discharge Guidance and Supervision Registers (Department of Health 1994). However, it must be said that there has been a lack of conceptual clarity regarding the CPA and that as the CSAG study on schizophrenia showed, several years after its introduction the CPA had not been implemented. We now know that, in order to make the CPA effective, patients need a variety of services and some, but not all, of these are provided by mental health services. The Department of Health guidance in *The Spectrum of Care* (Department of Health 1996) summarises the components of these services, including:

- 24-hour nursed care
- crisis services
- intensive home support
- assertive community treatment.

Recently, the Secretary of State for Health, Frank Dobson, announced a new vision and way forward for modern mental health services. The following summary of this strategy makes clear that the government has made mental health services a major priority. This is supported by a major new financial investment.

SUMMARY OF THE STRATEGY FOR MODERNISING MENTAL HEALTH SERVICES (DEPARTMENT OF HEALTH 1998)

- The government's commitment to a modern, decent and inclusive society provides the context for the vision for mental health services. The government is committed to working in new ways to tackle the problems of social exclusion.
- The government has set out clear proposals to modernise the NHS and social services:
  — the new NHS spelt out the need for health services to tackle the root causes of ill health, to ensure high standards of health care and to provide quicker treatment
  — modernising social services highlights three priorities for personal social services: promoting independence, improving protection and raising standards.

The government wishes the NHS and social services to work more in partnership to provide integrated services which will improve the quality of life for people using the services.

- The new vision for mental health services for adults will mean safe, sound and supportive services for patients and users. The government sets out how they will translate this into action at local level. Action is already being taken to improve mental health services for young people. The National Service Framework for Older People will consider the mental health needs of older people.
- This new vision will be supported by £700 million of new investment over 3 years, better treatment and care, and a modern framework

of law. The government will ensure this new investment is well spent by setting clear objectives, monitoring performance and by ensuring effectiveness and cost efficiency at every level.

Frank Dobson went on in this document to describe issues relating to failures of the past, modernising mental health and social care and investment for reform. These sections are quoted verbatim.

Failures of the past

- Although with staff dedication and commitment, the policy of care in the community has benefited many, there have been too many failures. Failure has been caused by:
  — inadequate care, poor management of resources and underfunding;
  — the proper range of services not always being available to provide the care support people need;
  — patients and service users not remaining in contact with services;
  — families who have willingly played a part in providing care have been overburdened;
  — problems in recruiting and retaining staff;
  — an outdated legal framework which failed to support effective treatment outside hospital.

Modernising mental health and social care

- We will modernise mental health services by providing safe, sound and supportive services:
  — services should be safe, to protect the public and provide effective care for those with mental illness at the time they need it;
  — services should be sound, ensuring that patients and service users have access to the full range of services which they need;

— services should be supportive, working with patients and service users, their families and carers to build healthier communities.

- Modern mental health services will assess individuals' needs, deliver better treatment and care whether at home or in hospital, enable 24-hour access to services, ensure public safety, and manage risk more effectively.
- Modern mental health services will have a firm base in primary care. Primary Care Groups will work closely with specialist teams to integrate service planning and delivery.
- Information systems will support the delivery of care and the management of resources, and there will be close partnerships with education, employment and housing.
- Patients, service users and carers will be involved in their own care, and in planning services.
- Services will be delivered in the most efficient and cost-effective way with clear guidance from the National Institute for Clinical Excellence.
- Secure hospital services will be improved. Public protection will remain our first priority at all times.

Investment for reform

- Reform will be underpinned by substantial new investment – £700m over 3 years. This new investment will be in return for reform and improvements in service delivery, efficiency and cost effectiveness.
- The new investment will provide extra beds of all kinds, better outreach services, better access to new anti-psychotic drugs, 24-hour crisis teams, more and better trained staff, regional commissioning teams for secure services, and development teams.
- Performance will be monitored through the new performance assessment frameworks for health and social care, complemented by external inspection through the Social Services Inspectorate, the Joint Reviews with the Audit Commission, and the new Commission for Health Improvement.
- A new mental health National Service Framework will determine service models

and national standards. Action is being taken to improve services for children and adolescents. The mental health needs of older people will be considered in the National Service Framework for Older People which will be published in 2000.

Where does this lead mental health nursing? Previous changes in policy have of course substantially altered the role of community mental health nurses, who have, across the country, de facto become case managers in many of the community mental health teams. This role has brought with it greater responsibility and autonomy, while at the same time nursing staff are realising that they have very important duties regarding joint working with other health and social care professions. As other chapters in this book show, nurses are acquiring a wider range of skills in social and psychological interventions, and there is no doubt that the role of the community mental health nurse is rapidly evolving. At the same time it has been recognised that the other professions involved in mental health care are also needing to address the twin demands of changing policy, and emerging evidence. In this context, the Sainsbury Centre undertook a review, chaired by Rabbi Julia Neuberger, to look at the roles of the various professions, and to examine training issues. The publication of the report *Pulling Together* (Sainsbury Centre 1997) has stimulated a great deal of debate. However, there is general agreement that, in order to make policy most effective, the recommendations of greater interdisciplinary training and working to produce practitioners with a number of core competencies are a priority. As far as community nursing is concerned, we have some idea of the changes which are occurring, having been informed of these by the latest quinquennial study of community psychiatric nursing (Brooker & White 1998).

What then of the future? Undoubtedly, the current proposals for changes in the commissioning of health services, and the shift to primary care, will have many implications. One of the major issues will be how primary care and mental health services address the needs of those who do not have schizophrenia, or other serious and enduring illnesses, but nevertheless are afflicted with depression, anxiety, phobias, obsessions and a range of other problems. These conditions produce not only a great deal of suffering for the individual but also a tremendous burden for their families and for society more generally. It needs to be said that, if untreated, some of the conditions which do not come under the broad umbrella of serious mental illness, do become chronic and intractable, and may well have the same impact on quality of life and economic burden as schizophrenia and major affective disorder. Some of the dilemmas regarding the targeting of these populations with effective interventions have been set out in a recent discussion document (Goldberg & Gournay 1997) and the Department of Health Review of Psychotherapy Services (Department of Health 1997) has suggested a typology for delivery of interventions. With regard to mental health nurses specifically, nurse therapists who have received specific training in effective interventions (ENB course no. 650) have been shown to provide a very cost-effective service (Marks 1985). The difficulty, however, is that the numbers of these nurse therapists is relatively small and a central challenge for the profession will be to develop courses which will provide larger numbers of such workers. Another solution to the problem is to strengthen the role of the general practitioner and the rest of the primary care team, something suggested by Michael Shepherd and colleagues more than 30 years ago (Shepherd et al 1966). In this regard, the Department of Health has recognised the importance of practice nurses in the detection and management of mental health problems and has funded a large study

to examine how this might be effected (Plummer et al 1997). This funding is most apposite, given the fact that a recent study reported that very significant amounts of practice nurse time are already given over to mental health tasks (Gray et al 1999). Other ways forward include a greater use of computer technology in both the assessment and treatment of mental health problems (Marks 1998). The developments in using computers as self-treatment aids in anxiety, depression, obsessions and phobias are currently being developed within the context of nurse-led clinics, and it seems entirely likely that, in time, the running of these clinics could be jointly managed by nurses and volunteers who may have had a mental health problem themselves.

It needs to be said that there are a number of areas of mental health nursing which have not received sufficient attention. These include services for the elderly and child and adolescent services. Both of these areas are currently being targeted by government. For example, the next NSF will focus on elderly people and we are awaiting the outcome of the Royal Commission on the Elderly. At the same time, we also know that certain aspects of caring for people with mental illnesses in whatever setting have also been relatively neglected. For example, although the standardised mortality ratios of people with schizophrenia are 2.5 that of the general population, attention to their physical health needs is often superficial, and problems such as smoking, weight gain (which is a particular problem with the new generation of atypical antipsychotic drugs) and sexual functioning are often not targeted. It is clear that interventions concerning physical health with these populations could lead to considerable health gain.

The final challenge is in the area of in-patient care, where it is recognised that nurses are now facing increasing difficulties, notably, pressure on beds, increased levels of violence, substance misuse, social deprivation, and poor education and training opportunities. Recently, the Standing Nursing Midwifery Advisory Committee (SNMAC) recognised this problem, and at the time of writing, a project commissioned by SNMAC is working on a report which will recommend the development of a range of initiatives in this area. As indicated above, current policy emphasises 24-hour nursed accommodation, and it is recognised that residential care will not necessarily be provided in the traditional district general hospital units, rather it will increasingly take place in properly staffed community residences. We also need to be cognisant of what seems to be a positive impact following

the setting up of psychiatric intensive care facilities. It seems clear that the provision of specific services for the patients in the most acute stages of their illness are important. However, it must be said that it is sometimes difficult to define exactly what an intensive care facility is.

In conclusion, policy in mental health care is currently developing at a breathtaking rate. The government is committed to seeing mental health as a priority for the foreseeable future. Nurses form the bedrock of modern services, and there is an imperative for continued attempts to strengthen, support and nourish this most valuable workforce.

REFERENCES

Brooker C, White E 1998 The fourth quinquennial survey of community psychiatric nursing. Department of Nursing Studies, University of Manchester, Manchester

Department of Health 1990 The Care Programme Approach for people with a mental illness referred to the specialist psychiatric services. HC(90) 23, LASSL (90)11

Department of Health 1994 Working in partnership: the review of mental health nursing. HMSO, London

Department of Health 1995a The report of the clinical standards advisory group on schizophrenia. HMSO, London

Department of Health 1995b Building bridges. HMSO, London

Department of Health 1996 The spectrum of care. HMSO, London

Department of Health 1997 Review of psychotherapy services in the NHS. HMSO, London

Department of Health 1998 Modernising mental health services: safe, sound and supportive. HMSO, London

Goldberg D, Gournay K 1997 The GP, the psychiatrist and the burden of mental health care. Maudsley Discussion Paper No.1. Institute of Psychiatry, London

Gray R, Parr A, Plummer S, et al 1999 A national survey of practice nurse involvement in mental health interventions. Journal of Advanced Nursing (In press)

Lewis G, Churchill R, Hotopf M 1997 Editorial: Systematic reviews and meta analysis. Psychological Medicine 27: 3–7

Marks I 1985 Nurse therapists in primary care. RCN, London

Marks I 1998 Computer aids to self treatment of anxiety. Progress in Neurology and Psychiatry 12: 35–37

Plummer S, Ritter S, Leach R, Mann A, Gournay K 1997 A controlled comparison of the ability of practice nurses to detect psychological distress in patients who attend their clinics. Journal of Psychiatric and Mental Health Nursing 4: 221–223

Sainsbury Centre for Mental Health 1997 Pulling together. Sainsbury Centre Publications, London

Shepherd M, Cooper B, Brown A, Kalton G 1966 Psychiatric illness in general practice. Oxford University Press, Oxford

CHAPTER CONTENTS

Key points 79

Introduction 80

The trouble with interviewing – a place to start 80

Questioning and advice-giving 81

Approaching the client 82
1. Each client is unique 83
2. Each client has skills 83
3. Each client interacts with the environment 83
4. Clients are like us 83
5. Clients are honest 83
6. Each client sincerely desires success 83
7. Clients desire interaction and negotiation and share responsibility with the interviewer 83
8. Each client knows what the problem is and when success has been achieved 84

Opening a consultation 84
Planning 84
Engaging with the client 85
Agenda setting 86

General assessment skills 86
Aims of assessment 86
Information-gathering 87

Alliance-building and treatment orientation 89
Orientation of the client and sharing information 89
Rewarding client information 91
Rewarding client attempts at coping 92
Offering a rationale for intervention 92

Goal-setting and planning 94
Working towards goals 97
Setting interim goals 97
Increasing the likelihood that clients will achieve goals 98

Conclusion 99

Exercise 100

Kay texts for further reading 100

References 100

6

General consultation skills

Robert Newell

KEY POINTS

- The job of skilled consultation is as complex as skilled interaction in ordinary social life, but differs in that the skills involved are applied systematically in a goal-directed way.

- The key goals involve eliciting information, emotion and behaviour change from the client.

- To meet these goals, the nurse:
  — employs appropriate general social skills
  — organises the consultation systematically
  — controls the flow of information using reinforcement
  — ensures the client is orientated during the consultation
  — rewards the client's attempts at coping
  — offers an appropriate rationale for treatment
  — sets mutually agreed summative and interim goals
  — uses reinforcement to help the client achieve these goals.

INTRODUCTION

The activity of interviewing is by no means confined to mental health nursing in particular or to nursing in general. Indeed, much of the empirical study of interviewing technique and effectiveness comes from other disciplines. Accordingly, the examples in this chapter will be drawn from fields as diverse as medicine, nursing, social science research interviewing and experimental and occupational psychology. The aim of the chapter is to present the reader with a viable approach to organising the general skills required in engaging with clients in mental health settings. Much of the information will, because of its general focus, be relevant to other areas of nursing. The chapter will rely, wherever possible, on insights drawn from actual studies of interviewing technique and will minimise reliance on other material which, while often quoted, has little empirical support. In certain instances, and in the absence of better evidence, the descriptive accounts of expert interviewers of their approach will be used.

The general approach of this chapter is to describe and define the *process* of interviewing, rather than the content. This specific content is influenced by the knowledge base and therapeutic orientation of the nurse, as well as the particular difficulties presented by a given client. Process, however, may be approached in a similar way across a wide range of settings. The approach to the process of interviewing outlined here is based on the cognitive–behavioural approach to interviews outlined in Newell (1994) (and, in particular, the role of reinforcement in controlling the flow of information and the therapeutic relationship) and draws on a range of empirical findings. It is this latter element that is, in many ways, the more important of the two. It is not necessary to accept the cognitive–behavioural approach to clinical practice (although this

is a very general, flexible and widely-accepted approach) in order to use this chapter to enhance your interviewing skill, merely to consider the implications for increasing interviewing skills of this approach and, in particular, the empirical studies which inform it.

THE TROUBLE WITH INTERVIEWING – A PLACE TO START

Mental health nursing relies heavily on the relationship between nurse and client and the forging of a therapeutic alliance. This, in turn, requires good communication skills on the part of the nurse. However, in a recent study of non-completion of community mental health interventions, Hostick & Newell (1998) found that the therapist was a major source of dissatisfaction for non-completers and that this seemed to be related to the therapist's ability to engage with the client. Moreover, dissatisfaction with the therapist was one of the most frequently cited reasons for discontinuing treatment. This dissatisfaction is common across disciplines. Thus, a major source of dissatisfaction during medical consultations is the clinician's poor interviewing skills (Ley 1977).

Newell (1994) has argued that these difficulties in engagement of the client occur, in part, because the clinician has a different world view from the client, which is kept a secret throughout the interview. The clinician has a particular agenda derived from the therapeutic standpoint, which leads the clinician to interact with the client in ways consistent with that standpoint. At its simplest, this may lead to the asking of a series of questions aimed at enabling the clinician to isolate particular areas of difficulty. Conversely, the interviewer who takes a non-directive approach may favour a free-flowing approach to the consultation, in which the client is simply encouraged to describe areas of concern, with little direction from the therapist. The problem, in each case, is that the therapist's agenda in structuring the interview is not shared with the client. A key complaint of clients is the lack of structure apparent in some interviews (Ley 1977). As a further complication, the client and clinician are likely to come from worlds which are literally different: different in education, income, class, specific knowledge and vocabulary. Although it is most likely that the clinician will be advantaged in all these spheres, it is, paradoxically, the client who has to make allowances for the clinician's differing background (Dillon 1990).

Imperfect questioning technique on the part of the clinician may have the result that such issues never reach the surface. This in turn may, in some respects, work to the short-term advantage of the clinician (e.g. by allowing greater control of aspects of the interview such as length, content and emotional material). Moreover, clinicians who are unaware of flaws in their interviewing run the risk of defending themselves by ascribing non-compliance to the client. This may indeed be the case, given that compliance, client satisfaction and interviewer skill are closely linked (Ley 1979). The point at issue here is that such non-compliance is now generally recognised as being within the control of the clinician. Given the greater power of the clinician during the consultation process, including the ability to control the way in which information is elicited and transmitted and the ability to reinforce appropriate client behaviour, it may be argued that adherence (or compliance) in interview situations is, in fact, primarily the *responsibility* of the clinician. Similarly, it is argued in this chapter that the clinician who gains poor information during assessment, or achieves poor adherence from the client to the therapeutic strategies they have arrived at together, does so primarily because of inappropriate interviewing behaviour.

QUESTIONING AND ADVICE-GIVING

The cognitive–behavioural approach to interviewing which underpins this chapter is highly focal and relies on direct questioning of the client in order to establish key elements of client difficulties. It is argued that these elements need to be established, regardless of the therapeutic orientation of the clinician. The use of questioning is by no means confined to the cognitive–behavioural approach. For example, Egan's model of skilled helping (1990) requires the use of some questioning in helping clients to clarify their difficulties. Nevertheless, some schools of thought in counselling deny the usefulness of asking questions of the client, often claiming that the chief role of the interviewer is in facilitating clients in coming to their own solutions to their problems, by the use of verbal statements and non-verbal behaviours indicative of warmth, genuineness and empathy with the client. Questions are seen as impeding this process (Rogers 1951).

Cognitive–behaviour therapists also offer a good deal of direct advice to clients. It has become traditional to suggest that nurses avoid advising the client directly, particularly where personal problems are concerned. Newell (1994) identified the following reasons why advice is supposed to be problematic:

- advice prevents clients from identifying and pursuing their own chosen course of action
- advice blocks the client from exploring emotional issues
- advice protects the clinician from feelings of inadequacy
- advice leads to premature closure of debate
- advice allows the possibility of manipulation of the clinician by the client (Sundeen et al 1989).

Despite these apparent problems, cognitive–behaviour therapy (CBT) has an extraordinarily sound record of therapeutic success (Fonagy & Roth 1996, Parry, 1996, Rachman & Wilson 1980). This apparent contradiction between some of the traditional teachings of counselling as transmitted into nurse training and the cognitive–behavioural approach is, however, capable of resolution.

Cognitive–behaviour therapists ask a great many questions, but seek to do so within the context of an open agenda which keeps the client orientated to the interview process throughout. As a consequence, questions do not become threatening or inhibiting, but allow the client to explore important areas in a highly focal manner. This agenda and structure are central to the approach described in this chapter.

Turning to advice, it should be noted that the offering of very general tactics is unlikely to be successful. A cognitive–behavioural approach to consultation skills does not advocate this. By contrast, advice-giving is best seen as an interactive, changing process of negotiation between client and therapist, in which both strive to find the best course of action. The therapist uses specialist knowledge to offer specific information which the client can apply to the process of trying to cope. This will doubtless involve, on occasion, straightforward, didactic information-giving, at one extreme, but can equally involve clients in an examination of their own thoughts, behaviours and feelings in a way which leads them to be able to create their own advice. In this second instance, the specialist knowledge provided by therapists resides in their skill in leading and encouraging the client towards the most potentially rewarding solutions. Thus, in the cognitive–behavioural approach, advice is any tactic which seeks to offer clients *skills or knowledge* to use in confronting and conquering their difficulties. Clearly, the imparting of such skills and knowledge must be handled in ways which maximise the likelihood of the client successfully

using them. Successful advice-giving, in this sense, is a complex range of skills involving not only the provision of information but, crucially, the use of reinforcement to cement a therapeutic relationship which motivates and supports the client in the use of this information. In the absence of these process skills, adherence is likely to be poor. This lack of skill may itself account for the bad name advice-giving has in health care.

It is also worth noting that some of the assertions made by counselling orthodoxy have received little support in the literature. There is, for example, little clear evidence to demonstrate that Rogers' (1957) 'necessary and sufficient conditions' for effective therapy (warmth, empathy and genuineness) are either necessary or sufficient (e.g. Lambert et al 1978, Rachman & Wilson 1980). Indeed, much of the content of this chapter both assumes that mental health nurses possess these characteristics and offers concrete ways of demonstrating them to clients. However, without clear and appropriate advice, based on the best available evidence, such characteristics alone are unlikely to be sufficient to enable clients to address their difficulties effectively.

APPROACHING THE CLIENT

In CBT, the emphasis is on the client as an active partner in care and this emphasis is likewise seen in the cognitive–behavioural approach to general consultation skills. Cognitive–behaviourists stress the uniqueness of individual experience and the continuity between problematic and non-problematic behaviour. As a consequence, the interviewer seeks to make the consultation as normal as possible for the client, approximating as far as possible to the client's experiences of social discourse in daily life, so that the client experiences as little distraction as possible from the business to be covered in the consultation. The following assumptions are derived from the cognitive–behavioural approach and may be thought of as guiding the nurse in all interactions with the client.

1. Each client is unique

Egan (1990) writes of helping clients to tell their stories, and this is at the heart of the effective consultation. Clinicians need to know this story in detail in order to develop the treatment interventions which are most appropriate to the client's needs and goals. Thus clinicians' behaviour at interview should seek to maximise the likelihood that the story will be told.

2. Each client has skills

Only small parts of clients' lives are generally concerned with their problems. An effective consultation also focuses on client strengths. These strengths can later be enlisted in constructing effective interventions.

3. Each client interacts with the environment

Effective consultations seek to place clients in the context of their lives away from the interview.

4. Clients are like us

Notions of 'pathology' have little place in the cognitive–behavioural approach to treatment or consultation. Effective consultation involves interviewers in accepting the similarity of their experiences with those of the clients, in terms of genetic inheritance and learning opportunities. Much of the consultation will be directed towards discovering the specifics of those learning experiences as they relate to the clients'

difficulties. Since cognitive–behavioural approaches accept the similarity between the genesis and maintenance of problematic and non-problematic behaviours, thoughts and feelings, it is also regarded as highly likely that clinicians can understand and empathise with client difficulties and build therapeutic relationships with them which facilitate advice-giving and performance motivation.

5. Clients are honest

The notion that clients are concealing information, either wilfully or because of putative unconscious motivations, has no place in the cognitive–behavioural consultation. As a general rule, clients are giving us the best information they can and poor histories are regarded as a consequence of poor history-taking.

6. Each client sincerely desires success

Clients often experience difficulty in adhering to the interventions they have agreed with therapists, but do not generally deliberately sabotage their treatment. The consultation seeks to optimise the conditions available to achieve appropriate adherence and the clinician is highly active and responsible in seeking to achieve collaboration.

7. Clients desire interaction and negotiation and share responsibility with the interviewer

The interviewer is more familiar with the consultation process and its consequences for treatment than is the client. Clients rarely welcome purely didactic instruction and this form of advice-giving is rarely useful. The effective consultation involves clients in each stage of the process.

8. Each client knows what the problem is and when success has been achieved

Effective consultation does not consist of a detective story which seeks clues as to mysterious causes. The effective interviewer simply attends closely to what clients say about their difficulties, their maintaining factors, their impact upon life and the desired changes.

OPENING A CONSULTATION

The beginning of an encounter is highly important, and is well-remembered by participants (Newell 1994). As a consequence, starting consultations merits particular attention. Appropriate beginnings offer the clinician the opportunity to begin the therapeutic relationship well and to orientate the client to the material that is to follow, with consequent improvement in information transmission. Goldberg et al (1984) studied the interviewing behaviour of trainee psychiatrists and found a number of basic skills were lacking. They initiated a training programme to address these deficits. Some elements of the programme were aimed at specific elements of a particular mode of psychotherapy and so are not relevant here. It should be noted, however, that the clearest deficits related to simple social behaviours involved in opening the interview and orienting the client. These deficits were also those areas most successfully addressed by the training programme and form the basis for the structure for starting consultations shown below. In more recent years, this approach has formed the backbone of teaching of consultation skills to nurse behaviour therapists, a group of clinicians whose practice is amongst the most extensively investigated in nursing (e.g. Ginsberg & Marks 1977, Marks et al 1977, Newell & Gournay 1994). The approach is further described in Richards & McDonald (1990) and Newell (1994).

Planning

Effective consultations are planned encounters for which the clinician aims to be as well prepared as possible. In this way, as little as possible is left to chance, and the clinician is freed to devote maximum concentration to clients and their stories.

Timing of the consultation is a basic consideration in good practice and is related to good case management. Hurried interviews are rarely successful. Thus, the effective interviewer attempts to maintain a caseload which allows for appropriate time to be devoted to each consultation.

Aims and objectives are at the heart of cognitive–behavioural intervention (which is highly goal directed) and are valued by consumers of education as well as of health care. Aims are broad statements of interviewer intent, while objectives are narrower, and may generally refer to both interviewer and interviewee behaviour at the end of the interview (Jarvis & Gibson 1985). We will examine goal-setting with clients as a consultation skill later in this chapter. In the context of preparation for a consultation, effective interviewers consider their likely goals during the consultation, in the context both of what they already know about the client and their more general goals for every consultation. Attending to the aims of the meeting has been shown to be associated with greater quality of information (Dzurec & Coleman 1997)

Referral data is an important source of preparatory information and should always be examined prior to a consultation. Nevertheless, such information should be examined in an analytical, critical and sympathetic manner. The collection of this data may well be biased owing to systematic distortion by time, personality and the expert's own interviewing style (Newell 1992, Thompson 1984a). Moreover, referral information may well contain irrelevant opinion about the client, which the clinician will do well to filter, particularly where it is clear a client is unpopular with the referring agent.

Resources of the clinician are an important potential constraint in the consultation. Most particularly, the interviewer may be able to assess, from the referral data, whether it is possible that the client will present difficulties which represent a significant challenge to the interviewer's current level of therapeutic expertise. In this case, the clinician will want to take care to have appropriate sources of professional advice and supervision which will be readily accessible. Practical issues such as caseload mix, distance and availability of co-therapy should also be considered.

Records and recording are important considerations prior to consultation, particularly if unusual forms or other recording devices are likely to be required. As well as ensuring that such equipment is ready to hand, the clinician may need to make provision for the gaining of consent from the client for its use.

Possible outcomes are, by their nature, difficult to predict if the clinician is pursuing a flexible consultation strategy which is sensitive to individual client needs. Nevertheless, some tentative consideration of likely outcomes is not only possible but also advisable, since the clinician will wish to be prepared for a range of eventualities resulting from the consultation.

Setting of the consultation has potential consequences which should be considered by the interviewer. Distracting, even unpleasant physical surroundings are, unfortunately, not always avoidable, but these practical limitations can be minimised if the interviewer explains the difficulty to the client. The presence of other people is an important aspect of setting which potentially requires careful handling. Dealing with group interviews is a skill which is beyond the scope of this chapter to examine. However, the clinician will certainly wish to consider the likely impact of interviewing the client in the presence of significant others.

Engaging with the client

Greeting is the first element of both engaging the client and orienting the client to the consultation.

The interviewer establishes the client's name, introduces himself or herself by name and explains the interviewer's role – behaviours which the majority of Maguire & Rutter's (1976) group were unable to perform with any consistency. Of these simple introductory elements, role statement is perhaps the most time-consuming, but is also of critical importance in orienting the client. First, the client may be quite unaware of the specific nature of the referral, with regard either to its reason or the person in the interviewer's role. Certainly, most people will have at best a sketchy idea of what mental health professionals, mental health nurses and counsellors actually do. For this reason, the effective interviewer explains, albeit briefly, precisely what the interviewer can generally be expected to do, both with clients *in general* and the individual client.

Scene-setting should attempt to recognise with the client any unusual aspects of the interview setting, such as the presence of others at the interview. In the case of professional colleagues, the interviewer will wish formally to seek permission for their presence and explain the rationale behind it. If others have accompanied the client, however, their role should be clarified, along with whether or not the client desires their presence.

Some interviewers begin a consultation with inconsequential small talk. There is, however, no evidence that, in clinical settings, this performs any useful role in setting the client at ease. Given that the client is there, in all likelihood, to discuss distressing or otherwise problematic material, small talk may, in fact, *heighten* anxiety, by delaying the time before which such material can be raised. Setting a friendly atmosphere for the interview can be done without recourse to small talk, through the use of appropriate orientation and non-verbal behaviour.

Agenda setting

The effective interviewer states the likely duration of the interview, thus allowing the client to prioritise the issues to be discussed, orientating the client to the likely demands which will be made on the client's attention and decreasing potential anxiety by rendering this element of the encounter predictable.

The content of the consultation, from the interviewer's viewpoint, is also stated. As well as orienting the client to the interviewer's agenda, this is also an offer of initial negotiation, through which the interviewer both seeks to give the client an experience of how treatment itself will involve collaboration and to build the therapeutic relationship more generally.

Through seeking client involvement, the agenda statement also aims to increase the likelihood that the client will adhere to any treatment instructions which are later offered, since the client will feel greater 'ownership' of the intervention process (Thompson 1984b). As well as content, the setting of the agenda should also discuss the likely *process* of the interview, including, for example, questioning style, the possibility of touching on difficult material and the opportunity for questions from the client. This can lead to inquiry about the client's own goals from the interview. The overall aim of this part of the interview is to reduce client uncertainty and increase the likelihood of the client making the best possible use of her attention, and, ultimately, the time set aside for the interview (Ley 1982).

GENERAL ASSESSMENT SKILLS

Cognitive–behavioural approaches both recognise the importance of a precise assessment of the client's difficulties and stress the integration of this process with orientation to treatment and the negotiation and measurement of outcome goals (Richards & McDonald 1990). The use of goal-setting during assessment suggests that, at its best, assessment is an important part of the process of treatment itself, rather than simply an information-gathering exercise.

Aims of assessment

The information-gathering element of successful assessment will embody the characteristics of *sufficiency* and *necessity*. Sufficient information should be gathered to allow the nurse to gain a clear picture of all elements of a client's life which bear upon the problem and help to either maintain it or cope with it, but *only* such information which is necessary to gain such a picture should be gained. The issue of sufficiency is self-explanatory, since effective intervention is unlikely to occur with insufficient detail regarding the nature of the client's difficulties. The notion of necessity is, however, equally important. Gaining information from the client which has no clear relationship to the maintenance of the client's difficulties is wasteful of time and disrespectful of client privacy. Moreover, such irrelevant information is a potential distraction for both client and nurse and may serve to dilute focus or divert attention from the central issues which surround the client's difficulties. Clearly, sensitivity, experience and a grasp of the knowledge base from which the nurse's interventions are derived are required in order to sift relevant from irrelevant information.

The notions of sufficiency and necessity provide the first aim of the assessment consultation

– *to gain the information necessary and sufficient to arrive at an understanding of the client's difficulties.*

The second aim of the assessment interview is the *commencement of the therapeutic liaison*. This includes *orientation* of the client to the nurse's therapeutic approach. This helps the client's later understanding of what is likely to be required during treatment, and so aids adherence. It also enables the client to offer informed consent to treatment.

The final aim of the assessment phase is *to assist the client to set achievable treatment goals*. Goal-setting and planning serve several purposes: the client's treatment is given focus; the client gains an opportunity to participate in and negotiate future care; the balance between nurse activity and client activity alters, with client participation increasing.

Each of these elements of the assessment consultation is also present in subsequent interviews, to varying degrees. Thus, further information-gathering (usually about the client's progress in treatment) continues throughout the client's and nurse's collaboration together. Similarly, the alliance needed for this collaboration continues to be built, with orientation to treatment becoming increasingly important as the therapist seeks to refine the guidance to the client in the light of continuing attempts to address the client's difficulties and in response to feedback received from the client. The client, in the effective consultation, comes to take an increasing lead in the way in which this guidance is translated into action. As part of this process, evaluation of goals occurs, along with the setting of *interim goals* which are aimed at guiding the client towards the eventual treatment goals and optimising reinforcement for completion of goal-directed tasks along the way.

We will now examine how each of these three aims – information-gathering, alliance-building and treatment orientation, setting and monitoring of treatment goals – are put into practice by the nurse. When we examine the offering of therapeutic instructions, the examples given will be from CBT, but these should be considered simply as illustrative, since nurses' therapeutic orientations will differ. The key issue to be considered throughout is the *process* by which these instructions are offered. While this is strongly derived from the cognitive–behavioural approach, and from learning and cognitive theories in education, it is practical as an effective process for offering therapeutic instructions during the course of *any* intervention, from counselling to medication monitoring.

Information-gathering

During this process, the nurse seeks to discover those things which are necessary and sufficient to define the client's main problem. Naturally, this occupies considerably more time during an assessment interview than on subsequent occasions. Nevertheless, the same general approach can be adopted during any interview, since any interview will require some element of information-gathering. In CBT, the approach to information-gathering is via a functional analysis of the client's difficulties (Richards & McDonald 1990). This often consists of a process of questioning guided by a 'three systems approach' (Lang 1971), examining the autonomic/physical, behavioural and cognitive components of a client's difficulties. These three systems are regarded as giving a comprehensive account of a person's experiences. Although a fourth element – affect or emotion – has been suggested as an addition to the three systems, this may not be necessary, since affect may be seen as being described in terms of the three systems themselves. For example, if I feel depressed (affect), I may express this through the three systems by thinking negative thoughts (cognitive system), social withdrawal (behavioural system) and diminished appetite (autonomic/physical system). While the three systems model has been particularly associated with CBT, there is no reason for its use to be restricted in this way, since a clear examination of these three aspects of human experience will provide a coherent structure through which to gather information about a client's difficulties, regardless of the nurse's therapeutic orientation.

Functional analysis is likewise derived from CBT, but does not need to be restricted to use by those who approach their work from this perspective. Cognitive–behaviour therapists seek to examine the antecedents of a particular problem episode, the precise circumstances surrounding that episode and the consequences of that episode because they contend that the contingencies surrounding a problem episode are responsible for maintaining it. In therapy, modification of these contingencies occupies a considerable amount of therapist and client energy. However, as with the three systems approach, the examination of antecedents, behavioural episode and consequences provides the nurse with an excellent structure for information-gathering, regardless of the nurse's personal approach to therapy with client difficulties. This is because functional analysis provides a clear, detailed picture of the circumstances of an individual's difficulties. This detailed information is essential for effective intervention, regardless of the type of intervention offered.

These two approaches are integrated by the nurse in order to provide a comprehensive account of the client's difficulties. Thus, the nurse asks questions which seek to gather precise information about the client's autonomic/physical state, behaviours and cognitions before, during and after a problem episode. Taking social anxiety as an example, we should expect responses similar to those shown in Box 6.1.

Box 6.1 Basic responses to three systems analysis of client with social anxiety

(A)NTECEDENTS: What does the client feel, do and think before entering the problem situation?

(A)utonomic/physical – racing heart, nausea, tremor
(B)ehavioural – take precautions (alcohol, tranquillisers), arrive late to social event, cancel appearance at event
(C)ognitive – 'People will laugh at me'; 'People don't want me to come'; 'I'll make a fool of myself'; 'I won't be able to think of anything to say'

(B)EHAVIOURAL EVENT: What does the client feel, do and think in the problem situation?

(A)utonomic/physical – racing heart, nausea, tremor
(B)ehavioural – avoid talking to others, talk only to people previously known, stay on the sidelines, use precautions (alcohol, etc.), leave early
(C)ognitive – 'People are looking at me, laughing at me'; 'I appear foolish'; 'I'm going crazy'; 'I can't think of anything to say'

(C)ONSEQUENCES: What does the client feel, do and think after the problem situation?

(A)utonomic/physical – reduction of physical symptoms
(B)ehavioural – tendency to avoid in future
(C)ognitive – 'I made a fool of myself'; 'I didn't cope'; 'People could tell I was nervous'; 'I won't be asked again'; 'I'll never be able to make friends'

(S)PECIFIERS

What?
Where?
When?
Who with?
What do others do?
Why?
(6 Ws)

How often do episodes occur?
How long ago did episodes begin?
How do episodes affect the client's daily life?
What goals does the client have from treatment?

The nurse uses this approach to examine a number of problematic episodes and draws common elements of the episodes together to arrive at a coherent picture of the factors maintaining the client's difficulties. The use of questions which further specify the nature of these difficulties (specifiers) offers a way of gaining precise information at each stage in this examination and gives an impression of how far the client's problem impacts upon her life. The principles of necessity and sufficiency are adhered to in that the nurse arrives, following information-gathering, at a point where an extremely rich picture of the client is gained *insofar as it relates to her difficulties*. By contrast, few questions which do not relate to those difficulties are pursued in depth. Elements of general history-taking are not emphasised in this approach, and such elements are simply scanned briefly by the nurse in order to ensure that issues relevant to the presenting difficulties have not been missed. This process of scanning may also follow the three systems approach, but should be client-led in order that unwarranted intrusion into possibly irrelevant aspects of the person's life is avoided. Clearly sensitivity is needed in order to be aware of the possible relevance of particular aspects of a client's story.

ALLIANCE-BUILDING AND TREATMENT ORIENTATION

This section is concerned principally with how the nurse develops and displays sensitivity to client needs during the consultation. The second aim of the assessment consultation involves the nurse much more in the process of effective interviewing, as the nurse begins to build an alliance with the client which will facilitate successful intervention. Thus, attention is now focused on the best process by which information may be gained from the client and transmitted to the nurse. These process skills involve a sympathetic, individualised approach to the consultation, which is tailored to client needs and responses. In order to ensure this, the following elements are suggested:

1. ensure the client is orientated during the interview
2. reward client information
3. reward client attempts at coping

4. offer an appropriate rationale for any intervention offered.

Orientation of the client and sharing the interview

Orientation seeks to set the client at ease, since uncertainty about the environment is associated with anxiety, which is in turn distracting from the business of the interview. Given that clients in mental health care settings may in any case be considerably anxious, it is doubly important to remove unnecessary sources of anxiety. Orientation of the client to what is happening during the interview is also a key method of showing the client that the nurse values the client's contribution and collaboration in the interview.

The following are key behaviours which the nurse can adopt in order to keep the client orientated during information-gathering sessions and beyond:

Proceeding from the general to the specific. The nurse moves from general open questions, through more specific open questions to closed questions which specify the required detail for each area of the client's difficulties. If you are uncertain about the distinction between these types of questioning, you may wish to examine an introductory text on communication skills (e.g. Burnard & Morrison 1991). For the purpose of orientation, the key aspect is that the questioning has *direction*. The movement from general to specific questions provides this direction and thus orientates the client. In the case of closed questions, although these are often necessary to gain precise information, the effective interviewer handles them sensitively, explaining to the client that such detailed questioning is likely to follow, and keeps them to a minimum. Too many closed questions inhibit disclosure of information (Maguire et al 1996)

This shift of focus from general to specific questions is the basic questioning sequence used in cognitive–behavioural consultations, and seeks to capitalise on our ability to remember specifics when they are set in the context of more general information. One recent study showed that clinicians tended to use too many closed questions, even in a highly emotionally laden situation (breaking bad news to cancer patients). This consultation style was associated with clinician domination of the consultation. Moreover, discussion of medical topics far outweighed any examination of psychosocial issues (Ford et al 1996). The general open questions asked for each component of assessment (autonomic, behaviours, cognitions; antecedents, behaviour, consequences, specifiers – ABCS) attempt to act as a cue for the more detailed questioning to follow. This tactic of presenting general information first can also be used when *transmitting* treatment information *to* the client.

Using statements as questions. An interviewing style which at times reframes questions as statements helps to avoid too threatening an interrogative style. Hobson (1984) has suggested that this is a particularly useful technique in eliciting emotion, but it can also be adapted for information-gathering. Moreover, as with much effective consultation technique, the use of statements as questions is by no means confined to formal interview situations, but reflects a conversational style which we employ in everyday life:

'It sounds like you might be keeping our date tomorrow.'

is really a *question*:

'Will you be keeping our date tomorrow?',

but is less threatening because it avoids the interrogative form.

Flexibility and cue-following. In the earlier sections of this chapter, we have noted the impor-

tance of certain set elements of format in the consultation, and the use of such a format indeed helps to orientate the client, particularly if this agenda is shared with the client at the beginning of an interaction. However, set formats are intended to be guidelines, rather than rules of discourse to be followed slavishly. It is not orientating for the client if the interviewer follows a personal agenda exclusively or interviews mechanically (Dillon 1990), since the client may be moved across topics in ways which make little sense to the client, because the client is not allowed to follow up a particular line of thought. Once again the analogy with informal conversation is useful. The effective consultation, like the relaxed conversation, involves the nurse in *being flexible and following client cues*. Through this, the nurse keeps the client orientated by *meaning* rather than structure. This tactic also helps to build the therapeutic alliance by demonstrating respect for the client, since it is *the client's* agenda which is now being followed. Striking the correct balance between structure and cue-following is a key skill to be practised. Emotionally laden material may be difficult for the client to describe directly, and so following of cues may be important in allowing the nurse to perceive clues as to an important line of questioning to follow. Since such clues (and even direct expressions of emotion) are often missed during consultations (Suchman et al 1997), effective interviewers will need to develop this skill as a conscious part of their consultation repertoire.

Redirecting the client. Part of developing this skill involves recognising that there are times when it is appropriate to redirect the client. Again, the analogy with everyday conversation is instructive here. Although some conversations, particularly between close friends, have a rambling, free-rolling quality, most interactions have some theme which is followed by the participants. Moreover, we certainly *do* redirect each other in social conversation, sometimes quite forcefully. Redirecting the client is orientating because it demonstrates the presence and importance of structure in the interview, and builds the therapeutic alliance because it shows that the nurse is concerned to help the client address personal difficulties in as focal a way as possible. Redirection is respectful of the client, provided it is handled sensitively. Avoiding redirection is actually *disrespectful*, because the nurse is allowing the client to waste valuable time in discussing irrelevant material.

Feedback. As part of respect for the client, the effective interviewer regularly *seeks feedback about both the content and process of the interview*. As well as the practical necessity to ensure that the interviewer has correctly understood the information gained, seeking feedback reinforces the therapeutic alliance by demonstrating respect.

Rewarding client information

Pursuing the analogy with everyday conversation further, it should be noted at the beginning of this section that reinforcement occurs naturally during almost every element of interpersonal interactions. As an example, the use of gaze during social interaction is so basic that we are generally unaware of it until it is disrupted. Thus, the physical interference with gaze caused by some facial disfigurements is regarded as a major component of the difficulties experienced by disfigured people in social situations, since the normal cues which regulate conversation are absent (Macgregor 1989). Indeed, some treatment for social difficulties among disfigured people specifically seeks to compensate for the non-availability of such cues (Robinson et al 1996), while the teaching of such mutual reinforcement skills as gaze is a mainstay of much social skills training (e.g. Ellis & Whittington 1981). We should not, therefore, regard the use of reinforce-

ment of client information as anything artificial. Indeed, at its best, reinforcement is a collaborative, interactive process, and several writers have written about the reciprocal relationship between participants in a reward setting (e.g. Bandura 1977, Egan 1990). The skilled consultation uses such reinforcement in a conscious, structured way in order *to increase the overall amount of information* the client gives and *to control the extent and nature* of the information the client gives on any given topic. Part of this latter process involves the use of reinforcement to *decrease* the amount of information offered about irrelevant material.

Reinforcement *controls information* from the client because the nurse is careful as to where reinforcing remarks from the interviewer occur. Thus the nurse uses such remarks as: 'I see'; 'Good'; and 'Go on' in a conscious way, rather than reinforcing the client's words indiscriminately. If the interview changes direction, and the change of topic is important, the frequency of reinforcing remarks by the interviewer should rise, aiming to increase the amount of information described. By contrast, the nurse can steer the client away from unfruitful avenues of investigation by decreasing or withdrawing such reinforcing remarks. With a reticent client, the use of reinforcement in a structured way is, of course, extremely important, in order to increase the flow of the client's account, but structured use of reinforcement is also a key skill with the garrulous client, since we may well want to be careful to reward only relevant information. In this last case, in particular, reinforcement also helps to orientate the client to the structure of the interview, by drawing the client's attention to those elements of the client's thinking (as revealed at interview) which are focal to the client's difficulties.

As with almost all elements of effective consultation, reinforcement also contributes to the development of the therapeutic relationship, since it is a way of demonstrating the nurse's respect for the client and the client's story. Moreover, reinforcement of the client should not be regarded as a simplistic manipulation. It would be strange if clinicians did not hold positive views of clients, their stories and their capabilities in addressing their difficulties. The structured use of reinforcement is merely a concrete way of making these positive views explicit to the client during the consultation.

Rewarding client attempts at coping

This notion of expressing respect for the client is developed further during effective consultation when we examine the client's previous attempts at coping and respond to them in a way which we intend will enhance further such attempts.

Two goals should be considered in this aspect of consultation. First, the nurse will wish to reinforce *all* previous attempts at coping. The purpose of this tactic is threefold: the nurse seeks to increase client confidence, to demonstrate respect for the client's efforts and to demonstrate that it is possible to cope with the client's difficulties, thus building hope for the future. Thus, all descriptions of previous attempts at dealing with the client's difficulties should initially be reinforced. This will be particularly important with the client who reports very limited attempts to address these difficulties in the past. From a behavioural standpoint, the process underlying this is *shaping* (Walker 1987), in which new, desired behaviours are learnt through a process of successive approximation. Reinforcement of any attempt at coping is the initial step in this procedure.

The nurse's second goal, when reinforcing client attempts at coping is to *differentially reinforce* only those attempts at coping which are most likely to be associated with client improvement. This represents later stages in the process

of shaping, in which reinforcement is not offered for steps towards the eventually desired behaviour which have already been achieved, but only for the *next* step towards that behaviour.

To return to our example of the disfigured person experiencing difficulties in social situations, we might, during the initial stages of the therapeutic relationship, offer considerable reinforcement for entering any social situation, even if the client avoided talking to others, used inappropriate camouflage tactics, or took alcohol to facilitate entry into the situation. As treatment progressed, we should almost certainly wish to cease these elements of the client's behaviour, and so would offer verbal reinforcement only for entry into social situations where some, or eventually all the undesired elements were absent. Even at an initial interview, we might follow a similar policy, reinforcing *all* descriptions of the client's previous attempts at coping, but reserving particular praise for those which most closely approximated to the client's desired eventual resolutions of difficulties. In CBT, such reinforcement is generally practised in an open, collaborative way, so that the client is entirely aware of which behaviours are being reinforced and why. Indeed, a major element of treatment often involves enabling clients to reinforce themselves for approximations to the desired goals. Appropriate reinforcement of *descriptions* of coping efforts by the client is the first step in this process.

Offering a rationale for intervention

The offering of an adequate rationale for treatment is not a one-off process, but continues throughout the therapeutic relationship. However, major elements of the course the nurse tends to pursue need to be delivered at an early stage. In this way, the client can give consent and is also most likely to possess sufficient information to begin to engage with treatment. As a result, adequate rationale-giving is both an ethical and a practical issue. While it may be the case, in some mental health settings, that clients lack sufficient appreciation of the nature or significance of their difficulties to understand either the nature of the intervention or the need for it, this situation is not only rare, but is simply a reason to be particularly painstaking in the way in which the rationale is offered. In most situations, some common ground between nurse and client can be found. It is on this ground that the offering of a rationale for intervention is begun. A full explanation of treatment should contain at least the following components:

Initial formulation of the client's problems

Clients are generally concerned about the causes of their difficulties. While some therapeutic orientations are, perhaps, largely uninterested in past causes of current difficulties (e.g. CBT), others are, arguably, over-concerned with such putative causes (e.g. biochemically or psychodynamically orientated interventions). However, in either situation, the effective consultation respects the client's concerns about cause and responds to them in a way which is relevant, particularly given that clients are very often concerned about how causes impact upon their everyday lives (Dillon 1990). Where our knowledge of causative and maintaining factors of a client's difficulties is not as complete as we should wish, this issue is shared with the client, sensitively but optimistically. In such situations, as in all aspects of effective consultation, the aim is to enlist the client as a partner.

Rationale underlying the nurse's proposed interventions for the problem

Naturally, for ethical and practical reasons, the client needs to know what the nurse proposes they will do together to address the client's difficulties. Providing a clear general rationale for why these proposed tactics might be useful not only begins to generate participation and adherence from the client but gives a general context into which to set later, more specific therapeutic instructions.

Examples of the nurse's expectations of the client

Almost every intervention will require some activity on the part of the client. In mental health care, this might range from the comparatively simple act of taking medication (although, even here, adherence is often extremely poor, as it is in general medicine and nursing (Thompson 1984b)), to learning a set of exercises, monitoring one's thoughts or entering situations which cause us distress and fear. Cognitive–behaviour therapists require a great deal from clients, and much of client activity is carried out without the supervision of a therapist. As a result, therapists have devoted considerable time to ensuring that clients are aware of what is likely to be required of them, as early in treatment as is possible, and usually at a first appointment. Only then can clients meaningfully give consent to participate in treatment. Equally, a clear idea of what is expected of the therapist is a key to motivation and participation during treatment (Ley 1982). Sufficient specific examples should be given to allow clients to be clear about the nature of what they will be required to do during treatment and questions should be actively sought. This procedure should be followed whenever a new element of treatment is introduced, and reinforced at each stage. The aim of this element of rationale-giving, in common with other aspects, is to enlist the client as an equal, knowledgeable partner in treatment.

Examples of what the client should expect of the nurse

Since equality within the therapeutic relationship is important, the nurse is also expected to behave in certain ways. These behaviours (explaining, coaching and consoling but also such practical elements as attending appointments, keeping in touch with the client, monitoring progress, negotiating the ending of treatment, emergency arrangements, re-referral) represent the nurse's commitment to the therapeutic process. Making them explicit to the client demonstrates this commitment to the client and also shows respect and decreases client uncertainty.

The likelihood of success

The level of accuracy with which a prediction can be made about outcome in mental health varies considerably, as it does in general medicine and nursing. Despite this, clients will legitimately be concerned about the likely outcome of the nurse's intervention, and the effective consultation responds to this honestly and in such a way as to maximise the likelihood of engaging the client with treatment. A minority of clients are likely to be knowledgeable about randomised controlled trials, non-randomised studies and expert opinion, still less about the arguments which underpin the assertion of different levels of reliability of these sorts of evidence in guiding interventions. This is, however, no reason to refrain from offering clients the best available estimate of likely success. This in turn places three burdens on the clinician: to develop and practise the skills required to evaluate research relevant to their area of practice; to be aware of the level of support for their interventions; and to transmit this information in understandable form to clients.

In many cases, the level of support for interventions in mental health care is low (Parry 1996). In such cases, we are required to rely on the expert opinion of others or on our own clinical experience. While this is an unhappy state of affairs, it is likely to continue for some years. The implication of this for rationale-giving is that the nurse must share the shortcomings of our knowledge frankly with the client. While this seems to present difficulties, this need not be so. In the absence of a clear body of knowledge in favour of a particular approach, it can be powerful to enlist the client as a collaborator in a process of experiment in search of the most effective approach, based on our clinical experience or the theoretical rationale behind our therapeutic orientation. Indeed, a great deal of cognitive–behavioural techniques were originally developed through the enlisting of clients in *single case experiments* (Yule & Helmsley 1977). Indeed, it has been suggested that this experimental approach to client difficulties is more clearly definitive of CBT than the behavioural and cognitive theories which are said to underlie it. As in much effective consultation, the key to useful predictions of outcome with the client is the practice of an open agenda, which allows for and responds to uncertainty.

Emphasis on negotiation

The idea of negotiation with the client has been stressed throughout this chapter. During the offering of a rationale for treatment, this emphasis is made explicit, with a view both to further ensuring that clients understand what is expected of them during treatment and to enlisting their active participation.

GOAL-SETTING AND PLANNING

So far, during this chapter, we have been considerably concerned with the process of intervention, as it is reflected in the consultation skills needed to gain and transmit information and build the therapeutic relationship. In the following sections, we shall shift our attention to *outcome*. Some form of behavioural, cognitive, emotional or physical change is desired in most health consultations, yet mental health nursing has, until recently, paid little attempt to the structured examination of client outcomes. A great deal of the material in later chapters of this book examines the effectiveness of tactics which aim to address a broad range of client problems. This section is not concerned with establishing which therapeutic interventions are or are not effective, but, instead, offers a general approach to the examination of outcomes in our clinical practice and relates this to the planning of treatment interventions to achieve those outcomes desired by clients.

While process skills are essential in all mental health consultation, they are not, by themselves, sufficient to ensure a positive outcome for clients. However expert the nurse becomes in managing the processes involved in skilful consultation, expert management of the tactics required to secure the outcomes desired by the client is also required, and the ability to quantify both these desired outcomes and the progress of the client towards them is an essential starting point in allowing nurses to examine the effectiveness of their own interventions. The single case experiments mentioned in the previous section represent one highly systematised attempt to determine the effectiveness of treatment. The level of technical sophistication required by such experiments is not generally seen in everyday clinical practice, but the general procedures of goal-setting and measurement which underlie it can be routinely used to guide treatment, regardless of the theoretical underpinning of that treatment. Goal-setting, as well as enabling client and nurse to examine the effectiveness of treatment together, can itself be therapeutic, both through allowing the clarification of often complex client difficulties and through helping the client to commit to change.

Cognitive–behavioural approaches to goal-setting have a long history in both the fields of education (e.g. Reilly 1975) and therapy (Shapiro 1961, Yule & Helmsley 1977). These approaches have been refined by successive clinicians and draw their credibility from their congruence with a body of psychological theory, the strength of the single case experimental approach as a research tool and the clinical effectiveness of the therapeutic interventions associated with explicit goal-setting and work towards such goals by client and therapists (Fonagy & Roth 1996, Rachman & Wilson 1980). This section represents a distillation of a broad range of cognitive–behavioural approaches to goal-setting, but is particularly associated with the work of Isaac Marks (Marks et al 1977) in nurse therapy.

Effective client goals contain the following elements and are intimately related to an individualised, detailed treatment assessment. First, goals should exemplify some gain related to the client's difficulties which the client *wishes to achieve*. This is more useful than a definition of improvement driven by particular theoretical views of mental health, and, likewise, more useful than goals driven by the desires of others, including people close to the client, such as friends and relatives, and the nurse. Therapists in particular have strong reasons for clients to get well (Ellis 1983), and there is no rationale for supposing that their estimates of improvement or definitions of appropriate goals are any more useful than those of anyone else. *Thus, effective goals are defined by the client.* They typically represent behaviours, thoughts and feelings which clients would wish to undertake or experience if they did not have their current difficulties.

Within this definition, however, the nurse takes responsibility for guiding the client towards goals which do, in fact, represent some significant change. Clients may have had debilitating problems for many months or years, and should be dissuaded from setting eventual targets which underestimate their own abilities and potential because they are currently dispirited by their difficulties. Careful, sensitive negotiation is required in order to identify the optimum target. Demonstrating to clients their own potential through negotiation of such targets is once again potentially therapeutic. *Thus, effective goals represent some significant change in the client's well-being.*

At the same time, negotiation of targets also seeks to deflect the client from targets which are clearly unrealistic. Clients who have had difficulties for a considerable time may retain a highly stylised idea both of what constitutes recovery and of their own state of happiness prior to the onset of their problems. This may lead to unrealistic expectations of interventions. *Thus, effective goals are realistic.*

Nevertheless, the process of goal-setting and measurement should not be allowed to become a substitute for active intervention and collaboration to address the client's difficulties. Too much goal-setting is likely to be an avoidance of beginning the often distressing process of tackling problems. In any case, the process of explicitly constructing goals relating to all areas of difficulties faced by a client is probably impossible, particularly with complex problems, and is certainly impractical, given time constraints. Cognitive–behaviourists describe the process of *generalisation*, by which learning in one situation is transferred to other similar situations. The process is well supported, both in the laboratory studies of animal behaviour which underpin operant conditioning (Walker 1987) and in the transfer of learning seen in clinical situations (Marks 1987). Since it may be expected that skills learnt by clients in addressing some areas of

difficulty may be equally useful in other, similar areas, different goals need only be set for clearly different problem areas (e.g. work and social life), and even here a considerable amount of similarity may be encountered. *Thus, effective goals are representative of improvements in other areas of the client's life.*

As well as these general characteristics, goals in cognitive–behavioural approaches to consultation also contain a number of specific attributes. Thus, effective goals state the *desired activity, frequency, duration, setting and additional criteria* of the eventual desired behaviours, thoughts or feelings. The reason for this explicitness is twofold. First, such explicit goal definition is useful *to drive the intervention* since both the client and therapist are clear about the eventual endpoint and the level of progress they have currently attained towards reaching it. Second, explicitness in goal definition *provides motivation* since it provides a mechanism through which feedback can be provided to the client. Indeed, in much CBT, this feedback is systematised in the form of numerical measurement of client goal attainment, often using scales individually tailored to the goals defined by the client (see Marks et al 1977, Marks 1987, Richards & McDonald 1990).

While frequency and duration are clear, some clarification of setting and additional criteria are required. Setting usually means the physical circumstances under which the desired activities are to occur – for the agoraphobic, this may be 'in the supermarket' and for the nervous student teacher 'in the classroom'. The additional criteria serve to further specify setting, and will often be quite detailed, for example – 'in the supermarket on Fridays, at lunchtime, without medication' and 'in the classroom, demonstrating at the flipchart, in front of my mentor, with a class of postgraduate students'. Together, these specific attributes contribute to the likelihood that both client and therapist will agree that the goals embody the general characteristics described above and will eventually agree that the desired change has or has not taken place. *Thus, effective goals allow client and nurse to agree the appropriateness of those goals and when they have/have not been achieved.* Box 6.2 reviews these elements of goal-setting and presents two specimen goals, one of which focuses on overt behaviour, while the other examines cognitions.

Box 6.2 Effective goal-setting

Effective goals
- are defined by the client
- represent some significant change in the client's well-being
- are realistic
- are representative of improvements in other areas of the client's life
- allow client and nurse to agree the appropriateness of those goals
- allow client and nurse to agree when those goals have/have not been achieved.

and contain the attributes of:
- desired activity
- frequency
- duration
- setting
- other criteria.

Case example 1
A specimen goal for a manager unable to speak assertively at meetings and tending to avoid these meetings as a consequence:

To attend (*desired activity*) team meetings (*setting*) twice weekly (*frequency*), staying till the end (*duration*) and to refuse unreasonable requests (*desired activity*) from colleagues (*other criteria*) whenever they occur (*frequency*) without raising my voice or making excuses (*other criteria*).

Case example 2
A specimen goal for a father with long-standing, unresolved grief:

To reduce unwanted thoughts (*desired activity*) of guilt about my dead son Gil (*other criteria*) which occur when I am alone (*other criteria*) in my car on the way home from work (*setting*), to once a month (*frequency*) for a maximum of 5 minutes (*duration*) without praying or driving the car fast to distract myself (*other criteria*).

Working towards goals

As noted earlier, it is beyond the scope of this chapter to set out in detail the specific therapeutic interventions the nurse may wish to employ with particular client difficulties, and subsequent chapters examine these interventions in detail. However, two general tactics will prove useful, regardless of the specific interventions employed. These tactics are the *setting of interim goals* which help the client to commit to treatment and achieve the ultimate goals that have been negotiated with the nurse, and the use of *appropriate approaches to client education* which empower the client to put into practice those techniques which lead towards improvement. This final section examines these two general tactics.

Setting interim goals

The goals we examined in the previous section represented general but explicit statements of improvement which the client would wish to achieve by the end of treatment. By their very nature, such goals are often unattainable by clients at the beginning of their collaboration with the nurse, and represent too large a step to be achieved all at once. Interim goals are constructed between the client and nurse in exactly the same way as these eventual treatment goals, but are more focal and short-term in nature. Indeed the chief aims of interim goals are *to motivate the client at each step in treatment* and *to demonstrate to client and therapist as each step towards improvement has been achieved*. Wherever possible, interim goals should share with outcome goals the qualities described in Box 6.2. However, it is unlikely that they will always have the same level of desirability as the eventual outcome of treatment, since they are merely a step towards such outcomes. The following guidelines will assist in the construction of interim goals which are optimally motivating for the client.

Wherever possible, interim goals should *clearly relate to outcomes*. It should be immediately clear to the client that such interim goals will facilitate the client in moving towards the eventual treatment goals. Where interim goals are exclusively concerned with the *process* of treatment (e.g. where a specific technique, such as relaxation, or monitoring negative thoughts, has to be learnt by clients *in order to address their difficulties*) careful verbal explanation from the nurse about how these goals link to achieving eventual outcome goals is required in order to facilitate adherence.

The *rewarding consequences* of adherence to process goals should be emphasised. The teaching tactics discussed later in this section will be useful here.

The *client should lead the process* of deciding on the next step in treatment and the interim goal associated with it, but the nurse should guide the client towards the *optimally rewarding interim goal*. This goal is that which gives the maximum benefit in terms of therapeutic improvement for the least input from the client, and the assistance of the nurse is required in selecting this goal because of the nurse's role as an expert consultant who understands the treatment process and most likely outcomes of particular elements of that process.

At the same time, at any given stage in treatment, *a variety of goals* should be set, at different levels of difficulty. As with identifying the optimally rewarding goal, the purpose of setting a range of goals is to maximise the likelihood of the client being successful at each stage in treatment, again generating motivation to continue.

Increasing the likelihood that clients will achieve goals

Throughout this chapter, we have returned to the central importance of reinforcement to a successful consultation process. While a detailed description of client education is beyond the scope of this chapter, it is worth noting that reinforcement is also a key aspect of helping clients to learn. The general tactics we have examined so far in looking at consultation skills (gaining appropriate information, enhancing the therapeutic relationship, goal-setting) are all important in setting the context for appropriate learning, but can be enhanced by the crucial addition of reinforcement of appropriate behaviours by the client in response to the therapeutic suggestions which the nurse makes.

In many treatment settings, it will be necessary for the client to perform some novel behaviours, whether these be overt or cognitive. Skilful consultation involves increasing the likelihood that such behaviours will be performed, and the principal behavioural technique here involves the use of operant conditioning, particularly the use of contingent reward. Learning occurs all the time and is, for the behaviourist, initiated and maintained by reinforcement, which may be of varying levels of simplicity or sophistication. This is viewed as a natural human process which occurs equally in formal and informal learning situations. The art of skilful consultation is to use reinforcement in a goal-directed, systematic way.

Nurses are potent sources of social reward for clients and may also be powerful models. Both these characteristics will be enhanced if the nurse is seen by the client as being generally similar to the client in status and abilities. In therapeutic situations, it is important to offer plenty of social rewards for the client's approximations to adherence to the agreed therapeutic programme. Appropriate recall of the elements of this programme is a prerequisite of adherence, and reinforcement of such recall is, in itself, a valuable tool in increasing recall, and, therefore, adherence. Much of this reinforcement will be at a simple verbal level, similar to that discussed during our examination of eliciting information. Once again, the key element is that reinforcement is applied *consciously and systematically*, increasing the likelihood that clients will be aware of precisely which elements of their behaviour are, in fact, being reinforced and, therefore, desirable. As in our earlier discussion of reinforcement of information-giving by the client, it is important to emphasise again that this is by no means an artificial process, since we spontaneously reinforce each other during everyday interaction.

Where the information is complex, checks on understanding (with appropriate reinforcement) will be frequent, guiding the client through each stage in the process. Reinforcement for achievement at each stage will be equally systematic and frequent. This process is referred to as shaping of the desired behaviours.

Additionally, modelling (or vicarious reinforcement), a technique derived from Bandura's (1977) social learning theory, has a demonstrable effect in increasing the frequency of desired behaviours. In some cases, the nurse will be involved in demonstrating particular skills for the client. The value of this tactic is increased if the nurse is then able to describe explicitly the likely rewards for demonstrating such a skill, since individuals are more likely to perform an action if they have seen others being rewarded for performing it. Where actual demonstration is impractical, the use of examples (e.g. other clients whom the nurse recalls) where the successful performance of a skill has been rewarded is a useful substitute. This becomes more powerful if clients can be encouraged to generate such examples from their own experience, thus acting as their *own* model, by remembering instances from their own lives where they have used skills similar to those required in treatment, been successful and been rewarded.

This principle of self-reinforcement can be carried into practical contexts, both during consultations and between the sessions. Such reinforcement may be covert, involving the clients in generating thoughts which remind them of their success and the likely advantages and rewards which will accrue from it, or in comparing their current successes with previous difficulties. Equally, tangible behavioural rewards may be generated, which clients themselves control and administer in return for performance of the desired behaviours. These tangible rewards may themselves be of two forms. Novel rewards may be generated, such as eating a meal in a favoured restaurant, or clients may be encouraged to examine their current behaviours and ensure that highly desired behaviours which they currently perform are made *contingent* upon successful performance of elements of the treatment programme. For example, a favourite television programme might be taped and played only after a part of the treatment has been performed.

Once again, this self-reinforcement is not at all artificial – just as we all set ourselves informal goals, so we all informally reinforce ourselves for achievement. For instance, in writing, I may set myself a target of so many words in a session. Having achieved this number, I might reinforce myself covertly (simply by congratulating myself, or by imagining how pleased I will be when the work is complete), or overtly (by eating a sweet or piece of fruit, or by deciding to have lunch only once the target number of words had been reached).

CONCLUSION

In treatment, this process of self-reward is rendered explicit, sometimes with the aid of the nurse, in the hope of maximising its effectiveness in helping clients achieve their goals. This process is similar to all aspects of the skilled interview. In such situations, the nurse seeks to use certain important but apparently automatic aspects of ordinary social interaction. The skilled interview is thus a structured social interaction in which the nurse uses a range of everyday social skills consciously, with foresight and in a goal-directed fashion aimed, ultimately, at enhancing client well-being.

Exercise

How do we reinforce each other? Tomorrow, keep a diary of as many occasions as you can on which you notice *you are rewarding yourself*. Take care not to overlook small instances. These are often extremely frequent. The following day, keep a diary of times *when others reinforce you*. Remember to include indirect verbal praise, non-verbal behaviour such as gaze, as well as obvious praise remarks such as 'well done'; 'I like you'. On the third day, keep a diary of occasions when *you reinforce others*.

Finally, examine ways in which each of these instances could have parallels in the organisation of consultation and treatment, applying them to your own clinical speciality.

KEY TEXTS FOR FURTHER READING

Richards D A, McDonald R 1990 Behavioural psychotherapy: A handbook for nurses. Heinemann, Oxford. *An excellent guide to behavioural interventions, with a strong emphasis on the nursing role and the development of good consultation skills.*
Newell R 1994 Interviewing skills for nurses: A structured approach. Routledge, London. *This book again takes a cognitive–behavioural approach as its starting point, but is* broader in focus than Richards & McDonald, being aimed at nursing in general, rather than those wishing to practise behavioural interventions.
Marks I M 1986 Behavioural psychotherapy: The Maudsley pocket book of clinical management. Wright, Bristol. *A source book of measurement tactics, rather than a reader, but with plenty of useful information about how to approach consultation.*

REFERENCES

Bandura A 1977 Social learning theory. Prentice-Hall, Englewood Cliffs, NJ
Burnard P, Morrison P 1991 Caring and communicating: The interpersonal relationship in nursing. Macmillan Education, Basingstoke
Dillon J T 1990 The practice of questioning. Routledge, London
Dzurec L C, Coleman P 1997 A hermeneutic analysis of the process of conducting clinical interviews. Journal of Psychosocial Nursing and Mental Health Services 35(8):31–36
Egan G 1990 The skilled helper: A systematic approach to effective helping. Brooks/Cole, Pacific Grove, California
Ellis A 1983 How to deal with your most difficult client: you. Journal of Rational-Emotive Therapy 1(1):3–8
Ellis R, Whittington D 1981 A guide to social skill training. Croom Helm, London
Fonagy A, Roth P 1996 What works for whom? A critical review of psychotherapy research. Guilford Press, New York
Ford S, Fallowfield L, Lewis S 1996 Doctor–patient interactions in oncology. Social Science and Medicine 42(11):151–159.
Ginsberg G, Marks I 1977 Costs and benefits of behavioural psychotherapy: a pilot study of neurotics treated by nurse-therapists. Psychological Medicine 7(4):685–700

Goldberg D P, Hobson R F, Maguire G P et al 1984 The clarification and assessment of a method of psychotherapy. British Journal of Psychiatry 144:567–580
Hobson R F 1984 The heart of psychotherapy. Tavistock, London
Hostick T, Newell R 1998 Follow up of non-completers of community mental health appointments. Report to Northern and Yorkshire Region NHSE
Jarvis P, Gibson P 1985 The teacher practitioner in nursing, midwifery and health visiting. Chapman and Hall, London.
Lambert M, deJulio S, Stein D 1978 Therapist interpersonal skills. Psychological Bulletin 83:467–489
Lang P 1971 The application of psychophysiological methods to the study of psychotherapy. In: Bergin A E, Garfield S L (eds) Handbook of psychotherapy and behavior change. Wiley, New York
Ley P 1977 Psychological studies of doctor–patient communication. In: Rachman S (ed) Contributions to medical psychology, vol I. Pergamon Press, Oxford
Ley P 1979 Improving clinical communication: effects of altering doctor behaviour. In: Oborne D J, Gruneberg M M, Eiser J R (eds) Research in psychology and medicine, vol II. Academic Press, London
Ley P 1982 Satisfaction, compliance and communication. British Journal of Clinical Psychology 21:241–254.

REFERENCES (*contd*)

Macgregor F C 1989 Social, psychological and cultural dimensions of cosmetic and reconstructive plastic surgery. Aesthetic Plastic Surgery 13:1–8.

Maguire P, Faulkner A, Booth K, Elliott C, Hillier V 1996 Helping cancer patients disclose their concerns. European Journal of Cancer 32(1):78–81

Maguire P, Rutter D R 1976 Teaching medical students to communicate. In: Bennett A E (ed) Communication between doctors and patients. Oxford University Press, Oxford

Marks I M 1987 Fears, phobias and rituals. Oxford University Press, Oxford

Marks I M, Hallam R S, Connolly J, Philpott R 1977 Nursing in behavioural psychotherapy. RCN, London

Newell R J 1992 Anxiety, accuracy and reflection: the limits of professional development. Journal of Advanced Nursing 17:1326–1333

Newell R 1994 Interviewing skills for nurses: A structured approach. Routledge, London

Newell R, Gournay K 1994 Nursing in behavioural psychotherapy: a 20-year follow-up. Journal of Advanced Nursing 20:53–60.

Parry G 1996 NHS psychotherapy services in England: Review of strategic policy. Department of Health, Wetherby

Rachman S J, Wilson G T 1980 The effects of psychological therapy, 2nd edn. Pergamon, Oxford

Reilly D 1975 Behavioural objectives in nursing: Evaluation of learner attainment. Appleton-Century-Crofts, New York

Richards D A, McDonald R 1990 Behavioural psychotherapy: A handbook for nurses. Heinemann, Oxford

Robinson E, Rumsey N, Partridge J 1996 An evaluation of the impact of social interaction skills training for facially disfigured people. British Journal of Plastic Surgery 49:281–289.

Rogers C R 1951 Client-centred therapy. Houghton-Mifflin, Boston.

Rogers C R 1957 The necessary and sufficient conditions of therapeutic personality change. Journal of Consulting Psychology 21:95–103

Shapiro M B 1961 A method of measuring psychological changes specific to the individual psychiatric patient. British Journal of Medical Psychology 34:151–155.

Suchman A L, Markakis K, Beckman H B, Frankel R 1997 A model of empathic communication in the medical interview. Journal of the American Medical Association 227(8):678–682.

Sundeen S J, Rankin G W, Rankin E A DeS, Cohen S A 1989 Nurse–client interaction: Implementing the nursing process. Mosby, St Louis

Thompson J 1984a Communicating with patients. In: Fitzpatrick R, Hinton J, Newman S, Scambler G, Thomson J (eds) The experience of illness. Tavistock, London

Thompson J 1984b Compliance. In: Fitzpatrick, R, Hinton J, Newman S, Scambler G, Thomson J (eds) The experience of illness. Tavistock, London

Walker S F 1987 Animal learning. Routledge, Kegan Paul, London.

Yule W, Helmsley D 1977 Single case method in medical psychology. In: Rachman S (ed) Contributions to medical psychology. Pergamon Press, Oxford

CHAPTER CONTENTS

Key points 103

Introduction 104
  The legislative framework 105
  Multidisciplinary working 105

What is assessment? 106

Nursing assessments 106
  Nursing models 107
  Psychosocial approach 107
  Behavioural approach 108
  Risk assessment 108
  Case study: risk assessment 110

The process of assessment 112
  The initial referral 112
  Primary information 113
  Secondary information 115
  Case study: initial assessment process 116

Guidelines for home visiting 116

Conclusion 118

Exercise 118

Key texts for further reading 119

References 119

7

Principles of assessment

*Wendy Maphosa   Mike Slade
Graham Thornicroft*

KEY POINTS

- The role of the community psychiatric nurse (CPN) has developed over the years, so that CPNs now use a range of specialist assessment skills and interventions to meet the needs of people suffering from severe mental health problems.

- The key goals of assessment are:
  — eliciting information about the client's physical, psychological and social well-being
  — formulating a picture of their problems, needs or difficulties
  — planning a tailored intervention to address these problems.

- The CPN will need:
  — to have knowledge of assessment models
  — to have knowledge of assessment methods
  — to decide which source(s) of information to consider
  — interview and listening skills
  — skills in interpreting assessment information
  — to be able to develop care plans on the basis of the assessment.

INTRODUCTION

Community psychiatric nursing started in Warlingham Park Hospital in 1954, where nurses were seconded to out-patient community duties in the Croydon community (White 1986). Their role was to provide a follow-up service to clients who had been discharged from a hospital ward following a psychotic episode or depression. Their work involved supervising and administering depot medication at the clients' homes, and assessing their mental health and functioning in their own environment. As clients were being seen and treated in their home environment, relapses were recognised earlier and interventions were implemented to help prevent hospitalisation. On evaluation, this service was found to be effective in reducing hospital admissions.

Following the Warlingham Park initiative, community psychiatric nursing services developed throughout the 1960s and 1970s. In 1968, there were still few community psychiatric nurses (CPNs) recorded in the UK because of the scarcity of mental health services. However, 2800 CPNs were recorded by 1985 (Simmonds & Brooker 1986). With the closure of large psychiatric hospitals and reduction in bed numbers, the numbers had doubled by 1990. The last quinquennial survey of CPNs showed that there were currently about 7000 CPNs across the country. The profession of community psychiatric nursing has been central to the transition of care from hospital to the community.

This move towards comprehensive and local mental health services has led to changes in the nursing-based care of people with mental health problems. These changes have been due to a number of reasons, including:

- developments and advances in pharmaceutical treatments, making rehabilitation possible even for those with severe mental illness

- closure of large psychiatric hospitals and the development of smaller units
- reduction in bed numbers
- recent government policies on community care.

The role of the CPN has also developed in line with these changes, shifting away from the traditional role of carrying out duties prescribed by medical doctors, towards being more autonomous practitioners. CPNs usually work within a multidisciplinary context to provide care and support for clients. In the last few years, there has been a gradual development of new and innovative services for people with serious and enduring illness. The role of the CPN has also developed, to include assessing and intervening with clients and their relatives, consultancy for other professions and monitoring the effects of a wide range of psychotropic medications. CPNs can also specialise in behavioural and cognitive therapy, psycho-educational interventions and working with families – areas of care traditionally associated with other professionals. CPNs are playing a central role as community-based clinical managers and are beginning to use a range of psychosocial interventions. Their role in contemporary interventions is highlighted by Gournay (1995, 1996).

The Sainsbury Centre document, *Pulling Together* (1997), looked at future roles and training of mental health workers in the community and identified the core knowledge, skills and attitudes required by these professionals to provide a comprehensive service for people with severe mental health problems. Recently, innovative training programmes have been developed in the UK to try to meet the education needs of mental health nurses. For example, the Thorn Programme based at Manchester University and the Institute of Psychiatry in London trains nurses with at least 2 years experience of working in the community. The programme aims to provide nurses with skills-based knowledge in working with people with mental health problems using problem-orientated case management. Topics covered include case management, cognitive–behavioural therapy, measuring symptom severity and family work. The goal of the initiative is to equip nurses with skills to conduct comprehensive assessments and interventions, using approaches that are often employed by other disciplines. Currently there are about 200 nurses who have completed the training, and there are now nine centres in the UK running the Thorn Programme or similar courses.

The legislative framework

There is continuing public anxiety concerning the care of the mentally ill people in the community. The numbers of suicides, homicides and other serious incidents have been the subject of great public as well as professional concern. Criticism about the lack of a comprehensive support network for clients discharged from hospital to community care and the lack of communication and integration of activities between agencies involved has led to several initiatives in community care legislation and government policy guidance. Nurses need to be familiar with the relevant legislation when working in the community.

The National Health Service and Community Care Act 1990 requires an assessment of need for people with mental health problems. Need is defined as:

> the requirements of individuals to enable them to achieve, maintain or restore an acceptable level of social independence or quality of life.
>
> Department of Health Social Services Inspectorate 1991:10

The Care Programme Approach (CPA) is a variation of case management, a model of care-

giving developed in America to help co-ordinate the activities of agencies. It was introduced in 1991, following the Spokes Inquiry (Spokes 1988). It requires inter-agency collaboration between health and social services to ensure that there is a co-ordinated safety net of care in place for people with severe mental illness. The goals were to clarify the complex issues surrounding the co-ordination of care, and to promote inter-professional communication and the effective targeting of resources by community mental health teams (CMHTs). The principles underlying the CPA are that care is provided by a multidisciplinary team and so most community nurses now work in teams with professionals from other disciplines. In summary, people with mental health problems need to be managed within a comprehensive system of care where both health and social needs are addressed sufficiently, and where all relevant agencies come together to produce a care plan intended to meet the needs of that individual client. More recent legislation, such as the Supervised Discharge Order and the Supervision Register, continues to change the working context for CPNs, further reinforcing the view that assessments should be carried out in the community by involving the multidisciplinary teams.

Multidisciplinary working

Nurses working in the community are normally members of a CMHT. CMHTs comprise professionals from different disciplines, who each bring a range of skills and experience in providing care. Multidisciplinary teams vary in their makeup, but typically consist of nurses, psychiatrists, occupational therapists, clinical psychologists, social workers and community support workers. The advantage of multidisciplinary working is the pooling together of different skills, expertise and ideas about providing the best possible care for an individual. The role of CPNs within a CMHT can be particularly important, since they often have more contact with clients than other professionals in the team.

One implication of multidisciplinary working is that nurses may undertake joint assessments with other professionals. Joint assessments may be conducted for a number of reasons, including the presenting problems of a client, and to ensure safety of the assessing staff. For example, a joint visit by a social worker and CPN may be conducted to assess a client who has both health and social needs, wheras one by a CPN and psychiatrist may be for mental health assessment and treatment. Joint assessments involving CPNs and other disciplines have increased and can provide an effective method of understanding a client's difficulties from a variety of perspectives.

Nursing assessments are used in collaboration with those of other disciplines to confirm the presence of psychological or family problems, for problem formulation or diagnosis, and to plan care for an individual.

WHAT IS ASSESSMENT?

Assessment has been defined 'as the collection and documentation of primary and secondary information about a patient, and the re-examining of this information in the light of outcomes of a care plan and intervention' (Whyte & Youill 1984). *Primary* information is that obtained from the client, and *secondary* information is that obtained from other sources (e.g. GP, formal and informal carers, referrer, casenotes). Assessment should involve the client and significant others involved with the client.

Other authors viewed assessment as a process of gathering information about a client using specialised knowledge and skills to identify and document the client's presenting problem(s) or mental state, with a view to offering an interven-

tion or referring the client on to appropriate services. For example, Barker (1997) suggested that assessment can be defined as 'the decision-making process based upon the collection of relevant information using a formal set of ethical criteria that contributes to an overall evaluation of a person and his circumstances.'

Central to assessments is the collection of information from different sources about the individuals, their mental health and their functioning. The information gathered will cover a wide range of areas, as shown in Box 7.1.

Box 7.1 Assessment of current circumstances and health status

- Personal details (age, sex, marital status, personal history)
- Family details (parents, siblings, family history)
- Current circumstances (accommodation, daytime activities, social network)
- Symptoms (intensity, duration, frequency, antecedents, consequences)
- Beliefs (cause of problems, what the solution is, delusions)
- Mood (depressed, grandiose, worried)
- Thinking (concentration, attention, formal thought disorder)
- Speech (disturbance, type of errors)
- Perceptual experiences (hallucinations, orientated to time, place and person)
- Current coping strategies (what helps and what doesn't help)
- Alcohol and drug use
- Physical health

NURSING ASSESSMENTS

For nurses, assessment of clients in the community is not just focused on diagnostic concerns but also investigates how individuals function in their social environment. The goal of assessing a client is thus to obtain a picture of the client's life, and inform decisions about what help (if any) to offer. This picture of the client's life should cover such areas as the client's personality, current circumstances and personal and social history. The client's perception of the nature and cause of problems being faced should be assessed, along with nursing assessments of any deficits and disabilities. Positive aspects should be identified, such as strengths, skills, assets, resources and coping strategies.

Traditional approaches to psychiatric nursing assessments have involved derivations of the diagnostic methods used by psychiatrists, which are used to make a psychiatric diagnosis. Nurses have been involved in assessing the client's mental state, with the information fed back at ward rounds and review meetings. For example, nursing staff might report to the team that a client was observed to be responding to auditory hallucinations, but not how the client was socialising, the client's level of activity or the client's social support (visits from family and friends). The mental state examination is a format used by psychiatrists to assess the mental functioning and current emotional state of a client. This medical model of assessing clients requires a clinician to collect data about an individual, analyse it and construct a treatment plan based on a diagnosis. Mental state assessments have the disadvantage that they do not emphasise the individual nature of the psychological and social difficulties that the client is experiencing.

An argument put forward by the Royal College of Nursing (1981) and Orem (1980) is that clients are best served if doctors use a medical model, concentrating on the diagnosis and treatment of illness, with nurses using a more holistic approach, helping the client to make sense of what is happening, and giving support and guidance. However, nursing assessments are eclectic and use approaches and ideas borrowed from other professions. Overall, nurses in multidisciplinary teams view clients as people who have certain problems or difficulties in life, ranging from the severely disabling to the mildly inconvenient. The goal of an assessment should

be to identify strengths as well as deficits, so that the resulting care plan will allow clients as far as possible to draw on these strengths in resolving their difficulties.

Nursing models

In order to address the needs of clients, nurses have developed nursing models – methods of assessing specific to nursing. Nursing models are well documented and have been widely used as an approach to assessing the needs of clients, identifying problems and formulating ways of helping them to improve their well-being. Examples include those of Peplau (1952), Orem (1980), Roy (1980) and Roper et al (1980).

Psychosocial approach

Another approach used in assessing clients has been to use the psychosocial framework. This takes into account the environmental theory which assumes that the person's behaviour is primarily a function of the individual's interaction with the environment and that people interact creatively with the world in which they live (Lewin 1951). Psychosocial assessment addresses factors such as:

- psychological and biological phenomena
- functional (behavioural) performance
- self-efficacy
- relationships with the family
- relationships with the wider social environment
- interpersonal communication
- social resources.

For example, when assessing the level of functioning, it is assumed that the CPN would interpret the levels of functioning obtained from the assessment within the context of the support currently available from the person's family, interpersonal and social environment.

Behavioural approach

This is a problem-orientated approach to assessing a client's difficulties. The assessment is approached in two stages: problem assessment and general assessment. *Problem assessment* involves interviewing clients, and helping them to define their problem as best as they can. Assessment concentrates on the here-and-now reality of the client's experiences, rather than the causes of the presenting problem (Richards & McDonald 1990). Behavioural analysis is used to gain an understanding of the problem behaviours. This involves an ABC analysis of behaviour:

- identifying the Antecedents
- recording the precise Behaviour
- examining the Consequences of the behaviour.

It is assumed no problem or behaviour exists in isolation, and that there will always be events and experiences that precede it (antecedents) and events that follow it (consequences). Both the antecedents and the consequences will help to explain the behaviour. This approach gives a framework in which to understand these difficulties. The second part of the assessment, *general assessment*, entails collecting information about the client's personal and family history, mental state, and past psychiatric and medical history.

Risk assessment

An area of particular concern for community nursing is the assessment of risk. Services have been criticised in the past for failing the mentally ill by not providing adequate follow-up and assessments, especially for those at risk of self-harm or harm to others.

With changes in the care of the mentally ill, there is more individual accountability of mental health care professionals for the client care they provide. Formal external inquiries about errors of treatment and clinical judgement now focus on the management of the client, and on the decision-making by the key clinicians (who may be nurses). Inquiries such as the Clunis Report (Ritchie et al 1994) have highlighted the need for all health professionals to be as rigorous and methodological in their assessments as much as possible.

Risk in the clinical sense can be defined as the likelihood of an event happening, whether the event is positive or negative. Risk is often associated with violence to others, but also refers to the risk of a relapse, unwanted side-effects or outcomes from treatment, verbal or physical aggression, self-harm or damage to property and sexual activity.

Risk assessment involves assessing the safety of a client and the risk the client poses to others. This is achieved by obtaining as much information as possible about the client's background, present and past mental state, social functioning and behaviour. This information informs decisions about the severity of the risk. CPNs have to ensure their clients' safety through continuous assessments, and by ensuring that other relevant disciplines are involved in their care and management. Therefore, it is important that CPNs make an assessment of risk in clients in the community.

Approaches to risk assessment are now being developed. Manchester University and the Department of Health published *Learning Materials on Mental Health* which addressed the whole topic of risk assessment. It consists of a series of modules for risk assessment to help clinicians gather information about potential risks of violence and develop a risk management plan. CANVAS (Clinical Assessment of Need: Violence Appraisal System) is a system that has been developed at the Institute of Psychiatry, London. It aims to help mental health professionals working in general adult services in gathering evidence to support a clinical decision about risk and its management. It consists of three modules:

1. a summary of the client's history of violence
2. potential risk factors for violence
3. a clinical plan to manage any risk of violence.

Initial risk assessment informs decisions about the level of urgency of a referral. Referrals can be for clients at risk of relapsing, self-harm, violence to others or suicide. On the other hand, the referral could be for a client who is experiencing a crisis because of confusion about benefit entitlements, housing or bills, and would benefit from advice about the benefit system. Therefore, the nature of the risk has to be identified. Relevant sources include the client, the client's referrer, casenotes, GP, family and friends, social worker, housing department and police.

Good practice in community nursing is to use a checklist to determine the risk and hence the urgency of a referral (see Box 7.2).

Once the initial risk is identified, further assessment should involve considering what meaning the client attaches to the behaviour and whether the client is motivated to avoid it (e.g. does the client believe it is quite appropriate to respond to verbal insults with physical aggression?), what are the controls on the client's behaviour (e.g. what stops a suicidal client from making the attempt?), how functional are the client's current coping strategies (e.g. drinking alcohol when depressed may increase the risk of an impulsive suicide attempt), and what is the history of the client's behaviour (e.g. has a previous suicide attempt been made? If so, how did the client feel when the attempt failed?).

Full risk assessment will inform decisions about whether the client needs to be admitted to hospital, and the development of a care plan to ensure that the risk is minimised and managed effectively. The care plan will involve liaison with other team members, and jointly devising a plan agreed by all those involved in the care of that client. Other members of the team may also be involved in the assessment, such as a psychiatrist to review the mental state and a social worker to address the carers' needs (in accordance with the Carers' Act 1996). Forensic CPNs may co-work clients with a history of violence or forensic history, or those where there are concerns about further risk of violence. The care plan might, for example, involve helping the client to identify relapses earlier, or educating the family about the illness and the best ways to manage difficult behaviour.

Case study 7.1 will be used to illustrate the purpose and outcome of a risk assessment.

Box 7.2 Checklist of factors to consider when assessing risk

- Can the referral wait for a week or longer? Does the client need to be seen immediately?
- What risk does the client pose to himself/herself or to other people?
- Has the client got adequate resources to support himself/herself and prevent the crisis escalating at home?
- Does the client need a place of safety? Has the person made threats to self-harm? Is there a history or family history of suicidal tendencies/behaviour?
- What is the mood of the client? If the client is depressed – how depressed? Is the client withdrawing or socially isolating himself/herself? Is there social support or social abandonment?
- Is the client's behaviour suggestive of someone who is at risk? What do family members think? Are they worried about the client and what is it that worries them? Has the client been saying things to make the family concerned about his/her safety?

Case study 7.1 Risk assessment

Referral letter to CMHT from GP practice.

Re: John Thimble

DOB 4.8.72

I would like to refer this young man to your team.

John is a 26-year-old man with a history of psychotic illness. He has had several in-patient admissions in Wales. He moved to London 2 years ago and has been working as a security guard in a local shop. He lives on his own in rented accommodation. His family are supportive and live nearby. He attends the surgery once a month for his prescription of chlorpromazine 100 mg bd. John abuses alcohol and non-prescribed drugs. His relapses in the past have been related to his drinking as well as his non-compliance with medication. These recent relapses have been characterised by aggressive outbursts directed at his mother. He has also made a suicide attempt while responding to auditory hallucinations, and slashed his wrist 3 days ago.

Assessment

The assessment checklist shown earlier was completed and it indicated that this referral needed urgent attention. From the referral letter, the following issues were identified:

Safety

John's condition was relapsing, and he was exhibiting threatening behaviour and being aggressive towards his mother. Questions about how safe it was for the CPN to visit John alone at home were raised and suggestions were made to have him initially assessed at the team base. As John was not willing to come to the team base and because of concerns about the safety of the assessor, a multidisciplinary decision was made to conduct a joint assessment at his home.

Lack of information

John was not known to the team or the local hospital. This lack of knowledge about him meant that more information needed to be collected from other sources. Background information obtained from his GP and more detailed background information including forensic history was obtained from hospital casenotes from the hospital in Wales.

Multiple problems

Not only did John have mental health problems, but he also had alcohol and drug problems. He was living in rented accommodation but it was unclear how secure his tenancy was. He had a job and there were concerns about how secure this was. In view of these factors, a wide-ranging assessment was required. A comprehensive multidisciplinary assessment was therefore conducted by a CPN and a psychiatrist. John was seen and assessed at his home address, with his family invited to be present for the assessment.

Client interview

The CPN and psychiatrist interviewed John initially and the purpose of the visit was explained. His GP had explained that he had referred him to the team. Initially he was asked questions about his personal history, work and interests and attempts were made to engage him in a dialogue with the CPN. This enabled him to relax and talk openly about himself. John was asked about his experiences and the difficulties he was experiencing. He was helped through sensitive questioning to identify those factors he thought had contributed to his relapse. He was asked about his aggressive behaviour and the factors that were leading to his aggressive outburst. He described hearing voices which he linked to his behaviour. He was questioned about how he controlled his anger, including what had helped in the past and what had not. His responses were helpful in the prediction of the likelihood of violent behaviour occurring, in identifying circumstances that had led to the violence occurring in the past, and in assessing whether similar circumstances were likely to occur again.

John talked about his reasons for not taking his medication. He believed the medication was not helping him and therefore he did not need to take it. His non-compliance had resulted in his symptoms worsening, but he found this difficult to acknowledge and believed if people left him alone to rest he would be fine. The assessors were aware that there is evidence to suggest that violence closely associated with acute episodes of a long mental illness can be anticipated when relapses are due to non-compliance with medication.

John's safety needs were taken very seriously, especially following the suicide attempt. When asked directly if he had any thoughts about harming himself or plans to do so, John admitted he felt suicidal at times and that these suicidal thoughts often coincided with the intensity of the voices and his lowered mood. He described the voices as instructing him to harm himself and his mother. He also believed his mother was trying to kill him by poisoning his food and that she was part of the conspiracy to harm him. Sutherby & Szmukler (1996) outlined factors associated with suicide risk (e.g. sociodemographic characteristics, medical, psychiatric and family history and behaviour which may be indicators of a suicide risk).

Family interview

John's mother and sister were also interviewed. They were given an opportunity to talk about their views of John's problems, and to give an explanation as to why they believed he was having these experiences, when they started and when they noticed the changes in his behaviour. It was also important to find out from the family about any transitional changes they were experiencing at the time. Usually information obtained from relatives and friends of the person who is seeking help will tend to complement the information given by the client. They disclosed that John had attended a religious festival and had come back believing he had been cured from all his worries, leading him to start working long hours, and to cease sleeping and eating. They had tried to encourage him to take the medication (especially his mother), but he would get angry saying he did not need it. The issue was therefore avoided and not discussed with him.

Particular focus in the family assessment was the relationship between John and his mother and other family members, their understanding of his illness, how it affected them and how they communicated with one another. Expressed

emotion studies indicate that family dynamics and relatives' behaviour have an effect on the well-being of the person with mental health problems. The way carers respond and communicate with the client can impact on the client's recovery (Leff & Vaughan 1985).

The problems identified from the assessment were:

- the return of positive symptoms
- anger problems exacerbated by alcohol and drugs
- suicidal thoughts and acts.

Outcome of the assessment

Once John's problems were identified, a decision was made about the immediate intervention to be implemented to help prevent his mental health deteriorating further. John reluctantly agreed to the help being offered to him and agreed to start taking his medication. He remained at his home with support from his family and agreed to work with the CPN. A social worker was involved to conduct a needs assessment on him and his mother (the main carer).

Short-term goals

A care plan involving John, his family and the CPN was formulated. It addressed issues about the early warning signs of his illness, with the aim of helping John and his family to identify relapses and to seek help early. Medication was prescribed for John to help alleviate some of distress he was experiencing from his symptoms.

Long-term goals

The family met regularly with the CPN to talk about their concerns, look at strategies for dealing with John's positive and negative symptoms and suicidal/aggressive threats and attempts, and to receive information about his illness. John was also referred to the team's psychologist for short-term intervention to help him with anger management. John's assessment is an ongoing process rather than a one-off exercise. The CPN will continue to assess him and develop a therapeutic relationship. Through face-to-face contact with his CPN, new information will be gathered.

THE PROCESS OF ASSESSMENT

The process of assessment involves a number of steps, and a framework suggested by Barker (1997) is shown in Box 7.3.

Box 7.3 A framework for a nursing assessment (after Barker 1997)

Method	Which method should be used?
↓	
Information	What has been elicited from the information?
↓	
Analysis	What is it that has been found out?
↓	
Picture	Nursing diagnosis/problem formulation.
↓	
Judgement	What care does the client need?

Assessment therefore involves deciding what information one wants to elicit (i.e. setting aims and objectives), choosing a method to collect this information, analysing and interpreting this information, formulating a picture of the client and the problem and deciding on the care the client will require.

Another approach suggested by Barker (1997) is for the assessor to ask the following questions about the purpose of the assessment, the assessment method to be used and how the information collected will be reviewed.

1. **Why** am I doing this assessment?
2. **What** is the aim of the assessment – what do I want to find out about referral?
3. **When** should I assess – is the referral urgent?
4. **How** will I get the information?
5. **How** will I judge what this information means (problem formulation)?
6. **How** might the client function differently if the problems are resolved?

The initial referral

The process of initial assessment by a nurse in a CMHT will now be discussed. However, it should be noted that assessment is not a one-off procedure, but an ongoing process of gathering information and reviewing the client's progress.

The *goal* of an initial assessment is to gather information which is necessary and sufficient to arrive at an understanding of the client's difficulties and to formulate a plan of care. Initial assessment should gain a clear picture of the client's current problems, from both the client's own perspective and the perspective of others. It should also cover the client's history, both to set the client in an individual context and to identify aspects of the client's history which have a particular bearing on the client's current difficulties.

Initial decisions about the assessment are made on the basis of the *referral*. Requests for assessments can come from a range of sources, such as general practitioners, accident and emergency departments, and other formal and informal carers. These are typically in the form of a letter, or a verbal referral by telephone or in person. Often there is only limited information contained in the referral and it usually represents only a portion of what the referrer has discovered about a client's experiences and difficulties. The information contained in a referral letter may therefore not necessarily represent a total or accurate picture of the client's problems, so there is a need for further assessment. Sometimes clients will refer themselves to a CMHT or emergency clinic when experiencing a crisis.

A decision needs to be made about *the urgency of the referral*, on the basis of information in the referral. Some CMHTs have a duty or crisis team to deal with referrals requiring an urgent response. They may consist of CPNs, social workers and psychiatrists who assess clients individually or jointly. Non-urgent referrals are discussed in team meetings, and depending on what the referrer is asking for and the needs of that client, a team member with particular skills to assess the client's needs is allocated to conduct the assessment.

There are *three sources* of information which can inform the assessment: the client, formal carers, and informal carers. Formal carers are those mental health professionals who deal with or have recently been involved with the client. Also within this category comes information in the referral letter (if the referrer is a mental health professional), casenotes and reports on the client. Informal carers include family, friends, neighbours and other members of the community who support the client (e.g. a priest). Typically, an assessment will involve the client, the main caregiver, the referrer and other involved professionals, and a review of casenotes.

The *multiple sources* of information for assessment can present a dilemma for nurses about how to conduct the assessment. If they assess formal or informal carers first, they run the risk of the client perceiving them as 'going behind their back'. If they assess the client first, they may miss areas of assessment which other sources would have indicated. Furthermore, the nurse may be unaware of factors indicating that the client may be a safety risk (e.g. a history of violence towards mental health staff), and so not take adequate precautions. It is therefore important for the nurse to think carefully about who and in what order to assess. A good compromise is usually to liaise in the first instance with the referrer (assuming the referrer is a formal carer).

It is important to clarify *what the referrer is asking for* – is the referrer asking for a comprehensive assessment and a care plan, or an opinion or advice on an aspect of care for the individual? The referrer should be asked for two specific items of information. First, information about

risk factors (e.g. paranoid or suicidal ideation, or a history of violence) will inform decisions about how to assess the client. This topic is discussed further in Section 3. Second, if the client is likely to be suspicious of the nurse (e.g. owing to paranoia or a history of aversive experiences with psychiatric services), it may be helpful to involve the referrer in the initial client assessment, if the referrer's relationship with the client is positive.

Another issue is *whether the client is aware of and in agreement with the referral*. If the client is unaware of the referral, why was the client not told? If the client does not believe there is anything wrong, then sensitivity is needed when interviewing the client. The goal is then to assess whether there really is a problem requiring help from mental health services. Does the client lack insight, or is the referrer misinformed? If the conclusion is that significant problems do exist, then the initial interview should lay the foundation for a therapeutic relationship, which may need to be assertively maintained in the absence of motivation from the client.

Two types of information are necessary for a comprehensive assessment: primary and secondary.

Primary information

Primary information is derived solely from the client, through what they say, and their actions, words, appearance and behaviour. Primary information for an initial assessment is usually gathered by interview.

Interviewing is a key skill in the CPNs repertoire, which ideally allows rapport with the client to be established, and the beginnings of a therapeutic relationship to be developed. Interviewing a client gives the assessor an idea of when to introduce other methods of assessing, such as rating scales to assess depression. The disadvantages of interviewing are the time involved, the demanding nature for the nurse, and the possibility that the assessment may have a negative effect on the client (and hence the subsequent nurse–client relationship) if clients experience the interview as involving too many questions being asked. Issues in community interviewing are explored further by Newell (1994), Parkman & Bixby (1996) and Barker (1997).

The way that an interview with the client is conducted can make the exercise more or less fruitful. It is therefore important for the assessor to decide on the best method that will allow for appropriate and sufficient information to be collected with least effort and cost for both the nurse and the client. There are a number of assessment methods that can be used to help clients give information about themselves, ranging from informal interviews to semi-structured and formal assessment schedules and questionnaires.

The interview may be an informal discussion with the client to give the client a chance to describe personal concerns and difficulties. Informal interviewing may be most appropriate for a client who is articulate and able to communicate well, or for one who would find a more formal approach to assessment intimidating. Alternatively, the nurse might use a semi-structured interview. This involves asking the client a range of exploratory questions on various topics relating to the client's difficulties or the reasons for seeking help. This approach is commonly used by CPNs because it provides some structure to the conversation.

Interviewing clients involves asking about feelings, thoughts, beliefs and behaviour, and relating the responses to the difficulties. Clients give information about themselves, which enables the assessor to isolate particular areas of difficulty or need, and to identify an intervention to meet these needs or difficulties.

Nurses are often called upon to assess new referrals (clients not known to the services) who may be acutely psychotic or in distress. The way clients present in a crisis varies from person to person. They may be confused, intoxicated, angry, violent, suicidal or uncommunicative (mute or catatonic). These factors present a particular challenge to nurses in their attempt to establish rapport with the client and elicit the necessary information. Psychotic symptoms can be particularly awkward to ask about. Some ways of opening up the topic are:

'Have you had any unusual experiences recently?' 'Can you describe them?'
'Do you ever hear voices when there is nobody around?'
'Do you ever have problems with your thoughts?'
'Do you find that people disagree with any of your beliefs?'
'Tell me what happens when you have these thoughts / voices?'

Formal assessment tools (e.g. questionnaires, validated schedules) are less used when conducting initial nursing assessments. This is because of the emphasis on developing a therapeutic relationship with the client which would help in working with the client to help resolve the difficulties. Highly structured questioning when meeting a client for the first time can appear impersonal and threatening, and may prevent a client from opening up or expressing their feelings. However, formal assessments such as symptom checklists are often useful in subsequent stages of assessing clients. They can be well structured and have been tested in research studies to ensure that they are reliable and valid tools. They are designed to assess particular areas, possibly providing a measure of severity. Formal approaches may be appropriate where the goal is to get a clear picture of the client's difficulties in a particular domain, or to take a baseline measure of severity. Some examples include:

- The Manchester Rating Scale – developed for people with enduring experiences of psychosis. The nurse needs to know the client and have developed a therapeutic relationship to allow the questionnaire to be completed (Kraweicka et al 1977).
- Camberwell Assessment of Need (CAN) – developed to provide a comprehensive assessment of the client's health and social needs, and the extent to which these are being met by the client's carers and services. A priority for the CAN is to identify rather than describe in-depth serious needs (Phelan et al 1995).
- Social Network Scale (SNS) – assesses the social support network of the client (Dunn et al 1990).
- Hopelessness Scale – developed to provide information about suicidal intent. It takes a few minutes to complete and may be given to the client on a regular basis to monitor the risk of suicide. It is based on the research finding that hopelessness is a better predictor of suicide than the level of depression (Beck et al 1974).
- Brief Psychiatric Rating Scale (BPRS) – uses a semi-structured interview, observation by the assessor and information given by carers. It measures presence and severity of psychotic symptoms (Overall & Gorham 1962).
- Beck Depression Inventory (BDI) – measures the severity of depression (Beck et al 1961).

Secondary information

Secondary information is the information obtained from the client's formal and informal carers. Information obtained from these sources often complements the primary information and is helpful in formulating a care plan. The first formal carer to be contacted is typically the referrer. Referrers will usually be able to give information about the nature, severity and duration of the client's current difficulties, details of similar problems that occurred in the past, interventions employed and their effectiveness, and the effect of the problem on the client and those around the client. They may also provide details of other professionals involved in the client's care, such as GPs, social workers, probation officers, and other health professionals who have worked closely with the individual. All of these sources of information may provide important information about aspects of the client's difficulties.

If the client has come into contact with services in the past, then *previous assessments* and interventions will have been documented by the relevant agency (such as medical notes, social services records or housing agency notes). Casenotes are therefore an important source of assessment information and may allow the assessment to focus on the client's current difficulties.

Informal carers are typically relatives or friends of a client. Their perspective is important, since they will often have the most contact with the client and know the client very well. They may provide valuable background information on the current episode of relapse, the patient's normal functioning and usual level of dependence. They may be the first to notice any changes in behaviour in their relative, and so are an important source of information on the early signs of relapse (Birchwood et al 1989).

Sometimes information given by the informal or formal carer does not agree with that given by the client. In such a case, on whose information should care plans be based? Two principles can inform this decision. First, the views of the client should be central to assessment. They may or may not be 'wrong', and indeed there is evidence to suggest that in some circumstances the view of the client is more reliable than the view of staff (MacCarthy et al 1986). However, an intervention which does not address the perceived problems of clients may be neither adhered to by the client nor successful. Second, a difference in perspective may be revealing in itself. For example, caregivers who emphasise how disabled the client is may be communicating their own need for support.

Case study 7.2 will be used to illustrate some issues in the initial assessment.

GUIDELINES FOR HOME VISITING

Clients can be seen in their homes, at the CMHT base, in the GP surgery, at a day centre, in an emergency clinic or in a voluntary sector setting. The decision about the location should be informed by two goals. First, the assessment process should be as enjoyable as possible for the

---

Case study 7.2 Initial assessment process

Joan is a 29-year-old, single woman. She lives at home with her parents and older sister. Her care has been managed by her GP and she has been diagnosed as suffering from a psychotic illness. Her relapses in the past were related to stressful events such as loss, exams and achievement pressure from her family, as well as non-compliance with her medication. Her family are very caring and supportive. Her mother is described as over-involved and her father denies any possibility of Joan having mental health problems and believes she puts on an act and is lazy. Her sister is doing well, has finished her college degree and has a job, a boyfriend and a network of friends.

Two weeks ago, Joan started behaving strangely. She stopped attending college, became hostile towards family members, especially her mother, refused to sit down and eat meals with them, neglected her self-care, talked to herself and would shout obscenities. At night, she paced up and down the stairs. Joan denied there was anything wrong with her and would get angry when asked how she was feeling. The atmosphere at home became increasingly tense with family members describing walking on egg shells in fear of upsetting her by doing or saying the wrong thing.

She was seen by her GP at the request of the family. She had become more distressed and attempted to stab herself in the stomach in response to the voices. She was referred to the local CMHT for further assessment.

Preparation for assessment

The referral was discussed in the team's referral meeting. From the referral letter, it was evident that Joan's behaviour had changed, causing concern to both her parents and the GP. The aim of the assessment was therefore to identify Joan's needs and problems, and to decide on the appropriate intervention that would help meet her needs. The following issues needed to be addressed by the team:

- What information should be obtained from the GP who had been involved with Joan and her family for the past 5 years?
- What are the possible precipitants to onset of relapse?
- What is happening in the family as a result of the changes in Joan's behaviour?
- What are Joan's experiences?
- Concerns are about her behaviour, and her and her mother's safety

A joint assessment by a CPN and a psychiatrist was organised, with Joan being assessed in her own environment so as to observe her functioning at home and her interaction with other family members. An appointment letter was sent to Joan and her family. The letter explained that her GP had referred her to the team, and that members of the team would like to meet with her to discuss ways of helping her with her difficulties.

Joan was not known to the mental health services and this was her first referral to the psychiatric services. Therefore, detailed information was obtained from the referrer, the GP, who had known

Joan for about 5 years, and was therefore able to give a clear picture of Joan's difficulties and how the family was being affected by her change in behaviour. Information about risk factors (i.e. suicidal ideation) and her awareness of the referral and likely response to meeting her assessors (suspiciousness towards strangers or health professionals from the psychiatric services) was also obtained. The GP was invited for the initial assessment.

Method of assessing
As this was an initial assessment, the assessment method of choice was to interview Joan and her family members. At this stage, it is important to establish rapport and trust and to facilitate the development of a therapeutic relationship. Because Joan is the index client, it is important to obtain as much information from her as possible by allowing her to describe her difficulties.

Sources of information
Four sources of information were used. Primary information was obtained from Joan, the client. Secondary information was obtained from the GP and family. The GP provided information about the severity of Joan's current problems and the effects on her family. Joan's family provided valuable information, because they knew her well and had the most contact with her. They discussed the current episode of relapse, her functioning, and significant changes or events which were

threatening to her and hence impacted on her mental state. In Joan's case, these included loss and change in the usual family routine (e.g. the presence of relatives in the family home, planned holidays away from her usual surroundings, social gathering, exams).

The problems identified from the assessment were:
- the presence of the positive symptoms, especially the voices that were instructing her to harm herself and her mother
- lack of motivation
- suicidal thoughts and intent
- worsening of symptoms and non-response to psychotropic medication.

Outcome of assessment
Joan was prescribed an anti-psychotic drug to help alleviate the distress she was experiencing. Concerns were raised about her safety while she remained with the family. Her family agreed to consider an admission to hospital if Joan's mental state worsened. They requested support and information to deal with her experiences. As part of her care plan, family work was negotiated with the family.

A CPN was allocated to monitor her mental state and review progress, and an occupational therapist to address her level of activity and functioning. The referrer was informed by letter of the outcome of the assessment and action plan.

client. This may mean that the home is the best setting for assessment, so that the nurse is on the client's 'territory'. Assessment of clients in their own environment also allows extra information to be gathered by observation, such as whether the home is clean, the type of food that is eaten, and the social niceties observed by the client. Alternatively, the client may not want psychiatric staff coming to the home, for fear of the neighbours finding out. This can best be ascertained in negotiation with the client when setting up the interview.

The second goal is to maintain the safety of the mental health worker and minimise the vulnerability of staff working in the community. If there is evidence that the client poses a potential safety risk to the nurse, the client should be assessed in a more controlled environment (e.g. CMHT base) where back-up can be provided by other team members if necessary. If this is not possible, the client should be interviewed by two members of the team in a neutral setting away from the home. At the very least, other team members should be aware of who is being seen and the expected time of return. Good practice is to have agreed guidelines for home visiting, which should include ways of notifying other team members of the expected time of return, and the procedure to be followed if this deadline is exceeded. An example of guidelines for home visiting (devised by a team working in an inner city area) is given in Box 7.4.

Box 7.4 Sample guidelines for home visiting

Before the visit
- Check the referral details. Gather as much information about the client before you decide on the visit. Decide whether it is safe to visit alone, or if a joint visit is required. If uncertain, discuss with the team.
- Check details for any history of violence or aggressive incidents (threatening behaviour). **Do not visit alone** if there is any known or suspected history or you are in doubt about your personal safety.
- Be aware of other agencies involved, such as social services, probation services or housing services, and liaise with them prior to the visit. Be aware of the presence of children in the home and especially those at risk.
- Ensure a team member knows your whereabouts (complete movement sheet on board giving name of client you are visiting, address, expected time of return and contact number (mobile number)).
- Carry your identification badge and do not carry any valuables.

During the visit
- When you receive an answer at the door, ask for the client you have called to see. Introduce yourself and explain the purpose of your visit.
- Make an assessment of the environment, without being too intrusive or interfering.
- Confirm who else lives with the client, any children, and if you could talk privately. Involve significant others if the client is comfortable with this.
- Should you feel unsafe (client making sexual advances or becoming distressed or angry and you feel this will lead to violence), **leave**. Arrange to visit with someone else the next day.
- If the client asks you to leave their home, **leave without hesitation**.

After the visit
- Inform your colleagues of your return.

If you are going on to another visit or somewhere else (e.g. home), **inform the team about your movements and your safety by telephone**.

CONCLUSION

This chapter has highlighted some of the principles underpinning community nursing assessments. Careful consideration needs to be given to the purpose of the assessment, its urgency, who to assess, and how the assessment is to be carried out. Risk assessment is especially important. For initial assessments, where the client is not known to the service, decisions are needed about whose views are to be given primacy when there is disagreement – the client, the formal carer or the informal carer? Safety when undertaking community-based assessments needs to be prioritised, with agreed team guidelines for interviewing.

The 'centre of gravity' of mental health care has shifted from institutional to community settings. This has provided an opportunity for the profession of psychiatric nursing to develop new roles in the multidisciplinary team. In particular, assessment in the community gives CPNs a distinct and more autonomous role than their institutional predecessors, and allows them to take the lead in the development of good practice.

Exercise

Think of a patient who has just been referred to you.
1. Why do you need to assess them?
2. How do you decide the urgency of the initial assessment?
3. How will you decide who to speak to?
4. What types of information will you gather?
5. Will you use any formal assessment tools? If not, what baseline measures will you use to allow evaluation of the patient's progress?
6. How will you decide whether to see the patient at home or at your place of work?
7. How will you know when the *initial* assessment is complete?

KEY TEXTS FOR FURTHER READING

Thornicroft G, Tansella M (eds) 1996 Mental health outcome measures. Springer, Heidelberg. *Describes formal assessment schedules for a range of purposes, including quality of life, social disability, satisfaction with services, and measures of global functioning. An excellent resource for the nurse who wants to use formal assessment schedules in clinical practice.*

Phelan M, Slade M, Thornicroft G et al 1995 The Camberwell assessment of need: the validity of an instrument to assess the needs of the seriously mentally ill. British Journal of Psychiatry 167:589–595. *Describes the Camberwell Assessment of Need (CAN), a reliable and valid schedule for the comprehensive assessment of the health and social needs of the severely mentally ill. The clinical version and the short version of the CAN are intended for routine clinical use.*

Wing J, Beevor A, Curtis R, Park S, Hadden S, Burns A 1998 Health of the nation outcome scales (HoNOS). British Journal of Psychiatry 172:11–18. *Describes the development of HoNOS, a schedule to assess the health and social functioning of mentally ill people. HoNOS is intended for routine clinical use.*

Onyett S 1992 Case management in mental health. Chapman and Hall, London. *Discusses the impact of case management, with consideration given to the central role of assessment. Key features of assessment are identified, and case studies are used throughout the book to illustrate the practical issues of case management.*

Falloon I, Fadden G 1993 Integrated mental health care. Cambridge University Press, Cambridge. *Provides an extended case study, based on experiences in Buckingham, England of providing comprehensive mental health services. The description of how community care was implemented includes problem-based assessment of functioning, a behavioural approach to assessment which directly informs treatment goals. Also covers other aspects of community care, such as therapeutic strategies, crisis interventions and home-based intensive care.*

REFERENCES

Barker P J 1997 Assessment in psychiatric and mental health nursing. Stanley Thornes, Cheltenham

Beck A T, Ward C H, Mendelson M 1961 An inventory for measuring depresssion. Archives of General Psychiatry 4:561–571

Beck A T, Weissman A, Lester D, Trexler L 1974 The measurement of pessimism: the Hopelessness Scale. Journal of Counselling and Clinical Psychology 42:861–865

Birchwood M, Smith J, Macmillan F et al 1989 Predicting relapse in schizophrenia: the development and implementation of an early signs monitoring sytem using patients and families as observers. Psychological Medicine 19:649–656.

Department of Health Social Services Inspectorate 1991 Care management and assessment: Practitioners' guide. HMSO, London

Dunn M, O'Driscoll C, Dayson D, Wills W, Leff J 1990 The TAPS Project 4: an observational study of the social life of long stay patients. British Journal of Psychiatry 157:852–858

Gournay K 1995 Mental health nurses working with serious and enduring mental illness – an international perpective. International Journal of Nursing Studies 4:341–352

Gournay K 1996 Mental health nursing : issues and roles. Advances in Psychiatric Treatment 2:103–109

Kraweicka M, Goldberg D, Vaughan M 1977 A standardised psychiatric assessment scale for rating chronic psychotic patients. Acta Psychiatrica Scandanavica 55:299–308

Leff J P, Vaughan C 1985 Expressed emotion in families. Guilford Press, New York

Lewin K 1951 Field theory in social science. Harper, New York

MacCarthy B, Benson J, Brewin C 1986 Task motivation and problem appraisal in long-term psychiatric patients. Psychological Medicine 16:431–438

National Health Service and Community Care Act 1990. HMSO, London.

Newell R 1994 Interviewing skills for nurses and other health care professionals. Routledge. London

Orem D 1980 Nursing: Concepts of practice, 2nd edn. McGraw-Hill, New York

Overall J E, Gorham D R 1962 The Brief Psychiatric Rating Scale. Psychological Reports 10:799–812

Parkman S, Bixby S 1996 Community interviewing: experience and recommendations. Psychiatric Bulletin 20:72–74

Peplau H E 1952 Interpersonal relations in nursing: A conceptual frame of reference for psychodynamic nursing. Putnam, New York

Phelan M, Slade M, Thornicroft G et al 1995 The Camberwell assessment of need: the validity of an instrument to assess the needs of the seriously mentally ill. British Journal of Psychiatry 167:589–595

Richards D, McDonald B 1990 Behavioural psychotherapy: A handbook for nurses. Heinemann, Oxford

Ritchie J, Dick D, Lingham R 1994 (North East Thames and South East Thames Regional Health Authorities) 1994 Report of the inquiry into the care and treatment of Christopher Clunis. HMSO, London.

Roper N, Logan W, Tierney A 1980 The Elements of nursing. Churchill Livingstone, Edinburgh

Roy C 1980 The Roy adaptation model. In: Rienl-Sisca J P, Roy C Conceptual models for nursing practice, 2nd edn Appleton-Century-Crofts, New York

Royal College of Nursing 1981 A structure for nursing. RCN, London

Sainsbury Centre for Mental Health 1997 Pulling together: The future roles and training of mental health staff. Sainsbury Centre for Mental Health, London

Simmonds S, Brooker C 1986 Community psychiatric nursing: A social perspective. Heinemann Nursing, London

REFERENCES (*contd*)

Spokes Inquiry 1988 Report of the community inquiry into the care and after-care of Miss S. Campbell. HMSO, London

Sutherby K, Szmukler G 1996 Emergency mental health services in the community : Community assessment of crisis. Cambridge University Press, Cambridge

White E 1986 Surveying CPNs. Nursing Times 86(51):62–64.

Whyte L, Youill G 1984 The nursing process in the care of the mentally ill. Nursing Times 1:49–51.

CHAPTER CONTENTS

Key points   121

Historic background   122

Evidence-based practice   123

Why focus on training?   124

How should we analyse training?   124

Issues in training   125
Is it effective?   125
How does effective supervision work?   128

Evaluation of training in mental health nursing –
    an illustrative literature review   130
Internal validity   130
Internal validity in a sample of the nurse training
    literature   132
Dependent variables   134
Clinical significance   134
External validity   135
Efficiency   136

Application – conducting evaluations   137
Task 1 Identifying service goals   137
Task 2 Analysing service actions   138
Task 3 Describing and standardising nursing
    services   138
Task 4 Measuring the amount of change that
    occurs   138
Task 5 Determining whether change is due to the
    nursing service   138
Task 6 Assessing the relative effectiveness of
    modified services   140

Conclusions   140
Introduction section   140
Method section   140
Results   141
Discussion   141

Exercise   141

Key texts for further reading   141

References   142

8

Evaluation in mental health nursing

Derek Milne

KEY POINTS

- Training and evidence-based practice are key elements of mental health care.

- Training is an essential method of developing evidence-based practice, and a number of brief training issues have been prioritised by the NHS (e.g. comparing the relative value of different educational strategies).

- Past research on training has generally been of poor quality and has led to dubious conclusions about the benefits of training.

- Five studies of the training of mental health nurses (working with clients who have enduring mental health problems) were reviewed critically. The studies indicated clear benefits for the nurses and their clients, though a number of ways to improve this kind of research were identified (e.g. more rigorous research designs and the measurement of the clinical significance of the results). There is also a marked need to improve the transfer and maintenance of training.

KEY POINTS (*contd*)

- Six tasks face the evaluator:
  - identify the service goals
  - analyse what the service does
  - describe and standardise the service
  - measure the amount of change that occurs
  - determine whether any change is due to the service
  - assess the relative effectiveness of modified services.

- A 'good' evaluation (of training or any other topic) includes a clear basis in relevant theory, appropriate objectives or hypotheses, a rigorous research design, varied treatments and multiple measures of outcome.

Evaluation has played a decisive part in the development of mental health nursing. Tracing its role from the pioneering work of Florence Nightingale, this chapter highlights a number of different forms of evaluation activity that have been dominant at different times through history. It follows these streams of activity to the current research and development initiative in the NHS, clarifying the different purposes that the different forms of evaluative research can serve and the tasks that need to be tackled.

HISTORIC BACKGROUND

Evaluation has presumably always attended human affairs, given that human beings are prone to judging the worth of things. Certainly, nursing has a long history of pursuing evaluation, most dramatically illustrated by the impressive way in which Florence Nightingale exposed the low standards of medical care in the army during the Crimean War. During this period and subsequently, she also developed a system of hospital statistics which anticipated performance indicators and the quality assurance approach.

Evaluation within the modern health services can be traced back to the 19th century, beginning with the collection and analysis of population data. Problem areas such as early childhood mortality placed great pressure on governments to assess the nature and extent of problems, so that appropriate therapies could be introduced (Holland 1983). At that time, however, the methods of evaluating nursing and other practices were still at an early stage of development, so that the data were unreliable and there was a high probability that false conclusions would be drawn about the success or otherwise of the various governmental interventions. A classic example is that mortality and other indications of the health of a population turned out, on later and more systematic evaluation, to be due to improvements in environmental factors alone (McKeown & Lowe 1966).

Latterly, a number of increasingly well-defined and developed systems of evaluation have come into operation, including action research, quality assurance, audit, organisational development, research and development, operational research and total quality management. These terms have been summarised by Parry (1992) and overlap in some important respects with service evaluation and basic or 'laboratory' research. For example, certain forms of service evaluation share with basic research a commitment to the publication of findings, and a value base concerning the importance of rigour and various aspects of methodology, such as the importance of objective measurement instruments. By contrast, they do not share a common purpose, in that basic research is intended to generate new knowledge, while service evaluation is intended to improve decisions about resources and services (Milne 1987). More recently, Russell & Wilson (1992)

Table 8.1   Relationships between the three research activities recognised in the research and development initiative (Russell & Wilson 1992)

	Explanatory research (also referred to as 'pure' and 'biomedical science' or *'efficacy'* research)	Pragmatic research (also referred to as 'technology'; ' applied clinical science'; *'effectiveness'* and 'development' research)	Audit (assessing the *'effects'*)
1. Purpose	To generate knowledge (e.g. the pharmacology of a drug)	To improve decisions about resource allocation (e.g. which drug to use)	To improve quality of care (e.g. adherence to standards as specified in clinical guidelines)
2. Method	RCTs ('explanatory trials')	Reproduce/simulate clinical conditions ('pragmatic trials')	Audit cycle (set standards, compare with performances, introduce changes)
3. Features	• Rigid control of the independent variable (IV) • Participants' eligibility/entry defined in advance • Statistical testing of hypotheses	• Flexible definition of IV (adapt to patients) • Eligibility based on judgment by clinician • Use statistical estimation (e.g. confidence intervals)	• Local interpretation of IV (the standard) • All patients seen are included • Statistics and hypotheses not common – graphs of descriptive statistics the norm
4. Example	Beta-blockers protect against myocardial ischaemia	Effects translate into substantial clinical benefit	Standard that 90% of patients receive appropriate medication and the results fed back to clinicians

have addressed themselves to this, at times, confusing overlap between the different research paradigms, distinguishing helpfully between what they term 'explanatory' research, 'pragmatic' research and 'audit'. Table 8.1 summarises the relationship between these three different kinds of research activity.

Evaluation in mental health nursing is therefore likely to be a blend of pragmatic research and audit, both being based on the traditional methods of service evaluation, although the boundaries are by no means clear cut. In essence, explanatory research is about establishing how things work under ideal conditions, whereas pragmatic research is about the extent to which such findings transfer successfully to service settings. These issues are traditionally regarded as related to internal and external validity, respectively, and are discussed in some depth later when the concepts are applied to a sample of illustrative studies of nurse training. Another useful concept to bear in mind when considering

the nature of different forms of evaluation or research is the issue of implementation; that is, the conditions under which new approaches for which there is evidence of effectiveness from either explanatory or pragmatic research (preferably both) are introduced in routine practice (Russell & Wilson 1992). This final implementation stage recognises an organisational or 'change management' aspect to research within the new NHS. This forms an integrated programme, designed to improve patient care so as to:

> secure a knowledge based health service in which clinical, managerial and policy decisions are based on sound and pertinent information about research findings and scientific development. This provides the basis for maximising the effectiveness, efficiency and appropriateness of patient services.
>
> Department of Health 1994:1

EVIDENCE-BASED PRACTICE

It has been argued that the NHS encompasses a

vast range of professional practices, some of which are 'indefensible' and others which are provided with an 'unacceptable variation in the quality of treatment delivered by different clinical teams' (Peckham 1991:367). To counter this diversity, a research and development programme has been implemented, designed to provide the new knowledge needed to improve the performance of professionals, and so contribute to 'evidence-based practice' (EBP). This is defined as the conscientious, explicit and judicious use of current best evidence in making decisions about the care of individual clients (Sackett et al 1996). Furthermore, the 'best evidence' is to be critically evaluated as part of the research and development programme, leading to practical clinical guidelines. As a result, it is anticipated that the procedures that professionals use will become more effective, acceptable and efficient.

In addition to supplying professionals with the best available evidence to guide their practice, the NHS intends to use audit to determine whether or not the desired changes take place, and to support service commissioners in implementing the evidence (e.g. in incorporating EBP guidelines into service contracts). It is recognised that other strategies, including training interventions (Grimshaw & Russell 1994), will be necessary to effect such a major change in the behaviour of mental health professionals.

WHY FOCUS ON TRAINING?

The broad purpose of the NHS is to improve the health of the population. More specific priorities have been identified in the Health of the Nation White Paper (Department of Health 1992), including community care of the severely mentally ill, mental health of the NHS taskforce, devising ways to assess the mental health needs of a population and training packages for use in primary care and community settings. From these priorities a larger number of topics have been identified for research funding by the NHS. Since in this chapter I propose to focus on just one of these priorities – the training packages – I now provide some examples of specific topics to be funded in this area (Department of Health 1995). As I also wish to restrict our focus to mental health nursing, some of the relevant examples include:

- training professionals to improve recognition of depression (including applying screening techniques)
- establishing the relative efficacy of psychological treatments, such as cognitive therapy in the treatment of anxiety
- evaluating the effectiveness of staff training for residential care of the elderly
- comparing the different educational strategies on staff knowledge, staff practice and effect on morale and staff turnover
- assessing the impact of training community psychiatric nurses (CPNs) to deliver psychosocial interventions with the severely mentally ill (especially short training courses).

In summary, the current government policy is to prioritise some key areas of mental health nursing practice, and a major way to develop such practice is through training. The NHS's research and development programme is designed to ensure that this policy directs research activity, leading in turn to clear recommendations for practice (Peckham 1991).

HOW SHOULD WE ANALYSE TRAINING?

Training is therefore one of a range of interventions designed to foster EBP. It is also clear that training itself should be studied carefully, so as to establish its effectiveness and efficiency. But how should such studies be conducted? Once again, there is central guidance available, in this instance on the research aspects in most need of attention (Department of Health 1996). Table 8.2 provides a summary of some of these issues.

Table 8.2 Better research practice, as anticipated in the research and development programme (Department of Health 1996)

Research aspect	Proposed improvements
1. Skill-sharing	Can generic mental health staff with a specific training provide brief therapies? How does effective supervision work?
2. Internal validity	Urgent need for controlled research into analytic and eclectic psychotherapies (e.g.measures of change mechanism); what are the critical process factors predicting benefit in any therapy? Careful selection of dependent variables
3. Clinical significance	Supplement statistical significance with measures of the practical importance of outcomes (e.g. reduced GP attendance/improved functioning)
4. External validity	Discover extent to which approaches supported by research evidence, i.e. with evidence of 'efficacy' (e.g. CBT) are'effective' (e.g. apply to clients with a dual diagnosis, ERMI). Longer term outcomes
5. Efficiency	To what extent can such approaches be delivered effectively in a brief form? What are the relative costs and benefits?

CBT, cognitive–behaviour therapy; ERMI, enduring and recurrent mental illness

These aspects will form the basis of the remainder of this chapter, in that I will analyse a small sample of the training literature in mental health nursing using the Table 8.2 dimensions. This is intended to illustrate the methods that can be employed to evaluate mental health interventions. While the training literature will provide the bulk of my examples, I will also introduce illustrations from other interventions with other professional groups, to fill out the range of applicable evaluation methods. As a result, I aim to produce an evidence-based summary of effective training approaches, together with guidance on evaluating mental health nursing more generally.

ISSUES IN TRAINING

Is it effective?

Before summarising the specific studies concerned with staff training, let me attempt to provide a summary of the main skill-sharing issues. One of these concerns the wider question facing all professional groups, namely whether training for mental health staff is effective. I then proceed to the question of the specific conditions under which training can be effective, focusing in particular on what makes supervision effective.

In a classic review, Ford (1979) evaluated studies on professional training conducted between 1960 and 1978. He highlighted the lack of sophistication in the field of professional training, including the tendency for studies to focus on teaching just one or more discrete skills in the context of very brief or poorly described interventions. Additional methodological problems included the use of unvalidated measures of training and the use of undergraduate students as 'trainees', as opposed to trainee mental health practitioners. As a result, he concluded that there was:

> no evidence that any one training intervention is capable of instilling sufficient cognitive, interpersonal, or technical therapist skills in trainees to guarantee that the trainees are (or can be) effective therapists.
>
> Ford 1979:112

This was a surprising summary of the training literature, partly because of the enormous time and resource poured into the preparation of professionals like mental health nurses, and partly because it seems self-evident that such industry must pay dividends. However, a subsequent review by Alberts & Edelstein (1990), which evaluated those therapist-training studies published subsequent to Ford's 1979 review, indicated that while some better quality studies had been conducted, in general researchers needed to aspire to higher standards of basic research design and measurement if we were to advance our understanding of how training works. These reviews therefore raise some fundamental evaluation questions, to which I will return.

Let us now consider an example of the kind of study reviewed by Ford (1979) and Alberts & Edelstein (1990) so as to try to explain the rather damning conclusions that they reached. Carkhuff et al (1968) conducted one of the reviewed studies on the effects of training. Counsellors were trained in the use of empathy, positive regard, genuineness, concreteness and self-disclosure (the 'core conditions'). Tape recordings were then made of 54 interviews conducted by clinical and non-clinical trainees (the 'trainees' were actually first-year clinical psychology graduate students), each of whom was instructed to be 'as helpful as you would ordinarily be if a client came to you seeking help'. They were instructed to explore problems with clients. These 'clients' were also trainees, drawn from another clinical psychology programme. They were instructed to present problems that were 'presently very real'.

The 45-minute interviews were taped and rated by three experienced clinicians who applied a scale measuring the above 'core conditions' of counselling. Each of these conditions, such as empathic understanding, was rated from level one (in which the expressions of the counsellor either do not attend to or detract significantly from expressions of the client) to level 5 (in which the counsellor's responses add

significantly to the feeling and meaning of the client's expression). Similar ratings were made for the other core conditions and indicated that overall there was a non-significant *decline* in the rated levels of empathy, regard, genuineness, concreteness and self-disclosure when tapes from the beginning and advanced stages of training were compared (i.e. a comparison between first and final year trainees was made). By contrast, Carkhuff et al (1968) found that a group of eight trainees who came from a completely separate and non-clinical programme, and who were exposed to proper training in providing these counselling conditions, were able to communicate and discriminate them at significantly better levels than the professional clinical trainees.

In discussing their findings, Carkhuff et al (1968) concluded that, overall, the results failed to establish the effectiveness of professional training. At best, the results indicated to them that there was no improvement on the key dimensions that were assessed; at worst, they perceived trends which suggested that there were actual deteriorations in the level of counselling provided by the trainees. The only clear and consistent benefit that seemed to follow from professional training was that the more senior trainees became better able to rate the core conditions of counselling, an unsatisfactory and somewhat secondary outcome for a programme of intensive training.

A parallel line of research on the effectiveness of training has contrasted studies focusing on professional and non-professional helpers. For example, Hattie et al (1984) reviewed earlier studies which had concluded that the clinical outcomes achieved by non-professionals were equal to or even significantly better than those obtained by professionals. While the studies using these findings had numerous methodological deficiencies and limitations (as per Carkhuff et al 1968, above), there was nonetheless a sense of disbelief in the training community. This led Hattie et al (1984) to re-examine the earlier review work (e.g. Durlak 1979). A key part of Durlak's analysis was the definition of 'professional' and 'non-professional': professionals were defined as those who had received formal clinical training through a professional programme of psychology, psychiatry, social work or psychiatric nursing. By exclusion, those who had not received such training were deemed to be non-professionals. It follows that the study discussed in some detail above (Carkhuff et al 1968) would be classed as a study of non-professional training, in contrast to its title. However, despite adopting a more graduated approach in which different levels of training were separated out, Hattie et al (1984) still concluded in accord with Durlak that:

> clients who seek help from non-professionals are more likely to achieve resolution of their problem than those who consult professionals.

Hattie et al 1984:534

These results, while alarming to the professional communities and to those who run training programmes, did however provide fuel for those who were keen to extend skill-sharing to non-professionals. A range of methods were used to teach non-professionals to use psychological techniques, and the effects that this had upon clients were reviewed in optimistic terms by the end of the 1980s (Harchik et al 1989).

More recent analyses of the effectiveness of professionals and non-professionals have continued to find in favour of the non-professionals. This is despite taking account of numerous methodological weaknesses in the comparative studies that had been analysed, which had been thought to produce systematic biases against the professionals. To illustrate, Faust & Zlotnick (1995) examined the major criticisms within a very careful re-analysis of the research literature,

focusing on such methodological problems as lack of proper controls and insensitive measures of outcome. But they found that there is still no evidence from the available literature to favour professionals over non-professionals. This conclusion does not, therefore, seem to be attributable to the methodological rigour in the studies, since the outcomes did not show any systematic relation to the soundness or weakness of the particular research study. Faust & Zlotnick's conclusion was that formal training in general does not predict successful therapy practice.

Countering this sobering trend in the evaluations of the effectiveness of professional training, the special series in the *Journal of Consulting and Clinical Psychology* (Volume 63 1995) explored the research evidence for the value of professional training in its own right. These articles suggested that professional training does indeed enhance clinical effectiveness, especially if the type of training, the setting in which the practice is conducted and the nature of the clients' problems are considered (Beutler & Kendall 1995). The reason for this more upbeat interpretation of the effectiveness of professional training is due to recognising and taking into account many of the inherent methodological problems touched on above (e.g. defining students as professionals).

Beutler & Kendall (1995) point out that many studies of professional training have oversimplified the issues, failing either to attend to differences in levels of experience and training required to use various specific skills, or omitting to address the distinctive effects that might accrue for each intervention with different types of problems, disorders and client groups. On the assumption that a failure to take due account of these more complex considerations may have led previous researchers (such as Faust & Zlotnick) to reach factually inaccurate conclusions, Beutler & Kendall highlighted the fact that most prior studies have used naturalistic research designs in which various undescribed 'therapies' are pooled together in some single category. In these studies, the nature of the therapies is given little attention and the characteristics of the client group are not analysed. They suggest that the results of studies with these flaws may tell us little or nothing about the effectiveness of professional training in relation to procedures that are specific to a particular problem or client group. A second problem they highlight is that expertise is defined in terms of experience. As they point out, experience in professional practice is not necessarily related to competence. Therefore, Beutler & Kendall (1995) concluded that professional training may well enhance clinical effectiveness, but that there was still insufficient knowledge of what specific aspects of professional training best contributed to clinical outcome. They suggested that amongst the many areas where research is needed, training should in particular focus on:

• identifying specific areas of clinical practice
• pinpointing the specific skills that are associated with benefits in that particular practice
• validating methods for identifying levels of therapist proficiency.

These points will be discussed in more detail below, when I focus on the literature review of training mental health nurses in the use of evidence-based ways of working with clients who have a severe mental illness.

How does effective supervision work?

To return to Table 8.2, the above review therefore suggests that training for mental health staff in psychological therapies can be effective, although conflicting evidence abounds. A subsequent question concerns the value of supervision, following initial training for mental health

nurses. How does effective supervision work and what contribution does it make to the provision of evidence-based care? Broadly speaking, the definition of supervision is that it is an ongoing educational process in which one person in the role of supervisor helps another, in the role of supervisee, acquire appropriate professional behaviour, through the examination of the supervisee's professional activities (Hart 1982). Numerous models exist to suggest how supervision should be provided, but for convenience these can be divided into three models, as summarised in Box 8.1.

Box 8.1 Three fundamental approaches to supervision (Hart 1982)

1. Apprentice–Master (didactic)
Supervisor believes that theory, techniques and professional practice must be conveyed to trainee, hence uses teaching skills

2. Therapist–Client (experiential)
Supervisor believes that insight into own attitudes and feelings should be fostered in trainee, hence uses therapy skills

3. Colleague (integration)
Supervisor believes that trainees' skills and self-awareness are adequate, so focuses on facilitation

---

As Box 8.1 suggests, the 'apprentice–master' model of supervision is most relevant for skill enhancement, whereas a 'therapist–client' model is relevant when the purpose of supervision is to facilitate attitudes or insight in the trainee. Finally, a 'colleague' model, which integrates to some extent the apprentice–master and therapist–client models, is typically more appropriate when the trainee is at a more senior level in general terms, or when the trainee has particular expertise in a specific area. Literature reviews covering the qualities of effective supervision suggest that there are similarly four main dimensions. The first consists of personal qualities such as empathy, flexibility, concern and a supportive, non-critical relationship to the trainee. Second, the ideal supervisor has certain professional qualities, such as an advanced knowledge base and an ability to be concrete in the presentation of material. Third, good supervisors also include appropriate use of teaching methods (e.g. goal-setting) and provide timely and appropriate feedback. Fourth, another distinctive quality of good supervision is a clear awareness of the boundaries that should exist around the material discussed in supervision. That is, the effective supervisor does not attempt to turn supervision into personal therapy (Carifio & Hess 1987).

A variant of these models is the so-called developmental model, which proposes that different methods of supervision are appropriate at different stages of training. For example, Slevin (1992), in discussing teaching and supervision in relation to Project 2000, distinguished between the 'mentoring' role (that was appropriate for a supervisor to adopt in relation to a new student) from later roles, such as 'preceptor', 'facilitator' and finally 'role model', towards the culmination of training. In this final developmental phase of supervision, the trainee is thought to pick out someone whom they respect, admire and who is available to help them.

Running through these different models of supervision is the theme that good supervisors apply what they know from therapy to the supervision process, without turning it into personal therapy. The following quote illustrates this:

> supervisors judged to be excellent, were empathic and focused upon the immediate concerns of the trainee. They had an experiential orientation and tailored their comments to the resident's concerns ... they frequently synthesised and reframed material for the resident (trainee) and made comments in depth. They were teachers who reflected with

trainees on their actions as therapists and supervisors.

> Shanfield et al 1992:355

While there is considerable consensus concerning what effective supervision entails, the scientific evaluation of supervision has produced discouraging results. In one review, the following rather depressing conclusion was stated:

> while there is an abundant literature consisting of theoretical, impressionistic, and anecdotal reports, scientific investigations of the procedures used by psychotherapy supervisors are practically non-existent ... studies that have attempted to assess the impact of supervision on trainee performance in actual therapy settings have had discouraging results.

> Binder 1993:304

In a discussion paper, Ellis et al (1996) systematically analysed the methodological status of research on supervision, so as to clarify where the literature is scientifically weak, as highlighted by Binder (1993). Box 8.2 summarises Ellis et al's (1996) account of the 'aggregate' study of supervision, noting a number of major research problems.

However, the relatively poor standing of research on supervision does not mean that we have no clear picture of how effective supervision works. It appears that it primarily functions by enhancing the knowledge base of the trainee, by sharpening role definitions, by raising proficiency in the use of complex therapy procedures and by increasing the trainees' ability to facilitate therapy (Holloway & Neufeldt 1995).

In contrast to these sweeping methodological reviews, more detailed accounts of effective methods of supervision are available in the literature. For example, in a book edited by Jacobs (1996) there are accounts of different approaches to supervision. In one of these, Fennell (who directs a part-time, post-qualification and multi-professional course in cognitive therapy in

Box 8.2 The 'aggregate study' of supervision as compiled by Ellis et al (1996) to highlight several strengths and several serious weaknesses

Introduction
- Multiple measures used
- A theoretical/exploratory investigation
- Vague or absent hypotheses
- Constructs under investigation not fully explicated

Method
- 'Field' context
- Measures include a host imported from other contexts (vast majority have poor psychometric status)
- Self-report method dominates
- Non-random allocation to treatments
- Independent variable (i.e. supervision) not manipulated
- Suitable sample size

Results
- Appropriate statistical procedures
- No correction for multiple tests
- Homogeneity assumption not tested
- Non-significant findings omitted

Discussion
- Couple of threats to external validity acknowledged
- 20 serious threats ignored
- Results considered credible and strongly supportive of the original purpose of the study

Oxford) describes how she would supervise one of the trainees, called Michael. Her account emphasises how in the cognitive model the supervisor looks for structure, clear goals and a pattern of systematic interventions. These are agreed between therapist and client and are designed not simply to clarify recurring patterns but also to work up a collaborative approach towards change. The change would be based on a mixture of cognitive–behavioural strategies, resulting in alterations to the way that the client perceives his or her world. As a consequence, Michael is able to modify his ways of coping both cognitively and behaviourally, so as to reduce distress. As well as providing a clear and detailed account of this form of effective supervision (one that embodies many of the principles already outlined), Fennell's account is also evidence-

based; that is, she makes extensive use of cognitive therapy methods, with their solid research base, in pursuit of effective supervision.

EVALUATION OF TRAINING IN MENTAL HEALTH NURSING – AN ILLUSTRATIVE LITERATURE REVIEW

The criteria for better research practice, as summarised in Table 8.2 above, are now applied to a small sample of empirical studies of nurse training in relation to severe mental illness. This is not a systematic review, but is rather intended to illustrate how evaluations in the staff training facet of mental health nursing have been conducted. The studies included are all concerned with services to people with enduring or recurrent mental illness, whether in receipt of in-patient or out-patient care. In addition, studies are included where nurses are the recipients of the training intervention, and where the studies are empirical evaluations of the training effort. As the literature review is not systematic (e.g. it is not based on all papers meeting the above criteria), no definitive conclusions are drawn. Rather, this review will provide an outline of the important criteria in evaluating practice, together with a profile of the current status of this form of nurse training. In the concluding part of the chapter, a parallel profile for future evaluations will be provided. The difference between these 'real' and 'ideal' profiles can serve to highlight the kind of evaluations that are required in the future, if mental health nursing is indeed to be developed through educational and training efforts.

Internal validity

Good research, including evaluation research, must be valid if the findings are to be treated with any confidence. A number of different forms of scientific validity have been distinguished, including 'internal', 'external', 'statistical conclusions' and 'construct' validity (Campbell & Stanley 1963). Of these different forms of validity, the two most fundamental ones are the first two and these will therefore be discussed in this section. *Internal validity* refers to the degree to which we can infer causality from a study. It deals with whether we can say with confidence that the treatment (or 'independent variable') is indeed responsible for producing observed changes (the 'dependent variable'). *External validity* refers to the extent to which the results from a study can be generalised across time, settings, behaviours or persons. It fundamentally concerns whether or not an intervention is realistic and likely to prove effective under routine service conditions. We will return to the topic of external validity later.

One of the core dilemmas in conducting evaluative research is that there is often a trade-off to be calculated between internal and external validity. That is, while it is possible to achieve high internal validity in a very controlled situation, such as a laboratory or a research centre, the findings from such tightly controlled situations are unlikely to transfer to a 'real world' context, such as the NHS. Classical examples of this problem were some of the early analogue studies of treatments such as behaviour therapy, which were conducted under artificial conditions with volunteer clients. By comparison, so-called 'field research' is conducted in natural settings with clinical populations, which gives studies high external validity, but at a great cost in terms of low internal validity (i.e. experimental control is much more difficult to obtain in the field settings: e.g. see Barker et al 1994).

The work of Campbell & Stanley (1963) provided an indispensable guide to the different kinds of research design that can be used within evaluations of mental health nursing, together with a systematic breakdown of their strengths and weaknesses. In essence, some simple designs such as a one group, pre-test/post-test design (in which an assessment is made before and after a treatment of a single group) are uninterpretable. This is because a number of threats to the internal validity of the study are not capable of being checked or controlled, such as historical events, the reactivity of the group to the act of measurement, or 'third variables' which confound the results. For this reason we need stronger internal validity (i.e. evaluation designs which build in some level of control over these threats) in order to permit the confident interpretation of the findings of a study.

To return to the example above, were we to add a second group assessed at the same point in time, but not receiving the treatment (i.e. a control group) we would be able to assess the extent to which some of those threats were present and so reach a firmer conclusion about the impact of a treatment. Better still, we could randomly allocate participants to the two groups, which would rule out selection biases and allow the use of statistical theories. The same threats to internal validity apply to other kinds of research designs (i.e. correlational, descriptive or single subject designs), so they should always be taken into account. While the 'perfect study' is impossible, nurses can still adopt approaches that contribute to solid and useful research (Milne 1987).

In addition to these general considerations about validity, the recent advice from the Department of Health on the needs for better research practice (see Table 8.2) emphasised that we also need to measure the intervention. This refers to actually describing, observing and recording the given treatment, as opposed to assuming (e.g. from the qualifications of the therapist) that a given treatment is being introduced as claimed. Another term for this assessment of the independent variable is a 'manipulation check', a good example of which was provided in the Sheffield psychotherapy project (Shapiro & Firth 1987). In that project, instead of assuming that therapists were providing either the exploratory or prescriptive therapy that was pre-scribed within the research design, the researchers directly observed and recorded the two forms of therapy, using the Helper Behaviour Rating Scale (HBRS, Hardy & Shapiro 1985). The HBRS assesses 12 different categories of therapists' speech, such as interpretation, exploration and reassurance. Some of these are expected to be much higher in the exploratory therapy (i.e. interpretation and exploration) whereas others should be much higher if a thera-pist is indeed conforming to the prescriptive mode of therapy (e.g. asking more questions and providing advice on how to cope with things out of session). As predicted, the Sheffield psy-chotherapy project did indeed demonstrate that therapists were implementing the two approaches as outlined in a manual, and so were adhering to the treatment that was believed to be responsible for beneficial therapy outcomes. This also pro-vides the basis for clarifying those factors within the therapy process that lead to benefits (mecha-nisms of change).

Internal validity in a sample of the nurse training literature

Next I consider how a sample of literature on mental health nurse training compares to these standards for internal validity. The five studies selected to illustrate these evaluation features are Milne (1984a), Rogers et al (1986), Brooker et al (1992), Brooker et al (1994) and Corrigan et al (1995). All of these studies met the above inclu-sion criteria (i.e. they were empirical evaluations of the training of mental health nurses in relation to enduring and recurrent mental illness). My own study (Milne 1984a) analysed why nurses

had only implemented training that they had received in behaviour therapy to a very small extent within the ward environment. The design was a simple comparison between an experimen-tal group that had received the 1-week 'core course' of ward-based behavioural therapy train-ing (n = 24), as opposed to a group of their prede-cessors (n = 41), who had received a standard, classroom-based training package.

Those 24 nurses attending the new, ward-based course were found to achieve much better results in terms of significantly higher levels of implementation of the behavioural methods with their patients following training. An earlier part of the study had included a classical comparison between an experimental and a control group (although these participants were not randomly assigned to the respective groups: Milne 1984b). The subsequent study was based on a 'waiting list control group', in which the 24 nurses who received the revised course were in effect a wait-ing list group, while the earlier sample of 41 mental health nurses received the initial class-room-based training programme. This is a rela-tively weak design, although the results can be interpreted with some confidence.

By comparison, the study by Rogers et al (1986) was a simple 'before and after' evaluation in which the impact of training staff from nine mental health agencies in recent technologies of psychiatric rehabilitation was assessed. The innovative part of this study was that the trainers themselves received intensive follow-up support to assist them in implementing the new pro-grammes in their own agencies, so the evaluation was in effect a study of the impact of training nurses to acquire and apply skills in psychiatric rehabilitation. Only two of the instruments used to assess the effectiveness of the training were administered before and after the training, which makes the design a very limited before and after study. Thus, although a number of very positive changes were obtained on the measures, in essence the results cannot be interpreted with any confidence. The internal validity of the study is quite weak in that a number of threats to valid conclusions about the effectiveness of training cannot be ruled out (such as a 'Hawthorne effect' in which the novelty of the study may have led to changes in staff behaviour which were not in fact due to the training intervention).

Brooker et al (1992) trained CPNs to deliver a psychosocial intervention to clients with a diagnosis of schizophrenia who were living at home with their relatives. Like the Milne (1984a) study, Brooker et al used a design in which some of the families were allocated to a control group, while others were placed in the experimental group. Assessments of seven different measures of change were then administered before and after the psychosocial intervention, and there was also a 12-month, follow-up assessment. This range of assessments (and, in particular, the use of a follow-up) makes this study an exceptionally sound evaluation, at least in relation to the literature on the training of mental health nurses. Owing to the fact that the design excluded a number of threats to the internal validity of a study, Brooker et al were able to conclude with some confidence that the favourable outcomes observed for the experimental group (such as improvements in their symptoms, functioning and social adjustment) were indeed due to the intervention, and not to other possible explanations (such as a Hawthorne effect, or simply the passage of time).

In a second, related study, Brooker et al (1994) carried out an analysis in which the same psychosocial intervention for families caring for a relative with schizophrenia was conducted by means of a within-subjects design. This entailed the CPNs acting as their own control groups, one sample forming an initial, waiting list, control group and the second a delayed intervention group. This design therefore took into account

the threats mentioned immediately above (i.e. Hawthorne effect and history) and provided a more valid research design than the earlier study (Brooker et al 1992).

In the final example, Corrigan et al (1995) studied the effectiveness of what they termed 'interactive staff training', being a blend of sound training methods with the principles of organisational psychology. This package was therefore expected to result in higher levels of implementation. Three conditions were analysed within the research design, a no-training baseline, a planning phase and a full, interactive, staff training programme, all within a multiple baseline design. The measures taken included staff participation in a token economy programme and their involvement in a social skills training programme. These indicated a dramatic increase in staff participation only following the full interactive staff training phase. That is, very low frequencies of participation were observed in both the baseline and the preparation phases. This is also quite a strong research design, in that, as per the Brooker et al (1994) study, it allows the authors to exclude various threats to internal validity. They were therefore able to report with considerable confidence that the interactive staff training led to significantly increased staff and patient participation in rehabilitation programmes, as well as decreasing rates of physical restraint and aggression.

These five illustrative studies of staff training provide a fairly representative picture of the range and rigour of designs used in evaluation research more generally. They go from the uninterpretable (Rogers et al 1986) to the fairly rigorous (e.g. Brooker et al 1992) but all provided helpful information to fieldworkers on how best to develop their services. They therefore provide a good set of designs for evaluating mental health practice in the future. More rigorous designs are obviously desirable, but are probably only feasible with the help of seasoned academic researchers. Details of what such more rigorous designs would look like can be found in Barker et al (1994) or, for those who prefer a gentle introduction, in Milne (1993).

Dependent variables

Internal validity depends on the selection of appropriate instruments to measure the effects of an intervention, just as much as it depends on a rigorous research design. The studies reviewed above provide some good examples of carefully selected dependent variables, as in recognising that instruments should reflect different perspectives (such as those of the nurse and of the carer), different symptom domains (such as thoughts, feelings and behaviours) and different domains of functioning (such as social and interpersonal relations: Roth & Fonagy 1996). Within each of these dimensions, 'good' dependent variables have the following characteristics:

- they are valid and reliable for the characteristic that is expected to change
- they are sensitive to change on the characteristics measured
- they provide a defined unit of measurement (unlike a coarse or categorical measure)
- they do not suffer from floor or ceiling effects in the range of expected responses
- the measures are administered in a consistent way
- the measurement is timed to coincide with peak response to treatment
- measurement is made of the more proximal effects, as well as the distal ones (e.g. symptoms and family functioning).

In providing this list, Lipsey (1990) also wrote a marvellous introduction to some of the key issues in designing good quality research, which is recommended.

Clinical significance

It has often been lamented that research has insufficient impact on clinical practice. One of the possible explanations for this is the fact that research is primarily concerned with reporting statistical significance. Such accounts are based on average improvement scores for all clients, and so provide no information on the effects of a treatment for specific individuals. This significance may also bear little or no relation to the clinical relevance of the change, and hence clinicians lose interest in the research. One solution to this impasse is to encourage researchers to report both statistical and clinical significance. The latter has been defined in a number of different ways, but is essentially concerned with some assessment of change expressed in terms of its practical importance. Examples include the proportion of clients improving, a change which is large in magnitude, an improvement in the client's everyday functioning, a change which is recognisable to peers and significant others, eliminating the presenting problem, and attaining a level of functioning which is no longer distinguishable from the client's non-deviant peers (Jacobson et al 1984). In essence, these authors defined clinical significance as a change that moves the client from the dysfunctional to the functional range during the course of therapy, on whatever variable is being used to measure the clinical problem. In a later paper, Jacobson & Truax (1991) provided examples of how clinical significance could be applied to clients.

The concept of clinical significance can also be applied to the training of mental health nurses, either in the obvious sense that one applies it to their clients and asks about the benefits of training for them in terms of clinical significance; or by applying similar rules to the benefits gained by nurses themselves as a result of the training that they have received. I next examine our five illustrative studies to see how they have assessed clinical significance in either or both of these respects. Table 8.3 summarises this mini-review, indicating that all five studies included at least one measure of clinical significance. Equally heartening were the range of variables assessed, including clinically significant changes in nurses and clients, as well as a range of ways of assessing the practical importance of the training effort.

Table 8.3 Examples of 'clinical significance' measures in the illustrative sample of nurse training studies

Clinical significance variable	Study
Proportion of nurses applying the training to their clients	Milne (1984b)
'Social validity' (i.e. perceptions of the practical value of the training)	Milne (1984b)
Client benefits large in magnitude	Milne (1984b)
Nurses using skills in psychiatric rehabilitation much more following training	Rogers et al (1986)
Clients' medication usage decreased	Brooker et al (1992)
No group difference between clients on hospital admissions	Brooker et al (1992)
Relatives' satisfaction with client functioning higher for those receiving psychosocial intervention	Brooker et al (1992)
Length of hospital stay longer for control group	Brooker et al (1994)
Clients' social functioning/adjustment higher for psychosocial intervention group	Brooker et al (1994)
Use of client restraints was reduced by 41% following staff training	Corrigan et al (1995)
Aggressive incidents also decreased (by 13%) following this training	Corrigan et al (1995)

External validity

External validity (sometimes called ecological validity) refers to the extent to which the results of a study can be generalised beyond the study context (e.g. over time or to different settings, as in transferring findings from a special research centre to an NHS clinic). In the language of the new research and development initiative in the NHS, the question is whether those treatments with evidence of 'efficacy' have also got 'effectiveness' (Peckham 1991). This is a topic that has attracted considerable interest in relation to mental health nursing for severe mental illness. For instance, Hughes et al (1996) provided an account of family-based intervention approaches in schizophrenia within a routine clinical service over the past 10 years in South Glamorgan. They reported that although the service developed out of the early published, family intervention studies to carers of schizophrenia sufferers, the focus of the service changed over the years, partly in response to clinical need, but also as a result of the clinical experience developed by the team. That is, the service broadened its scope to include all sufferers of severe mental illness, and they have also found that education alone is of limited value, by contrast with the emphasis they now place on the role of the family in promoting the active rehabilitation of the sufferer.

The Hughes et al (1996) account indicates the modest external validity of the original, family-based intervention package, and other related studies indicate why this might be the case. Corrigan et al (1994), for example, emphasised that for treatments to be transferred, it is important to ensure that staff are adequately surveyed regarding their perception of the needs for training. For example, McDonald (1991) identified three additional factors to take into account if one is to be successful in transferring training (i.e. administrative support, external agency support and incentives). Even allowing for these considerations, Corrigan & McCracken (1995) argue that is inappropriate to attempt a faithful, external validation of a treatment technology. Rather, they suggest formation of a programme committee to address some of the factors identified by McDonald (1991), amongst other efforts made by a staff group to determine which elements of a treatment should be transferred to a local mental health service. Unless such sensitive and organisationally based approaches are introduced, it is likely that external validity will be low. To illustrate, Kavanagh et al (1993) found that although a research team invested considerable effort in training mental health workers in a cognitive–behavioural approach to family intervention, few of the trainees actually engaged families for any length of time. Discussing this saddening finding, Birchwood & Tarrier (1994) suggest that one of the reasons for the poor finding (by comparison with the relative success of the Brooker et al studies) was that there was no continuity in clinical supervision for the trainees.

Having outlined some general examples of external validity problems and solutions, I now assess how the five illustrative studies tackled the external validity issue. Milne (1984a) addressed external validity by including a 9-month, follow-up assessment of the learning achieved during the initial phase of training. Additionally, ecological analysis of change following the training was carried out across people (i.e. influence of the trained staff on student nurses), across behaviours (i.e. from behaviours targeted in training to untargeted behaviours), and across settings (i.e. written care plans in either the training environment or the ward environment) and indicated some significant signs of external validity (Milne 1986b). In addition, the course of training that was developed was set out in a manual and disseminated to other interested hospitals, leading to its being implemented in six other settings by a mixture of course leaders, including nurses and a psychiatrist. The results of these 'replications' of the course were very similar to those obtained originally, indicating that it had high external validity (Burdett & Milne 1985).

In the Rogers et al study (1986), the transfer of training was a prime focus, so extensive follow-up support was organised in a systematic way to ensure that the new technology was implemented. They also went out of their way to ensure that the technology itself was highly acceptable (characterised as credible, relevant, giving relative advantage, being easy to understand and install, and compatible with the existing practice). The effectiveness of this package of strategies was indicated by improved nursing practice (e.g. skills in reaching a rehabilitation diagnosis, planning an intervention and implementing it) over periods of up to 2 years following training. Long follow-ups were also reported in the two Brooker et al studies (i.e. up to 12 months' post-training). In summary, the external validity of the illustrative sample of nurse training studies is quite impressive and varied.

Efficiency

In any service where there are limited resources, a pressing issue is whether either more can be achieved with the same resources or the same can be achieved with fewer resources. In terms of staff training work, this would include demonstrating that shorter courses of training yield results comparable to those obtained following longer courses, measured in terms of relative costs and benefits. Although this has much appeal, there appear to be very few analyses in which short versions of training are contrasted with longer programmes. As already outlined, in my own research (Milne 1984a, 1986b) a comparison was made between a classroom-based course and a patient-centred one, located partly in the classroom and partly in the nurses' ward. Although the total duration of the course remained constant at 5 days, the number of learning steps in the respective courses reduced from 16 to 12. This allowed nurses to spend more time attempting to practise material from the course in their own routine work environment. The question was whether this change, intended to increase the external validity of the training, would actually result in significantly less favourable learning in relation to the measures of the nurses' thoughts, feelings and behaviours, as administered before and after the training. However, comparisons between the two forms of training indicated that the new 'patient-centred' approach yielded equally good results by the end of training, in terms of nurses' learning. Indeed, it was actually superior in terms of both the nurses' rating of the value of the course and in terms of the number of care plans conducted following training (75%, as compared to 26% in the case of the classroom-based course). In summary, the patient-centred approach could be judged to be more efficient, in that for the same 5-day input greater benefits were derived for both the mental health nurses and their clients.

While there may have been few such comparative studies in the past, it is highly likely that these will increase in the future, given that the research and development initiative in the NHS has targeted efficient training as one of its priority areas.

APPLICATION – CONDUCTING EVALUATIONS

In the preceding section, several examples were given of the key tasks in conducting an evaluation in mental health nursing, in relation to training. For instance, it is necessary to have a clearly defined intervention (the independent variable) and to measure the effectiveness of introducing such an intervention on a number of appropriately selected measures of outcome (the dependent variables). In this section, I add a summary of the fundamental tasks that need to

be undertaken in carrying out an evaluation, fleshing these out with examples that complete a more rounded picture of the range of options than it was possible to provide from the small, illustrative sample of studies in the preceding section.

Task 1 Identifying service goals

The initial evaluation task is to specify objectives for a programme or nursing service in a sufficiently clear form for them to serve as a basis for evaluation. This is of paramount importance, since the definition of evaluation hinges on the extent to which treatment goals have been achieved (Milne 1987). In the parlance of audit, such objectives would be standards, which illustrate one overlap between service evaluation and audit. (By contrast, basic or explanatory research would have hypotheses rather than objectives or standards.)

One way to set goals is to consider the kind of improvements discussed in the previous section under clinical significance, such as an improvement in an individual client to such an extent that the client is able to function more independently. One may also set objectives or standards for a whole service, as is now common practice. A particularly helpful example in mental health nursing, from my experience, has been to use the Ward Atmosphere Scale (Moos 1974). The scale can provide a general orientation to the way that nurses and clients perceive a service, resulting in a profile of the 'real' ward atmosphere. Completion of the 'ideal' sister form of the scale then provides a second profile which is usually higher than the real one. The ideal profile can then serve as the goals for a service, such as improving programme clarity. The use of the scale in this way, allied to some changes that nurses decide to introduce in order to reduce the real–ideal discrepancy, has been shown to be helpful in improving nursing services and illustrates nicely the role that clear goal-setting and evaluation can play in improving mental health nursing practice (see Milne 1986a).

Task 2 Analysing service actions

Having defined goals or standards for a service, the next issue is to be clear about what the service has to do in attempting to achieve the goals. The classic illustration in mental health services concerns being clear about which therapeutic orientation or nursing model should be implemented. In addition to such questions about how a task might be tackled, there is also the issue of what a service should be addressing. In this latter instance the task is to conduct assessments of client need, according to the prevailing model, so that the service actions can be specified clearly. In addition to structured interviews, need can also be defined helpfully through the use of published questionnaires or observational systems, or through ratings made by clients or significant others. To encourage use of such instruments, some publishers have started to produce portfolios of assessment instruments, which provide photocopiable versions of the scales with clear instructions for the scoring and interpretation of the results (e.g. see Milne 1992).

Task 3 Describing and standardising nursing services

Given some statement of clients' need and an approach to be followed, the next task is to be consistent in providing the service that is to meet these needs. Once again, audit provides a helpful example of this aspect of evaluation, in that a number of service standards would normally be specified and help to govern the way in which a service is provided. A more challenging issue for the evaluator is to try to define and standardise

individual therapy, in that it is quite apparent that even though we may use terms that indicate some kind of shared activity (such as 'reality orientation' or 'cognitive therapy') the evidence suggests that what we each do under these headings is much more variable. For this reason, a good evaluation would include such features as a manual, detailing precisely what is to be done in the name of such interventions, and then would observe carefully whether or not the therapist adhered to the manual. As mentioned earlier, the Sheffield psychotherapy project (Shapiro et al 1990) is a good example of carrying out this kind of task.

Task 4 Measuring the amount of change that occurs

Having clarified what is to be done and demonstrating that it is done consistently in a particular way, the next task is to assess whether or not it achieves the intended results. The illustrations from the nurse training literature provided earlier actually afford a fairly full range of examples of how such assessments can be made in relation to a therapy. The service can be assessed by means of the Ward Atmosphere Scale; by assessing staff stress, coping and distress (e.g. by means of the Occupational Stress Indicator: Cooper et al 1988); or again through assessment based on audit of the extent of which standards for a nursing service have been achieved.

Task 5 Determining whether change is due to the nursing service

The preceding steps are relatively straightforward and arguably could be conducted fairly much within an audit framework, with possibly a touch of the more rigorous service evaluation methods. This next step is more challenging as it requires the introduction of scientific method, particularly the use of research designs. A research design is a way of planning an evaluation so that we are clear about such issues as when information will be collected, on whom such data will be collected (e.g. nurses and/or clients?) and whether there will be some kind of experimental design, involving a control group, for instance. It therefore provides a logical structure, guiding data collection in an evaluation. This structure will have major consequences for whether or not we can claim with any confidence that a service is indeed responsible for any changes that we may obtain on the dependent variables. As illustrated earlier, studies which simply measure before and after a service is provided cannot actually be interpreted, since there are so many alternative possible explanations for any observed improvement. For this reason more rigorous research designs are needed, such as those in which clients are randomly allocated to two or more conditions and in which one group (i.e. the experimental group) receives the treatment.

Such a design is actually very difficult to organise and implement in routine NHS practice, and thankfully there are some more manageable alternatives available. One range of alternatives is the non-experimental designs, such as descriptive studies of a population or correlational analysis of whether two or more variables are associated (e.g. the correlation between schizophrenia and community tenure). Such designs do not allow one, however, to tease out cause and effect, although they can be useful in highlighting certain correlates of a situation. To proceed to judging whether or not there is indeed cause and effect, one needs to adopt an experimental design (again, several useful illustrations were provided earlier). The reader is referred to Barker et al (1994) or any of the many other relevant textbooks for detailed accounts of experimental designs.

Fortunately for practitioners with an interest in the question of whether or not their nursing practice is helpful, there is a new breed of research designs available, ones that are much more manageable. These are referred to as 'single subject' (n = 1) designs and need not be impractical or time-consuming. In particular, they are helpful in assessing how the individual uniqueness and complexity of the client interacts with the therapy and the nurses' approach. Such designs can vary considerably in terms of their rigour, just as much as can the traditional group designs. For example, one could simply assess an individual client's functioning on some symptomatic questionnaire before and after a period of nursing care. This, however, could not actually be interpreted with any confidence, since any improvement in the score may be due to all sorts of other factors (see the threats to internal validity mentioned above). But other kinds of n = 1 design can be every bit as rigorous as a true experimental design, such as the multiple baseline and multiple phase designs. A multiple baseline design takes a number of problems or clients, typically only three or four, and provides the treatment successively to the different problems or clients. What makes this design rigorous is that it allows one to interpret with some confidence whether or not the treatment is actually causing the change that is observed. The multiple phase design is similar in rigour, but differs in having a measure of a problem related to a number of phases, starting with the baseline and going on to an intervention before, for example, repeating the baseline (referred to as an ABA or 'withdrawal' design). More commonly, nurses would wish to conclude their analysis with the re-instated intervention, referred to as an ABAB design ('reversal'). Such single subject designs have grown in popularity, especially amongst clinicians who value the individual focus and convenience of this approach. More detailed accounts can be found in Herson &

Barlow (1976), and will probably now be located also in most modern texts on research design.

Task 6 Assessing the relative effectiveness of modified services

Whether or not a service has been found to be effective through an n = 1 outcome evaluation, a time may come when nurses wish to assess the relative benefit of modified programmes of care. Particularly in the current cost-conscious NHS, more efficient ways of deploying scarce resources are at a premium. For example, are there other duties that can be carried out perfectly competently by nursing assistants? Would this free up more highly qualified and experienced nurses for more specialised activities? Regardless of the characteristics of the provider of nursing care, can some aspects of care be either removed or reduced without diminishing the benefit? Questions of these kinds are relevant in this final evaluation task, which is essentially whether there is a better way of doing things.

Often the answer to these questions will be suggested by more straightforward evaluations dealing with some of the early tasks. For example, an outcome evaluation concerning the effects of a service may indicate that some people benefit far more than others, and in turn that the service is actually inappropriate for some people. This could lead to a much more focused or targeted service, freeing up resource for other attempts at dealing with the unmet need. In essence, in a 'learning organisation', the information from previous phases of activity are studied in order to learn lessons about better ways of doing things in the future. This is now generally subsumed under the heading of audit and quality assurance.

CONCLUSIONS

To return to the specific issue of staff training in

mental health, what would a 'good' evaluation of training include? The following are some of the main conclusions:

Introduction section

- Based on prior research, set out a clear theory or model which suggests how the training is expected to prove effective (e.g. by enhancing specific coping skills in nursing)
- Formulate clear hypotheses.

Method section

- Randomly allocate nurses to different experimental conditions or use single subject designs
- Collect relevant demographic data
- Manipulate more than one form of training (the independent variable)
- Ensure that the training is provided according to a manual and is provided in the most effective and thorough-going form (a 'strong' treatment, akin to a high dosage of medication)
- Assess the training (adherence and competence)
- Construct or adapt measures to provide sensitive, timely (peak response) and psychometrically sound assessments of the impact of training (i.e. reliable and valid)
- Assess the impact at different 'levels', as in the effect of supervision on the nurse and in turn on clients (i.e. 'proximal' and 'distal' effects)
- In particular, assess the transfer or 'generalisation' of training across time (maintenance), across behaviours, across settings and across persons
- Use multiple measures of outcome, covering different domains and using different methods (e.g. self-report, observation and archival data).

Results

- Analyse only those data that are directly related to the hypotheses
- Test for violations of statistical assumptions
- Assess the clinical significance of the training.

Discussion

- Evaluate the study against the threats to its validity
- Identify rival explanations for the findings
- Report the major flaws and confounds, not just the strengths
- Interpret the data accordingly (i.e. probably fairly cautiously).

These requirements are very exacting ones, based on an outstanding methodological review of clinical supervision research (Ellis et al 1996). However, they are not unattainable standards for evaluation and in pursuing them nurses and other mental health professionals will be moving in step with the research and development initiative (Peckham 1991). This will be necessary for nurses and others working outside the special research centres to maintain an active involvement in the range of evaluative research undertakings and to promote evidence-based nursing.

Acknowledgements

I am indebted to Partrick Corrigan for copious information on his training work and to Jan Fife for excellent secretarial support.

Exercise

In relation to a particular nursing service, try to define and measure:

a. the goals of the service
b. how the service attempts to achieve these goals
c. the extent to which these goals are achieved.

For question (a) the goals (or objectives/standards) of a nursing service are normally written down somewhere, or can be obtained by interviewing key personnel. Are all nurses aware of these goals? Do other staff (e.g. managers) accept these goals? A structured interview format or questionnaire could be used to address these questions.

Question (b) above is equivalent to defining the 'independent variable', namely the treatment/s that a service provides to its clients. Examples could include individual counselling or groups intended to develop clients' coping skills (e.g. anxiety management). This could be measured by direct or participant observation, as in recording systematically what is taking place in a part of a unit every few minutes; or by following a few clients through their typical sequence of activities and recording the service that they receive.

Question (c) could be measured by a wide range of research methods, including ratings of client satisfaction or staff evaluations of their own service.

KEY TEXTS FOR FURTHER READING

Barker C, Pistrang N, Elliott R 1994 Research methods in clinical and counselling psychology. Wiley, Chichester
Campbell D T, Stanley J C 1963 Experimental and quasi experimental designs for research. Rand McNally, Chicago
Lipsey M W 1990 Design sensitivity: Statistical power for experimental research. Sage, London

Milne D L 1987 Evaluating mental health practice: Methods and applications. Routledge, London
Roth A, Fonagy P 1996 What works for whom? Guilford Press, London

REFERENCES

Alberts G, Edelstein B 1990 Therapist training: a critical review of skill training studies. Clinical Psychology Review 10:497–511

Barker C, Pistrang N, Elliott R 1994 Research methods in clinical and counselling psychology. Wiley, Chichester

Beutler L E, Kendall P C 1995 Introduction to the special section: the case for training in the provision of psychological therapy. Journal of Consulting and Clinical Psychology 63:179–181

Binder J L 1993 Is it time to improve psychotherapy training? Clinical Psychology Review 13:301–318

Birchwood M, Tarrier N 1994 Psychological management of schizophrenia. Wiley, Chichester

Brooker C, Tarrier N, Barraclough C, Butterworth A, Goldberg D 1992 Training community psychiatric nurses for psychosocial intervention. British Journal of Psychiatry 160:836–844

Brooker C, Falloon I, Butterworth A, Goldberg D, Graham-Hole V, Hillier V 1994 The outcome of training community psychiatric nurses to deliver psychosocial intervention. British Journal of Psychiatry 165:222–230

Burdett C, Milne D L 1985 'Setting events' as determinants of staff behaviour: an exploratory study. Behavioural Psychotherapy 13:300–308

Campbell D T, Stanley J C 1963 Experimental and quasi experimental designs for research. Rand McNally, Chicago

Carifio M S, Hess A K 1987 Who is the ideal supervisor? Professional Psychology: Research and Practice 18:244–250

Carkhuff R R, Kratochvil D, Friel T 1968 Effects of professional training: communication and discrimination of facilitative conditions. Journal of Counselling Psychology 15:68–74

Cooper C L, Sloan S J, Williams S 1988 Occupational stress indicator. ASE/NFER Nelson, Windsor

Corrigan P W, McCracken S G 1995 Refocusing the training of psychiatric rehabilitation staff. Psychiatric Services 46:1172–1177

Corrigan P, Holmes E P, Luchins D et al 1994 The effects of interactive staff training on staff programming and patient aggression in a psychiatric in-patient ward. Behavioural Interventions 10:17–32

Department of Health 1992 The health of the nation: A strategy for health in England. HMSO, London

Department of Health 1994 Research and development in the NHS. NHS Executive, Leeds

Department of Health 1995 National mental health R & D programme: Progress report. NHS Executive, London

Department of Health 1996 NHS psychotherapy services in England: Review of strategic policy. NHS Executive, Wetherby

Durlak J A 1979 Comparative effectiveness of paraprofessional and professional helpers. Psychological Bulletin 86:80–92

Ellis N V, Ladany N, Krengel M, Schult D 1996 Clinical supervision research from 1981 to 1993: a methodological critique. Journal of Counselling Psychology 43:3550

Faust D, Zlotnick C 1995 Another dodo bird verdict? Revisiting the comparative effectiveness of professional and paraprofessional therapists. Clinical Psychology and Psychotherapy 2:157–167

Fennell M 1996 Cognitive behaviour therapy. In: Jacobs M (ed) In search of supervision. Open University Press, Buckingham

Ford J D 1979 Research on training counsellors and clinicians. Review of Educational Research 69:87–130

Grimshaw J M, Russell I T 1994 Achieving health gain through clinical guidelines II: Ensuring guidelines change medical practice. Quality in Health Care 3:45–52

Harchik A E, Sherman J A, Hopkins B L, Strouse M C, Sheldon J B 1989 Use of behavioural techniques by paraprofessional staff: a review and proposal. Behavioural Residential Treatment 4:331–357

Hardy G E, Shapiro D A 1985 Therapist response modes in prescriptive vs exploratory psychotherapy. British Journal of Clinical Psychology 24:235–245

Hart G M 1982 The process of clinical supervision. University Park Press, Baltimore

Hattie J A, Sharpley C F, Rogers H J 1984 Comparative effectiveness of professional and paraprofessional helpers. Psychological Bulletin 95:534–541

Herson M, Barlow D H 1976 Single case experimental designs: Strategies for studying behaviour change. Pergamon, New York

Holland W W (ed) 1983 Evaluation of health care. Oxford University Press, Oxford

Holloway E L, Neufeldt S A 1995 Supervision: its contribution to treatment efficacy. Journal of Consulting and Clinical Psychology 63:207–213

Hughes I, Hailwood R, Abbati-Yeoman J, Budd R 1996 Developing a family intervention service for serious mental illness: clinical observations and experiences. Journal of Mental Health 5:145–159

Jacobs N 1996 In search of supervision. Open University Press, Milton Keynes

Jacobson N S, Truax P 1991 Clinical significance: a statistical approach to defining meaningful change in psychotherapy research. Journal of Counselling and Clinical Psychology 59:12–19

Jacobson N S, Follette W C, Revenstorf D 1984 Psychotherapy outcome research: methods for reporting variability and evaluating clinical significance. Behaviour Therapy 15:336–352

Kavanagh D, Clark D, Piatkowska O et al 1993 Application of cognitive behavioural family intervention to schizophrenia in multidisciplinary teams: what can the matter be? Australian Psychologist 28:1–8

Lipsey M W 1990 Design sensitivity: Statistical power for experimental research. Sage, London

McDonald R M 1991 Assessment of organisational context: a missing component in evaluations of training programmes. Evaluation and Programme Planning 14:273–279

McKeown T, Lowe C R 1966 An introduction to social medicine. Blackwell Scientific, Oxford

Milne D L 1984a Improving the social validity and implementation of behaviour therapy training for psychiatric nurses using a patient centred learning format. British Journal of Clinical Psychology 23:313–314

Milne D L 1984b The development and evaluation of a structured learning format introduction to behaviour therapy for psychiatric nurses. British Journal of Clinical Psychology 23:175–185

REFERENCES (*contd*)

Milne D L 1986a Planning and evaluating innovations in nursing practice by measuring the ward atmosphere. Journal of Advanced Nursing 11:203–210

Milne D L 1986b Training behaviour therapists: Methods, evaluation and implementation with parents, nurses and teachers. Routledge, London

Milne D L 1987 Evaluating mental health practice: Methods and applications. Routledge, London

Milne D L 1992 Assessment: A mental health portfolio. NFER Nelson, Windsor

Milne D L 1993 Psychology and mental health nursing. Macmillan, London

Moos R H 1974 Evaluating treatment environments: A social ecological approach. Wiley, London

Parry G 1992 Improving psychotherapy services: applications of research, audit and evaluation. British Journal of Clinical Psychology 31:3–19

Peckham M 1991 Research and development for the National Health Service. The Lancet 338:367–371

Rogers E S, Cohen B F, Danley K S, Hutchinson D, Anthony W A 1986 Training mental health workers in psychiatric rehabilitation. Schizophrenia Bulletin 12:709–719

Roth A, Fonagy P 1996 What works for whom? Guilford Press, London

Russell I T, Wilson B J 1992 Audit: the third clinical science? Quality in Health Care 1:51–55

Sackett D L, Rosenberg W M C, Gray J A M, Haynes R B, Richardson W S 1996 Evidence-based medicine: what it is and what it's not. British Medical Journal 312:71–72

Shanfield S B, Mohl P C, Mathews K L, Hetherly V 1992 Quantitative assessment of the behaviour of psychotherapy supervisors. American Journal of Psychiatry 149:352–357

Shapiro D A, Firth J 1987 Prescriptive v exploratory psychotherapy: outcomes of the Sheffield psychotherapy project. British Journal of Psychiatry 151:790–799

Shapiro D A, Barkham M, Hardy G E, Morrison L A 1990 The second Sheffield psychotherapy project. British Journal of Medical Psychology 63:97–108

Slevin O 1992 Teaching and supervision in Project 2000. In: Slevin O, Buckenham M (eds) Project 2000: The teachers speak. Campion Press, Edinburgh

Mental health care: approaches to client problems

SECTION CONTENTS

9. Schizophrenia   147

10. Disorders of mood: depression and mania   165

11. Suicide and self-harm   187

12. Phobias and rituals   207

13. Somatisation and inappropriate illness behaviour   225

14. Eating disorders   243

15. Anger and impulse control   265

16. Post-traumatic disorders   291

17. Children's and adolescents' difficulties   313

18. Mental disorders of older people 341

CHAPTER CONTENTS

Key points   147

Introduction   148

Clinical presentation and types   148

Causation   149

Drug treatments   150
   Traditional antipsychotic drugs   151
   Atypical antipsychotic drugs   151
   Depot injections   152
   Nursing roles in medication   152

Models of service delivery for people with
schizophrenia   153

Cognitive–behaviour therapy and psychological
interventions   154

Early intervention   155

Family interventions   157

Dual diagnosis   158

Training   159

Conclusion   160

Key texts for further reading   161

References   161

9

Schizophrenia

Kevin Gournay

KEY POINTS

- Schizophrenia is an umbrella term to cover a number of different conditions which share common clinical features.

- Schizophrenia is the most severe and enduring of all the functional illnesses; only one-third of patients make a complete recovery.

- While the basic causation is certainly biological, social and psychological factors are important in the triggering and maintenance of the condition.

- Effective drugs have been used for 40 years, but they often have very disabling side effects.

- New drugs called atypical antipsychotics are now being used. These seem to have better clinical outcomes, and have a much lower incidence of side effects.

- There is a need for people with schizophrenia to have consistent input, and they should not be allowed to drop out of services.

- Treatment approaches should be comprehensive, addressing physical, psychological and social needs.

KEY POINTS (*contd*)

- There are a range of behavioural interventions which improve daily living skills.

- There are a range of cognitive–behavioural interventions which help the sufferer cope with symptoms.

- Families bear tremendous burdens.

- There are now interventions which focus on the family. These consist of education, problem-solving and changing family atmosphere.

- Schizophrenia is often complicated by drug and alcohol use. We are now developing ways of helping people who have this 'dual diagnosis'.

- The UK is leading the way in developing training for the mental health workforce.

- There is a need for a great deal of research into which models of training are most effective.

- Research needs to cover both skill acquisition and patient outcome.

INTRODUCTION

The Mental Health Nursing Review (Department of Health 1994) recommended that the focus of mental health nursing should be on people with serious and enduring mental illness. The most important diagnostic group in that category is schizophrenia. As this chapter will show, schizophrenia is in fact an umbrella term for a number of disorders which cause very significant levels of distress and in many cases lifelong handicap

for the sufferer. Furthermore, schizophrenia also produces a considerable burden on both carers and the health care system. The evidence regarding the nature and treatment of this condition is growing rapidly. This chapter will provide a comprehensive account of various aspects of the condition, but will particularly highlight the evidence which is most relevant to mental health nursing. The main areas covered will be:

- clinical presentation and types
- causation
- drug treatments
- models of service delivery
- cognitive–behaviour therapy and other psychological interventions
- early intervention
- family interventions
- dual diagnosis
- training.

CLINICAL PRESENTATION AND TYPES

As research into schizophrenia progresses, it is becoming clear that the term is in fact an umbrella for a large number of related disorders. Over the years, the classification of schizophrenia has changed and even the leading experts in the field cannot agree wholeheartedly on a way of defining the various sub-types. In addition, we have two systems of classification – the International Classification of Diseases, which is currently in its 10th revision, and the Diagnostic and Statistical Manual of the American Psychiatric Association, which is now in its fourth edition. Notwithstanding these difficulties, it is clear that the group of disorders which come under the umbrella term schizophrenia is certainly the commonest of the severe and enduring illnesses. In turn, schizophrenia accounts for more pain and suffering than any group of mental health problems, both in terms of those afflicted and their families and carers. Davies & Drummond (1994) calculated that the total cost of treating schizophrenia is equivalent to 1.6% of the total health care budget for the country and the indirect annual costs of this illness are in excess of £1.7 billion annually.

Schizophrenia is seen in all cultures and has recently been studied extensively within a World Health Organisation study which examined the occurrence of the illness in 10 different countries (Jablensky et al 1994). This study found that overall the lifetime risk is about 1%, but there was considerable variation across all of the countries in incidence. Research shows that men are likely to develop schizophrenia about 5 years earlier than women, although the incidence is roughly the same. In industrialised societies, there are more people with schizophrenia in the lower socioeconomic classes, but this may be accounted for by 'social drift' wherein people with schizophrenia become socially disadvantaged. Nevertheless, as Gournay (1996) has pointed out, the consequences of social deprivation, and hence maternal undernutrition, may be a factor in causation. As noted above, there are a number of ways of classifying the disorder. However as Frangou & Murray (1996) describe, there are a number of common clinical features:

- abnormal thoughts
- disorders of thought process and speech
- abnormal perceptions
- abnormal affect
- passivity phenomena
- motor abnormalities
- cognitive deficits
- lack of volition
- lack of insight.

The purpose of this chapter is not to provide a detailed account of the phenomenology of schiz-ophrenia, but to examine issues connected with the problem and its treatment which are relevant to nurses. For this reason, the reader is referred to other texts (e.g. Gournay 1996) which describe some of the issues in more detail. The course of schizophrenia is extremely variable. There is general agreement that about one-quarter of patients will suffer one episode of the illness and will recover completely; one-third of patients suffer multiple episodes, but in between episodes remain 'largely well'; and approximately 40% will suffer a lifetime impairment, which will either show a pattern of continuing deterioration, or otherwise remain on a plateau. There is a great deal of research (Frangou & Murray 1996) which shows that certain characteristics correlate with a better outcome. These include being married, being female, having good social relationships and work record, and the disorder itself is characterised by an acute florid onset which responds well to medication.

CAUSATION

Many of the considerable advances in knowledge of the last 10 years are accounted for by research carried out with new technologies. The work on genetics has been greatly developed because of monumental advances in recombinant DNA technology, and this approach has revolutionised our understanding of not only schizophrenia, but other disorders such as alcoholism, anxiety, Alzheimer's disease and Huntington's chorea (see McGuffin et al 1994). The emerging picture is of schizophrenia being a very heterogeneous disorder with some subtypes being much more inheritable than others. Sham et al (1995) have argued that there may be an increased genetic loading in female and early onset schizophrenia. However, as noted above, there is evidence that environmental factors, such as maternal undernutrition (Susser & Lin

1992) or viral infection (Eagles 1992) may also be implicated in causation. The second area where knowledge has greatly increased is in the use of brain-imaging techniques. Computerised tomography now gives us much better X-ray pictures of the brain, but magnetic resonance imaging is now replacing traditional X-rays. There are also other advances which enable us to study the working brain, for example positron emission tomography (PET scanning) and single photon emission tomography (SPET scanning). These methods allow a detailed study of blood flow and glucose metabolism and researchers are now able to carry out very carefully controlled experiments looking at individuals over the course of time, or comparing groups of individuals with various disorders, including schizophrenia, with control populations.

There are now numerous studies which report the structural abnormalities in the brain of people with schizophrenia. These have highlighted various pathologies such as increased ventricular enlargement, abnormalities in the temporal lobes, frontal lobes, basal ganglia, thalamus, corpus callosum, and hippocampal formation (Liddle 1994, Royston & Lewis 1993, Van Horne & MacManus 1992).

In addition to these biological abnormalities there has been an increased focus on research which considers psychological function in people with schizophrenia. This research has very important implications for mental health nursing practice. Neuropsychologists have systematically tested the processes of memory, attention and problem-solving, and shown that, overall, people with schizophrenia may have very marked abnormalities in cognitive function and that some of these abnormalities link with certain symptom types (Heinreich & Awad 1993). Various detailed reviews of this area have been carried out and more detail can be found in Corcoran & Frith (1994) and Gournay (1996).

The new research findings in neuropsychology have many implications for mental health nursing practice. First, it is clear that many people with schizophrenia suffer serious deficits of attention and memory. There is therefore a need for nurses to take these deficits into account when carrying out assessments and interventions. For example, people with a poor attention span should be seen for short periods of time, of say 10 to 15 minutes. For the many people with schizophrenia who have problems processing information, educational material should be given to them in various ways, for example reinforcing the verbal message with written accounts and repeating the message several times over. In medication management this is particularly important. A study carried out by Corrigan et al (1994) examined the various difficulties involved in teaching people with schizophrenia self-management skills in medication, and showed quite clearly that skill-learning was impaired by the memory deficits which were so common in this condition. Thus the rehabilitation process needs to monitor both skill acquisition and attention. In the future, it seems likely that there will be much more emphasis placed on attempting to rehabilitate people with schizophrenia in the same way that people with brain injuries are rehabilitated. This work is now continuing at several centres across the world and details of research carried out can be found in Gournay (1996).

DRUG TREATMENTS

At the time of writing, the treatment of schizophrenia by drugs is undergoing something of a minor revolution. Since 1996 at least four new drugs have been marketed and the general expectation is that these products will make significant contributions to improvement in the management of this condition.

Traditional antipsychotic drugs

Chlorpromazine was introduced in the 1950s and over the next 30 years, a number of other related compounds were marketed. Carlson & Lindquist (1963) proposed that this group of drugs worked by blocking dopamine receptors in the brain, preventing messages being transmitted across the synapse by the neurotransmitter. We now know that there are at least five different types of dopamine receptor in various parts of the brain. Chlorpromazine and similar drugs seem to block receptors in the parts of the brain known as the mesolimbic system and work effectively on the positive symptoms of schizophrenia, that is hallucinations, delusions and thought disorder. However, these drugs also block dopamine in parts of the brain called the striatum and this causes the so-called extrapyramidal side-effects (Sandberg 1980) which can cause so much distress and discomfort. The most common extrapyramidal side-effects, which may occur in up to 75% of patients (Mortimer 1994) are parkinsonism, dystonia, akathisia and, more seriously, tardive dyskinesia. In addition, traditional antipsychotic drugs block other receptors, including serotonin and histamine and the so-called anticholinergic side-effects such as dry mouth, blurred vision and constipation may also occur. These drugs may also impair concentration and cognitive processing, cause undue sedation and lead to blood pressure changes (Gray 1999). Recently some authors (e.g. Day & Bentall 1996) have suggested that the side-effects on the endocrine system may cause many patients a great deal of distress. The most commonly observed endocrine effects of these drugs are related to the increased production of prolactin and may lead to impotence and the development of breasts in men, and menstrual disturbances in women. A comprehensive account of drug treatment is out of place here, but Gray et al (1997) provide detailed references for further reading. Suffice it to say, the traditional antipsychotic drugs, while beneficial in modifying the symptoms of schizophrenia, are for many patients unacceptable because of their side-effects and non-compliance affects up to 80% of the population who take them (Bebbington 1995).

Atypical antipsychotic drugs

These drugs are now providing a great deal of hope for sufferers, both in terms of possible increase in efficacy and in a much lower incidence of side-effects (particularly in the newer compounds). The first step in producing a new generation of drugs was in fact made more than 30 years ago when clozapine was first released. Initially there was a great deal of enthusiasm for this drug, as it produced marked improvement in a number of patients who were deemed to be 'treatment resistant'. An additional benefit was that these gains occurred without the drug producing the classic extrapyramidal side-effects. However, 20 years ago several patients taking this drug developed agranulocytosis (a severe and potentially fatal reduction in white blood cells) and the drug was withdrawn. However, a research group in the USA (Kane et al 1988) continued to research the therapeutic effects of clozapine and noted that some patients who had not responded to the traditional antipsychotic compounds showed dramatic response to clozapine therapy, with improvements in both positive and negative symptoms. Because of the very encouraging data from this research group's efforts, clozapine was re-introduced in 1990 under strict rules regarding regular blood monitoring for use with people who had treatment-resistant schizophrenia.

Subsequently, a number of studies (e.g. Cleghorn et al 1987, Clozapine Study Group 1993) have shown that clozapine is superior to traditional drugs in its effect on both positive and negative symptoms. Furthermore, there are now widespread reports of patients who have, for many years, led impoverished lives in hospital, and because of treatment with clozapine have shown such improvement that it has been possible to discharge them into the community in a much improved state. Apart from the blood side-effects which are relatively rare, clozapine does lead to an increase in salivation, weight gain and, most seriously, a risk of seizures. Since the introduction of clozapine, researchers have continued their attempts to develop compounds which, like clozapine, have a low incidence of extrapyramidal side-effects and increased efficacy but without the other serious problems. Clozapine seems to work by blocking both serotonin and dopamine receptors, the latter in a different way to the traditional antipsychotic drugs. The new compounds which have been marketed in the past few years seem to work in the same broad fashion.

The first drug in the new series to be launched was risperidone in 1993 and although in high doses this drug does produce extrapyramidal side-effects, for most patients the side-effect profile is excellent. The efficacy is such that it is now used as a first-line treatment in many parts of the USA and now in some services in the UK.

Quetiapine was launched in 1997 and in clinical trials it is as effective as haloperidol in treating both the positive and negative symptoms of schizophrenia. The main treatment emergent side-effects associated with quetiapine are constipation, dyspepsia and headache. Limited weight gain is associated with quetiapine, but appears to be transient. Significantly, across the full dose range quetiapine is associated with a low level of sexual dysfunction and proclactin-related side-effects, and does not require regular ECG or blood pressure monitoring. Unlike other novel antipsychotics, the risk of EPS is not emergent at higher doses.

Olanzapine was launched in October 1996 and is very similar in its chemical structure to clozapine. It has been shown to be effective in treating both the positive and negative symptoms of schizophrenia (Beasley et al 1996) and seems to have a low incidence of all side-effects. One of the benefits of olanzapine is that it requires only a single daily dose.

Depot injections

The traditional antipsychotic drugs have been produced in depot form, requiring an injection of a long-acting compound, to be given every 2 to 4 weeks. One of the reasons for producing drugs in depot form is to increase compliance; and it might therefore be argued that if the newer compounds produce fewer side-effects, compliance might be less of a problem. However, if one sets aside the issue of side-effects, one must also remember that schizophrenia is, almost by definition, a condition where motivational levels are low and depot forms of the new drugs may still be necessary. It is thought that some, but not all, of the new atypical compounds may be developed in this form; however, it is likely that these depot versions will be many years away.

Nursing roles in medication

The nurse's role in medication management was central to the original development of community psychiatric nursing services in the 1950s and 1960s. However, several studies have shown that there is a need for nurses to develop more medication management skills and knowledge (Bennett et al 1995, Sandford 1996, Turner 1993). While there is obviously a need to help nurses develop an increase in skill in monitoring side-effects and using structured measures for detecting these (e.g. the Liverpool University Neuroleptic Side-Effect Rating Scale (LUNSERS), Day et al 1995), it is also important to develop skills in providing education to users and carers, as well as dealing with poor compliance, using cognitive–behavioural techniques such as motivational interviewing. A randomised controlled trial carried out by Kemp et al in 1996 demonstrated that compliance can be improved by providing patients with a package of treatment which includes education and motivational interviewing. This innovation is now being taught to nurses on the Thorn Initiative at the Institute of Psychiatry and the teaching of these methods is being tested within a randomised controlled trial, also run at the Institute.

MODELS OF SERVICE DELIVERY FOR PEOPLE WITH SCHIZOPHRENIA

The method of delivering mental health services for people with schizophrenia and other severe and enduring mental illnesses has changed considerably in the last two decades. Case management has now become the overall method for delivery. This approach was originally developed by a research team in Madison, Wisconsin in the 1970s (Stein & Test 1980) who originally set up a 'ward in the community' and organised services around the principle of providing treatment and care within a natural community setting. However, a recent Cochrane Review (Marshall et al 1996) highlighted the fact that case management may be applied in an ineffective way by some providers. There are now several reviews (Andrews & Teesson 1994, Muijen et al 1994, Santos et al 1995) that show that certain methods (notably those that come under the headings of Assertive Community Treatment and Home-Based Care) provide an effective approach, producing gains in clinical, social and quality of life outcomes. These approaches

involve case managers who have a range of clinical skills in various psychosocial methods and who work with small caseload sizes. In the UK such case managers are predominantly nurses, but in the USA these case managers may be more likely to come from a social work or non-professional background. The recent review of roles and training in mental health care (Sainsbury Centre 1997) has highlighted the great overlap in roles between professions and placed an emphasis on the need to develop multidisciplinary models of training and education.

Essentially, case managers are the workers to whom the patient relates most. It is the case manager who develops a continuing relationship with the patient and, if appropriately trained, may carry out most of the standard assessments of clinical state and need. The patient will initially have been assessed by a qualified psychiatrist, who will, with the case manager, provide overall responsibility for that patient's care and treatment over time and this may amount to a responsibility throughout the remainder of the patient's lifetime. The psychiatrist will provide an overarching authority for that patient's care and be responsible for reviewing the patient's medication and physical health needs. However, on a day-to-day basis, all of the main treatment and care tasks will be delegated to the case manager. According to the patient's needs, this case manager may provide cognitive–behaviour therapy for symptoms, or may manage issues of medication side-effects and non-compliance. The case manager should always be ready to help patients and their families and carers with information about the illness and the treatment, and also assist with practical issues such as benefits and entitlements. Patient and carer education may be a complex and long-term task. For several reasons, not least in effecting an increase in social support, educational initiatives are best managed in groups. In many cases, the case manager may work actively with voluntary sector organisations, such as National Schizophrenia Fellowship and MIND. Case managers, particularly from a nursing background, are responsible for ensuring that the patient's physical health needs are met and that there is a regular monitoring of basic measures of health, such as weight and blood pressure. In addition, because people with schizophrenia have much higher standardised mortality ratios than the general population (Department of Health 1995), there is a need to ensure that the patient is given relevant health education, for example in the areas of smoking and HIV infection.

In modern services, case managers are responsible for networking with a whole range of agencies in both the public and voluntary sector, with the aims of ensuring that first of all, communication between all those involved in the patient's care is satisfactory, and second, that all possible service options are explored. In turn, the case manager will generally be responsible for making sure that these services are, where necessary, purchased and that the patient takes advantage of them. These brokering and networking roles are not easy, and modern case managers need to have an intimate knowledge of the workings of the criminal justice system, social security, housing and employment as people with mental illnesses such as schizophrenia are frequently in contact with these agencies. There is certainly a role for case management aides and many teams are now employing support workers who can assist patients with some of the more mundane, but nevertheless important, areas of daily living, such as laundry, cleaning and cooking. Furthermore, there is an increasing recognition that some of these case manager aide functions could be easily carried out by persons who have themselves experienced mental health problems. This model of service delivery has been in use for a number of years in the USA and Sherman &

Porter (1991) set up a comprehensive project for user case managers training 11 years ago in Denver, Colorado. This programme has been thoroughly researched and shows that user case management aides have the added value of increasing compliance among the people they care for. The health status of these aides also seems to benefit from the involvement in a very useful occupation which is recompensed at the full market rate for such work. Services in the UK have much to learn from this approach.

COGNITIVE–BEHAVIOUR THERAPY AND OTHER PSYCHOLOGICAL INTERVENTIONS

Effective psychological interventions are, of course, not new in the treatment of schizophrenia. Ayllon & Azrin (1968) developed a behavioural approach to schizophrenia based on the use of reinforcement. These treatments were applied in in-patient settings and focused on increasing socially desirable behaviours and improving daily living skills. The system became operationalised using tokens as the central method of reinforcement and the whole treatment system became known as the 'token economy'. Token economy systems were developed in England during the 1970s and the most well-known of these were in hospitals in Wakefield, Yorkshire and Hellingly, East Sussex. The system required very intensive staffing and the in-patient units often used a ratio of one member of staff to one patient (at any one time). Obviously this method of treatment was very expensive and is certainly beyond the resources available to the services of the present day. However, a second problem with the token economy system was that while there were major changes in the patient's behaviour, it was very difficult to generalise these positive gains beyond the token economy setting. Eventually, therefore, these systems were abandoned. However, experience with the token economy taught us much about the functional analysis of behaviour, and the principles of applying reinforcement which we learned during these programmes hold as true today as ever.

One other approach, social skills training, has endured to the present day and there is considerable evidence that social skills training for schizophrenia is at least as effective as family interventions (Smith et al 1996). Social skills training targets the social skills problems which are so common in schizophrenia and which may be caused by either the illness itself or arise as a consequence of the inability to practise certain behaviours because of long periods of institutionalisation (Brady 1984). Social skills training comprises a number of components, central of which are:

- role-play of specific behaviours by the patient
- feedback, preferably using video tape from the therapist and other patients
- modelling by the therapist or another patient
- repeat of the role-play following feedback and modelling
- real-life practice
- feedback of real-life experience
- more role-play.

Social skills training is often delivered in groups, and this approach makes for cost-effectiveness. Practitioners should however be aware that social skills training is very time consuming with some patients requiring literally dozens of sessions. In addition, therapists need a considerable level of skill.

Cognitive–behavioural techniques have been developed in the last few years and most recent research has focused on targeting hallucinations and delusions for intervention. However, one should also note that people with schizophrenia suffer a number of other mental health problems, including anxiety states, depression and phobias

and there is no reason why the techniques which are used for such conditions when they develop in a primary way should not be used with people with schizophrenia.

Most of the techniques used for hallucinations and delusions are simple, and many involve behavioural strategies such as the use of distraction and alternative activity. There are also a number of cognitive techniques, which come under the heading of reattribution, where the patient is asked to consider, for example, alternative explanations for a particular delusional idea. Overall most of these approaches also emphasise more adaptive methods of coping. For a fuller discussion of cognitive–behavioural approaches, the reader is referred to Birchwood & Tarrier (1994) or Haddock & Slade (1996).

EARLY INTERVENTION

Early intervention in schizophrenia is now becoming an important topic in its own right. Early intervention takes two forms:

- recognising schizophrenia early and initiating effective treatment
- intervening early in the case of psychotic relapse.

Although schizophrenia often seems to begin suddenly, there are often a range of signs and symptoms which may begin in childhood and early adolescence. Often, by the time the disease is diagnosed formally and treatment initiated, the patient may have come to considerable harm. Very often bizarre, hostile or impulsive behaviour leads to the breakdown of social and family relationships, the loss of occupation, and the sufferer may drift into homelessness. Obviously, recognising the disease at an early point and initiating appropriate treatment could prevent many of these consequences. Thus, early intervention in the sense of recognising and responding to the disease has many facets. First of all, there is a need for the education of health professionals so that more skill can be developed in picking up early indicators of the condition. Second, early intervention requires very skilled management by appropriate medication. Third, early intervention also needs to provide for supporting the family at what is often a very distressing time. This family support may involve education, but more often than not families need someone to listen to their concerns and provide appropriate responses. Family members may often blame themselves as being responsible for the problem, and may be afraid of stigma. The general public lack an awareness of the various services that may be provided, and are often bewildered by the array of mental health professionals who may become involved. Thus, in a sense, early recognition is part of a wider public health problem.

With regard to early intervention in psychotic relapse, this is something which has now been studied by groups of workers across several continents. In the UK, a group in Birmingham, led by Professor Max Birchwood, has been the most prolific, while in Australia, Professor Pat McGorry in Melbourne, has pursued this area relentlessly, so that it is now one of Australia's national priorities in mental health.

Early intervention in relapse is underpinned by several simple strategies. First and foremost, one must listen to the patient and gather information about the signs and symptoms that have preceded previous episodes. Several studies, e.g. Kumar et al (1989), have shown that many individuals suffering from schizophrenia not only recognise early warning signs, but take remedial action by seeking professional help, changing their medication themselves, or engaging in various other activities. Similarly, several pieces of research have shown that relatives often recognise early warning signs of an impending

relapse. For example, Birchwood et al (1989) and Herz & Melville (1980) have reported that relatives identified symptoms such as anxiety, depression and sleep problems. Nevertheless, as Birchwood et al (1998) have pointed out, the process of relapse is something which needs a great deal of further research, and while paying closer attention to patients' own reports of changes in their emotional and behavioural state is important, there is no absolutely foolproof way of predicting relapse.

What then are the appropriate responses to relapse? First, it needs to be said that the patient's treatment plan should include a plan for what will happen if a relapse does occur, and if at all possible the patient must be central to the drawing-up of such a plan. Indeed there are now several schemes which ask patients to identify their preferred treatment in the case of relapse. These plans are drawn up when the patient is in a stable state and can give carers an account of treatment strategies which have been in the past helpful, or conversely those which have caused distress. At the Maudsley Hospital, these patient-centred treatment plans have been defined on a 'crisis card' which the patient carries around, and which can be used should a relapse occur.

There is no doubt that, while medication is the mainstay of treatment, and the dose of this may be varied if the patient's state deteriorates, other social and psychological strategies are important in reducing the impact of the condition, or even preventing a relapse. Obviously, some relapses are precipitated by stress in the environment, and attention given to the patient's anxiety or modification of environmental stresses may be possible. Some of these environmental stresses may involve the responses of family members who may be instructed to use different strategies and tactics for coping with the sufferer. Stress may come from an inability to deal with certain social situations, and in such cases social skills training and anxiety management strategies may be used.

Early intervention is likely to become an increasing priority in the care and treatment of people with schizophrenia. However, it must be pointed out that early intervention will only work if there exists a good relationship between the patient and key-worker, and other people in the team. Good relationships, where the patient feels they can trust and confide in their key-worker, will lead to patients being able to disclose their previous experiences, and to be able to tell their key-worker or carer about the distressing symptoms which may precede a full relapse.

FAMILY INTERVENTIONS

Family interventions in schizophrenia were developed from the research on expressed emotion in families (Leff et al 1982) and initially the approach targeted those aspects of family interaction which were seen as important in the triggering of relapse. These approaches have been developed within a more behavioural framework by others (e.g. Tarrier et al 1988), and across the world, family interventions are now used in different forms. A recent systematic review of family interventions in schizophrenia (Mari et al 1996) concluded that family intervention reduces the rate of relapse in hospital admission as well as improving compliance with medication. However, one should be aware that this systematic review covered a number of different family interventions (some more behavioural than others) and comprised only 12 studies. In addition, the review also showed surprisingly that family interventions did not reduce family burden or expressed emotion. Thus, in a sense, while family interventions are effective, the current picture is that the overall approach has very significant limitations. Solomon (1996), in a consideration of

the limitations of family intervention for schizophrenia, argued quite convincingly that brief, focused family education might actually be a much more effective strategy and reach much larger populations than traditional, expressed emotion-type approaches. Readers should therefore be aware that this is an area which may evolve and some of the current practices may change in light of research findings.

There is general agreement about the successful ingredients of family intervention, and more detail can be found in Mari et al (1996). These ingredients can be summarised as follows:

- Professionals, the patient and carer need to agree on a working model of schizophrenia. This is generally called the Stress Vulnerability Model which accepts a biological underpinning of the condition, but notes that psychological and social factors are important in the maintenance of the condition, and the triggering of relapse.
- Family interventions can only be successfully employed when an appropriate medication is being used, and when a comprehensive system of clinical case management is in place.
- There needs to be a very positive alliance between patient, the family and the therapist.
- The patient and family need to be seen together for at least some of the sessions.
- There needs to be an emphasis on education about the condition and its treatment, including practical information.
- Family problem-solving skills should be targeted.
- Family communication is also targeted, with the aim of reducing less negative emotion and hence reducing negative family atmosphere.
- Families, patients and therapists need to work on clear and realistic goals.

- Interventions need to be maintained after initial input over an indefinite period, albeit in many cases the time involved need not be great.

DUAL DIAGNOSIS

The term 'dual diagnosis' refers to the co-existence of severe mental illness (notably schizophrenia) and the use of drugs and/or alcohol. This phenomenon is without doubt a rising tide which may become one of the most important challenges for mental health services in the next few years. There is clear epidemiological evidence, both from the USA (Regier et al 1990) and the UK (Menezes et al 1996) showing that up to 40% of people with psychosis have such a problem. The reader is referred for more detailed study to a review of literature (Gournay et al 1997), which gives an account of prevalence, the relationship of dual diagnosis with other conditions, the impact on services and models of management.

A number of reasons for substance abuse in schizophrenia have been put forward, including self-medication for extrapyramidal side-effects and depression, cultural factors and the possibility that the taking of substances may improve social interactions. While there are some reviews of which substances may be used by people with psychosis (e.g. Cuffel et al 1993, Lehman et al 1994) there is no easy way to describe the picture. We know anecdotally that patients may take a range of substances (polyabuse) and that the substances taken may vary according to availability of the drugs on the street. While there is no definitive evidence, there is wide agreement among clinicians that some substances, for example crack cocaine, produce many more problems for the sufferers than others. There is also some alarming evidence (e.g. Swanson et al 1990) which suggests that there are very high rates of violence among this population, perhaps as much as 15 times that of the normal population. It is also noteworthy that substance abuse emerges time and again in the enquiries into homicide by mentally ill people. While one of the major challenges for mental health services is the recognition of substance abuse among the mentally ill, there are also problems within the mental health system itself. Recently, Sandford (1995) reported the results of a survey of 400 mental health nurses across the UK who were randomly selected from membership records. The majority of respondents reported illicit drug use in the psychiatric unit where they worked and, more worryingly, 13% of respondents suggested that medical and/or nursing staff were also involved in the taking of illicit substances. Even within Special Hospitals, substance abuse by patients is a significant problem (McKeown & Liebling 1995); this study highlighted the lack of training of nurses in this area.

There is no research whatsoever on efficacy of treatment approaches to this population in the UK. However, there has been considerable research undertaken in the USA, particularly in New Hampshire. Drake & Noordsy (1994) described the development of services for people with co-existing, severe mental disorder and emphasised the importance of approaching each problem (i.e. mental illness and substance abuse) in an integrated way, that is, applying treatment for both problems concurrently. The New Hampshire work emphasised the need to approach people with this problem in a graduated, non-confrontational fashion, and identified four central stages in the intervention process:

- engagement
- persuasion
- active treatment
- relapse prevention.

In view of the prevalence of substance abuse in

society, it is extremely unlikely that the problems associated with dual diagnosis will reduce. This places an onus on all those involved in mental health services and in training and education to recognise that schizophrenia and other mental illnesses will co-exist with substance abuse problems in a very large proportion of cases and that one cannot separate treatment approaches to the respective problems.

TRAINING

1997 saw the publication of *Pulling Together*, a review of roles and training for all mental health professionals. This was instigated by the influential Sainsbury Centre for Mental Health as a response to a realisation that there were many difficulties and dilemmas concerning the training of the mental health workforce. The review pointed to problems in psychiatry, social work and nursing and suggested that a much more unified approach to training was necessary, with emphasis on defining core competencies for all mental health professionals. The view endorsed the need to set up more multidisciplinary training. Unfortunately, there is very little research evidence on the outcomes of training – the notable exception is the extensive work carried out by Professor Isaac Marks on the evaluation of nurse therapy (e.g. Marks 1985, Marks et al 1977). One recent training development, which is currently being evaluated, is the development of a programme which was initially for nurses, but which is now multidisciplinary, the Thorn Initiative. This initiative was pump-primed by a generous donation from the Sir Jules Thorn Trust, with the explicit aim of developing a training in research-based interventions for schizophrenia. Funding allowed for the development of the programme, a 3-year piloting in two sites and an evaluation. The team that developed this programme comprised individuals from psychi-

atry, psychology and nursing and latterly the programme has involved voluntary sector organisations such as the National Schizophrenia Fellowship. The basic elements of this programme are:

- a focus on psychosis
- the adoption of a Stress Vulnerability Model (Zubin & Spring 1977) to underpin the total approach
- the use of cognitive–behavioural approaches
- the linkage of clinical practice to training
- the use of structured clinical supervision; in turn, the Thorn Programme which runs on a part-time basis, has three equally weighted modules:

    clinical case management, which includes training of students in the use of valid and reliable assessments of mental state, the use of medication management, brokering and networking and a range of other clinical skills

    behavioural and cognitive behavioural interventions for symptoms

    family interventions, including family education and family stress management training.

The programme was originally set up at the Institute of Psychiatry and the University of Manchester, but by late 1997 new courses were either beginning, or in a process of being set up, in Nottingham, York, Gloucestershire, Belfast, City and Hackney Trust, the Royal College of Nursing Institute and several other centres. Since the programme began in 1992, it has gradually become the model for training nurses in community approaches. The Thorn Initiative has been evaluated with the outcome of training being determined by using repeated patient measures (Lancashire et al 1977) and on trainee skill and knowledge. Overall, the results are encouraging, with a general trend evident of patients, who have been case managed by Thorn graduates, showing improvements in clinical and social function. However, we are gradually becoming aware that not all students carry on practising their clinical skills once training is over, or that they practise their skills in a diluted or infrequent fashion. These impressions are much in accord with the results of research carried out in New South Wales by Kavanagh et al (1993) which showed that fidelity to the training model was a substantial problem. There are currently various efforts being made to address this issue, for example by giving more attention to preparation of the work-setting that the graduates will return to. This approach is currently much in evidence in the training programme delivered by the Sainsbury Centre for Mental Health which has now begun various training initiatives with complete mental health teams throughout the UK. In addition to Thorn, several Masters Programmes, using the same clinical skills focus have developed – the first of these was set up by the author at Middlesex University in 1992 and this was followed by programmes at Birmingham and Sheffield.

Training is certainly one of the biggest challenges for our mental health system, and ranks alongside the task of ensuring that research findings are put into everyday practice. One of the difficulties of course in mental illness is that the effectiveness literature in this area is small by comparison with other areas of medicine and as Lewis et al (1997) remarked: 'the task of producing a complete comprehensive effectiveness literature for mental health problems is truly Herculean.'

CONCLUSION

Schizophrenia is an umbrella term for a group of disorders which account for a huge amount of distress and suffering. It is a condition which can be found in every corner of the globe. Although there is some variation in different settings, a majority of sufferers will, using current treatment approaches, always have a degree of social and psychological handicap. In many cases this is such that independent living is not possible. There is a great deal of hope that research will uncover the causation of this condition; however, it is likely that the causation is likely to be complex and variable across the different sub-types. The new medications called 'atypical antipsychotics' are offering new hope. It is likely that, because these medications have fewer side-effects, compliance with treatment will be improved, and thus there will be an ensuing reduction in distress and burden. The last quarter of a century has seen an evolution of approaches which are based on the social and psychological aspects of the condition, and on the delivery of effective services. These have been crystallised in the last few years in a method known as assertive community treatment, where patients are treated in their natural setting with a comprehensive and integrated range of treatment strategies. However, one of the great obstacles to ensuring that this more effective method of care and treatment is delivered to all is the issue of training. Currently, there are models of training which promise a great deal. However, it is likely that it will be many years before sufficient numbers of the workforce have received this training, and thus the ideal of every patient receiving a comprehensive and effective pattern of care and treatment is many years away. For the mental health nurse, schizophrenia probably represents one of the most daunting challenges. Although there are skills which can be developed, schizophrenia is nevertheless a very difficult condition to deal with on a day-by-day basis. In contrast with phobic and obsessional states, where patients return, in all senses of the word, to normality, success in the treatment of patients with schizophrenia sometimes means keeping their level of symptoms and handicap constant. Nevertheless, the contribution by nurses to a quality of life with people with schizophrenia and their families cannot be underestimated, and therefore, for the foreseeable future the nurses' role in the care and treatment of this condition must be seen as a priority over all others.

KEY TEXTS FOR FURTHER READING

Chadwick P, Birchwood M, Trower P (eds) 1996 Cognitive therapy for delusions, voices and paranoia. Wiley, Chichester. *This is one of the best books on psychological approaches to schizophrenia so far published. It contains a rich variety of case information which allows the reader to become acquainted with the internal experiences of sufferers of delusions and voices. In turn, the book sets out a range of strategies for dealing with these phenomena, while at the same time highlighting the need for working with the sufferer as a collaborator. The one criticism of this book is that it is perhaps overly optimistic about the impact of a psychological approach for this condition. Nevertheless, it is a scholarly, but readable account of the area, and one which would give any student a good feel for not only the current situation, but also how the area might develop in future.*

Fadden G 1998 Family intervention. In: Brooker C, Repper J (eds) Serious mental health problems in the community. Baillière Tindall, London. *This chapter provides the reader with a comprehensive overview of the research so far carried out on the family and schizophrenia, and describes the various attempts to develop family intervention skills. In turn, the chapter pays a great deal of attention to how those skills can be acquired in the workforce, and what measures are necessary to ensure that, once these skills are acquired, they are maintained at a high level. In particular, there is a focus on supervision and the way that family interventions fit within other areas of clinical intervention.*

Gournay K 1996 Schizophrenia: a review of contemporary literature and implications for mental health nursing theory, practice and education. Journal of Psychiatric and Mental Health Nursing 3(1):7–12. *This review was specifically written for mental health nurses, and covers the main aspects of research findings in causation. The bibliography in this article consists of many other review articles where detailed source material may be obtained. However, as an overview, it would probably suffice for any student who wishes to cover the area for an undergraduate degree.*

Gournay K, Sandford T, Johnson S, Thornicroft G 1997 Dual diagnosis of severe mental health problems and substance dependence: a major priority for mental health nursing. Journal of Psychiatric and Mental Health Nursing 4:89–95. *This paper is a review specifically written for nurses covering all aspects of dual diagnosis: definition, prevalence, causation, treatment approaches and training. The specific implications for nursing are discussed in some detail. Each of the authors of this paper has carried out research in dual diagnosis, and this includes a fascinating study by Tom Sandford of the prevalence of drug use in in-patient units in the UK.*

Marshall M, Lockwood A 1998 Assertive community treatment for people with mental disorders. The Cochrane Library. BMJ Publications, London. *This is a systematic review of studies on assertive community treatment, and looks at this method as an alternative to standard community care, traditional hospital-based rehabilitation, and more general case management. Although some of the conclusions of the review may be debatable, it is nevertheless a most comprehensive document as it lists and describes all of the major research studies carried out in this article over the last two decades. For the reader who wishes to become acquainted with main findings, this article provides those in a reasonably simple form. However, for those who wish to examine some of the subtleties of this area, this is a rich source of material. This might be the case for a student who is wishing to write a dissertation or literature review on the area. The review is obtainable in all medical libraries in compact disc form, which has the advantage of allowing reprints to be easily made.*

REFERENCES

Andrews G, Teesson M 1994 Smart versus dumb treatment: services for mental disorders. Current Opinion in Psychiatry 7:181–185

Ayllon T, Azrin N 1968 The token economy: A motivational system for therapy and rehabilitation. Appleton-Century-Crofts, New York

Beasley C M, Tollefson G, Tran P et al 1996 Olanzapine versus placebo and haloperidol. Acute phase results of the North American double-blind olanzapine trial. Neuropsychopharmacology 14(2):111–123

Bebbington P E 1995 The content and context of compliance. International Clinical Psychopharmacology 9 (Suppl 5):41–50

Bennett J, Done J, Harrison-Read P, Hunt B 1995 Developing a rating scale/checklist to assess the side-effects of antipsychotics by community psychiatric nurses. In: Brooker C, White E (eds) Community psychiatric nursing: A research prospective, vol 3. Chapman and Hall, London

Birchwood M, Tarrier N 1994 Psychological management of schizophrenia. Wiley, London

Birchwood M, Smith J, MacMillan F 1989 Predicting relapse in schizophrenia: the development and implementation of an early signs monitoring system using patients and families as observers. Psychological Medicine 19:649–656

REFERENCES (*contd*)

Birchwood M, Smith J, MacMillan F, McGovern D 1998 Early intervention in psychotic relapse. In Brooker C, Repper J (eds) Serious mental health problems in the community. Baillière Tindall, London

Brady J 1984 Social skills training for psychiatric patients I: concepts, methods and clinical results. American Journal of Psychiatry 141:333–340

Carlson A, Lindquist M 1963 The effect of chlorpromazine and haloperidol on formation 3-methoxtyramine and normetanephrine in mouse brain. Acta Pharmacologica et Toxicologica 20:140–144

Cleghorn J M, Kaplan R D, Szechtman B et al 1987 Neuroleptic drug effects on cognitive function in schizophrenia. Schizophrenia Research 3:211–219

Clozapine Study Group 1993 The safety and efficacy of clozapine in severe treatment-resistant schizophrenic patients in the UK. British Journal of Psychiatry 163:150–154

Corcoran R, Frith C 1994 The neuropsychology and neurophysiology of schizophrenia. Current Opinion in Psychiatry 7(1):47–50

Corrigan P W, Wallace C J, Schade M L, Green M F 1994 Learning medication self-management skills in schizophrenia: relationship with cognitive deficits in psychiatric symptoms. Behaviour Therapy 25(1):5–16

Cuffel B, Heithoff K, Lawson W 1993 Correlates of patterns of substance abuse among patients with schizophrenia. Hospital and Community Psychiatry 44:247–251

Davies L, Drummond M 1994 Economics and schizophrenia: the real cost. British Journal of Psychiatry 165(Suppl 25):18–21

Day J, Bentall R P 1996 Neuroleptic medication. In: Haddock G, Slade P (eds) Cognitive behavioural interventions with psychotic disorders. Routledge, London

Day J C, Wood G, Dewer M, Bertall R P 1995 A self-rating scale for measuring neuroleptic side-effects. British Journal of Psychiatry 166(5):650–653

Department of Health 1994 Working in partnership: The review of mental health nursing. HMSO, London

Department of Health 1995 Report of the Clinical Standards Advisory Group on Schizophrenia. HMSO, London

Drake R, Noordsy D 1994 Case management for people with co-existing severe mental disorder and substance abuse disorder. Psychiatric Annals 24:427–431

Eagles J 1992 Are polio viruses a cause of schizophrenia? British Journal of Psychiatry 160:598–600

Frangou S, Murray R 1996 Schizophrenia. Martin Dunitz, London

Gournay K 1996 Schizophrenia: a review of contemporary literature and implications for mental health nursing theory, practice and education. Journal of Psychiatric and Mental Health Nursing 3(1):7–12

Gournay K, Sandford T, Johnson S, Thornicroft G 1997 Dual diagnosis of severe mental health problems and substance abuse/dependence: a major priority for mental health nursing. Journal of Psychiatric and Mental Health Nursing 4:89–95

Gray R 1999 Antipsychotics, side-effects and effective management. Mental Health Practice 2(7):14–20

Gray R, Gournay K, Taylor D 1997 New drug treatments for schizophrenia: implications for mental health nursing. Mental Health Practice 1(1):20–23

Haddock G, Slade P 1996 Cognitive behavioural interventions with psychotic disorders. Routledge, London

Heinrich R, Awad A 1993 Neurocognitive subtypes of chronic schizophrenia. Schizophrenia Research, 9:49–58

Herz M, Melville C 1980 Relapse in schizophrenia. American Journal of Psychiatry 139:801–812

Jablensky A, Sartorius N, Cooper J, Anker M, Korten A, Bertelsen A 1994 Culture and schizophrenia. British Journal of Psychiatry 165:434–436

Kane J, Honigfeld G, Singer J et al 1988 Clozapine for the treatment resistant schizophrenic. Archives of General Psychiatry 45:789–796

Kavanagh D, Clark D, Piatkowska O et al 1993 Application of cognitive behavioural interventions for schizophrenia: what can the matter be? Australian Psychologist 28:1–8

Kemp R, Hayward P, Applewaite G et al 1996 Compliance therapy in psychotic disorders. British Medical Journal 312:345–349

Kumar S, Thara R, Rajikumar S 1989 Coping with symptoms of relapse in schizophrenia. European Archives of Psychiatric Neurological Science 239:213–215

Lancashire S, Haddock G, Tarrier N 1997 Effects of training in psychosocial interventions for community psychiatric nurses in England. Psychiatric Services 48(1):39–41

Leff J, Kuipers L, Berkowitz R et al 1982 A controlled trial of intervention in the families of schizophrenic patients. British Journal of Psychiatry 141:121–134

Lehman A, Myers C, Dickson L, Johnson J 1994 Defining sub-groups of dual diagnosis patients for service planning. Hospital and Community Psychiatry 45:556–561

Lewis G, Churchill R, Hotopf M 1997 Editorial: Systematic reviews and meta-analysis. Psychological Medicine 27: 3–7

Liddle P 1994 The neurobiology of schizophrenia. Current Opinion in Psychiatry 7(1):43–46

McGuffin P, Owen M, O'Donovan M, Thepar A, Gottesman I 1994 Psychiatric genetics. Gaskell, London

McKeown M, Liebling H 1995 Staff perceptions of illicit drug use within a special hospital. Journal of Psychiatric and Mental Health Nursing 2:343–350

Mari J, Adams C, Streiner D 1996 Family intervention for those with schizophrenia. The Cochrane Library. BMJ Publications 23 February 1996

Marks I 1985 Nurse therapists in primary care. RCN, London

Marks I, Connolly J, Hallam R, Philpott R 1977 Nursing in behavioural psychotherapy. RCN, London

Marshall M, Gray A, Lockwood A, Green R 1996 Case management for severe mental disorders. Cochrane Collaboration, Oxford (February 1996)

Menezes P R, Johnson S, Thornicroft G et al 1996 Drug and alcohol problems among people with severe mental illnesses in south London. British Journal of Psychiatry 168:612–619

Mortimer A 1994 Newer and older antipsychotics: a comparative review of appropriate use. CNS Drugs 2(5):381–396

REFERENCES (*contd*)

Muijen M, Coone Y, Strathdee G 1994 Community Psychiatric Nursing teams: intensive care versus generic care. British Journal of Psychiatry 165:211–217

Regier D, Farmer N, Rae D 1990 Co-morbidity of mental disorders with alcohol and other drugs of abuse: results from the epidemiological catchment area (ECA). Journal of American Medical Association 264:2511–2518

Royston M, Lewis S 1993 Brain pathology in schizophrenia: developmental or degenerative? Current Opinion in Psychiatry 6:70–73

Sainsbury Centre 1997 'Pulling together'. A review of roles and training in mental health care. Sainsbury Centre Publications, London

Sandberg P 1980 Haloperidol induced catalextrapyramidal side-effects. Nature 254:472–473

Sandford T 1995 Drug use is increasing. Nursing Standard 9:16–17

Sandford T 1996 Users' perceptions of a depot clinic. In: Sandford T, Gournay K (eds) Perspectives in mental health nursing. Baillière Tindall, London

Santos A, Scott W, Burns B et al 1995 Research on field based services: models for reform. American Journal of Psychiatry 152(8):1111–1123

Sham P, Jones P, Russell A et al 1995 Aged onset, sex and familial psychiatric morbidity in schizophrenia. British Journal of Psychiatry

Sherman P, Porter R 1991 Mental health consumers as case manager aides. Hospital and Community Psychiatry 42(5):494–498

Smith T, Bellack A, Lieberman R 1996 Social skills training for schizophrenia: review and future directions. Clinical Psychology Review 16(7):599–617

Solomon P 1996 Moving from psycho-education to family education for families of adults with serious mental illness. Psychiatric Services 47(12):1364–1370

Stein L, Test M 1980 Alternative to mental hospital treatment. Archives of General Psychiatry 37(4):392–397

Susser E, Lin S 1992 Schizophrenia after prenatal exposure to the Dutch hunger winter of 1994/1995. Archives of General Psychiatry 49:983–988

Swanson J, Holzer C, Ganju V 1990 Violence and psychiatric disorder in the community: evidence from the epidemiological catchment area survey. Hospital and Community Psychiatry 41:761–770

Tarrier N, Barraclough C, Vaughn C et al 1988 The community management of schizophrenia: a controlled trial of a behavioural intervention with families to reduce relapse. British Journal of Psychiatry 153:532–542

Turner G 1993 Depot medication. In: Brooker C, White E (eds) Community psychiatric nursing research, vol 2. Chapman and Hall, London

Van Horne J, MacManus I 1992 Ventricular enlargement in schizophrenia. British Journal of Psychiatry 16:687–697

Zubin J, Spring B 1977 Vulnerability: a new view of schizophrenia. Journal of Abnormal Psychology 86:260–266

CHAPTER CONTENTS

Key points 165

Introduction 166

The concept of affective disorder 166

The continuum of affective disorders 168
Main presenting symptoms and epidemiology
168
Prognosis and outcome 169
Suicide and parasuicide 169
Aetiological theories 171
Treatment approaches 176
The role of self-management in depression and
mania 178

The current role of the mental health nurse 179
The therapeutic relationship 179
Early warning signs 180
The promotion of psycho-education and self-
management 181
Suicide prevention strategies 181

The future role of the nurse 182

Exercise 182

Key texts for further reading 183

References 183

10

Disorders of mood: depression and mania

Robert Gareth Hill   Geoff Shepherd

KEY POINTS

- Disorders of mood cover a spectrum from minor emotional disturbances (mixed anxiety/depression) which are common and generally transient, through to profound emotional disturbances ('psychotic' depression/manic–depressive disorders) which are less common, but may be persistent and/or recurrent, and have major effects on other aspects of social and psychological functioning.

- Most mood disorders have some kind of biological 'substrate' (i.e. physical manifestations) which probably reflects genetic vulnerability. There is therefore usually a role for medication in symptomatic treatment (except in the most transient cases).

- The timing, impact, course and outcome of mood disorders are shaped by psychological and social factors such as life events (loss, social support), coping ability, quality of social supports and opportunities for social re-integration through work.

KEY POINTS (*contd*)

- Effective treatment and management must take into account these biological, psychological and social factors and attempt to deliver a comprehensive 'package' of care which will not only provide effective symptom relief but will also contain a range of psychological and social interventions to improve maintenance and prevent (or at least postpone) relapse.

- Research evidence is now beginning to appear on the prodromal signs in bi-polar disorder and factors associated with relapse in severe depression.

- The more serious forms of depression carry a high risk of suicide. The factors generally associated with increased risk are well known and there should be systems in place to identify those at highest risk and ensure close monitoring.

- Nursing staff have a key role to play in detection, early treatment and management of mood disorders. They have an especially important contribution to make in terms of the provision of information, encouraging self-management, help with social problems, risk identification and management.

INTRODUCTION

Psychotic depression and bi-polar disorder (manic–depression) are separate, but related, forms of affective disorder. Both are often persistent and recurrent in nature and should be viewed as *potentially* chronic conditions (Thase 1993). The central feature of these disorders is an abnormality of mood.

It is the aim of this chapter to provide an up-to-date, research-based account of these conditions as they present in adults aged 18 to 65. Specifically, we will:

- introduce the concept of affective disorder and describe the continuum of mood changes
- examine the main symptoms of these disorders and their epidemiology
- outline current theories of causation
- describe the impact on social and occupational functioning
- discuss the main types of treatment currently on offer and their effectiveness
- discuss the role of the mental health nurse both in the hospital and the community.

We hope to provide sufficient detail to enable the mental health nurse (and other relevant professionals) to recognise these disorders accurately and improve their management approaches in both hospital and community settings.

THE CONCEPT OF AFFECTIVE DISORDER

The concept of affective disorder owes its origins to Kraeplin who introduced the category of 'manic–depressive psychosis'. More recently, a separation was proposed into a 'bi-polar group' (depressed patients with a history of manic episodes) and a 'unipolar group' (patients with depressive episodes only). Cassano et al (1994) note that approximately 15 to 20% of individuals suffering from psychotic depression fall within the bi-polar disorder group and the remaining 80 to 85% within the unipolar group. There are therefore good reasons to distinguish between 'bi-polar' disorder and severe depressive or psychotic disorder, although it is important to note that the depressive episodes in bi-polar disorder are generally indistinguishable from episodes of unipolar depression (Bond & Lader 1996). Before

Table 10.1   The continuum of mood disorders

	'Mixed' anxiety and depressive disorder	'Mild to moderate' depression	'Psychotic' depression/bi-polar disorders
Main presenting symptoms	• mixed anxiety and depression • good social functioning • often transient (< 6 mths) • may be 'masked' by physical symptoms • onset often linked to ongoing social stress or 'loss' life event	• persistent lowered mood • sleep disturbance (usually initial insomnia) • reduced energy • impaired concentration • recurrent intrusive thoughts • reduced libido • social functioning may be affected • onset often linked to ongoing social stress or 'loss' life event	• persistent lowered (and/or periodically elevated) mood • sleep disturbance (usually early morning waking) • impaired concentration • reduced appetite (may be life threatening) • depressive delusional thinking • reduced libido • social functioning profoundly affected • relationship between onset and life events
Epidemiology (lifetime risk)	not available	5–10%	0.5–1.5%
Where likely to present?	primary health care (GP)	specialist psychiatric out-patients	in-patient
Pharmacological treatments	• nothing • antidepressants (particularly SSRIs)	• antidepressants (preferably combined with CBT)	• antidepressants • antipsychotics • ECT
Psychological treatments	• bried, focused counselling (providing a psychological model for distress) • self-help • education/information	• CBT (combined with medication to prevent relapse) • relationship interventions (IPT- or EE-based) to improve quality of social support • self-help • education/information	• self-help • education/information • 'early signs' monitoring • self-management
Social management	• practical help to relieve social or interpersonal stresses (e.g. housing/financial/work problems)	• practical help (housing, work, money) • special importance of work and occupation	• practical help (housing, work, money) • special importance of work and occupation
Role of community mental health nurse	• brief counselling • addressing practical problems	• providing CBT-, IPT- or EE-based interventions if trained • addressing practical problems • providing information on medication and other treatments	• early diagnosis • risk assessment and management • liaison with prescribing doctor, GP or psychiatrist • providing information on medication and other treatments • encouraging 'early signs' monitoring and self-management

CBT, cognitive–behaviour therapy; EE, expressed emotion; IPT, interpersonal therapy; SSRI, selective serotonin reuptake inhibitor.

we consider these disorders in more detail, it may be helpful to differentiate *severe* mood disorders from less severe and 'mixed' affective disorders and neurotic depression. These are set out in Table 10.1.

THE CONTINUUM OF AFFECTIVE DISORDERS

It is clear from Table 10.1 that psychotic depression and bi-polar disorder have the most serious symptomatic and social consequences. In the most severe cases, individuals may require hospitalisation and the social effects of the disorders tend to occur over a longer period. Of particular importance in this respect are the effects upon self-esteem, confidence and work prospects (see pp 172–176).

Main presenting symptoms and epidemiology

Bi-polar disorder

Bi-polar disorder is a recurrent, episodic, long-term illness which tends to have a number of negative effects for the sufferer, family members and society as a whole (Lish et al 1994). The disorder can be divided into two distinct types: bi-polar I and bi-polar II. Manic episodes interspersed with depressive episodes are referred to as bi-polar I; depressive disorder with hypomania, as bi-polar II (Vieta et al 1997). The data on such a separation are by no means clear cut (Coryell & Winokur, 1992) although Keller (1989) recommends the separation of bi-polar I patients from bi-polar II patients for purposes of clinical practice and research. There have also been attempts to introduce 'bi-polar III' as a separate category for those individuals who experience antidepressant-induced mania (Klerman 1981).

Bi-polar I disorder is generally recurrent in nature, with well over two-thirds of patients having repeat manic episodes. These tend to decrease as the individual gets older. Mood lability and functional difficulties are seen in 20 to 30% of people between episodes of bi-polar I disorders and in around 15% of those with bi-polar II disorders. Bi-polar II disorders with rapid 'cycling' (i.e. four or more episodes per year) have a particularly poor prognosis and this presentation accounts for 13 to 20% of bi-polar patients (Healy & McKeon 1997).

The clinical features of mania are euphoria and/or irritability; overactivity; distractibility; socially inappropriate behaviour; reduced sleep; increased appetite and libido; flight of ideas; expansive ideas; grandiose delusions; hallucinations and impaired insight. The disorder usually manifests itself between the ages of 20 and 25 and is equally distributed between men and women.

In terms of the epidemiology of the disorder, it is important to note that in the case of major affective disorders 'the fundamental statistic of epidemiology, frequency of a defined condition in a defined population, is hard to capture with precision and assurance in the field of affective illness' (Rawnsley, 1982:129). This is due in part to the dependence upon the classification system used and the conceptual standpoint adopted.

In the USA, the National Institute of Mental Health (NIMH) figures for 1-year prevalence rates are 1.2% for bi-polar I and bi-polar II disorders combined (Regier et al 1993). Lifetime risk is estimated at between 1 and 2%. In the UK, the National Psychiatric Morbidity Survey (Meltzer et al 1995) found that 0.4% of adults in private households were suffering from a psychotic mood disorder or schizophrenia. However, as this study included more than one disorder under the label 'psychotic', it is difficult to assess the precise prevalence of bi-polar disorder. Notwithstanding this difficulty, it would appear that the prevalence of bi-polar disorder is higher in the USA than in the UK (see Zarate et al 1997). This may be due to a variety of factors including diagnostic or cultural differences and mode of presentation.

Psychotic depression

Severe depressive disorder (sometimes called 'psychotic depression') shares many features with neurotic depression, although obviously to a more severe degree. However, there are also a number of additional features which characterise psychotic depression, particularly delusional thinking (Gelder et al 1996). The main themes of such delusions are usually worthlessness, guilt, ill-health, poverty, nihilism and persecution. Sometimes auditory hallucinations (and rarely visual) will also occur. It is possible to differentiate the nature of the delusional thinking as either mood congruent (delusion based on thoughts of guilt, ruin, misery and repentance) or incongruous (delusion based on ideas of persecution, influence from external forces and poisoning). Cassano et al (1994) point out that many patients may be unaware of being ill. Loss of interest in eating (and in some cases drinking) can be a considerable problem and may be life-threatening, requiring early identification and prompt action.

The epidemiology of psychotic depression in the UK is far from clear or consistent, again because of difficulties with clinical definition and classificatory status (Parker et al 1997). In the USA, the NIMH study suggests a 1-year prevalence rate for severe depression of around 5% (Regier et al 1993) and it is estimated that in the USA, psychotic depression accounts for 25% of hospitalised cases of depression. Lifetime risk of major depression is between 10 and 25% for women and 5 and 12% for men, with an average age of onset in the mid-20s (American Psychiatric Association 1994a).

Prognosis and outcome

Bi-polar disorder

Bi-polar disorder is a recurrent condition with over 90% of individuals having repeated manic episodes, but the frequency of episodes generally declines as individuals grow older. Hypomania occurs in 60 to 70% of bi-polar II patients after a major depressive episode. It also has high levels of relapse (42 to 55% in 1 year). Mood lability/functional disabilities are seen in 20 to 30% bi-polar I and in 15% bi-polar II individuals and there can be high levels of psychosocial impairment. High rates of alcohol abuse/dependence are not uncommon and high levels of non-compliance with medication are also frequently reported. Both these factors tend to be associated with poor outcomes. There is a high suicide risk, particularly amongst bi-polar II patients and the mortality rate is two to three times greater than in the general population. There is some limited research to suggest that there is a 2- to 4-week prodromal period and 'early signs' of relapse include increased motor activity, bizarre thoughts and disrupted sleep pattern.

Psychotic depression

Psychotic depression has a more variable course. The number of previous episodes is the strongest predictor of future episodes. Symptoms tend to stabilise through subsequent episodes. Onset tends to be associated with negative life events and frequently leads to hospitalisation. There may be high levels of psychosocial impairment. There is a high risk of suicide (15%), particularly if there have been previous suicide attempts. Other risk factors for suicide include male sex, being single, living alone and older age (female). Outcome tends to be worst if associated with an underlying chronic anxiety disorder, substance abuse, or poor quality close, social relationships (e.g. with partner or spouse).

Suicide and parasuicide

One of the targets of *The Health of the Nation*

(Department of Health 1994) is to reduce the suicide rate of severely mentally ill people by at least one-third by the year 2000. This would reduce rates from an estimate of 15% in 1990 to no more than 10%. Although suicide or parasuicide is not a presenting 'symptom' of either psychotic depression or bi-polar disorder, there is a clear association and the lifetime completion rate of suicide for all forms of affective disorder varies between 15 and 19% (Goodwin & Jamison 1990, Guze & Robins 1970). This amounts to an approximately 30-fold excess risk compared with the general population (Hawton 1992). For bi-polar disorders the risk appears to be greatest relatively early on in the illness. For example, Johnson & Hunt (1979) found that the median time between onset of illness and suicide attempt was 5.5 years, with males more likely to attempt suicide early after illness onset. Isometsä et al (1994) also suggest that suicides are more likely to occur early in the illness and emphasise the association with alcohol dependence. While suicides are common during the depressed phase of the illness, there is also a raised likelihood of risk-taking behaviour in the manic phase, particularly if it remains untreated.

In a study of members of a national, self-help group (the Manic Depression Fellowship – MDF) Hill et al (1996) found that 47% of respondents reported at least one suicide attempt. Alcohol abuse, a family history of manic depression and female gender all contributed to a significantly enhanced risk. As indicated, this is consistent with previous research.

Clearly not all cases of parasuicide can be seen as deliberate and determined attempts at death (Bancroft et al 1979). It is estimated that only 1% of parasuicides will go on to kill themselves in 1 year (Hawton & Catalan 1987, MacLeod et al 1992). However, a Danish study of attempted suicides found that about 10% do go on to kill themselves within a 5-year period (Nielsen et al

1990). It is also important to note that a high proportion of individuals who go on to kill themselves will have been in contact with health professionals shortly before their death. Thus, in the Nielsen et al study, 75% of suicides were committed less than 6 months after the last contact with the psychiatric ward. Similarly, Bancroft et al (1977) found that 30% of all suicides and parasuicides visited a primary care physician in the month prior to their attempt. Suicide and deliberate self-harm are discussed in detail in Chapter 11.

Psychotic depression

The risk of suicide in psychotic depression is estimated at between 11 and 17% (Black et al 1987, Pitts & Winokur 1964) with no difference between endogenous and non-endogenous sub-types. Thus, it carries a fairly similar risk to that of bi-polar disorder. The Royal College of Psychiatrists in their 'Defeat Depression' campaign noted that depression is a major factor in the estimated 4000 suicides in the UK each year.

The most important risk factor for suicide is a diagnosis of depression combined with a previous history of attempted suicide (Goldstein et al 1991). The highest risk remains in untreated depression (Isometsä et al 1994). Other factors associated with risk are insomnia, self-neglect, impaired memory, hopelessness, loss of pleasure and mood cycling, male sex, older age (females), history of suicide attempts, being single and living alone. It is also important to note that suicide among in-patients is also common (Hawton 1978).

The assessment of suicide risk is not an exact science. As the Health Advisory Service (1994) noted, risk factors tend to predict risk in the long term, rather than in the immediate future. Risk factors are also more useful in highlighting risk in groups, rather than in making predictions about individuals. However, they should still represent an important element in routine clinical assessment and nurses, GPs and other health professionals need to 'manage' individuals at high risk of self-harm in a more informed and effective manner (see pp 181–182).

Aetiological theories

Major affective disorders are, like other psychoses, complex conditions with biological, psychological and social causes. A 'bio-psychosocial' model of aetiology (and treatment) is therefore required. No one explanation can account for all the evidence on its own and different explanations may address the same phenomena (e.g. depressive delusions) at different 'levels' (e.g. biological vs psychological). A working knowledge and acceptance of a number of theoretical explanations are therefore necessary.

Biological and genetic explanations

Bi-polar disorder is recognised to have, at least partly, a partial genetic cause. Reich (1995:3) notes that, 'classical population, family, twin, and adoption studies, when combined, support the hypothesis that genetic susceptibility genes are important determinants of bi-polar disorder.' There have been numerous studies of physiological correlates of bi-polar disorder, including neuroendocrine functioning, neuropeptides, sleep studies and changes in circadian rhythm. (See McFarland et al (1997) for a summary of this research in relation to nursing.) Much of this detailed research lies outside the practical, day-to-day demands of nursing staff. Nevertheless, it is important for nurses to be aware of the general direction, if for no other reason than that some patients (particularly those who belong to specialised self-help groups) may be specifically interested and knowledgeable in this area.

Psychological theories

While there are a number of psychological theories (e.g. psycho-analytic and psychodynamic theories, cognitive theories and learned helplessness theory) that attempt to explain the cause of bi-polar disorder, most focus on the depressive side of the illness. Psychological explanations of mania remain weak.

Psycho-analytic and psychodynamic theories. Traditional psycho-analytic explanations tend to treat depression and mania as separate entities, regarding mania as a 'defence' against depression. Thus, Freud viewed depression as resembling the process of mourning and suggested that depressed patients have regressed to an earlier developmental stage (the oral phase). Lund (1997:26) suggests that psychodynamic approaches are 'rarely, if ever, the single mode of treatment for a manic depressive' although they may be useful as part of an overall management strategy.

Cognitive theories. Cognitive theories have tended to focus almost exclusively on the depressive side of bi-polar illness. For instance, Beck (1976) suggests that depression occurs because individuals have dysfunctional attitudes towards the world resulting in automatic thoughts that distort their perceptions. A number of logical errors can occur such as arbitrary inference, all-or-nothing thinking, over-generalisation and selective abstraction. Such errors increase the frequency of automatic negative thoughts, leading to depression. Similarly, Gelder et al (1996:219) note 'depressive cognitions are associated with negative biases in information processing'. What is not clear is whether such biases are cause or effect (although if psychological treatment is effective, perhaps it does not matter).

Learned helplessness. Seligman (1975) has suggested that individuals, faced with negative life events that they cannot control, literally 'learn' how to be helpless. The problem with the theory is that it does not provide a sufficient explanation as to why certain individuals are more likely to be affected. For example, Frankl (1959) observed that those who coped best with arbitrary punishment and abuse in the Nazi concentration camps had a strong sense of meaning or purpose in their lives. Perhaps 'learned helplessness' may therefore be mediated by certain personality factors. As indicated, it is also possible that there are differences in terms of genetic susceptibility.

Life events

Brown & Harris (1978) have shown the triggering effects of life events – mainly those involving loss – in relation to depressive disorders and it has been suggested that life events affect both severe depression and bi-polar disorder (Ellicott et al 1990, Hunt et al 1992). Furthermore, there seems to be more of an effect on first episodes (Post 1992). However, there are also data which do not support any connection. For example, Pardoen et al (1996:160) found no clear association between life events and the onset of recurrent depressive episodes and they conclude that 'the causal association between life events and the onset of depression, shown to be relevant in non-chronically depressed subjects, does not apply in chronic affective disorders.' While the connection between life events and depression is stronger than that for bi-polar disorder (Paykel 1994), one therefore has to agree with Sclare & Creed (1990) that definitive data have yet to be produced.

Pardoen et al also found that the quality of ongoing close personal relationships had an impact on the onset of recurrent hypomanic and manic episodes and this is consistent with Hooley et al (1986) who found that patients with a severe depressive disorder relapsed at lower levels of criticism (high 'expressed emotion')

compared with people with schizophrenic symptoms.

To summarise, this brief overview highlights the contribution of biological and genetic processes, interpersonal stressors and external life events in the course and outcome of major depressive disorders. In the current situation, where the contribution of each area seems to be important, a multifaceted approach is therefore necessary.

The social effects

We will now examine the social and occupational impact of severe depressive disorders in more detail. There is clear evidence that psychotic depression and bi-polar disorder have a negative impact upon the individual's quality of life. Moreover, the negative effects on self-esteem and confidence do not necessarily disappear even when the symptoms are in remission. In this section, we will report on a large postal study of the MDF (Hill et al 1996) in which we surveyed over a thousand individuals with reported manic–depression. The questionnaire data were supplemented by focus group discussions.

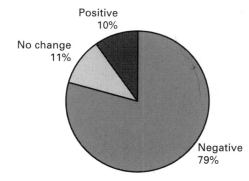

Figure 10.1 Work and work prospects since illness onset (n = 1367).

Work and occupation. Scott (1995:581) notes that 'it is estimated that an adult developing bi-polar disorder in his/her mid-20s loses on average '9 years of life, 12 years of normal health and 14 years of work activity.' In our study we found that nearly 80% of individuals reported a 'slight' or 'very' negative impact on their work or work prospects since the onset of the illness (Fig. 10.1). This was in the context of a highly educated group (47% had 'A' levels, 37% a first degree and 14% were postgraduates).

Of those individuals not currently working, 83% thought their illness had played a part. There was a significant difference between males and females with men more likely to judge that the illness had affected their work prospects than women. There were a number of significant differences at the 5% level between those currently in work and those who were unemployed (Table 10.2).

Table 10.2 Summary of significant differences by employment status

	% Employed (n)	% Unemployed (n)
Women	56 (260)	45 (177)
Married/stable relationship	51 (235)	21 (82)
With occupational qualifications	57 (255)	35 (127)
Attempted suicide	38 (176)	53 (205)
Stopped by the police	31 (139)	53 (204)
Problems with alcohol	17 (78)	23 (89)
Problems with drugs	5 (24)	10 (39)
'Totally' self-manage the illness	24 (71)	10 (22)
Admitted to psychiatric hospital	84 (387)	92 (354)
Admitted to hospital once	19 (74)	13 (46)
Admitted under section	46 (177)	58 (205)
Admitted in the past 2 years	33 (123)	58 (186)

As can be seen in Table 10.2, those currently in work were more likely to be women, married or in a stable relationship and were more likely to have occupational qualifications. Those who were currently employed were *less* likely to have had problems with alcohol or drugs, to have been stopped by the police during a period of their illness, or to have attempted suicide.

Although only a small number of the overall sample had not been admitted to hospital, those in work were less likely to be in this category. They were also less likely to have been admitted under a section of the Mental Health Act.

In the focus groups, individuals spoke of work as important in order to avoid certain negative experiences: 'I've done some pretty grotty jobs … part of my motivation was always to remain in work, everything else had been taken away from me … if I had lost work I would have disappeared from the face of the earth'.

A minority saw work as a positive factor in itself: 'For some of us work was therapeutic, my problems were not in the job, but in the home, I love working.' However, for most people it was not work itself that was important, but having something meaningful to do. As one person said, 'I'm quite happy and contented now because I'm doing what I want … I have no desire to work for someone. Financially I'm all right, if I had worries, my views may be different.' For many, work remained an economic necessity. Both men and women recognised there was more stigma for men in not working: 'I thought I would kill myself if I couldn't work' (male); 'I've accepted I can't work' (female). Many of the participants had also experienced profound problems surrounding the issue of whether or not to disclose their mental health history to prospective employers. As one person said: 'As we all know, to return to a job after even 2 years history of mental illness is virtually impossible, unless you tell lies or evade leading questions.' Most individuals felt uncomfortable about lying on application forms, not only because of possible future legal consequences, but also because of the added pressure of having to hide their illness.

A related issue regarding work concerned the inflexibility of the current Department of Social Security (DSS) benefit regulations with regard to part-time or voluntary work. One individual, who approached the DSS in order to undertake some local invigilating of exams, reported that the delay was so great that the exams were over before a decision was made! This inflexibility, both in terms of what is permissible and in terms of speed of decisions, was not an isolated example.

Once in work, most people recognised that there would be periods of difficulty both for themselves and for the employer during episodes of illness. However, few employers seemed willing (or able) to meet the challenge of employing someone with a major mental health problem. Most individuals knew that it was 'difficult to carry on as if nothing was happening'; one person put it like this, 'It's a problem of concentration, sometimes I can't think rationally. In most jobs you have to communicate, with manic–depression it can be difficult for other people and for yourself ... I couldn't hold a conversation.'

For others, the problem was not the work itself, but the attitudes of employers and workmates. One individual in a senior, professional job stated that: 'Although I was kept on at the same rate as before, I was made to feel the inferior member of the department.' Another had to write down every task she performed on a daily basis and explain any discrepancy between her daily timings. She said that this 'took all my confidence and enjoyment away'. A few employers were helpful in keeping jobs open and being supportive, but not many. For some, work simply proved too much: 'I was completely incapable of fulfilling my role. My psychiatrist said keep plodding away, but it just got worse and worse.' Another stated: 'I've returned to work a good few times and kept becoming ill through pushing myself.'

In general, there was therefore a sense of pessimism about the impact of the illness upon the person's ability to work and also regarding the attitudes of employers. The majority of respondents felt that the problems could be explained by the attitude of employers – and sometimes employees – towards people with mental illness and the inflexibility of the benefits system which made partial return to work very difficult. Such comments clearly reflect the experiences of a large number of people with manic–depression and, while we have no data on individuals with psychotic depression only, there is no reason to believe that the issues raised would be different.

Work is an important activity in all our lives and the deleterious effects of unemployment on mental health are now well documented (Warr 1987). There is also an increasing recognition of the role that supportive work schemes can play (Nehring et al 1993, Pozner et al 1996) although, as Fulford (1997) notes, there is still a long way to go. The importance of work for people with major mental illness therefore needs to be clearly understood by practitioners and unambiguously communicated to purchasers and commissioners. Employers must also be helped to take a more positive role and encouraged to exploit, rather than ignore, a large pool of skilled and motivated workers.

Self-esteem and confidence. The impact of manic–depression on self-esteem and confidence is of central importance. In our study, 71% assessed the impact as overwhelmingly negative, a minority (20%) assessed the impact as positive and a further 9% reported no change (Fig. 10.2).

On the negative side, one person talked about the 'dramatic change, which comes out of the blue'. It was recognised that self-esteem was also tied up with general social attitudes towards the mentally ill. As one person stated: 'People have no knowledge of mental illness and are not equipped to deal with what is going to be difficult anyway ... There is also loss of self-esteem in realising you have a mental illness.

This ties into a society that stigmatises mental illness.' Positive self-esteem appeared to come about through a process of acceptance and social support. One person stated: 'When first diagnosed, it's negative; if you then take positive action, it is possible to increase self-esteem/confidence ... Being open and honest myself has been of great help.'

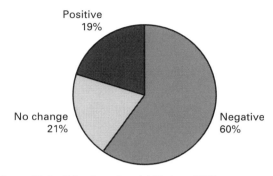

Figure 10.3   Friends and social life (n = 1399).

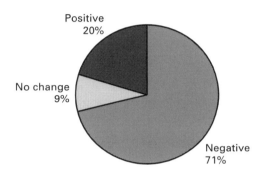

Figure 10.2   Self-esteem and confidence (n = 1408).

The loss of a sense of personal control was obviously central to people's experiences. Almost half of the survey did not seek help of their own volition first when they became ill, but rather as a result of pressure from family and friends. Moreover, more than half the respondents had been admitted to hospital under a section of the Mental Health Act and a substantial proportion (38%) had been questioned or detained by the police during a period of their illness. It is easy to see how such experiences would affect an individual's sense of being 'in control' and underlies the importance of attempts to combat this through various self-management techniques.

Friends and social life. The majority of respondents viewed the impact on friends and social life to be negative (60%), although 40% saw it as positive or neutral. This can be seen in Figure 10.3.

In the focus groups a number of themes emerged such as the difficulty of making commitments owing to the illness, the alienating effects of mania, over-protection by friends ('I don't want to be questioned every time I crack a joke'), the lack of anything in common with contemporaries, the temptation to socialise only with manic–depression sufferers, and the fact that some people had to change their social life in order to cope with their illness.

As with the question of self-esteem, there was a recognition that a diminished circle of friends or social life could result either from, 'a moving away by other people, or a moving away yourself'. There was a significant difference between men and women with regard to their social life, with women seeing their friends and social life as changing more positively than men since the onset of the illness. Many people felt that if there was some benefit from the illness, it was in terms of allowing them to find out who their *real* friends were and for this they were grateful. But stigma and ignorance still seemed to be central issues: 'Knowledge is the key thing. I took some friendships to the very edge; they have been restored because we know what the illness is. When you are struggling around in the dark, friendships break up.'

It is a truism to state that what individuals with manic–depression want is a better quality of life. Like anyone else, they would like an increase in their self-esteem and confidence, to have improved relationships with their family, better friendships and social life, and to be given the opportunity for work. These are completely understandable desires, but are very difficult to realise. For many individuals with serious depression, their quality of life tends to deteriorate over time (Welner et al 1977). Doing something about this, by intervening early to promote positive attitudes, better relationships and less disrupted work patterns must therefore be central to the better management of the disorder.

Treatment approaches

As indicated in Table 10.1, people with bi-polar disorder and psychotic depression are most likely to receive some treatment within a hospital setting. Other forms of treatment will almost inevitably occur in the community, with involvement from the primary care team and possibly a community psychiatric nurse (CPN) or psychologist. There is also likely to be some specialist care from a consultant psychiatrist. In the MDF survey cited earlier these professionals, psychiatrists, CPNs and GPs were rated as very helpful by about half of the sample. Psychologists and psychotherapists were rated by far fewer people and were rated as less useful (Fig. 10.4).

Individuals generally spoke very positively of the supportive relationships they had developed with their CPN, although some felt that they were not always readily available, especially in a crisis. Some noted that they tended to deal with more minor illnesses. Friends and relatives also noted the positive benefits of CPNs in terms of practical help, their ability to communicate in everyday language and the frequency of visits. The CPN, while being a relatively scarce resource, thus clearly has a central role to play for both individuals with bi-polar disorder and their friends and relatives.

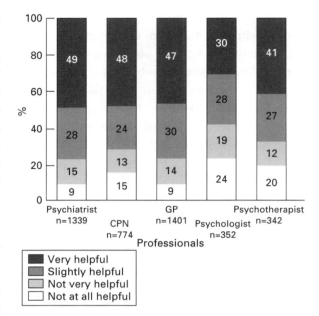

Figure 10.4 Helpfulness of professionals.

Pharmacological treatments

Supervision of medication is one of the key roles for CPNs. Lithium is probably the most widely used drug in the treatment of bi-polar disorder and is effective in terms of both treatment and prevention (American Psychiatric Association 1994b). It protects about 25 to 50% of individuals from further episodes and is effective in preventing relapse in both mania and major episodes of depression (Goodwin & Jamison 1990). Side-effects are common and lithium levels need to be regularly monitored because of the dangers of toxicity (Jefferson et al 1987). Toxic levels are uncomfortably close to the therapeutic dose. Side-effects of lithium can be neurological (tremor), gastrointestinal (nausea, diarrhoea), renal (polyuria, polydipsia), thyroid function (goitre, hypothyroidism) and weight gain (Bond & Lader 1996).

Carbamazepine is also used as a mood-stabilising treatment, both in the treatment of acute mania and acute bi-polar depression, although it is not formally licensed for this indication because of lack of systematic data (Bond & Lader 1996). As with lithium, there is a high risk of side-effects and potentially serious adverse reactions. Toxicity also needs to be closely monitored, since carbamazepine may be fatal in overdose.

Antidepressant medication is almost always indicated for individuals with moderate to severe depression. Tricyclic antidepressants are generally the first choice for patients with severe depression (Potter et al 1991) while selective serotonin reuptake inhibitors are administered where tricylics are contra-indicated because of their anticholinergic side-effects or because of pre-existing cardiac disease (Gelder et al 1996). Where there is a psychotic element to the depressive disorder, an antipsychotic drug such as chlorpromazine or risperidone may be given as well.

Medication compliance. Medication compliance is seen as a major issue in the management of bi-polar disorder and thus identifying and prescribing the appropriate drug are only the start of the pharmacological approach to treating the illness; clearly, patients also have to take the medication. Scott (1995) and Jamison & Akiskal (1983) report non-compliance rates of 25 to 50% and this may be a particular problem for those individuals who miss their 'highs'.

The reasons underlying non-compliance vary. Clearly the fact that 75% of patients on lithium report one or more side-effects must be an important factor (Goodwin & Jamison 1990). However, this is not the only explanation. Concern about not wanting mood to be controlled and the attitudes of significant others may also play a part.

There is some evidence that psycho-education programmes can improve medication. For example, Cochran (1984) found that patients in a cognitive–behaviour therapy (CBT) programme were less likely to be rated as having major problems with compliance and less likely to terminate lithium against medical advice, or to suffer an episode of illness precipitated by non-compliance, than were control patients.

The role of electroconvulsive therapy. Electroconvulsive therapy (ECT) is used for patients with either bi-polar disorder or psychotic depression. ECT generally is given on an in-patient basis, since the severity of the condition generally warrants hospitalisation and it is easier to monitor fasting before anaesthesia.

There are a number of well-controlled trials indicating the effectiveness of ECT in severe depression (Janicak et al 1985) and some evidence for its superiority over antidepressant drug medication (Paykel 1989). Moreover, two studies have suggested the superiority of ECT for individuals with psychotic depression over both tricyclic antidepressants and antipsychotic medication (Perry et al 1982, Spiker et al 1985).

ECT has also been widely used in the control of mania and found to be effective in individuals who did not respond to antipsychotic medication (Mukherjee et al 1988). ECT has been shown to be particularly effective in the treatment of acute mania with an overall response rate of 80% (Mukherjee et al 1994). Thus Rasmussen & Hallstrom (1997:114) note that 'ECT may give the most rapid control of the most severe and psychotic episodes of either the manic or the depressive phases of the disease'. Despite such findings, ECT remains a controversial treatment, mainly because of the unwanted effects after the treatment, including short-term memory loss which means that despite its proven efficacy, it may not be acceptable to some individuals.

Psychological treatments. In one sense the effectiveness of drug treatments and ECT has limited research into other approaches for dealing with bi-polar disorder and severe depression. However, in the last few years, there appears to have been something of a cultural mood change, with individuals becoming far more interested and accepting of psychological approaches to the treatment and management of their illness.

Scott (1995:586) in a review article on psychological treatments for bi-polar disorder notes that 'the paucity of psychosocial research in bi-polar disorder has many parallels with the situation regarding schizophrenia 20 years ago.' She notes the finding by Bloch et al (1994) that 25 to 30% of the prognostic variance in bi-polar disorder is due to psychosocial factors and that, 'even under optimal research conditions, prophylaxis will protect fewer than 50% of patients against further episodes' (Scott 1995:581). As already noted, there is some research which suggests that combining lithium with CBT is more effective than just lithium on its own (Cochran 1984). Scott (1996:17) states that 'if CT is to be used with bi-polar disorder, a cognitive profile of these individuals will also be needed.' Jenaway & O'Leary (1997) suggest three potential (as yet unproved) benefits from using a CBT approach:

1. to shorten or lessen the severity of each manic or depressive episode
2. to prevent the development of further episodes
3. to modify other aspects of the patient's life which are causing problems. These potential benefits wait to be further explored.

While the majority of work using CBT has been with non-psychotic forms of depression, work is starting to appear dealing with more severe forms of the illness (Birchwood et al 1993). There is also some evidence for the efficacy of psychological interventions with delusions (Garety et al 1994). Such work is encouraging and while there is no suggestion that such interventions could entirely replace pharmacological treatments, they may well prove a useful, and in the future, routine adjunct.

The role of self-management in depression and mania

Although they may be knowledgeable about the signs and symptoms of a disorder, professionals usually lack insight into what it feels to experience the condition from the inside. Over the years, a number of writers and film makers have attempted to capture the experience of bi-polar illness. For example, John Custance's *Wisdom, Madness and Folly* (1951), David Wigoder's *Images of Destruction* (1987), Kay Redfield Jamison's *An Unquiet Mind* (1995) and the recent film *Mr Jones*. Out of such work there has grown up models of 'self-management' which have become increasingly popular as part of the self-help movement. The majority of work in this area has related to bi-polar disorder, as opposed to psychotic depression, and its popularisation is due in large part to the efforts of organisations like the Manic Depression Fellowship.

The term 'self-management' does not refer to one specific intervention, nor does it necessarily imply that individuals works entirely on their own. David Guiness of the MDF describes self-management as 'a process of taking increasing responsibility for your health. It entails learning about the illness and developing the skills to recognise and control mood swings. It is about taking charge and finding out what you can do to help your condition' (Guiness 1997:165). Thus, self-management can occur alongside both pharmacological and psychological treatments.

The following are all recognised forms of self-management:

- *self-medication* – in which individuals, in consultation with their doctor, agree the extent to which their drug dosage can be used flexibly

- *self-monitoring of mood* – through the keeping of diaries or using specific work logs of the type developed by Copeland (1992)
- *education* – and recording of illness 'triggers' and early signs of relapse (McKeon 1992).

Currently, there is little evidence to assess the effectiveness of self-management programmes. Survey data (e.g. Hill et al 1996) suggest that individuals who practise active self-management are less likely to have been admitted to hospital in the last 2 years, less likely to have negative self-esteem/confidence, and less likely to have attempted suicide, than those who self-manage less often. Intriguingly, these data also suggested that individuals who never self-managed had better outcomes than those who self-managed occasionally. We do not know if this is a simple reflection of less severe disorders. Those who regularly self-managed were also slightly older and were likely to have had their diagnosis for longer. While these results are tentative, they do highlight the possibility that self-management may be able to contribute to a better outcome. A randomised controlled trial of unselected individuals would now be extremely valuable.

Most work on self-management has been related to bi-polar disorder, but some attempt has also been made to specify a self-help programme for individuals with severe depression (Barker 1992). In this, Barker provides an outline guide to take individuals through the stages of examination, reflection and action. At the heart is a cognitive approach to depression, focusing on current and alternative constructions of the world. Usefully, Barker has ensured that the guide has been written at a level that 'acknowledges the motivational and cognitive deficits commonly shown by people who are depressed' (Barker

1992:181). It would be useful to evaluate this guide since it is one of the few UK self-help programmes which specifically focuses on severe depression.

THE CURRENT ROLE OF THE MENTAL HEALTH NURSE

To summarise, there are three areas where the role of the nurse is particularly (although clearly not exclusively) important:

1. the identification of early warning signs
2. psycho-educational strategies, including self-management
3. the identification and prevention of suicide.
   Underlying all of these areas is the therapeutic relationship.

The therapeutic relationship

Establishing and maintaining a good therapeutic relationship is not, of course, unique to the care of people with severe affective disorder. There is now a considerable literature on enhancing such relationships in nursing (McFarland et al 1997) and some general principles need to be borne in mind:

- First, many patients who are seen on the ward will be involuntary. In the case of someone who is manic, incarceration in a hospital may seem like an unjustified restraint and therefore to be challenged. This is hardly a good basis for fostering a therapeutic relationship. The nurse needs to accept that in such cases the relationship will need to be worked on and that they may have to try particularly hard to be honest and professional in a situation where their structural 'power' may interfere with their therapeutic aims.
- Second, nurses need not only to be aware of

current theories regarding illness states, but they must also be prepared to share this knowledge with the patients. 'Empowerment' through knowledge is a central goal.

- Third, they must ensure that their social interventions enhance the medical treatment. Symptom control is generally only a means to an 'end'. The 'end' is usually improvements or restoration of social functioning (work, friends, family and relationships). The nurse must therefore always keep these social goals in mind, especially as they are likely to be of great importance to the patient.
- Fourth, therapeutic relationships should stress the ability of patients to guide and manage their own care. It is not simply the case that a therapeutic relationship consists of a nurse doing something for the patient; rather, the nurse should act as a facilitator, helping, encouraging, and 'empowering' the patient. This is particularly important when the patient is struggling to achieve some level of self-management.

These are some of the general therapeutic aims that nurses need to bear in mind, but there are also specific factors that they need to focus on, in order to maximise their effectiveness.

Early warning signs

Given the serious effects that may occur as a result of relapse in both bi-polar and unipolar disorders, it is vital that any prodromal signs (early signs of relapse) are systematically recorded. While the majority of work on early signs monitoring has occurred in relation to schizophrenia, one study has focused on unipolar depression (Kupfer et al 1989) and work is beginning to emerge on bi-polar disorder (Molnar et al 1988, Smith & Tarrier 1992). These studies suggest that the prodrome in depression is shorter (11 to 19 days) than the manic prodrome (21 to 29 days),

although as with the majority of such studies the range was large. Prodromal signs were found to be similar across episodes and identifiable by both patients and relatives. Perry et al (1995) reviewing these studies note that four main symptoms tended in different combinations to characterise the individual 'relapse signature' (Birchwood et al 1992). These are shown in Table 10.3.

Table 10.3 Characteristic signs of relapse

Onset prior to:	Examples of prodromal signs/symptoms
1. Manic relapse	Racing thoughts, decreased need for sleep
2. Depressive relapse	Loss of energy, not wanting to see people
3. Both manic and depressive relapse	Feeling irritable, poor concentration
4. Idiosyncratic	Particular to the patient

Perry et al outline a useful format for identifying prodromal signs, comprising an initial interview, identification of prodromes, action planning, training in symptom monitoring and a final consolidation session.

There is some evidence that the monitoring of prodromal signs is effective in preventing relapse in schizophrenia (Jolley et al 1990) and, based on this work, a number of considerations need to be borne in mind. Prodromal signs need to be monitored over a period of weeks, the process must be 'patient led' and the action plan needs to be clearly articulated. Staff must be aware of the identified procedures and what has been agreed in the event of signs and symptoms emerging. Underlying the approach is a process of differentiation, by which patients, staff and relatives can distinguish normal mood variation from prodromal signs. This work is potentially of major importance and is currently being evaluated in a large-scale study at the University of Manchester (Perry, personal communication).

In relation to the prevention of major depressive episodes, Falloon et al (1992) describe a pilot study of a clinical approach that combines targeted biomedical and psychosocial strategies to reduce the severity of depressive episodes. Central to this was the complete integration of mental health services into primary care teams. Although there do not seem to be specific prodromal signs for major depression 'many patients and their family members are able to recognise specific features that are the earliest manifestations of their impending illness' (Falloon et al 1992:55). Although this was not a controlled study, there were indications that such an approach may be of use in reducing the severity of depressive disorder. A formal trial would now be extremely valuable.

The promotion of psycho-education and self-management

Involvement in the monitoring of relapse in severe mood disorder can be seen as part of the nurse's wider role in promoting psycho-educational strategies. Central to the notion of psycho-education is the belief that the delivery of knowledge can have a positive effect upon behaviour and mental state. Psycho-education programmes can be aimed at both carers (friends and relatives) and at the individuals with affective disorders themselves. Much of the emphasis for psycho-education in the latter group is centred around the principles of self-management.

Nursing staff have a key role to play in supporting, educating and learning from friends and relatives who are involved in supporting the individual. Such a process needs to have the full backing and co-operation of all involved to succeed and needs to be part of a long-term management strategy. Because affective disorders can be long term and recurrent, it is important to give attention to managing such areas as work and occupation, as well as the long-term maintenance of social relationships. For family and friends this involves both understanding the nature and course of the illness and coming to terms with the possible limitations that this may impose upon their own life and relationships. Relatives may also need to recognise the importance of monitoring their own emotional reactions and reducing criticism and hostility (low expressed emotion) in order to promote positive mental health in the sufferer. The CPN's knowledge of intervention strategies, from cognitive therapy to self-medication, makes them useful educators in the different methods of self-management (Hill & Shepherd 1996).

Suicide prevention strategies

Nurses have a key role to play both in the hospital and in the community in the prevention of suicide. As we have already seen, the risk of suicide amongst in-patients is high and strategies for monitoring risk among individuals with affective disorders should be acknowledged in any care planning. By far the greatest risk factor known is previous suicide attempt. Other important factors (already noted) are:

- active depressive symptoms
- substance abuse
- clear communication of suicidal intent
- early parental loss
- male gender
- adolescence (males)
- old age (females)
- unemployment
- severe negative life-events.

Many individuals in the community are frequently in touch with health professionals before suicidal attempts and vigilance by nurses and other health care professionals is therefore required. The nurse obviously needs to be attentive to those signs and symptoms which are closely associated with a high suicide risk.

While it is undoubtedly the case that family members (including friends) are often best placed to pick up on changes in mental health or behaviour, they may not be familiar with some of the particular cues that can precipitate a suicide attempt. It is therefore an important part of the nurse's role to educate family and friends and to agree what action should be taken in the event that they are concerned. Many professionals remain reticent about acting on 'suspicions' of risk, but, in the case of suicide, leaving things too late may mean the difference between a problem and a tragedy. Such an educational strategy can also be employed with non-health professionals such as police and probation officers, local authority staff and residential care workers.

At its most general level, nurses also have a role to play in educating the public about the risk factors associated with suicide. There is still a stereotype that individuals who commit suicide are generally withdrawn and uncommunicative. This is often far from the case and it may be argued that the knowledge we have about risk factors needs to be communicated more widely throughout the community as part of health education programmes. Suicide prevention is potentially everyone's business and neighbours, church officials and non-health professionals often play a key role in supporting people with major mental health problems living in the community (Rose 1996). Risk assessment is examined further in Chapter 11.

THE FUTURE ROLE OF THE NURSE

Nurses are the largest single group working in the field of mental health and, as such, will con-

tinue to play a key role in the management of severe depression and mania in the future. However, nursing roles are likely to change in the direction of greater emphasis on specific technical skills and the ability to deliver interventions of known effectiveness (Butterworth 1994). Nurses will therefore have to learn new skills and ways of interacting with their clients. This chapter has highlighted some of the areas that advanced nurse practitioners will need to focus on. Those involved in the training and education of nurses must now take up the challenge to equip nurses with the necessary skills.

Exercise

The following quotes come from a survey conducted with almost 2000 members of the Manic Depression Fellowship, a national self-help organisation. Either individually or as a group consider the most appropriate way to respond to the concerns expressed. Consider how you would respond as a health professional and what, if anything, society could do to aid this process:

1. 'The mentally ill shouldn't feel there is a shutter brought down because of the illness. They may need work more than most.'
2. 'I thought I would kill myself if I couldn't work.'
3. 'There is a loss of self-esteem in realising you have a mental illness. This ties into a society that stigmatises mental illness.'
4. 'What's confusing for our partners is knowing that we don't always want to be treated the same. They see how you are today, and they have to decide how you want to be treated.'
5. 'Knowledge is the key thing. I took some friendships to the very edge; they have been restored, because we know what the illness is. When you are struggling around in the dark, friendships break up.'
6. 'I don't want to be questioned every time I crack a joke.'

KEY TEXTS FOR FURTHER READING

General guidelines
American Psychiatric Association 1994 Practice guideline for the treatment of patients with bi-polar disorder. Supplement to the American Journal of Psychiatry 151(12):1–36

Major texts
Goodwin F K, Jamison K R 1990 Manic–depressive illness. Oxford University Press, Oxford
Paykel E S (ed) 1992 Handbook of affective disorders, 2nd edn. Churchill Livingstone, Edinburgh

Management, self-management and individual accounts
Barker P J 1992 Severe depression: A practitioner's guide. Chapman and Hall, London
Copeland M 1992 The depression workbook: A guide for living with depression and manic depression. New Harbinger Press, Oakland, CA
Jamison K R 1995 An unquiet mind: A memoir of moods and madness. Picador, London
McKeon P 1992 Coping with depression and elation. Sheldon Press, London
Perry A, Tarrier N, Morriss R 1995 Identification of prodromal signs and symptoms and early intervention in manic depressive psychosis patients: a case example. Behavioural and Cognitive Psychotherapy 23:399–409.

Varma V (ed) Managing manic depressive disorders. Jessica Kingsley, London

Social effects
Hill R G, Hardy P, Shepherd G 1996 Perspectives on manic depression: A survey of the Manic Depression Fellowship. The Sainsbury Centre for Mental Health, London
Lish J D, Dime-Meenan S, Whybrow P C, Arlen Price R, Hirschfeld R M A 1994 The National Depressive and Manic–Depressive Association (DMDA) survey of bi-polar members. Journal of Affective Disorders 31:281–294.

Suicide and suicide prevention
Hawton K 1992 Suicide and attempted suicide. In: Paykel E S (ed) Handbook of affective disorders, 2nd edn. Churchill Livingstone, Edinburgh
Health Advisory Service 1994 Suicide prevention: The challenge confronted. HMSO, London

Therapeutic approaches
Scott J 1995 Psychotherapy for bi-polar disorder. British Journal of Psychiatry 167:581–588
Scott J 1996 Cognitive therapy of affective disorders. Journal of Affective Disorders 37:1–11.
Varma V (ed) Managing manic depressive disorders. Jessica Kingsley, London

REFERENCES

American Psychiatric Association 1994a Diagnostic and statistical manual of mental disorders, DSM-IV, 4th edn. American Psychiatric Association, Washington, DC
American Psychiatric Association 1994b Practice guideline for the treatment of patients with bi-polar disorder. Supplement to the American Journal of Psychiatry 151(12):1–36
Bancroft J, Skirmshire A, Casson J, Harvard-Watts O, Reynolds F 1977 People who deliberately poison themselves: their problems and their contacts with helping agencies. Psychological Medicine 7:289–303
Bancroft J, Hawton K, Simkin S, Kingston B, Cumming C, Whitwell D 1979 The reasons people give for taking overdoses: a further enquiry. British Journal of Medical Psychology 52:353–365
Barker P J 1992 Severe depression: A practitioner's guide. Chapman and Hall, London
Beck A 1976 Cognitive therapy and the emotional disorders. International Universities Press, New York
Birchwood M, Macmillan F, Smith J 1992 Early signs of relapse in schizophrenia: monitoring methodology. In: Kavanagh D (ed) Schizophrenia: An interdisciplinary handbook. Chapman and Hall, London
Birchwood M, Mason R, Macmillan F, Healy J 1993 Depression, demoralisation and control over psychotic illness: a comparison of depressed and non-depressed patients with chronic psychosis. Psychological Medicine, 23:387–395
Black D W, Winokur G, Hasrallah A 1987 Suicide in subtypes

of major affective disorders. Archives of General Psychiatry 44:878–880
Bloch S, Hafner J, Harari E et al 1994 The family in clinical psychiatry. Oxford Medical, Oxford, p 92–108
Bond A J, Lader M H 1996 Understanding drug treatment in mental health care. Wiley, Chichester
Brown G W, Harris T O 1978 Social origins of depression. Tavistock, London
Butterworth T 1994 Mental health review. HMSO, London
Cassano G B, Tundo A, Micheli C 1994 Bi-polar and psychotic depressions. Current Opinions in Psychiatry 7:5–8
Cochran S 1984 Preventing medical non-compliance in the outpatient treatment of bi-polar affective disorder. Journal of Nervous and Mental Disorders 176:457–464
Copeland M 1992 The depression workbook: A guide for living with depression and manic depression. New Harbinger Press, Oakland, CA
Coryell W, Winokur G 1992 Course and outcome. In: Paykel E S (ed) Handbook of affective disorders, 2nd edn. Churchill Livingstone, Edinburgh, ch 7
Custance J 1951 Wisdom, madness and folly: The philosophy of a lunatic. Gollancz, London
Department of Health 1994 The health of the nation white paper. HMSO, London
Ellicott A, Hammen C, Gitlin M, Brown G, Jamison K 1990 Life events and the course of bi-polar disorder. American Journal of Psychiatry 147:1194–1198
Falloon I, Shanahan W, Laporta M 1992 Prevention of major

REFERENCES (*contd*)

depressive episodes: early intervention with family-based stress management. Journal of Mental Health 1(1):53–61

Frankl V E 1959 Man's search for meaning. Beacon Press, New York

Fulford M 1997 Foreword. In: Varma V (ed) Managing manic depressive disorders. Jessica Kingsley, London

Garety P, Kuipers L, Fowler D, Chamberlain F, Dunn G 1994 CBT for drug resistant psychosis. British Journal of Medical Psychology, 67:259–271

Gelder M, Gath D, Mayou R, Cowen P 1996 Concise Oxford textbook of psychiatry, 3rd edn. Oxford Medical, Oxford

Goldstein R B, Black D W, Nasrallah A, Winokur G 1991 The prediction of suicide. Archives of General Psychiatry 48:418–422

Goodwin F K, Jamison K R 1990 Manic–depressive illness. Oxford University Press, Oxford

Guiness D 1997 A guide to self-management. In: Varma V (ed) Managing manic depressive disorders. Jessica Kingsley, London

Guze S, Robins E 1970 Suicide and primary affective disorders. British Journal of Psychiatry 117:437–438

Hawton K 1978 Deliberate self-poisoning and self-injury in the psychiatric hospital. British Journal of Psychiatry 51:253–259

Hawton K 1992 Suicide and attempted suicide. In: Paykel E S (ed) Handbook of affective disorders, 2nd edn. Churchill Livingstone, Edinburgh

Hawton K, Catalan J 1987 Attempted suicide: A practical guide to its nature and management, 2nd edn. Oxford University Press, Oxford

Healy E, McKeon P 1997 Rapid cycling mood disorder: a review. Irish Journal of Psychological Medicine 14(1):26–31

Health Advisory Service 1994 Suicide prevention: The challenge confronted. HMSO, London

Hill R G, Shepherd G 1996 Manic depression and the role of the mental health nurse. Mental Health Nursing 16(1):18–20

Hill R G, Hardy P, Shepherd G 1996 Perspectives on manic depression: A survey of the Manic Depression Fellowship. The Sainsbury Centre for Mental Health, London

Hooley J L, Orley J, Teasdale J T 1986 Levels of expressed emotion and relapse in depressed patients. British Journal of Psychiatry 148:642–647

Hunt N, Bruce-Jones W, Silverstone T 1992 Life events and relapse in bi-polar affective disorder. Journal of Affective Disorders 25:13–20

Isometsä E T, Henricksson M M, Aillevi M A, Lonngvist J K 1994 Suicide in bi-polar disorder in Finland. American Journal of Psychiatry 151(7):1020–1024

Jamison K R 1995 An unquiet mind: A memoir of moods and madness. Picador, London

Jamison K, Akiskal H 1983 Medication compliance in patients with bi-polar disorders. Psychiatric Clinics of North America 6:175–192

Janicak P G, Davis J M, Gibbons R D et al 1985 Efficacy of ECT: a meta-analysis. American Journal of Psychiatry 142:297–302

Jefferson J W, Greist J H, Acherman D L, Carrol J A 1987 Lithium encyclopaedia for clinical practice, 2nd edn. American Psychiatric Press, Washington, DC

Jenaway A, O'Leary D 1997 What a cognitive behavioural

approach can do to help. In: Varma V (ed) Managing manic depressive disorders. Jessica Kingsley, London

Johnson G F, Hunt G 1979 Suicidal behaviour in bi-polar manic–depressive patients and their families. Comprehensive Psychiatry 20(2):159–164

Jolley A G, Hirsch S R, Morrison E, McRink A, Wilson L 1990 Trial of brief intermittent neuroleptic prophylaxis for selected schizophrenic outpatients: clinical outcome at one year. British Medical Journal 301:837–842

Keller M B 1989 Current concepts in affective disorder. Journal of Clinical Psychiatry 50(5):157–162

Klerman G L 1981 The spectrum of mania. Comprehensive Psychiatry 22:11–20

Kupfer D J, Frank E, Perel J M 1989 The advantages of early treatment intervention in recurrent depression. Archives of General Psychiatry 46:771–775

Lish J D, Dime-Meenan S, Whybrow P C, Arlen Price R, Hirschfeld R M A 1994 The National Depressive and Manic–Depressive Association (DMDA) survey of bi-polar members. Journal of Affective Disorders 31:281–294

Lund C 1997 What psychodynamic approaches can do to help. In: Varma V (ed) Managing manic depressive disorders. Jessica Kingsley, London

McFarland G K, Wasli E L, Gerety E K 1997 Nursing diagnosis and process in psychiatric mental health nursing. Lippincott, Philadelphia

McKeon P 1992 Coping with depression and elation. Sheldon Press, London

MacLeod A K, Williams J M G, Linehan M M 1992 New developments in the understanding and treatment of suicidal behaviour. Behavioural Psychotherapy 20: 193–218

Meltzer H, Gill B, Pettigrew M, Hinds K 1995 The prevalence of psychiatric morbidity among adults living in private households. OPCS, London

Molnar G, Feeney M G, Fava G A 1988 Duration and symptoms of bi-polar prodromes. American Journal of Psychiatry 145(12):1576–1578

Mukherjee S, Sackheim H A, Lee C 1988 Unilateral ECT in the treatment of manic episodes. Convulsive Therapy 4:74–80

Mukherjee S, Sackheim H A, Schnur D B 1994 Electroconvulsive therapy of acute manic episodes: a review of fifty years experience. American Journal of Psychiatry 151:169–176.

Nehring J, Hill R G, Poole L 1993 Work, empowerment and community. The Sainsbury Centre for Mental Health, London

Nielsen B, Wang A G, Bille-Brahe U 1990 Attempted suicide in Denmark. A five year follow-up. Acta Psychiatrica Scandinavica 81:250–254

Pardoen D, Bauwens F, Dramix M et al 1996 Life events and primary affective disorders: a one year prospective study. British Journal of Psychiatry 169:160–166

Parker G, Roussos J, Mitchell P, Wilhelm K, Austin M-P, Hadzi-Pavlovic D 1997 Distinguishing psychotic depression from melancholia. Journal of Affective Disorders 42:155–167

Paykel E S 1989 Treatment of depression: the relevance of research to clinical practice. British Journal of Psychiatry 155:754–763

REFERENCES (*contd*)

Paykel E S 1994 Life events, social support and depression. Acta Psychiatrica Scandinavica Supplement 377:50–58

Perry P S, Morgan D E, Smith R E, Tsuang M T 1982 Treatment of unipolar depression accompanied by delusions. Journal of Affective Disorders 4:195–200

Perry A, Tarrier N, Morriss R 1995 Identification of prodromal signs and symptoms and early intervention in manic depressive psychosis patients: a case example. Behavioural and Cognitive Psychotherapy 23:399–409

Pitts F N, Winokur G 1964 Affective disorders III: diagnostic correlates and incidence of suicide. Journal of Nervous and Mental Disease 139:176–181

Post R M 1992 Transduction of psychosocial stress into the neurobiology of recurrent affective disorder. American Journal of Psychiatry 149:999–1010

Potter W Z, Rudorfer M V, Manji H 1991 The pharmacological treatment of depression. New England Journal of Medicine 325:633–642

Pozner A, Ng M L, Hammond J, Shepherd G 1996 Working it out creating work opportunities for people with mental health problems: A developmental handbook. Pavillion / The Sainsbury Centre for Mental Health / Outset, Brighton

Rasmussen J, Hallstrom C 1997 In:Varma V (ed) Managing manic depressive disorders. Jessica Kingsley, London

Rawnsley K 1982 Epidemiology of affective psychoses. In: Wing J K, Wing L (eds) Handbook of psychiatry 3: Psychoses of uncertain aetiology. Cambridge University Press, Cambridge

Regier D A, Narrow W E, Rae D S, Mandersheid R W, Locke B Z, Goodwin F K 1993 The de facto US mental and addictive disorders service system: epidemiologic catchment area prospective 1–year prevalence rates of disorder and services. Archives of General Psychiatry 50:85–94

Reich T 1995 Genetic linkage studies of bi-polar disorder. Current Opinion in Psychiatry 8:3–6

Rose D 1996 Living in the community. The Sainsbury Centre for Mental Health, London.

Sclare P, Creed F 1990 Life events and the onset of mania. British Journal of Psychiatry 156:508–514.

Scott J 1995 Psychotherapy for bi-polar disorder. British Journal of Psychiatry 167:581–588.

Scott, J 1996 Cognitive therapy of affective disorders. Journal of Affective Disorders 37:1–11

Seligman M E P 1975 Helplessness on depression, development and death. Freeman, San Fransisco, CA

Smith J A, Tarrier N 1992 Prodromal symptoms in manic depressive psychosis. Social Psychiatry and Psychiatric Epidemiology 27:245–248

Spiker D G, Weiss J, Dealy R et al 1985 The pharmacological treatment of delusional depression. American Journal of Psychiatry 142:430–436

Thase M E 1993 Maintenance treatments of recurrent affective disorders. Current Opinion in Psychiatry 6:16–21

Vieta E, Gasto C, Otero A, Nieto E, Vallejo J 1997 Differential features between bi-polar I and bi-polar II disorder. Comprehensive Psychiatry 38:98–101

Warr P 1987 Work, unemployment and mental health. Oxford Scientific, Oxford

Welner A, Welner Z, Leonard M A 1977 Bi-polar manic–depressive disorder: a reassessment of course and outcome. Comprehensive Psychiatry 18(4):327–332

Wigoder D 1987 Images of destruction. Routledge and Kegan Paul, London

Zarate C A, Tohen M, Baraibar G, Zarate S B, Baldessarini R J 1997 Shifts in hospital diagnostic frequencies: bi-polar disorder subtypes 1981–1993. Journal of Affective Disorders 43:79–84

CHAPTER CONTENTS

Key points   187

Introduction   188

Why do people kill themselves?   188

Aetiology of suicide   189
   Background   189

Risk factors   190
   Psychiatric features   190
   Socioeconomic factors   192
   Other features   193

**Problems of translating risk factors into clinical
   assessment**   195
   General vs specific reasons   195
   Low base rate   195
   Alteration of risk over time   195
   Long-term vs short-term risk   195
   Risk is not universal   195
   Practical difficulties   196
   Suicide rating scales   196

Assessment of risk   197
   Formulating risk   198
   Clinical judgements based on an assessment
      of risk   198

Interventions   199
   Immediate risk   200
   Evaluated psychosocial interventions for
      individuals following DSH   201
   Longer term interventions   203

Conclusion   203

Exercise   204

Key texts for further reading   204

References   204

11

Suicide and self-harm

Sarah Kelly

KEY POINTS

- Mental illness is the feature most commonly associated with suicide, particularly affective–depressive disorder with symptoms of hopelessness.

- There are some difficulties in translating retrospective research into identifying individuals who are likely to commit suicide. However, research can be used to identify *groups* of individuals who are more likely to be at higher risk of suicide than the general population.

- There are a number of indicators that will assist in identifying current suicide risk, including symptoms of hopelessness, previous suicide attempts and current suicidal thoughts, opportunity, drug and alcohol use, social circumstances and recent events.

- When assessing an individual's risk of suicide, risk assessment scales should be used only in conjunction with a detailed clinical assessment.

- Where risk is identified, the clinician should consider both immediate and long-term clinical interventions.

INTRODUCTION

Suicide accounts for nearly 1% of all deaths annually in the UK (Department of Health 1994). The mental health nurse will be required to assess whether individuals who are receiving care are at risk of killing themselves or at risk of deliberate self-harming behaviour. The assessment may take place in different circumstances; the client may have been referred to a community mental health team, have been admitted into a psychiatric in-patient facility or have been discharged from such a facility, or the assessment may be part of ongoing assessment and treatment. Having assessed the degree of risk, the nurse will be required to use therapeutic interventions that reduce this risk. This chapter looks at research undertaken in the area of suicide risk factors and how these factors translate into clinical practice. The chapter examines some aspects of treatment that may be of value in reducing suicide risk and preventing future suicide.

A common mistake is to assume that acts of deliberate self-harm (DSH) equate with suicide. While many people commit acts of DSH, the vast majority do not go on to commit suicide. Suicidal behaviour can be described as a continuum which includes suicide, non-fatal attempts, gestures, indirect suicide, suicidal thoughts and, commonly, parasuicide. Suicide in this country is defined by determining the individual's 'intent' to kill themselves and the 'act' of doing so. While some acts of DSH also include the 'intent' and the intended 'act' which has failed, not all instances are a result of a deliberate intention to commit suicide. One difficulty in examining suicidal behaviour is that people who commit acts of DSH or complete suicide are individuals whose reasons and circumstances leading to the act will be varied and unique to that individual. We can examine factors that will help to understand common elements, and help in identifying those individuals who are more at risk than others, as well as reducing the possibility of suicide or further DSH. Translating this into clinical practice, however, does not always take into account the complexity of this area.

WHY DO PEOPLE KILL THEMSELVES?

Theorists have attempted to answer this question from many different perspectives and have tried to define different 'types' of suicide, developing theories that attempt to explain the general reasons why people commit suicide. Durkheim (1952) used a sociological perspective, dividing the reasons for suicide into three main areas: 'egotistic', 'altruistic' and 'anomic'. He described 'egotistic' suicide as a result of an individual's lack of integration into society, where the individual feels alienated and disconnected from community, family and friends. Durkheim referred to 'anomic' suicide as occurring when an individual fails to adjust to social change such as divorce or sudden change in standards of living. He described 'altruistic' suicide as happening when the individual's identity is governed by the group to which the individual belongs, and suicide results from the 'higher command' of the group, such as religious or political sacrifice.

Freud (1957) attempted to explain suicide by two different drives: eros and thanatos. Eros is the life instinct and thanatos the drive towards death, destruction and aggression, with a constant shifting of balance existing between the two. He described suicide as aggression turned against the individual him- or herself. Baechler (1979) argued that all suicides fell into the categories of 'escapist', 'aggressive', 'self-sacrificing' or 'lucid' (risk-taking). Menninger (1938) suggested suicides were motivated by a wish to kill, a wish to die as a result of depression, a wish to be killed because of guilt or a combination of these elements.

Schneidman (1992) lists a number of possible approaches to understanding suicide: life history, personal documentation, demographic systems, philosophical/theological, sociocultural, sociological relationships and family, psychiatric, psychodynamic, psychological, constitutional or biological. He argues, however, that regardless of which perspective one studies, there are a number of common features. One characteristic is that the purpose of suicide is to seek a solution to a crisis, real or perceived. Suicide is a problem-solving behaviour intended to reduce tension, where the goal is to cease consciousness, with an unwillingness to tolerate psychological pain and an active will to stop it. The stimulus is unendurable psychological pain for which the stressor is frustrated psychological needs. The most common emotion described by individuals is the feeling of hopelessness and helplessness. Schneidman describes the common cognitive state as ambivalence, with contradictory feelings of having to commit suicide while at the same time yearning for rescue. He describes the common perceptual state as constriction, where the perception of the individual has narrowed available life options down to 'all or nothing'. The common action is to escape. The common interpersonal act is that of communication of intent with others in some verbal or non-verbal fashion, and when the person's lifelong coping strategies are explored there will be indicators in the individual's previous acts of some form of escape, regardless of whether that involved a suicide attempt. What emerges from examining the work of theorists is that the picture is complex with many subtleties that are not easy to translate into the practical aspects of assessment and management of suicide risk.

AETIOLOGY OF SUICIDE

Background

In a much more pragmatic sense, our understanding of suicide comes from research work primarily undertaken with information about people who have committed suicide. Ethical and practical considerations of collecting information on future suicide often prevent the design of prospective studies. Therefore, the main type of research done in this area is in the form of retrospective studies which correlate information gathered after the event. Prior to reviewing the factors that have been identified through this research, it is important to note some of the difficulties in this type of research.

Identifying groups of people who have committed suicide

One aspect is the use of coroners' statistics in identifying general statistics about suicide. Pounder (1992) suggests two reasons why suicide statistics taken from coroners' verdicts may not be reliable: first, suicides may be inaccurately categorised as undetermined; second, the statistics reflect regional differences (and refer to England and Wales only). Some of the more recent studies have dealt with this potential source of bias by including undetermined deaths in their statistical analysis. The opposite difficulty in using undetermined deaths is, of course, that analysis may include individuals whose death was not suicide, but has been unintentional and has been categorised as undetermined.

Retrospective analysis

Another problematic aspect of suicide research using retrospective studies is the use of information following an individual's death, which may be problematic. One reason for this is the use of information, from relatives or professionals in close contact with the individual, that is collected following the suicide. Since the information on what caused the suicide does not come from the individuals themselves, symptoms or reasons for suicide may be inaccurately judged. In addition, the death of that individual may affect the perception of the individual giving information after the event, and therefore affect the reliability of that information. Information may come from records made prior to the suicide: data collected on a large scale from records may be incomplete or vague. These aspects may potentially bias the results and affect the reliability of outcome studies.

Effect of treatment

Research work is undertaken on people who have committed suicide. This does not take into account people who have not committed suicide as a result of successful treatment. The effect of treatment is difficult to quantify and it is therefore difficult to measure its impact on suicide.

However, despite design flaws, this type of research can identify groups of individuals who are at a higher risk. From retrospective studies, it is possible to identify general risk factors such as age, gender, employment, some psychiatric symptoms such as depression and schizophrenia, alcohol abuse, previous suicide attempts, and domestic circumstances. These can be of assistance in identifying risk factors for the individual being assessed.

RISK FACTORS

Psychiatric features

Mental illness is the feature most commonly associated with suicide. Many studies have indi-

cated that a large percentage of individuals who kill themselves have some form of mental illness. For example, King (1994) identified that 59% of completed suicides had a history of mental illness, while Barraclough et al (1974) showed 24% of individuals who committed suicide were receiving current psychiatric care and 93% were given a subsequent diagnosis of some form of psychiatric disorder. Previous psychiatric history with community or in-patient services has been shown to be associated with increased risk of suicide (King 1994), with the risk of suicide greater in the year after discharge from a psychiatric hospital, and in the first month in particular (Goldacre et al 1993).

Affective–depressive disorder

The most common psychiatric symptoms noted in individuals who complete suicide are those of depression (Barraclough et al 1974, Barraclough & Pallis 1975, Guze & Robins 1970, Holding et al 1977, King 1994). In a 7-year review of parasuicide in Edinburgh, Holding et al (1977) found that 40% of women and 28% of men were diagnosed as having depression. Barraclough et al (1974) found that 64% of 100 cases reviewed had symptoms of depression. Guze & Robins (1970) reviewed 17 follow-up studies and suggested that the risk of suicide for people with affective disorders was increased to approximately 30 times that of the general population, making the lifetime risk about 15%. In Barraclough & Pallis's (1975) study, they compared 64 people who committed suicide and were retrospectively diagnosed as having depression, with 128 living individuals with depression. The results showed that the distinguishing features of those who killed themselves were insomnia, impaired memory and self-neglect. Roose et al (1983) suggest that depressed patients with delusions were approximately five times more likely to commit suicide than non-delusional patients with depression. While other psychiatric disorders such as acute anxiety are also indicative of increased suicide risk (Coryell et al 1982), this is particularly the case when these are related to depressive features.

One of the most particular aspects within depressive disorder, which is associated with suicide, is hopelessness, as defined by an individual's attitude towards the future. Beck et al (1974) suggested that one of the distinguishing differences between those with depression who kill themselves and those who do not is the level of hopelessness (i.e. pessimism about the future and importantly, viewing one's life situation in a negative way). Beck suggested that these features relate not just to short-term risk but will also predict a longer-term risk to the individual.

Schizophrenia

Schizophrenia is also associated with increased individual risk of suicide. Miles (1977) reviewed existing studies and suggested that 10% of individuals with schizophrenia commit suicide. In his comparison of individuals with chronic schizophrenia who committed suicide with those who did not, Roy (1982a) noted that significantly more suicides had a chronic relapsing illness, had recently been discharged from hospital, had a history of depression, and were depressed in the last episode of contact. In addition to these main factors, Drake & Ehrlich (1985) suggested that suicide associated with schizophrenia occurs in a relatively non-psychotic phase of the illness. This study indicates that schizophrenics who commit suicide tend to have reached a higher educational standing than average within the population and have a realistic understanding of the prognosis of the illness. Drake's study indicated that fear of recurrence, suicide threats and

hopelessness were strong indicators of suicide in individuals with schizophrenia.

Personality disorder

A study by Ovenstone & Kreitman (1974) indicated that individuals who have personality difficulties will have increased risk, suggesting that up to 10% of individuals committing suicide will have some form of personality disorder. Difficulty with personality is particularly associated with DSH (Kreitman & Foster 1991) and is one of the distinguishing differences between the profile of people who complete suicide and those who deliberately self-harm.

Alcohol and drug use

It is often questioned whether the misuse of illicit drugs and/or alcohol can be classed as a psychiatric disorder. However, both are commonly associated with suicide and are also often associated with 'dual diagnosis'. El-Guebaly (1990) found a large percentage of people with alcohol problems, for example, also had formal psychiatric disorders.

In his research, Barraclough et al (1974) found that 15% of those committing suicide were retrospectively diagnosed as alcoholic. Symptoms of depression were also noted in this study. Other studies have identified distinguishing features that will further increase the risk of suicide in individuals with alcoholism. Motto (1980) identifies poor physical health, poor recent work record and previous suicidal behaviour. Although less research has been undertaken in the area of drug misuse, James (1967) suggests that addiction to heroin also significantly increases an individual's risk. His study of young male heroin addicts indicated that the risk might be increased to 20 times that of the general population.

Suicide in in-patients

Psychiatric in-patients have been identified as being at much higher risk than the general population, with the risk in acute settings being the highest. In his review of research work on suicide in hospital settings, Crammer (1984) suggested that alienation from staff and other patients had been noted as a precursor to suicide. In addition, increased suicide risk factors included fear of the future in newly admitted patients, poor communication, difficult environment for observation, reduced staffing levels, inexperienced nursing and medical staff and lack of medical audit.

Socioeconomic factors

While formal psychiatric disorders have an impact on the risk of suicide, non-psychiatric factors will also have an influence.

Gender

The UK ratio of male to female suicides averages 3.32:1 and this trend of men killing themselves more than women is reflected throughout the Western world. It has been shown that men tend to use more violent means (Department of Health 1994), with the most common methods being car exhaust fumes (accounting for 32%), and hanging and suffocation (accounting for 31%). The most common method for women was self-poisoning, accounting for 43% of all suicides, with the next most often used method being hanging (25%).

Age

The highest rates of suicide are shown among older people, particularly people over 75 years. While suicide rates in people of both sexes over the age of 45 years have decreased since the 1960s, there has been an increase in young males, with an increase of approximately one-third for males between 25 and 44 years in England and Wales and an increase of 85% for males between 15 and 24 years. Conversely, there has been a decrease in suicides for young females.

Employment

While employment is generally associated with lower risk of suicide, particular occupations carry a higher risk than others. These occupations include vets, pharmacists, dental and medical practitioners and farmers (Charlton et al 1994). Whether this trend is as a result of these particular occupations causing high stress levels or because they have easy access to lethal means is unknown. Platt & Kreitman (1984) found a definite association between an increase in unemployment and an increase in DSH, while Platt's (1984) study on unemployment and suicide offers substantial evidence to suggest unemployment increases risk among men, although the risk is less clear among women. One of the reasons for lack of clarity for women is that women may be masked on the unemployment register.

Physical health

Poor physical health also apparently contributes to a higher risk of suicide. Dorpat & Ripley (1960) showed at least 50% of the individuals in their study of suicide had relatively serious physical disorder, in particular neurological, gastrointestinal, cardiovascular and malignant disorders. The presence of epilepsy also appears to increase the risk of suicide. In his review of several follow-up studies, Barraclough (1981) estimated a fivefold increase in suicide risk and even greater risk of suicide in those with acquired temporal lobe epilepsy. An increased suicide risk has been found for people with acquired immune deficiency syndrome (AIDS), with a particular increase in suicide risk after individuals first learn they have a diagnosis of HIV-positive (Schneider et al 1990).

Family history and bereavement

An experience of bereavement in childhood appears to increase risk of suicide. Brown & Harris (1978) showed that death of a parent in childhood increased the risk of depression in adulthood, thereby increasing the potential risk of suicide. Several aspects of family relationships may also affect the individual's potential risk of suicide: bereavement, family history and relationship difficulties. McMahon & Pugh (1965) showed recent bereavement, particularly of a spouse or parent, increased the risk of suicide. Bunch (1972) showed that risk of suicide was increased in the first 4 to 5 years following bereavement. This risk was particularly increased in the first 2 years. Those most at risk had a formal psychiatric disorder and had showed suicidal behaviour before the bereavement. Roy (1982b) shows that a family history of suicide increases risk, although it is unclear whether this is because of learnt behaviour or predisposition to affective disorder.

Living circumstances

A sense of social isolation appears to be a factor for increased suicide risk (Vogel & Woldersdorf 1989), with marriage reducing risk of suicide for men, and single people more likely to kill themselves than those with a partner. Homelessness and increased suicide have also been correlated (Appleby & Desai 1985) and homelessness has also been shown to have an impact on suicide risk.

Other features

Contact with the health services and helping agencies

Although little is known about the content of contacts made by individuals prior to committing suicide, there is research-based evidence to suggest that a considerable percentage (up to 30%) of people who commit suicide have visited GPs or health professionals in the month prior to the suicide (Bancroft et al 1977, Barraclough et al 1974). In a study of contacts with helping agencies by people who made a parasuicidal act, Bancroft et al (1977) found that 82% of the 132 individuals studied had sought help in the month prior to the attempt: 62% of those individuals had sought help from the GP.

Suicidal ideation

Beck et al (1975) define suicidal ideation as the presence of thoughts, plans and urges to commit suicide. Suicidal ideation has been shown to precede a completed suicide on some occasions. Barraclough et al (1974) identified that over half the individuals included in their study had given some indication of suicidal intention prior to the suicide. According to Beck, this indication could be as short as 1 hour before acting on the intention. The content of the ideation may indicate the seriousness or lethality of the intention to commit suicide. So, for example, someone who has made specific plans to kill himself or herself would be considered a higher risk than someone who occasionally experiences passive thoughts of 'not wishing to be here' but has no concrete plans.

Previous deliberate self-harm

Research suggests that once individuals have made a suicide attempt, they are more likely to make a further attempt and/or to kill themselves than members of the general population. Nearly half the individuals committing suicide had made a previous act of DSH in Barraclough et al's (1974) study. Bancroft & Marsack's (1977) study indicated that approximately 18% of individuals who make a suicide attempt will re-attempt within the next 2 years. In a 3-year follow-up study, 62% of the re-attempts occurred within the first 6 months. This figure is generally similar to Buglass & Horton's (1974a) study that suggested that between 14% and 17% of individuals attempting suicide would re-attempt per year. While acknowledging the difficulties of prediction in the short-term with small numbers, Buglass & Horton's (1974b) study indicated that nearly 1% of individuals who were admitted to the Edinburgh Regional Poisoning Centre went on to kill themselves within a year of the index attempt. This study explores the prediction of re-attempts in the year following an index attempt. Once individuals have made an attempt, they are at increased risk of repetition of an attempt and completing a suicide. Within this higher risk group, Buglass & Horton (1974b) identify and define aspects which increase this risk further: sociopathy, problems in the use of alcohol (which includes 'excessive drinking' as well as an addiction to alcohol), previous psychiatric out-patient care, previous parasuicide admission and not living with a relative. Pierce (1977) suggests that individuals whose repeated attempts are increasingly severe appear to be at a higher risk of suicide. In the case of suicide, one of the best indicators is a previous episode of parasuicide.

Perception of risk

For individuals who have made a suicide attempt, another aspect of research in this area is the examination of the individual's perception of the degree of risk posed by the suicide attempt. Results from Beck et al (1975) suggest that when the individual has an accurate understanding of the potential lethality of the suicide attempt, the degree of danger from the suicide attempt is predictive of future suicidal intent (i.e. the more potentially lethal the method was, the higher the future suicide risk). However, if individuals do not have an accurate view, potential lethality of the attempt is not predictive of future suicide risk.

Deliberate self-harm

The greatest single reason for acute female admissions in England and Wales was drug overdose, exceeding 100 000 per annum (Department of Health 1994), while it was the second most common reason for male medical admissions (Hawton & Catalan 1987). As has already been discussed, individuals who commit an act of DSH are at increased risk of suicide. However, while there is a clear association between the act of DSH and subsequent completed suicide, the profile of those who deliberately self-harm is not the same as those who commit suicide. The characteristics of DSH are slightly different from suicide: while people who commit suicide tend to be male and older, people who tend to deliberately self-harm are younger and female.

Reasons people give for DSH. Several studies have examined this issue (Bancroft et al 1977, Williams 1986). Results from Bancroft et al (1977) found that only one-third of patients who made a parasuicidal act actually said they definitely wanted to die, and one-half of the patients in the Williams (1986) study said that at no stage had they wanted to die. Reasons rated highly by patients included 'I wanted to get relief from a terrible state of mind', 'The situation was so unbearable that I had to do something and I did not know what else to do', and 'I wanted to escape for a while from an impossible situation'. Other categories included 'I wanted to make people understand how desperate I was feeling' and 'I wanted to make things easier for others.'

Some studies have used information gained from those who have attempted to kill themselves in order to identify immediate risk factors. One of the major difficulties of using this sort of approach to understanding suicide is that the profile of individuals who make a suicide attempt is not the same as the profile of individuals who do kill themselves. From this research, however, we gain much more information about the complexities involved in the act of DSH, such as cognitive processing, personality, and reasons for attempt given by the individuals themselves. This research gives a more accurate impression of the immediate reasons why people deliberately self-harm and is therefore useful in identifying more immediate risk factors for DSH.

PROBLEMS OF TRANSLATING RISK FACTORS INTO CLINICAL ASSESSMENT

While much research has been undertaken to identify factors which will increase an individual's risk of suicide, translating this into risk identification is challenging for practitioners for a number of reasons.

General vs specific reasons

Research on suicide has generally been undertaken using retrospective studies examining factors after the event. These studies will offer information on general risk factors for groups of people, such as increased factors for men and people who are unemployed, but do not offer information concerning specific reasons why specific individuals kill themselves.

Low base rate

One difficulty is identifying a small group of people who commit suicide in comparison to the general population. As an illustration of this, Buglass & Horton (1974a) studied a group of individuals who were at a much higher risk than the general population (i.e. individuals who have already attempted suicide). This study suggested that only 1% of those making an attempt would kill themselves within a year of the index attempt. In this instance, the task of the practitioner is to accurately identify the one person in a hundred who is at a greater risk than the others and treat that person effectively in order to prevent that suicide.

Alteration of risk over time

Risk factors for individuals will alter over time. This may include change over a very short period of time (e.g. some people may be more at risk of killing themselves at particular times of the day or stages in their illness). Risk may also alter over a longer period of time, so someone identified as not being at risk on assessment may have an increased risk over a period of time through a change in circumstances such as loss or illness.

Long-term vs short-term risk

Mental health nurses need to predict and distinguish between long-term and short-term risk. The interventions used by the nurse are likely to vary, dependent on whether they consider that the individual they assess is at immediate risk or at risk at some point in the future.

Risk is not universal

Risk factors are not universal. It is useful to note, for example, that the profile of those who commit suicide while in-patients of the services is different from those not receiving in-patient care, and therefore different characteristics need to be identified in in-patient assessment of risk.

Practical difficulties

There are a number of practical difficulties for the practitioner assessing risk. The person being assessed may deny suicidal thoughts or behave in a way that makes assessment difficult. In addition, as noted with in-patients, there may be misleading signs of improvement leading to an inaccurate judgement of the severity of the risk.

Suicide rating scales

One of the issues for clinicians who are endeavouring to assess the degree of suicide risk is the use of rating scales or tests that have been designed to predict future suicide or suicidal behaviour and the relative value of these scales in the process of assessment. There are numerous rating scales that have been developed to assist in the identification of suicide risk in a variety of different contexts. The Scale for Predicting Subsequent Suicidal Behaviour (SPSSB, Buglass & Horton 1974b), for example, is used for screening in accident and emergency environments, while the Beck Hopelessness Scale (1974), which is used to identify hopelessness, is known to be a strong predictor of suicide, and is the best available at present.

When considering the use of scales or tests there are four aspects worth considering: reliability, validity, sensitivity and specificity. If a scale or test is reliable, then the results of the test will be consistent; so, for example, if a test was administered and gained an initial score of 4, but was then repeated to check the result and got a score of 10, this test would be unreliable. Validity is whether the test measures what it is supposed to measure. So if a test was administered to predict suicide potential, but did in fact predict a depressive illness rather than suicide potential, this test would be described as lacking validity. While these definitions do not cover different sub-types of validity and reliability, these general aspects are important when considering rating scales or tests. One way in which rating scales are evaluated is through examination of sensitivity and specificity, which are calculated by looking at 'positive' and 'negative' outcomes. There are four possible outcomes in any prediction of suicide:

- true positive (where suicide is predicted and subsequently occurs)
- false positive (where suicide is predicted and does not occur)
- true negative (where non-suicide is predicted and suicide does not occur)
- false negative (where non-suicide is predicted and suicide subsequently occurs).

Sensitivity is defined as the proportion of correctly identified positive cases, while specificity is the proportion of correctly identified negative cases. The ideal test would produce both high sensitivity and high specificity, and low false-positive and false-negative scores. Using an imaginary example, 4000 patients are tested using a scale that predicts future suicide and 60 subsequently commit suicide, producing the following results:

- true Positives = 30 (of 60) = 50% sensitivity
- false Positives = 1400 (of 3940)
- true Negatives = 2540 (of 3940) = 64.5% specificity
- false Negatives = 30 (of 60).

In this imaginary example, only half the subsequent suicides were predicted. In addition, the scale also falsely predicted that a further 1400 individuals were going to commit suicide but they did not. Such a scale is unlikely to be useful in clinical practice.

Not all published rating scales have evaluated sensitivity and specificity, and those scales where this type of evaluation has taken place show varying degrees of accuracy in both areas. So, for example, the Short Risk Scale (SRS, Pallis et al 1982), used to discriminate completed suicide from future suicide attempts with suicide attempters, was found to have a sensitivity and specificity of 83% and 67% respectively, in a follow-up study (Pallis et al 1984). The SPSSB (Buglass & Horton 1974b), however, found that the presence of one or more items on the scale was found to predict suicide repetition with 88% sensitivity and 44% specificity. Some rating scales have evaluated predictive validity (i.e. the current ability of the scale to predict future behaviour), but this does not always take account of false positives (individuals who have been rated as high risk who do not commit suicide). When translating this into clinical assessment, the result is that rating scales will not always accurately identify those who subsequently commit suicide or re-attempt. In addition to this, a high number of false positives will mean that clinicians still have to determine which individuals their efforts need to target.

There appears to be a general acknowledgement that while rating scales may offer a useful adjunct to clinical judgement, and are certainly useful for research purposes, they are not a substitute for detailed clinical assessment itself.

ASSESSMENT OF RISK

Research has given us indicators which will be of assistance in identifying suicide risk or risk of DSH and helping in a formulation of risk, leading to appropriate treatment. General factors such as age and gender need to be considered when formulating risk. The following list for inclusion in an assessment of risk is not comprehensive, but may be of value in formulating the degree of risk for the individual being assessed.

Is the client experiencing symptoms of hopelessness? How does the client see the future/life/self? Is the client optimistic or pessimistic about the future? Does the client feel hopeful or hopeless? Does the client feel positive about himself/herself or positive/negative about life?

Has the client made any previous suicide attempts? If so, how many suicide attempts has the client made and when was the last attempt? What was (were) the method(s) used and how harmful did the client believe the attempt(s) to be? What reasons does the client give for previous attempt(s) and how does the client feel about the attempt(s) now?

Is the client experiencing current suicidal thoughts? How strongly and how frequently is the client experiencing suicidal thoughts at present? Has the client made any plans? If so, what sort of plans has the client made? What reasons does the client give for current suicidal thoughts? Does the client have any reasons for not committing suicide? Are there times of the day or situations when the thoughts are stronger than at other times or in other situations? What would 'tip the client over the edge'?

Does the client have the means and opportunity to kill himself/herself?

If the client is verbally denying any suicidal thoughts, does the client's non-verbal communication indicate the same? Does other information from previous records or from relatives and friends suggest otherwise?

Is the client experiencing symptoms of mental illness, particularly depression or schizophrenia?

Is the client experiencing other symptoms of mental illness such as personality disorder?

Does the client have a previous or current psychiatric history?

Has the client recently been discharged from psychiatric in-patient service?

What are the client's current circumstances? Does the client live alone? Is the client employed? What type of support structures does the client use? How isolated is the client?

Is the client using alcohol above advised limits? If so, what is the pattern of drinking? How much is the client drinking? How long has the client been drinking above advised limits? Does the client have physical problems relating to alcohol use?

Is the client using illicit drugs and/or non-prescribed medication? If so, what type of drugs is the client using (cannabis, amphetamines, heroin)? How much is the client taking per day/week? What effect does this have on the client's mental health?

What are the recent life events for the client? Has the client experienced a recent loss, or traumatic experience that has had a psychological impact? What are the current stressors for the client?

Does the client behave in a way that suggests alienation from others?

What are the client's coping strategies? How does the client normally deal with life problems that arise? How safe does the client feel?

Formulating risk

When formulating the information available, it is necessary to remember that recent stressors may play an important part in the individual's present situation and degree of risk, and these will hold a different level of significance for each person. For example, while one person might be mildly sad at the recent death of a distant relative, this may be a much more significant event to another. Individuals also have different coping strategies that will influence their level of risk. In addition, the reasons why people wish to kill themselves will be personal to them. So while generally recognised suicide risk factors will play a role in assessing the level of risk and making decisions about treatment, the assessor needs to take the more personal elements into account.

Clinical judgements based on assessment of risk

The NHS Health Advisory Service's publication, *Suicide Prevention: The Challenge Confronted*, (Health Advisory Service 1994) lists a number of features where treatment within the community might be acceptable in managing risk. These include:

- when clinical judgement is that the degree of risk is manageable in the community and there have been no serious attempts in the recent past
- when good rapport has been established and individuals are able to give a commitment not to harm themselves and are compliant with the interventions offered
- when the individual prefers to be treated at home and can cope within the environment, both in terms of stressors and living skills, and where the appropriate levels of support are available
- when alcohol and drug use is under control and the individual has no history of impulsive behaviour.

Where interventions can be offered within the community there are opportunities for individuals to use and increase their coping skills, while maintaining responsibility and not losing contact with their environment. However, monitoring areas such as safety and medical and physical condition is more difficult than in a hospital setting.

The Health Advisory Service (1994) also identified a number of features in judging the degree of suicidal risk which might suggest that in-patient treatment is preferable:

- when the individual is not known and there is limited information from others about the person's history or of recent events
- When there is a previous history of suicide risk and recent DSH, particularly if it has been planned and there are continuing suicidal thoughts.

However, risk is also great if the individual denies suicidal thoughts even though there has been a recent serious episode of DSH. Clinical features indicating depression, particularly with feelings of hopelessness and morbid ideas, or the presence of other clinical features indicating a psychotic illness, impulsive personality, drug or alcohol misuse would also suggest in-patient treatment. In addition, failure to establish a good rapport with the individual, and where there is a sense of alienation towards others and difficulty in accepting support or help from others would suggest caution in offering community interventions.

The challenge for the mental health nurse will be to identify the level of risk and then make decisions on what intervention(s) will offer the most therapeutic course of action. However, clinical interventions will vary, dependent on the level of risk identified, how immediate that risk is and the underlying reasons for the suicide risk. There is no easy formula which will tell the practitioner whether the individual being assessed is going to make a suicide attempt or when it might happen. However, thorough, detailed assessment will be of value in making educated decisions about risk.

INTERVENTIONS

For mental health nurses, as with any profession, it is important, wherever possible, to use clinical interventions that have been evaluated and shown to be clinically effective with the difficul-

ties identified. However, this is particularly problematic when examining effective interventions specifically known to reduce suicide. There are a number of difficulties associated with the development of research-based interventions known to reduce suicide.

It is difficult to know whether individuals who otherwise would have killed themselves have not done so as a result of the clinical interventions they have received. It would be both ethically and morally inappropriate to design research studies using a control group who were denied treatment if they were identified as being at risk of suicide in order to act as a comparison for examining the effectiveness of the treatment offered.

As described earlier, the base rate for suicide is low. Longitudinal studies examining the effect of treatment over an extended period of time would suffer from bias resulting from extraneous factors other than clinical intervention having an effect on suicide.

Since individuals identified as being at risk of suicide are a heterogeneous group, presenting with many different reasons for being at risk, the type of clinical intervention used to treat those individuals will also be varied and unique to those individuals.

While much research has taken place to identify individuals who are at risk of suicide and DSH, much less research has been undertaken to evaluate effective treatments for preventing suicide. However, there have been studies to evaluate the impact of psychosocial interventions on individuals following an act of DSH, as will be described shortly. In addition, there are a number of good practice guidelines which have been developed for both in-patient and community treatment and which have been based on risk factors identified through research.

Another issue to be considered when examining practice designed to reduce suicide is short-term versus long-term risk. While the individual assessed may not present with immediate sui-cide risk, the assessment may indicate that they have a much higher long-term risk of suicide. For example, individuals with symptoms of schizo-phrenia may not present with immediate suicidal thoughts, or have made any previous suicide attempts, and may be in a current situation that suggests they are well supported in their social circumstances. Nonetheless, these individuals will still ultimately carry a higher risk of ultimate suicide than the general population. There are clinical interventions that have been shown to have a positive effect on mental illness and its impact on an individual's life. These interven-tions may well also have a positive impact in reducing suicide.

Immediate risk

In-patients

Some individuals will present with such a high degree of immediate risk of suicide or DSH that hospitalisation will be necessary. Approaches to treatment in this context are generally good prac-tice guidelines that have been developed through examination of research or audit of the factors that increase risk of suicide in this setting. Prerequisites to any treatment within a hospital environment are full assessment, agreed treat-ment plan and communication of this to all mem-bers of staff.

One aspect that seems self-evident is reduction of practical means which individuals might use to commit an act of DSH or suicide. It has been suggested that a ward's facilities may present practical risks such as high windows and stair-cases, and so an awareness of security and the environment itself will be an important aspect of care. In addition, practical means available to the individual, such as ties or belts, should be removed.

One intervention that offers immediate man-agement of suicide risk is the use of observation. Observation should be seen as an opportunity to develop a therapeutic relationship with the indi-vidual rather than as custodial care. A good description of guidelines for observation in a hospital setting is given in *Suicide Prevention: The Challenge Confronted* (Health Advisory Service 1994). Recommendations are made on different levels of observation which may be used in dif-ferent circumstances varying from constant observation of the individual to 'known place' observation, advising that levels of observation should be agreed between both medical and nursing staff and should be reviewed on a regu-lar basis.

Research has suggested that signs of improve-ment prior to suicide can mislead staff. Becoming increasingly alienated from both staff and other patients has also been shown to be indicative of increased suicide risk. Therefore, staff awareness, both of individuals becoming alienated and showing misleading signs of improvement, will be an important part of continuing assessment within this setting.

Leave from the ward environment has been indicated as a high-risk period (Crammer 1984). Therefore, plans for leave need to include an assessment of potential risks and this should be judged to be manageable, and a plan similar to that for management of suicide risk in the com-munity should be made. Research has also shown that the immediate period after discharge is a high-risk period for individuals (Goldacre et al 1993). Therefore, good planning for follow-up on discharge is essential to ensure that commu-nity support is available during this time.

Community

For individuals whose risk of suicide or DSH has been identified as being manageable within the community, 'crisis' style interventions may assist in the management of more immediate risk. Like the management of in-patient risk, some of the interventions are based on good practice guidelines from research.

The client agrees to and receives regular contact from the clinician and is continually re-assessed during the period of crisis. This contact may well initially be on a daily basis, and will be gradually reduced as the crisis subsides.

The client needs to be able to contact others in case of emergency. Developing a list of contact points for emergencies such as friends, GP, Samaritans, may be useful.

Plans of what clients will do over the immediate period should be negotiated, clearly identifying periods of increased risk such as time when they will be on their own and agreeing strategies for dealing with risk periods. So, for example, clients could agree to visit friends during a time of day when they are likely to be on their own.

'Availability of means' (e.g. arrangements for others to keep medication) should be reduced.

One method which is recommended is the use of contracts (Health Advisory Service 1994). In essence, this is a written and signed contract made between the individual and the clinician that acts as a sign of commitment on the part of both the clinician and the client. The contract will include emergency alternatives if the client becomes acutely suicidal. One particular aspect in the use of contracts is in deciding what will happen if the client is unable to honour the contract. Inability to keep to the contract should not be seen as failure either on the part of the client or the clinician.

Problem-solving strategies (described below) can be used to help the client identify the immediate problems leading to suicidal behaviour, increase the ability to solve problems and therefore reduce the long-term risk.

As with in-patient care, good communication is an essential element of treatment. Keeping all people involved in the care of the individual is extremely important. GPs and other professionals involved need to be aware of both the risks and the treatment of the individual.

Evaluated psychosocial interventions for individuals following DSH

Despite a general lack of research on interventions reducing suicide risk, a number of randomised controlled trials have taken place to evaluate the impact of psychosocial interventions for individuals who have attempted suicide. Therefore, it is useful to offer a brief overview of these particular studies.

Hawton et al (1981) evaluated domiciliary and out-patient treatment by medical and non-medical staff of patients admitted to the psychiatric service at the general hospital following deliberate self-poisoning. The interventions used were the same for both groups and used brief, problem-solving counselling, emphasising the present and future, with measures to prevent further self-harm. Treatment took place within a 3-month period and both medical and non-medical staff were trained in using the approach. Results showed that twice as many patients offered treatment at home kept their appointments and while social improvements were noted for both groups, they were higher for the domiciliary group. Results also showed that fewer of the domiciliary group repeated attempts although this difference did not attain significance.

In a second study, differences between out-patient counselling and general practitioner care following overdoses were compared (Hawton et al 1987). The out-patient counselling group received brief problem-orientated counselling (Hawton & Catalan 1987). Training included exploration of the meaning of the overdose, clarifying problems and agreeing treatment goals, designing strategies to promote communication between the patient and significant others, planning tasks to be performed between sessions and attempts by the counsellor to link past experiences or those occurring in other contexts to the patient's current situation. Assessment of mental state during these sessions became less formal as contact progressed. All the counsellors taking part in the study had been trained in using this approach. For patients allocated to the GP group, a discharge summary was sent which included recommendations for the GP to provide or arrange further care (examples given included marital or individual therapy) and these recommendations were also discussed with the GP by telephone prior to discharge. There was no statistical difference in rates of repeated attempts although 15.4% of the GP group repeated in comparison to 7.3% of the out-patient group in the period of the year. An increased benefit in the out-patient group was noted with regard to resolution or improvement in targets after a 4-month period, and improved results with regard to leisure role.

Salkovskis et al (1990) explored the difference in outcome between patients considered to be a high risk in terms of repetition of parasuicidal acts, who were offered brief cognitive–behavioural sessions or 'treatment as usual'. Treatment of the experimental group was again based on a problem-solving approach, with five sessions of treatment, which were completed within 1 month of the index attempt. In the study, the main elements of the approach included teaching patients how to identify problems and priorities; teaching patients how to generate a wide range of solutions through brainstorming techniques and narrowing these down to achievable goals; developing strategies for realising these goals; and jointly considering ways of monitoring

success. The patients in the 'treatment as usual' group were referred back to their GP with a discharge letter. Results showed evidence of improvements on ratings for depression, suicidal ideation and target problems at the end of treatment and at the end of 6 months.

McLeavey et al (1994) examined the effectiveness of training on a specific problem-solving programme with a 'treatment as usual' control group for 39 patients admitted to a casualty department after a suicide attempt involving poison. The experimental group received treatment from staff who were trained in the use of interpersonal problem-solving skills (McLeavey & Daly 1988), while the control group patients were offered a brief problem-orientated approach based on the principles of crisis intervention (Hawton & Catalan 1982). Results indicated that both groups showed a reduction in symptoms of hopelessness and the number of presenting problems. However, there were significant improvements in the experimental group compared with the control group on measures of interpersonal cognitive problem-solving (Platt & Spivack 1977), on the self-rating, problem-solving scale (McLeavey et al 1994).

In the final study reviewed here, Van der Sande et al (1997) examined individuals making a suicide attempt in the Netherlands. They compared 'treatment as usual' with intensive psychosocial intervention following a suicide attempt. The treatment group was offered a short admission to a unit specialising in people who have made suicide attempts, with psychiatric staff whose role was to encourage the patient to discuss problems leading to the suicide attempt. During this stay, a CPN was assigned to develop a therapeutic relationship, using treatment based on Hawton & Catalan's problem-solving approach (Hawton & Catalan 1987). Following discharge, appointments were made on a weekly basis and the patient was encouraged to contact the unit in times of crisis. The control group received the routine clinical service with 25% hospitalised in a psychiatric unit and 75% discharged, of which 90% were referred to an outpatient clinic. In this study, no significant differences were found in repeated suicide attempts or on hopelessness (Beck et al 1974), although the experimental group attended significantly more out-patient appointments.

While these studies have not shown significant differences in further suicide attempts or reduction in suicide, they have indicated that problem-solving interventions may be of value in reducing suicide risk for individuals who are at risk. Problem-solving is an approach that often works within a cognitive–behavioural framework. The aims of the problem-solving process are to help clients identify both problems and resources available to solve those problems, as well as teaching clients systematic methods for solving both present and possible future problems while improving the individuals' sense of control over their difficulties. Hawton & Kirk (1989) describe the key stages of a problem-solving strategy that is integrated into a cognitive–behavioural approach as:

- helping clients to define the problems they are experiencing
- helping clients to recognise the resources they have to deal with the difficulties
- teaching clients a systematic method of overcoming the problems they experience
- enhancing clients' sense of control over their problems
- equipping clients with a method for tackling future problems.

Longer term interventions

As people with mental illness are at much higher risk of suicide than others, effective treatment for the particular illness they experience is likely to be an important aspect of overall reduction of risk. Cognitive therapy, for example, has been shown to be have a positive effect in the treatment of depression (Fennel & Teasdale 1987) and may be more effective than antidepressant medication in preventing relapse (Kovacs et al 1981). Similarly, a family approach to schizophrenia has been shown to have a positive impact (Falloon 1984). It has to be remembered that individuals with longer term mental health needs are likely to go through periods of crisis when their risk of suicide or DSH will be much greater and that assessment and management of risk are not simply one-off events. Therefore, longer-term treatment of mental illness and support for those individuals will be important in reducing the risk of ultimate suicide, with continuous assessment and evaluation. Longer-term treatment may need to be interspersed with periods of 'crisis' management when the individual is particularly at risk.

CONCLUSION

It is important to acknowledge that suicide is unlikely to be completely eradicated and that, regardless of every effort, some suicides will not be prevented. However, within this chapter is the implicit assumption that some suicides are preventable and that mental health nurses can play a role in this prevention. Assessment and management of suicide risk and DSH continue to be extremely important aspects of clinical practice for mental health nurses, regardless of whether this is in an in-patient or community setting. As has been illustrated in this chapter, the factors that influence individuals to commit suicide or an act of DSH are complex. Research which has been undertaken to identify factors that increase risk is fraught with methodological difficulties and sometimes of limited value to the clinician presented with the challenge of assessing a particular individual. While psychological tests may prove a useful adjunct to assessment, they are not always good predictors of risk and can only be used with caution.

There are clinical interventions that have been evaluated and indicated to be of value with this client group. However, in a recent review of clinical effectiveness in community mental health nursing, Brooker et al (1996) comprehensively reviewed the literature available on the use of randomised controlled trials specifically undertaken by community mental health nurses in the UK since 1966 and discovered only 10 such trials. While this is not the only method of evaluating

clinical practice, it indicates a general lack of evaluation in mental health nursing, including the use of interventions to reduce suicide potential. The future of mental health practice needs to include further evaluation of clinical interventions with clients presenting with risk of suicide or DSH.

Exercise

Consider a client you have nursed who was at risk of suicide. Examine the general risk factors described in this chapter and note *both* how far each might have applied to this client *and* what management consequences, *if any*, knowing that these risk factors were present, there might have been.

KEY TEXTS FOR FURTHER READING

Department of Health 1994 The prevention of suicide (Jenkins R, Griffiths S, Wylie I, Hawton K, Morgan G, Tylee A (eds)). HMSO, London

Hawton K, Catalan J 1987 Attempted suicide: A practical guide to its nature and management. Oxford University Press, Oxford

Hawton K, Kirk J W 1989 Problem-solving. In: Hawton K, Salkovskis P M, Kirk J W (eds) Cognitive–behavioural treatment of adult psychological disorders. Oxford University Press, Oxford

NHS Health Advisory Service Thematic Review 1994 Suicide prevention: The challenge confronted. HMSO, London

---

REFERENCES

Appleby J, Desai P N 1985 Documenting the relationship between homelessness and psychiatric hospitalisation. Hospital Community Psychiatry 36 (7):732–737

Baechler J 1979 Suicides. Basic Books, New York

Bancroft J, Marsack P 1977 The repetitiveness of self-poisoning and self-injury. British Journal of Psychiatry 131:394–399

Bancroft J, Skrimshire A, Casson J, Harvard-Watts O, Reynolds F 1977 People who deliberately poison or injure themselves: their problems and their contacts with helping agencies. Psychological Medicine 7:289–303

Barraclough B 1981 Suicide and epilepsy. In: Reynolds, Trimble (eds) Epilepsy and psychiatry. Churchill Livingstone, Edinburgh

Barraclough B, Pallis D 1975 Depression followed by suicide: a comparison of depressed suicides with living depressives. Psychological Medicine 5:55–61

Barraclough B, Bunch J, Nelson B, Sainsbury P 1974 A hundred cases of suicide: clinical aspects. British Journal of Psychiatry 125:355–373

Beck A, Weissman A, Lester D, Trexler L 1974 The measurement of pessimism: the hopelessness scale. Journal of Consulting and Clinical Psychology 42:861–865

Beck A, Beck R, Kovacs M 1975 Classification of suicidal behaviours: I. Quantifying intent and medical lethality. American Journal of Psychiatry 132(3):285–287

Brooker C, Repper J, Booth A 1996 Examining effectiveness of community mental health nursing. Mental Health Nursing 16(3):12–15

Brown G W, Harris T 1978 Social origins of depression. Tavistock, London

Buglass D, Horton J 1974a The repetition of parasuicide: a comparison of three cohorts. British Journal of Psychiatry 125:168–174

Buglass D, Horton J 1974b A scale for predicting subsequent suicidal behaviour. British Journal of Psychiatry 124:573–578

Bunch J 1972 Recent bereavement in relation to suicide. Journal of Psychosomatic Research 16:361–366

Charlton J, Kelly S, Dunnell K, Evans B, Jenkins R 1994 Suicide deaths in England and Wales: trends in factors associated with suicide deaths. The prevention of suicide. HMSO, London

Coryell W, Noyes R, Clancy J 1982 Excess mortality in panic disorder: a comparison with primary unipolar depression. Archives of General Psychiatry 39:701–703

REFERENCES (*contd*)

Crammer J L 1984 The special characteristics of suicide in hospital in-patients. British Journal of Psychiatry 145:460–476

Department of Health 1994 The prevention of suicide (Jenkins R, Griffiths S, Wylie I, Hawton K, Morgan G, Tylee A (eds)). HMSO, London

Dorpat T L, Ripley H S 1960 A study of suicide in the Seattle area. Comprehensive Psychiatry 1:349–359

Drake R E, Ehrlich J 1985 Suicide attempts associated with akathisia. American Journal of Psychiatry 142(4):499–501

Durkheim E 1952 Suicide: a study in sociology. Routledge and Kegan Paul, London

El-Guebaly A M 1990 Substance abuse and mental disorders; the dual diagnosis concept. Canadian Journal of Psychiatry 35(3):261–267

Falloon I R H 1984 Family care of schizophrenia. Guilford Press, London

Fennel M J V, Teasdale J D 1987 Cognitive therapy for depression: individual differences in the process of change. Cognitive Therapy and Research 11:253–271

Freud S 1957 Mourning as melancholia. Hogarth Press, London

Goldacre M, Seagroatt V, Hawton K 1993 Suicide after discharge from psychiatric In-patient care. The Lancet 342:283–286

Guze S B, Robins E 1970 Suicide and primary affective disorders. British Journal of Psychiatry 117:437–438

Hawton K, Catalan J 1982 Attempted suicide: A practical guide to its nature and management, 1st edn. Oxford University Press, Oxford

Hawton K, Catalan J 1987 Attempted suicide: A practical guide to its nature and management, 2nd edn. Oxford University Press, Oxford

Hawton K, Kirk J W 1989 Problem-solving. In: Hawton K, Salkovskis P M, Kirk J W (eds) Cognitive–behavioural treatment of adult psychological disorders. Oxford University Press, Oxford

Hawton K, Bancroft J, Catalan J, Kingston B, Welch N 1981 Domiciliary and out-patient treatment of self-poisoning patients by medical and non-medical staff. Psychological Medicine 11:169–177

Hawton K, McKeown S, Day A, Martin P, Kreitman N 1987 Evaluation of out-patient counselling compared with general practitioner care following overdoses. Psychological Medicine 17:751–761

Health Advisory Service Thematic Review 1994 Suicide prevention: The challenge confronted. HMSO, London

Holding T A, Buglass D, Duffy J C, Kreitman N 1977 Parasuicide in Edinburgh – A seven year review 1968–1974. British Journal of Psychiatry 130:534–543

James I P 1967 Suicide and mortality amongst heroin addicts. British Journal of Addiction 62:391–398

King E 1994 Suicide and the mentally ill: an epidemiological sample and implications for clinicians. British Journal of Psychiatry 165:658–663

Kreitman N, Foster J 1991 The construction and selection of predictive scales with particular reference to parasuicide. British Journal of Psychiatry 159:185–192

Kovacs M, Rush A J, Beck A T, Hollon S D 1981 Depressed outpatients treated with cognitive therapy or pharmocotherapy; a one-year follow-up. Archives of

General Psychiatry 135:525–533

McLeavey B C, Daly R J 1988 Interpersonal problem-solving training. Unpublished manuscript, University College, Cork

McLeavey B C, Daly R J, Ludgate J W, Murray C M 1994 Interpersonal problem-solving skills training in the treatment of self-poisoning patients. Suicide and Life Threatening Behaviour 24:382–393

McMahon B, Pugh T F 1965 Suicide in the widowed. American Journal of Epidemiology 81:23–31

Menninger K 1938 Man against himself. Harcourt Brace & World, New York

Miles P 1977 Conditions predisposing to suicide: a review. Journal of Nervous and Mental Disorders 164:231–246

Motto J A 1980 Suicide risk factors in alcohol abuse. Suicide and Life Threatening Behaviour 10:230–238

Ovenstone I M K, Kreitman N 1974 Two syndromes of suicide. British Journal of Psychiatry 124:336–345

Pallis D J, Barraclough B M, Levey A B, Jenkins J S, Sainsbury P 1982 Estimated suicide risk among attempted suicides: I. The development of new clinical scales. British Journal of Psychiatry 141:37–44

Pallis D J, Gibbons J S, Pierce D W 1984 Estimating suicide risk among attempted suicides: II. Efficiency of predictive scales after the attempt. British Journal of Psychiatry 144:139–148

Pierce D 1977 Suicidal intent in self injury. British Journal of Psychiatry 130:377–385

Platt S 1984 Unemployment and suicidal behaviour: a review of the literature. Social Science and Medicine 19:93–115

Platt S, Kreitman N 1984 Trends in parasuicide and unemployment among men in Edinburgh, 1968–1982. British Medical Journal 289:1029–1032

Platt J, Spivack G 1977 Measures of interpersonal cognitive problem-solving for adults and adolescents. Hahnemann Medical College and Hospital, Philadelphia

Pounder D J 1992 Classifying suicide. British Medical Journal 305:472

Roose S P, Glassman A H, Walsh T, Woodring S, Vital-Herne J 1983 Depression, delusions, and suicide. American Journal of Psychiatry 140(9):1159–1162

Roy A 1982a Suicide in chronic schizophrenia. British Journal of Psychiatry 141:171–177

Roy A 1982b Risk factors for suicide in psychiatric patients. Archives of General Psychiatry 39:1089–1095

Salkovskis P, Atha C, Storer D 1990 Cognitive–behavioural problem-solving in the treatment of patients who repeatedly attempt suicide. British Journal of Psychiatry 157:871–876

Schneidner S G, Taylor S E, Hammen C 1990 AIDS-related factors predictive of suicidal ideation of low and high intent among gay and bi-sexual men. Suicide and Life Threatening Behaviour 21(4):313–328

Shneidman E S 1992 What do suicides have in common? Summary of the psychological approach. In: Bongar B (ed) Suicide: guidelines for assessment, management and treatment. Oxford University Press, Oxford

Van der Sande R, Van Roojen L, Buskens E et al 1997 Intensive in-patient and community intervention versus routine care after attempted suicide – a randomised

REFERENCES (*contd*)

controlled intervention study. British Journal of Psychiatry 171:35–41

Vogel R, Woldersrdorf M 1989 Suicide and mental illness in the elderly. Psychopathology 22:202–207

Williams J M G 1986 Differences in reasons for taking overdoses in high and low hopelessness groups. British Journal of Medical Psychology 59:369–373

CHAPTER CONTENTS

Key points 207

Introduction 208

Phobic states 209

Panic disorder 209
  Management of panic 210
  Treatment of panic disorder 210

Specific phobias 212
  Treatment 213

Social phobias 214
  Treatment 215

Agoraphobia 216
  Treatment 216

Obsessive–compulsive disorder 217
  Treatment 217
  Outcome of treatment for obsessive ruminations vs
    obsessive rituals 219
  Obsessive slowness 219
  Obsessive–compulsive disorder with and without
    tics 220
  Measures in the assessment and treatment of
    obsessive–compulsive disorder 220

Nurse therapists 221

Exercise 223

Key texts for further reading 223

References 223

12

Phobias and rituals

Kevin Gournay   Lindsey Denford

KEY POINTS

For twenty-five years, nurses have been trained as autonomous therapists, to provide behavioural and cognitive psychotherapy to patients with anxiety disorders. In order to deal with such patients, nurses need to acquire skills in a framework which consists of assessment, interventions, measurement of symptoms, evaluation of outcome, and the ability to work within cognitive and behavioural models.

To meet these goals, the nurse must:

- Understand the nature of the conditions, i.e. phobias and obsessions.

- Undertake assessment of the patient's state using multiple reliable measures of change.

- Engage the patient in a collaborative relationship.

- Develop a set of interventions based on the initial assessment.

- Help the patient apply those interventions to their problem.

KEY POINTS (*contd*)

- Gradually make the patient more responsible for the intervention.

- Involve the family, carers, etc., as co-therapists.

- Audit the care of the individual patient and groups of patients within the service.

- Keep up to date with the evidence-based literature.

- Undertake regular re-education and refresher training.

- Use clinical supervision as an integral part of practice.

INTRODUCTION

The treatment of phobic and obsessional states is important for many reasons, not least the fact that phobic states are ubiquitous and most of us can relate to a fear of spiders, heights, flying, confined spaces, speaking in public, dentists and the sight of blood. However, the majority of people who suffer phobias do not need or seek treatment as these conditions do not interfere in any substantial way with their lives. Nevertheless, phobias which are severe enough to warrant treatment are still very widespread and, as we shall see below, conditions such as agoraphobia can cause the sufferer handicaps as severe as those that accrue to people with illnesses such as schizophrenia. Obsessional states are much commoner in society than was previously thought and, without doubt, these conditions can also cause very significant handicaps for both sufferer

and family. The nature and treatment of phobias and obsessions will be explored in more detail below. However, it must be said from the outset that these conditions are particularly pertinent for nursing practice.

25 years ago Professor Isaac Marks, a psychiatrist working at the Maudsley Hospital, set up the first training programme which enabled nurses to become competent in the practice of behavioural psychotherapy. This innovation proved to be a landmark event in the development of autonomous nurse practitioners and these nurse therapists became the first nurses to become responsible for the entire assessment, treatment and follow-up of patients with significant psychiatric conditions. The programme has continued to develop and evolve, responding to developments in the field of behavioural and cognitive psychotherapy.

In particular, nurse therapists spend many weeks learning the skills of interviewing and individual assessment. This process begins with the detailed gathering of information, enabling a functional (behavioural) analysis of the individual's presenting problem. Subsequent to therapist and patient agreeing a definition of the main current problem(s), a treatment plan is negotiated. The plan is subject to ongoing re-evaluation during treatment and follow-up.

This chapter will provide an overview of the nature and treatment of phobic and obsessional disorders and emphasise the evidence related to effective treatments. For the purpose of clarity, problems are presented under diagnostic clusters. However, it is worth remembering that overlap of features of the different conditions can sometimes occur. Following these accounts, the concluding part of the chapter will provide an overview of nurse therapy training and summarise the benefits of this approach for mental health care in general.

PHOBIC STATES

Phobic states are of course a variety of anxiety disorders and many anxiety states have considerable overlap. This chapter will concentrate on the treatment of phobic states including social phobia and agoraphobia. However, it should be noted that phobic states are often linked with panic disorder, which is defined within the Diagnostic and Statistical Manual of the American Psychiatric Association (DSM-IV) as a discrete entity. For this reason, panic disorder and its treatment will be described first. The reader should be aware that although the treatment of panic disorder and phobias are described separately, in practice treatment often involves an approach which blends both sets of treatment. Each patient presents a unique challenge and although many patients may share common symptoms, patients need to have a treatment programme tailored to their own problem. Thus, this chapter should be read with this principle in mind. We begin with panic disorder, as panic is perhaps the most overt and severe manifestation of anxiety. All mental health nurses need to be aware of both the nature and management of panic attacks.

PANIC DISORDER

Panic disorder itself is defined in DSM-IV as:

A condition in which there are:

- recurrent unexpected panic attacks
- at least one of the attacks has been followed by 1 month or more of one (or more) of the following:
  — persistent concern about having additional attacks
  — worry about the implications of the attack or the consequences (e.g. losing control, having a heart attack, going crazy)
  — a significant change in behaviour related to the attacks.

The DSM-IV definition also makes the point that in order to make a diagnosis of panic disorder, one should ensure that the panic attacks are not attributable to the direct physiological effects of a substance, for example, an amphetamine, or a general medical condition, for example, hyperthyroidism. The definition also states that panic attacks are often associated with direct exposure to a phobic object/situation. In order to meet the criteria for having a diagnosis of panic disorder, it has to be shown that these panic attacks occur independently of direct exposure to phobic objects/situations, for example, they appear spontaneous in nature and come 'out of the blue'.

Panic is quite difficult to define. In many ways there is still a great deal of difficulty differentiating between panic attack and extreme anxiety. Simply put, different people may label the same experience in different ways. However, the DSM-IV manual defines panic as 'a discreet period of intense discomfort in which four or more of the following symptoms developed abruptly and reached a peak within ten minutes'. The symptoms are:

1. palpitations
2. sweating
3. trembling or shaking
4. sensations of shortness of breath or smothering
5. feelings of choking
6. chest pain or discomfort
7. nausea or abdominal distress
8. feeling dizzy, unsteady, light-headed or faint
9. derealisation (feelings of unreality), or depersonalisation (feelings of being detached from oneself)
10. fear of losing control or going crazy
11. fear of dying
12. numbing or tingling sensations
13. chills or hot flushes.

One must also bear in mind that the above description of a panic attack applies as much to those of us who experience isolated attacks at say a time of great personal stress as to those who suffer the regular and repeated episodes that amount to the condition known as 'panic disorder'. There is considerable evidence (Gournay 1996, Marks 1987) that single episodes of panic are extremely common in the population, with one in four of us experiencing a panic attack in our lifetime. Of course, most people who suffer panic attacks do not seek or receive treatment. However, sufferers of panic disorder often lead miserable and restricted lives, and unfortunately many do not receive treatment because of the shortage of suitably skilled and trained therapists.

Management of panic

Most nurses will encounter a patient with a panic attack early in their career. If one works in an accident and emergency department, panic attacks are commonly seen. Patients may present following the shock of a life trauma or may be taken to the department because of the sudden overwhelming physical symptoms which lead the patient or others to believe that the patient is about to die, have a heart attack or another catastrophic and immediate life-threatening event. Obviously in such circumstances it is important to establish that physical disease is not present. The management of a panic attack essentially comprises following certain simple rules. It is worth emphasising that one may make the condition worse if the rules in Box 12.1 are not followed.

Treatment of panic disorder (rather than an isolated panic attack)

If an individual experiences panic attacks which continue for more than a few weeks, and which

---

Box 12.1 Simple rules for managing a panic attack

- Panic attacks will subside naturally over minutes rather than hours. (Panic is a state of extreme 'fight or flight' and the body can only maintain the highest levels of arousal for short periods.)
- Panic attacks do not lead to death or heart attacks – therefore stay calm.
- Stay calm yourself, speak slowly and quietly.
- Sit or lie the patient down, and explain that continuing to rush around will make the anxiety worse.
- Ask the patient to try to slow his/her breathing and to breathe from the diaphragm (during panic attacks, overbreathing – sometimes called hyperventilation – makes symptoms worse because this causes the loss of too much carbon dioxide from the body).
- In extreme cases, where hyperventilation leads to muscle spasm, the old remedy of re-breathing expired air from a paper bag is effective within minutes. Remember, even extreme hyperventilation will cause no real harm.
- If at all possible, avoid administering tranquillising medication or alcohol. The panic will probably pass before these substances have time to act.

---

do not seem to respond to simple measures (e.g. dealing with work stresses, paying more attention to physical relaxation and exercise) professional treatment may be warranted. Treatment follows a simple process:

- assessment
- intervention(s)
- evaluation.

Assessment

Assessment has a number of components. First of all, one needs to simply listen to the patient's account of the main current problem. This then needs to be put in the context of an historical perspective: that is, a history of the patient's background and the life and history of the presenting complaints. We will not cover this background history in detail, other than to say that it is important to understand the context of the problem and to bear in mind individual factors relating to the patient's past treatment experiences and cultural perspectives. Panic symptoms themselves may be measured by the use of rating scales and questionnaires. For example, the Panic Cognitions Inventory identifies thoughts associated with the panic, and attempts to quantify their severity. The therapist will also wish to identify whether the panic attacks lead to avoidance and, in this respect, the Fear Questionnaire (Marks & Matthews 1978) is particularly useful in defining situations which are avoided because of fear or other unpleasant feelings. It is also wise to measure more general anxiety, using one of several available instruments, for example, the Beck Anxiety Inventory and to measure mood. The commonest measure of mood is a self-report scale, the Beck Depression Inventory. However, the process most central to all cognitive and behavioural assessment is functional analysis (Fig. 12.1). This very simply requires a description of the central event, in this case the panic, and the definition of which factors precede the event, and which factors follow the event.

Figure 12.1 shows a simple ABC representation of functional analysis:

A – *the antecedents*, i.e. the thoughts or physical feelings which act as triggers
B – *the event itself* with attendant thoughts and physical feelings
C – *the consequences*, which are usually avoidance or escape.

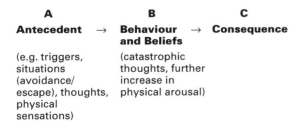

A		B		C
Antecedent	$\rightarrow$	**Behaviour and Beliefs**	$\rightarrow$	**Consequence**
(e.g. triggers, situations (avoidance/ escape), thoughts, physical sensations)		(catastrophic thoughts, further increase in physical arousal)		

Figure 12.1 Functional analysis.

The antecedents can of course be a variety or combination of factors. Thus, for example, a particular thought may trigger a panic in the case of someone who has illness fears; a thought about physical illness may lead to a panic being triggered. However, in the case of someone who has agoraphobic fears, being in a closed situation, such as a supermarket or underground train, may trigger the panic. Thus, in this case, the antecedent is the situation. As far as consequences are concerned, the consequence in the case of someone who has illness fears may be to go to a doctor to seek reassurance, or in the case of someone who has panic in a supermarket or underground train, to avoid that situation. Obviously, consequences of panics may lead to more antecedents. Thus, for example, the person with illness fears who goes to the doctor to seek reassurance may obtain temporary relief, but then experience more anxiety because of the uncertainty that this reassurance seeking gave! Thus the vicious circle begins again.

As part of the assessment process, the therapist will usually ask the patient to keep a diary, recording the occurrence of panics, and noting the antecedents and consequences. Over a period of time, the therapist will be able to obtain a true representation of how the problem affects the patient, and based on this pattern, a treatment plan can be established. One of the central tasks for the therapist is to define the components of the panic attack, and generally speaking, the patient will complain of physical feelings which are caused by general anxious arousal hyperventilation, and anxiety thoughts which are often catastrophic; for example, 'I am going to die', 'I am going to pass out', 'I am going to faint', and 'I am going to collapse'. The diary is the most reliable way of collecting comprehensive information about both the panic attacks and their context.

Interventions

The therapist will target both the thoughts and the physical feelings with specific interventions. Obviously, detailed accounts of these interventions are out of place here, but suffice it to say that research shows that a combination of strategies to deal with catastrophic thoughts and physical feelings is necessary. If the patient shows avoidance behaviour, it is very important that the therapist helps the patient to deal with avoidance by a programme of helping the patient to face up to the fears in graduated doses of difficulty. Exposure treatment is detailed below, under the treatment of specific phobias. The therapist will also deal with the pattern of catastrophic thoughts by teaching the patient to deal with these more rationally. The patient's diary may reveal that innocent symptoms such as one's heart beating fast will lead to thoughts that a heart attack is imminent. The therapist will, over a number of sessions, focus on this and other examples to help the patient challenge this irrational process and substitute new patterns of more logical, rational reasoned thinking. These strategies are at the core of what is generally known as 'cognitive therapy'. Other interventions may include the banning of reassurance-seeking and more general anxiety management methods such as relaxation training. For more detailed accounts of intervention the reader is referred to Hawton et al (1989) or Gournay (1996).

Evaluation

All therapeutic interventions demand evaluation. For the patient the simplest measure is probably: how many panic attacks have I had this week compared with this time 6 months ago? Indeed, this may also be the central measure for the therapist. Generally speaking, however, evaluation should involve various measures of change.

Therefore for panic attacks one should include, apart from number and frequency of panic attacks, the patient's scores on the various assessment measures (e.g. Fear Questionnaire, Panic Cognitions Inventory) and the patient's evaluation of problem severity (e.g. on a scale of 0–8). These evaluations should be repeated at various times during treatment (e.g. every five sessions), at the end of treatment and, if appropriate, during continuing follow-up. Obviously it is important to rate the patient on the same measures at all these points. Such evaluation is important to provide an objective assessment of the individual patient's progress. However, it is also important to collect such data so that the efficacy of the overall service is also measured. Finally, if one collects this information on all patients, clinical supervision becomes much more focused and effective. With difficult-to-treat patients who may not readily respond to intervention, this evaluation information will assist the supervisor when considering what advice is to be offered to the supervisee.

SPECIFIC PHOBIAS

Specific (also known as simple) phobias are defined in DSM-IV as:

- a marked or persistent fear that is excessive or unreasonable, cued by the presence or anticipation of a specific object or situation
- exposure to the phobic stimulus almost invariably produces an immediate anxiety response
- the person recognises the fear is excessive or unreasonable.

Simple phobias include common fears of spiders, flying insects, small animals, heights, enclosed spaces, flying and thunder. They are rarely of inanimate objects. The fears often have a tendency to generalise to associated objects/situations: for example, a wasp phobic may experience anxiety when seeing black and yellow colour combinations. Generalisation of fears may obscure initial problem identification unless assessment is sufficiently detailed.

In simple phobias, contact or anticipated contact with the feared object or situation is feared above all, but in social phobia the key fear is frequently the perceived negative evaluation by others and its consequences. Generally, in simple phobia, overt avoidance is the patient's main coping strategy, while in social phobia avoidances often involve a range of overt and subtle avoidances and props (i.e. alcohol) to cope with situations.

Social phobias are defined within DSM-IV as:

- A marked or persistent fear of one or more social or performance situations in which the person is exposed to unfamiliar people, or to possible scrutiny by others. Individuals fear that they will act in a way (or show anxiety symptoms) that will be humiliating or embarrassing.
- Exposure to the feared social situation almost invariably provokes anxiety which may take the form of the situationally bound or situationally disposed panic attack.
- The person recognises that the fear is excessive or unreasonable.
- The feared social or performance situation is avoided, or is endured with intense anxiety.
- The avoidance, anxious anticipation or distress interferes significantly with the person's life.

Treatment

Simple phobias are so common that it is not practical to treat everyone who is referred. Specialist treatment, particularly by nurse therapists, should be reserved for people whose problem

causes serious life handicaps. However, it should be said that in the great majority of cases, simple exposure is the treatment of choice and produces very significant gains.

The principles and practice of simple exposure must incorporate the following conditions:

- planned and graded to individual's most therapeutic pace
- regular/repeated
- engagement and proactive
- practised as homework
- of adequate duration to ensure reduction of anxiety occurs during exposure.

To cite a simple example, it is possible for someone with a spider phobia to be gradually exposed to live spiders over a couple of sessions of 2 to 3 hours each. At first, the therapist exposes the patient to small live spiders in a closed container several feet away, and then encourages the patient to continue with this exposure until the patient's anxiety falls. At a pace which is acceptable to the patient, the therapist continues with exposure, graduating to open containers, until finally the patient is able to handle large, live spiders with little or no anxiety. More often than not, the patient requires much less treatment than the patient anticipates, but of course effective treatment by a therapist is reinforced with home practice. The therapist should ask the patient to record homework in a diary and report back after a reasonable period.

Some phobic problems may require far more graded exposure which may take more sessions of shorter duration over a longer period of time. For example, some patients have a phobia about becoming incontinent of urine and this may or may not stem from an experience when bladder control was lost. Such a potentially distressing event, for example, stress incontinence in females, or finding oneself in a situation where one has no access to a lavatory may have been the cause of the problem. However, in many cases, no obvious cause can be detected, and in any case the management is likely to be the same. Sufferers have usually reduced their fluid intake, and restricted journeys away from home. Patients with this phobia may often plan any trips or excursions very carefully, so that they can map out lavatories en route and inappropriately use pads 'just in case'.

Treatment for such a problem would consist of asking the patient to gradually increase fluid intake, and at the same time not to respond immediately to the perception of a full bladder and thus increase the time spent away from toilets. The therapist's main task therefore is that of assisting patients with the planning of their treatment programme and meeting them to monitor progress. Patients will generally keep a behavioural diary, including data concerning the amount of fluid consumed, the number of urinations, and places visited, together with a rating of anxiety for each task undertaken. Such treatment usually has an excellent outcome, but it may take several weeks or months for patients to retrain themselves appropriately.

Some phobias are difficult to treat because exposure is not easily arranged. One example would be thunder and lightning phobia. On occasion, patients will go to extraordinary lengths to avoid thunderstorms, and one patient spent several thousand pounds building himself a sound-proof room in his house. Other patients may resort to drugs or alcohol to help them deal with the distress of an impending thunderstorm, and may obsessively telephone for weather forecasts. When real-life exposure is impractical, undesirable or difficult, the therapist has to be more creative in generating effective exposure opportunities. Examples of these would be the use of exposure in imagination, using audio- and/or video-taped simulations (i.e. thunder soundtracks, films of storms) and multimedia packages. In addition, the therapist would also ask the patient to rehearse more appropriate behaviour during thunderstorms (i.e. to ban the continual checking of a weather forecast or to ask the patient (often with the assistance of a friend or relative who acts as a co-therapist) to leave the house during such a storm).

Thus, in treatment of phobias:

- degree of handicap/distress determines specialist intervention
- principles and practice of simple exposure are the treatment of choice
- need to be creative in facilitating exposure with feared objects/situations that are difficult to replicate
- grading of exposure may depend on extent of generalisation of phobic fears.

SOCIAL PHOBIAS

Social phobias are very common in the general population. Indeed, it is difficult to define where everyday shyness and embarrassment end and where social phobia begins. Probably the guiding principle should be to ask whether the problem upsets and/or interferes with one's life to a significant degree; if the problem does it can be called a phobia. Social phobias are often characterised by fears of 'making a fool of oneself' and there may be associated fears of some inappropriate behaviour, an oversensitivity to blushing, not knowing what to say in certain situations, being embarrassed about making eye contact and fears about being 'rejected' by friends or members of the opposite sex. The associated avoidance behaviour often leads to social isolation, which leads, in turn, to feeling dejected. Panic attacks and depression commonly accompany social phobia and it is, unfortunately, common to see sufferers leading very miserable, isolated lives. Nevertheless, treatment can be very effective.

Treatment

As with all other phobic avoidance, the central treatment for social phobia is exposure to the situation the person avoids, which, as in the case of simple phobias, should be implemented in gradual doses of increasing difficulty with patients understanding that they will need to confront the situation repeatedly for long periods of time before the fear declines. In social phobia, there is frequently a persistent underlying concern about others judging one. Thus, for example, people with social phobia often have these pervasive negative thoughts in combination with high levels of physiological arousal, which includes sweating and rapid heartbeat. Some patients may become concerned about this arousal in itself. For example, some patients become completely preoccupied about sweating in social situations, and may go to great lengths to hide this. Other patients fear blushing or drawing attention to themselves in some other way. Individuals frequently will negatively rehearse the feared situation prior to entry which will maintain avoidance and, if they do enter, will persistently self-monitor their arousal symptoms, focusing on themselves rather than the situation.

These problems can be approached in several ways; for example, some patients respond well to trying to change their thinking about such situations by gradually adopting a 'so what' attitude with the therapist reinforcing the view that few people other than the patient will notice such a symptom and if they do, for example, notice the patient sweating they will either think nothing of it or, if they do realise the person is anxious, feel sympathetic towards them. This may assist to de-catastrophe the patient's fears and encourage engagement with effective exposure. Another helpful therapeutic technique is sometimes called 'paradoxical intention'. In this, patients are instructed to try to bring the symptom on, and quite often, if they really attempt to do this, they find that (paradoxically) the symptom recedes or goes away completely.

Social phobia can also be complicated by other factors which need intervention. For example, some patients with social phobia may have deficits of social skill. Thus, for example, they may avoid eye contact or stand rather awkwardly. These problems in themselves can compound the anxiety – in the case of poor eye contact, by depriving the person of any feedback from the other person. Thus, a vicious cycle can develop between the phobic component of the condition and the social skill part.

The obvious initial treatment approach is to help patients to improve their social skills. This can be done as treatment in the clinic, either on an individual or group basis. The patient is asked to role-play the difficult situations and, if possible, this role-play is video-taped. The therapist and patient look at the video tape and decide on various strategies to change the behaviour. The therapist or another person may 'model' an appropriate behaviour, and following both feedback and modelling, the patient will then attempt to try the new behaviour in a further role-play. Sometimes one needs to repeat this sequence of events several times prior to asking the patient to try to practise this in real life. Often one works on one or two behaviours at a time, gradually building a new repertoire. Social skills training will lead to exposure to previously avoided situations which is in itself therapeutic. It should also be noted that video feedback can also be extremely useful in assisting people to recognise that how they believe they appear is a subjective perception and often not the case. Video feedback may facilitate a more objective evaluation of oneself.

AGORAPHOBIA

Agoraphobia is a very interesting, if complex, condition. The term was originally coined by Westphal, a German neurologist, more than 130 years ago, to describe a condition that he had observed in four men. Since then there have been many descriptions of the condition, and many names have been attached to it; for example another German neurologist, Benedikt, used a term that literally translates as 'dizziness in public places'. It has also been called *peur d'espace*, phobic anxiety depersonalisation syndrome, endogenous anxiety and street fear.

However, it is now defined in DSM-IV as:

> Anxiety about being in places or situations from which escape might be difficult or embarrassing, or in which help might not be available in the event of having a panic attack or panic-like symptoms. Agoraphobic fears typically involve characteristic situations including being outside the home alone, being in a crowd or standing in a queue, being on a bridge or travelling in a bus, train or car. The situations are either avoided or else endured with considerable anxiety and many sufferers will rely on being accompanied by others to attempt to enter situations.

Thus, agoraphobia involves a whole range of situations where the patient develops fear or other unpleasant feelings, and because the avoidance is so widespread, patients are often very handicapped. Agoraphobic fears are very common in the population, and up to 1 in 8 people are concerned about specific situations where escape might be difficult, for example tube trains, but the full agoraphobic syndrome is probably present in only about 1% of the population (Gournay 1989).

Treatment

Although simple exposure principles and practice are paramount, the application in many cases of agoraphobia is not as straightforward as it may seem. The question for many therapists is, if a patient has numerous avoidance behaviours, where does one start? In attempting to answer this question, there are several guiding principles. The first is to ask the patient about the behaviour which the patient most desires to be changed. Sometimes this is obvious to all concerned; for example, the person with a fear of the tube may only be able to travel to work by this route. Another principle is to target behaviours which are easily repeatable, if possible on a daily basis. Another principle which seems rather obvious, but this needs pointing out, is to ensure that the situation reliably produces an anxiety response. There are some patients who have variable anxiety in certain situations, and it is usually best not to target these as a treatment priority, since occurrence of anxiety and, therefore, exposure and habituation to it will be less frequent.

Exposure is clearly the most effective approach, but what has research told us about treatment method? There are a number of variables which are important in considering the effectiveness of exposure treatment. We know that long sessions (i.e. more than 2 hours) are more effective (e.g. Stern & Marks 1973); treatment in cohesive groups may be better than individual treatment (e.g. Hand et al 1974) and self-help is usually very effective (see Chapter 19 in this book). However, there are many more variables which are connected with effective exposure treatment. Since detailed discussion is out of place here, the reader is referred to Gournay (1989), Hawton et al (1989) and Gournay (1996).

OBSESSIVE–COMPULSIVE DISORDER

Obsessive–compulsive disorder (OCD) is a condition which may affect up to 2% of the population (Marks 1987). As the name implies, the condition is characterised by obsessions or compulsions, or more commonly, a mixture of both. DSM-IV defines obsessions as:

- recurrent and persistent thoughts or impulses or images that are experienced at some time during the disturbance as intrusive and inappropriate and cause marked anxiety or distress
- the thoughts, impulses or images are not simply excessive worries about real-life problems
- the person attempts to ignore or suppress such thoughts, impulses or images, or to neutralise them with other thought or action
- the person recognises that the obsessive thoughts, impulses or images are a product of his or her own mind, and not imposed from without, as in the thought of insertion found in schizophrenia.

Compulsions are defined as:

- repetitive behaviours (e.g. handwashing, ordering, checking) or mental acts (e.g. praying, counting, repeating words silently) that the person feels driven to perform in response to an obsession or according to rules that must be applied rigidly
- the behaviour or mental acts are aimed at preventing or reducing distress, or preventing some dreaded event or situation. However, these behaviours or mental acts are either not connected in a realistic way with what they are designed to neutralise, or prevent, or are clearly excessive.

The DSM-IV definition goes on to qualify the definition of obsessions and compulsions by making the point that in this condition the person has recognised that the obsessions or compulsions are excessive or unreasonable (this does not however apply to children with the condi-

tion). In addition, in order to make such a diagnosis it needs to be clear that the obsessions or compulsions cause the individual not only distress, but are time consuming or significantly interfere with the individual's normal activities.

Treatment

The point must be made that before the advent of behavioural treatments for this condition, patients with OCD did not appear to respond to any of the available psychological treatments (which were mainly psycho-analytic) or to medications. Many patients with OCD became long-stay patients and many endured ineffective and often barbarous 'psycho-surgery'. However, behavioural treatments for this condition were developed nearly 30 years ago and used two central methods. These were, first, exposure to the feared stimulus and second, prevention of the ritualistic response (response-prevention). One of the first accounts of this treatment was described by Meyer (1966) who published an account of two cases in which patients were exposed to their anxiety-evoking situations and then prevented from performing their rituals. This treatment was applied in an in-patient setting.

Since that time, behavioural treatment has become the mainstay of psychological approaches to OCD. Meyer's approach has been gradually refined over the years and now patients with rituals are gradually exposed to their feared situations and taught to prevent their normal ritualistic response. The efficacy of this approach has been supported by several clinical trials (e.g. Abel 1993, Marks et al 1975, Mawson et al 1982). Since the original development of behavioural treatment, which was in in-patient settings, the vast majority of patients are now managed as out-patients, and increasingly assisted by a range of self-help methods, including books and computer programs (e.g. Ghosh & Marks 1987). There is evidence that patients may be effectively treated by behavioural methods in groups (Fals-Stewart et al 1993). This is obviously also effective from an economic point of view, but group methods have not been taken up in a widespread way by clinical services. Treatment may be lengthy, and many patients may require 15 to 20 sessions, including treatment in the home setting.

The predominant approach is exposure; ritual-(response-) prevention enables the individual to engage and stay with exposure. For example, if the patient has a contamination fear, the therapist may help the patient, if it is appropriate, to touch a wastebin, and then encourage the patient to resist the urge to wash the hands. There is substantial evidence (e.g. O'Sullivan et al 1991) that patients are considerably helped if the therapist demonstrates the exposure, before asking the patient to follow suit; this approach is called 'modelling'. The therapist often needs also to help patients to learn once again to wash their hands in a reasonable way (many patients may not only wash their hands very frequently but wash them in a very ritualistic and prolonged fashion). It is not uncommon to see patients whose skin has become infected because of washing hands for prolonged periods, or using harmful detergents and disinfectants which cause burns or ulceration.

In between the sessions of exposure and response-prevention, patients will be asked to undertake 'homework exercises', which consolidate the gains they have made in the session with the therapist. Home sessions are often important, and the involvement of close friends or family members is helpful, as they can be trained to act as 'co-therapists'. Co-therapists may be able to encourage and supervise homework treatment tasks. It is also important to involve the family so as to break the pattern of reassurance-seeking which often builds up with such problems. By the time patients are referred for treatment, they may have developed a habit of asking reassurance continually. While this reassurance is usually forthcoming from the patient's family and friends and may comfort the patient in the short term, the reassurance itself often, in the long term, makes the problem worse. This is because reassurance-seeking is a type of behavioural avoidance of anxiety and is, in consequence, associated with maintenance of such anxiety. The therapist will therefore ask the patient to stop reassurance-seeking and to instruct the family and friends with more appropriate responses, should the patient continue to seek such reassurance.

The treatment of obsessive ruminations is often more problematic. As noted above, the patient may have a constant intrusive preoccupation with a particularly aversive theme which may be connected to a theme of violence, obscenity, or death. By definition, the patient will try to resist these intrusive, anxiety-provoking thoughts and attempt to avoid them, often by using thought (cognitive) rituals which are aimed to reduce the anxiety generated.

Therapy involves helping patients to 'face up' to their thoughts in a gradual and systematic fashion and to do this, the therapist may use several methods. These may include having patients record their anxiety-provoking thoughts on audio tape, and playing them continuously until the anxiety evoked by such thoughts subsides, without using the cognitive ritualising previously referred to. Alternatively, the therapist may expose the patient to particular situations which may give rise to the ruminations occurring. For example, a patient, whose obsessive ruminations centre around violent actions, may be asked to watch a violent film and to continue watching this film until the obsessive thoughts which are triggered no longer occur or occur at a much lesser frequency and with much less anxiety. Such treatment is often very distressing for the patient and the therapist needs to ensure that each step of the treatment programme is properly graduated so that the patient is able to tolerate the anxiety evoked. The simple rule of thumb is for patients to be exposed to their fears or obsessive thoughts in not only a graduated way, but also to use the central principle that each exposure task should be 'difficult, but manageable'.

The treatment of obsessions (both rituals and ruminations) often presents one of the greatest challenges for therapists. However, as noted above, trained nurse behaviour therapists produce excellent treatment outcomes with this group, and there are now several studies which have lengthy post-treatment follow-up (see Gournay 1995 for an extended review). It is worth noting that Steketee (1994) examined 25 open and controlled studies representing 500 patients with OCD from various countries, and overall 85% of patients were at least improved, and 55% of patients treated were much improved.

Many patients do however have residual problems and behavioural treatment does not help everyone. The use of medications, with or without behavioural treatment, has been dominant over the last 20 years. In the first, randomised controlled trial (RCT), which compared a tricyclic antidepressant, clomipramine, and exposure, and which reported a 2-year follow-up (Mawson et al 1982), the benefits of exposure treatment alone were clear. However, the benefits of adding clomipramine to exposure were not entirely obvious and the controversy concerning treatment with this group of drugs continues (e.g. Kozak 1994).

The newer antidepressant drugs, the selective serotonin reuptake inhibitors, do also seem to help this group of patients (e.g. Montgomery et al 1993) and there is clearly a need to continue evaluating treatment of patients with OCD by behavioural and pharmacological methods, both alone and in combination.

Outcome of treatment for obsessive ruminations vs obsessive rituals

There is an overall view (e.g. Marks 1987) that psychological treatment for rituals yields better outcomes than that for obsessive ruminations. However, the reality is that many patients have a mixture of both rituals and ruminations and there is some evidence (e.g. Duggan et al 1993) that patients treated by nurse therapists for obsessive ruminations have, over the years, shown better outcomes than previously. This may simply reflect the refining of exposure techniques over the period studied (1978–1991).

Obsessive slowness

Rachman (1974) described a condition he called 'primary obsessional slowness' in which patients were described as taking hours to carry out routine tasks. It was suggested that the term be used because the activities concerned were not rituals and there was no apparent reduction in anxiety or euphoria before or after the activity, and the slowness seemed to occur in the setting of a relative absence of obsessional thoughts.

This view has recently been challenged by Veale (1993) who argues that the slowness observed is not primary and is part and parcel of a more general network of rituals and ruminations. Veale has argued that the condition should be treated with exposure, and that drug treatments may be helpful as an adjunct.

Obsessive–compulsive disorder with and without tics

In the last decade, it has been recognised that obsessive–compulsive symptoms may be linked with tics, which have a neurological basis. Furthermore, Pauls (1990) has pointed out that obsessive–compulsive symptoms are much more prevalent among patients with Gilles de la Tourette syndrome, and a higher proportion of patients with OCD and their first degree relatives have tic symptoms. More recently, researchers (e.g. McGuire et al 1994) have highlighted the possible biological basis of OCD and the condition is probably best conceptualised as one with a mixture of psychological and biological factors in its causation.

Measures in the assessment and treatment of obsessive–compulsive disorder

Effective psychological treatment is of course underpinned by the use of measurement. Measurement enables the therapist first of all to assess the problem in an objective fashion, and then to use these instruments to detect change during and after treatment. There are standardised interviews that reliably diagnose OCD, for example, the Structured Clinical Interview (Spitzer et al 1987). However, there is now an extremely useful assessment instrument which was developed specifically for OCD, the Yale Brown Obsessive Compulsive Scale (YBOCS). The YBOCS represents the most comprehensive measure of OCD so far developed. It examines five aspects of the disorder (time spent, interference, distress, resistance and perceived control) and it is now recognised as the gold standard; nurse therapists are increasingly using this measure. However, one should also remember that,

as well as the specific measures of obsessional rituals and rumination, one may need to measure more general phenomena, such as anxiety, fears and phobias, and depression. In addition, the therapist will need to work in collaboration with the patient to define treatment targets which should cover a wide range of areas.

As with other treatments, any approach to OCD must include the use of an assessment battery which is repeated during and after treatment. If the patient needs to be seen for a large number of sessions, it is usually advisable to rate the patient's progress every five sessions. Most therapists will find that the treatment strategies for a particular patient will need adjusting and it is only careful measurement of various aspects of the problem which will allow the therapist to determine whether a particular therapeutic strategy needs continuing, adapting, or abandoning to be replaced by another intervention.

In conclusion:

- While OCD problems often present a complex picture, the importance of intrinsic cognitive–behavioural psychotherapy principles applies. The fear is maintained in the long term by the short-term reduction in fear achieved by active attempts (rituals) to reduce it. In general the obsession (intrusion) is followed by compulsion (urge to perform ritual) which is intended to reduce anxious arousal. Therefore, in order to achieve effective duration of exposure, ritual- (response-) prevention must be incorporated.
- Behavioural approaches continue to be demonstrated as the psychological treatment of choice with or without the use of medication.
- Measurement and evaluation are therapeutic tools and their use within OCD problems is no exception.

NURSE THERAPISTS

Marks recognised that the rapid development of behavioural treatments for a range of conditions which was occurring in the 1970s would lead to a demand for behavioural psychotherapy services which the traditional professions of psychiatry and psychology could not meet. Marks drew from the experience of 'barefoot doctors' (i.e. doctor's assistants working in remote areas) to argue that individuals with a nursing background could, with the correct training, be very effective deliverers of psychiatric services. The first programme, which involved a 3-year, full-time training for five nurses between 1972 and 1975, led to the inauguration of an 18-month intensive course which continues to the present day. The original centre at the Maudsley has now provided continuous training for 25 years. Other centres have been established and some have closed, but several hundred nurses have now been trained and there are probably 200 equivalents in practice in England and Wales (Gournay et al 1999).

The nurse therapy programme is underpinned by the following general principles of cognitive–behavioural psychotherapy:

- detailed behavioural (functional) analysis
- evidence-based practice
- explicit negotiation and planning
- plentiful real-life practice of assessment and treatment skills
  - the use of multiple, reliable measures of change
- a pragmatic approach.

The general skills acquired by nurse therapists are in the following areas:

- interviewing
- problem-orientated record-keeping and communications

- caseload management and planning
- supervisory and training skills
- understanding and addressing ethical issues
- liaison, i.e. interprofessional collaboration
- an ability to recognise the limits of competence.

Training methods include formal didactic teaching, but the bulk of the programme is given over to skills acquisition. Skills are developed by a number of experiential and evaluable methods, including:

- demonstrations, which involve both live patients and via video tape
- role rehearsal by trainees of interviewing and treatment procedures
- monitoring and feedback using close circuit television and other methods
- the use of a highly focused model of clinical supervision.

Nurses spend 12 months in an intensive training period when they assess and treat a number of patients. The core categories of problems addressed are as follows:

- agoraphobia and panic disorder
- specific phobias
- social phobias
- social skills problems
- sexual problems
- obsessive–compulsive disorder
- other conditions which have been shown to be amenable to behavioural and cognitive–behavioural psychotherapy, including post-traumatic stress disorder and somatisation problems.

After the initial period of intensive training, nurse therapists then complete the rest of their course by practising their skills with expert supervision from experienced clinicians who may be psychologists, psychiatrists or trained nurse therapists in other settings. Therefore, by the end of the 18 months, students are experienced in the treatment of a range of conditions which have been shown to be amenable to behavioural and cognitive–behavioural psychotherapy. They will also have had experience of treating these patients in home, hospital and out-patient settings. In addition, trainees will have had considerable experience of working with families.

Nurse therapy training is recognised to be at a level which is sufficient to enable the graduate of the course to be accredited by the British Association of Behavioural and Cognitive Psychotherapy. In turn, graduates of the programme are also then able to register with the United Kingdom Council for Psychotherapy and be given full registration as behavioural/cognitive psychotherapists.

Marks tested the efficacy of nurse therapists within an RCT conducted in primary care (Marks 1985). This study showed that nurse therapists working with phobic and obsessional problems achieved significant clinical gains in patients, compared with patients provided with routine care from their GPs. In addition, an economic analysis conducted within the context of this study showed that nurse therapy treatment produces economic gains for both the patient and the health care system. The efficacy of nurse therapy has been tested further in audits of large numbers of patients treated by nurse therapists (Duggan et al 1993) and a number of nurse therapists have conducted, or have taken part in, RCTs of treatment which all testify to the benefits of nurse therapist intervention. For example, Deale et al (1997) carried out an RCT using cognitive–behaviour therapy delivered by a nurse therapist for chronic fatigue syndrome, and showed substantial improvement over a placebo treatment. Lovell (1997) demonstrated the benefits of nurse therapy treatment for post-traumatic stress disor-

der, within an RCT. Gournay (1991a, 1991b) showed, within a large RCT with follow-up to 2 years after treatment, that nurse therapists treat people with agoraphobia with great effect. Marks et al (1980) reported an RCT of the treatment of OCD with substantial gains being attributable to behavioural treatment.

There are many more examples of nurse therapists developing innovations in behavioural and cognitive–behavioural treatment. For example, Newell & Shrubb (1994) developed techniques for managing body image disorder, while Gournay et al (1997) developed this work further, in a study which used a cognitive–behavioural package for people with body image disorder and compared this approach with a waiting list control. The outcome of this study showed that the cognitive–behavioural package produced very significant gains for the patient, while those patients in the waiting list condition did not improve at all.

The nurse therapy programme, although small, has been incredibly influential in the development and innovation of British mental health nursing with nurse therapy graduates holding the most senior posts in practice, education, commissioning, management, research and public policy.

What of the future? Clearly the experiment started by Marks 25 years ago has been a great success. However, the time has surely come to develop training and education programmes which will disseminate nurse therapy skills more widely at pre- and post-registration level, to other disciplines and in in-patient as well as community settings. At present, there are very large numbers of patients who could benefit, but who are currently deprived of treatment because of the serious shortage of therapists. This situation should obviously not be allowed to continue and extending nurse therapy models of service delivery provides the obvious answer.

Exercise

The treatment of phobias and rituals is a highly practical skill. To gain a clear idea of what is involved, go through the following steps:

1. Identify some situation which causes you anxiety. This could be an everyday situation such as speaking in public, or a mild phobia (perhaps, for example, you find it difficult to dispose of spiders you find in the house).
2. Read one of the books in the key texts for further reading section, paying particular attention to the material concerning the treatment of phobias, and make careful notes on the principles and practice of conquering common fears.
3. Work systematically at examining and confronting the anxiety you have identified in step 1.

This experiential exercise will prove a valuable insight into the experience of both normal and, by extension, clinical anxiety, and their treatment.

KEY TEXTS FOR FURTHER READING

Marks I M 1987 Fears, phobias and rituals. Oxford University Press, Oxford. *This is a definitive text which describes every aspect of fears, phobias and rituals, and remains the best source of background information. There is no other book which comprehensively addresses the background of research, and although more than a decade has passed since the book was published, much of the material still holds true. However, readers will need to be aware that they should update their knowledge on treatment approaches.*

Hawton K, Kirk J, Clark D, Salkovskis P 1989 Cognitive behaviour therapy for psychiatric problems. Oxford University Press, Oxford. *This is still the best basic text for training in cognitive–behaviour therapy, setting out an introduction to this therapeutic approach for a range of problems. The material in this book on approaches to anxiety disorders will help the reader understand the whole basis of the general approach, and to acquire some specific knowledge regarding interventions and evaluation.*

Steketee G, White K 1990 When once is not enough: help for obsessive compulsives. New Harbinger Publications, Oakland, California. *This book is written for both sufferers of OCD and for therapists. It presents a great deal of background knowledge concerning the basis of OCD. It also provides some excellent advice about planning treatment, reducing obsessive fears, exposure therapies and the role of medication. Therapists can use this book, both as a resource for themselves and to help patients with the augmentation of their therapy.*

Gournay K 1996 No panic. Asset Books, Guildford. *This text is primarily written as a self-help manual for sufferers of panic attacks, and describes the background concerning causation of panics, and then deals with the range of strategies which can be used by sufferers, including all of the effective behavioural and cognitive interventions.*

REFERENCES

Abel L 1993 Exposure with response prevention and serotonergic antidepressants in the treatment of obsessive compulsive disorder: a review and implications for interdisciplinary treatment. Behaviour Research and Therapy 31:463–478

Deale A, Chalder T, Marks I, Wesselly S 1997 Cognitive behaviour therapy for chronic fatigue syndrome: a randomised controlled trial. American Journal of Psychiatry 154:408–414

Duggan C, Marks I, Richards D 1993 Clinical audit of behavioural therapy training of nurses. Health Trends 25:25–30

Fals-Stewart W, Marks A, Schafer J 1993 A comparison of group therapy and individual behaviour therapy in treating obsessive compulsive disorder. Journal of Nervous and Mental Disease 181:189–193

Ghosh A, Marks I 1987 Self treatment of agoraphobia by exposure. Behaviour Therapy 18(1):3–16

Gournay K 1989 Agoraphobia: Nature and treatment. Routledge, London

Gournay K 1991a The base for exposure treatment in agoraphobia: some indicators for nurse therapists and community psychiatric nurses. Journal of Advanced Nursing 16:82–91

REFERENCES (*contd*)

Gournay K 1991b The failure of exposure treatment in agoraphobia: implications for the practice of nurse therapists and community psychiatric nurses. Journal of Advanced Nursing 16:1099–1109

Gournay K 1995 The treatment of obsessive compulsive disorder: approaches using behavioural psychotherapy alone or in combination with other treatments. Journal of Serotonin Research Suppl 1:37–47

Gournay K J M 1996 No panic. Asset Books, Guildford

Gournay K, Veale D, Walburn J 1997 Body image disorder: pilot randomized controlled trial. Clinical Effectiveness in Nursing 1:38–46

Gournay K, Denford L, Parr A, Newell R 1999 British nurses in behavioural psychotherapy. Journal of Advanced Nursing (in press)

Hand I, Lamontagne Y, Marks I 1974 Group exposure *in vivo* for agoraphobics. British Journal of Psychiatry 124:588–602

Hawton K, Salkovskis P, Kirk J, Clark B 1989 Cognitive behaviour therapy for psychiatric problems. Oxford University Press, Oxford

Kozak M J 1994 Obsessive compulsive disorder. Current Opinion in Psychiatry 7:474–479

Lovell K 1997 The nature and treatment of post-traumatic stress disorder. Unpublished PhD thesis, Institute of Psychiatry, London

McGuire P K, Bench C, Frith C, Marks I, Frackowiak R, Dolan R 1994 Functional anatomy of obsessive compulsive phenomena. British Journal of Psychiatry 164:459–468

Marks I 1985 Nurse therapists in primary care. RCN Publications, London

Marks I M 1987 Fears, phobias and rituals. Oxford University Press, Oxford

Marks I M, Hodgson R, Rachman S 1975 Treatment of chronic obsessive compulsive neurosis in vivo exposure, a two year follow-up in issues in treatment. British Journal of Psychiatry 127:349–364

Marks I, Matthews A 1978 Brief standard self rating for phobic patients. Behaviour Research and Therapy 17:263–267

Marks I, Stern R, Mawson D, Cobb J, McDonald R 1980 Clomipramine and exposure for obsessive compulsive rituals. British Journal of Psychiatry 135:1–25

Mawson D, Marks I, Ramm E 1982 Clomipramine – an exposure for chronic obsessive compulsive rituals: 2 year follow-up. British Journal of Psychiatry 140:11–18

Meyer V 1966 Modification of expectations in cases with obsessional rituals. Behaviour Research and Therapy 4:273–280

Montgomery S A, McIntyre A, Osterheider M et al 1993 A double blind placebo controlled study of fluorexetine in patients with DSMIIIR obsessive compulsive disorders. European Neuropsychopharmacology 3:143–152

Newell R, Shrubb S 1994 Attitude change and behaviour therapy in body dysmorphic disorder: two case reports. Behavioural and Cognitive Psychotherapy 22:163–169

O'Sullivan G, Noshirvani H, Marks I, Monteiro W, Lelliott P 1991 Six year follow-up after exposure and clomipramine therapy for obsessive compulsive disorder. Journal of Clinical Psychiatry 52:150–155

Pauls D 1990 Gilles de la Tourette syndrome, an obsessive compulsive disorder familial relationships. In: Jeniike M, Baer L, Minichiello W (eds) Obsessive compulsive disorders, 2nd edn. Year Book Medical Publishers, New York

Rachman S 1974 Primary obsessional slowness. Behaviour Research and Therapy 12:9–18

Spitzer R, Williams J, Gobbon M 1987 SCID: Structured clinical interview for DSMIIIR. New York State Psychiatric Institute, New York

Steketee G 1994 Behavioural assessment and treatment planning with obsessive compulsive disorder. Behaviour Therapy 25:613–634

Stern R, Marks I 1973 Brief and prolonged flooding: a comparison in agoraphobic patients. Archives of General Psychiatry 28:270–276

Veale D 1993 Classification and treatment of obsessional slowness. British Journal of Psychiatry 162:198–203

CHAPTER CONTENTS

Key points   225

Introduction   226

Epidemiology – the extent of the problem   226
   Primary care   226
   Secondary care   227

Concepts and definitions   227
   Mind–body dualism   227
   Terminology – disease and illness   227
   Psychosomatic and somatisation   227
   Hysteria   228
   Medically unexplained symptoms   228
   Functional   228
   Classification   229
   Somatoform disorders   229
   Chronic fatigue syndrome   230
   Illness behaviour   230

Aetiology and model for understanding somatic
      syndrome   231
   Predisposing factors   231
   Precipitating factors   232
   Perpetuating factors   232
   Summary   233

Cognitive–behavioural treatment   233
   Treatment process   234

Evidence-based practice   239

Conclusions   239

Exercise   240

Key texts for further reading   240

References   240

13

Somatisation and inappropriate illness behaviour

Trudie Chalder

KEY POINTS

- Somatic symptoms are extremely common in primary and secondary care.

- Physical symptoms without clear-cut organic pathology are real and have a physiological component.

- A variety of labels are used to describe them.

- Associated disability can be marked.

- A variety of behavioural and cognitive techniques can be used to improve symptoms and disability.

- There are a number of randomised controlled trials demonstrating the effectiveness of cognitive–behavioural therapy for these problems.

INTRODUCTION

Physical symptoms without organic pathology have been referred to by a variety of labels such as medically unexplained symptoms, hypochondriasis and somatisation. These labels will be described and discussed. Everyone experiences physical symptoms not related to specific aetiology from time to time. However, when the symptoms become the focus of an individual's attention, the severity of the symptom often increases and varying degrees of disability result. Clearly, different people cope with symptoms in different ways. However, when the degree of disability is in excess of what is expected, patients often find themselves in conflict with health professionals in general, and doctors in particular. It is in this context that the concept of abnormal illness behaviour is used. Although the term can be applied to any patient who is responding to illness or disease in a way which does not match expectations, this chapter will focus on those patients with symptoms not associated with organic pathology.

Abnormal illness behaviour will be defined, although it will be argued that it is an unhelpful term which is often used in a pejorative way by health professionals when talking about patient behaviour. This unhelpful labelling is the result of being caught in a dualistic framework in which the mind and body are seen as separate entities. Given that this model is all pervasive in our society, it is not surprising therefore that when patients present with symptoms not easily explained by the traditional medical model they are inadvertently blamed for not getting better. An alternative model, which transcends mind–body dualism, takes into account cognitive, behavioural and physiological aspects of illness, and which makes a distinction between precipitating and perpetuating factors will be described. This more comprehensive model of understanding somatic symptoms leads on to flexible, pragmatic management approaches and can be applied in either primary or secondary care. The example of chronic fatigue syndrome (CFS) will be used to illustrate the approach.

EPIDEMIOLOGY – THE EXTENT OF THE PROBLEM

Everyone experiences physical symptoms not related to specific aetiology from time to time. Prevalence rates vary considerably depending on the setting and the specific symptom being studied. However, despite the fact that 90% of the population experience at least one symptom per week (Andersen et al 1968, Hannay 1978), only a minority result in consultation. The prevalence of somatisation disorder in a UK primary care sample was about 2 per 1000 (Deighton & Nichol 1985), while data from the North American Epidemiological Catchment Area Study, suggests a lifetime prevalence of somatisation disorder within the general population of 0.4% (Swartz et al 1986). Particular symptoms (e.g. chest pain) are more likely than others (e.g. headache) to arouse concern and result in consultation behaviour (Banks et al 1975), which implies that factors other than the symptom itself affect whether people interpret bodily sensations as a sign of illness (Craig & Boardman 1990).

Primary care

Up to one in five new consultations in primary care is related to somatic symptoms for which no specific cause can be found (Bridges & Goldberg 1985). The impact of these symptoms can be enormous and consequently affects the individual's ability to carry out normal activities. Given that the medical model operating in the health service works on the premise that physical symptoms have organic causes, it is not surprising that many patients feel dissatisfied with both the lack of a diagnosis and the advice given.

Secondary care

Physical symptoms with no obvious cause are amongst the commonest reasons for out-patient referral in the UK (Bradlow et al 1992). Typically, patients present with a specific symptom or set of physical symptoms. They have an expectation that investigations carried out will lead onto a medical diagnosis and effective treatment. This does not always happen. In many patients, investigations are normal and the patient is left feeling dissatisfied with the outcome. As a result the patient continues to consult, constantly requests further investigations and uses considerable amounts of NHS resources without gaining any benefit (de Gruy et al 1987, Katon et al 1990).

CONCEPTS AND DEFINITIONS

Mind–body dualism

Our society tends to view illness and disease in a *dualistic* way: that is to say that problems are seen as being either physical or psychological. If there is an obvious physical cause, then the problem is perceived as being real whereas illnesses without demonstrable organic pathology are viewed as being 'all in the mind' or psychiatric and therefore potentially not real. The model inherent in our society and therefore our health service is inadequate. It assumes that because we cannot find specific organic pathology to account for the symptoms that the symptom does not exist and cannot be treated. This is reflected in the attitudes and behaviour of some doctors. Largely speaking, the doctor has internalised the current scientific approach to disease. A linear cause–effect model in which aetiological pathogenic agents lead to bodily pathology is assumed (Singh et al 1981).

This split between mind and body has been traced back to Rene Descartes' dualistic philosophy of the 17th century, but these ideas were not entirely new. They evolved from earlier ideas espoused by the Greeks. For example, Plato saw man as being divided between the soul, of divine origin, and the body, its fleshly prison. Clearly, this presents the patient with a problem. The patients referred to in this chapter have real physical symptoms but on the whole do not have demonstrable organic pathology to account for the symptoms. Some will have an obvious psychiatric disorder such as depression or anxiety but many will not. The patient senses that something is wrong and tries to make sense of the experience. As taught from childhood, a visit to the doctor seems to be a sensible course of action. There is an expectation that after an adequate assessment, the doctor will reveal the cause of the symptoms and will then state clearly what needs to be done in order to get better (Singh et al 1981). Simply reassuring the patient that everything is normal does not work. The patient will understandably feel that the doctor is refusing to regard them as ill.

Terminology – disease and illness

The terms disease and illness are often used synonymously. However, while *disease* implies the presence of organic pathology, *illness* usually refers to the presence of symptoms, usually physical, which cause the sufferer concern but may not be related to demonstrable organic pathology. In this chapter, then, it is assumed that patients have an illness but not necessarily a disease.

Psychosomatic and somatisation

Physical symptoms which are not easily explained have been given a variety of labels. This probably results from the considerable confusion surrounding how they are caused and subsequently managed. The term *psychosomatic* is a term pertaining to that which is presumed to have both psychic (mental) and somatic (bodily) components. The usual implication here is that these two separate aspects interact, each having impact on the other. A psychosomatic disorder is a general label used for any disorder with *somatic* (bodily) manifestations that are assumed to have at least a partial cognitive or emotional cause (i.e. they are to some degree psychological) (Reber 1988.)

Somatisation, a term frequently used, implies that psychological distress is expressed in the form of physical symptoms (Kellner 1990, Lipowski 1988). Thus defined, it encompasses a wide spectrum of symptoms related to various organs or systems, appearing acutely or chronically and mimicking a wide variety of diseases. It is usually assumed that somatisation occurs in the context of psychosocial stress in a person who is vulnerable in some way. Such stresses may not be recognised or acknowledged by the patient.

These terms are not only dualistic but they can also be unhelpful; to the patient whose model of illness differs from that of the professional and to the doctor who is left not knowing how to treat the patient. From the patient's perspective, the main concern is getting rid of an unpleasant or painful symptom which is interfering with the ability to carry out normal activities. Patients cannot necessarily make the link between physical symptoms and distressing events in their life and even if they could the link might be neither useful nor accurate. From the professional's point of view, a psychological reason as to why the patient should be feeling unwell cannot always be found, and even if it could, the patient may not make the same connection. Making links between symptoms and causative factors does not always lead onto pragmatic management strategies.

Hysteria

The term *hysteria* is often used in a neurological setting where symptoms suggestive of neurologic disease are present but unaccounted for by organic pathology. This label is particularly unhelpful because it has multiple meanings (Kendell 1972) and is not a label which can be shared with patients without repercussions. It is a term which is often used synonymously with the label *conversion disorder*. Implicit in the diagnosis of conversion disorder is the idea that unconscious, unresolved conflicts are converted into a somatic symptom (Breuer & Freud 1955). The resolution of the conflict, rendered harmless by the conversion was assumed to be the *primary gain*, while the advantages resulting from the assumption of the sick role were known as the *secondary gain*. These terms are frequently used by health professionals looking after patients with these difficulties, but in the author's view are judgemental, and, even if they did have any validity, are largely unhelpful in terms of managing patients.

Medically unexplained symptoms

Medically unexplained symptoms (Smith et al 1986), unexplained medical symptoms (Escobar & Canino 1989) and medical symptoms not explained by organic disease (Creed et al 1992) are all descriptions often used by liaison psychiatrists. However, these labels make the assumption that somatic symptoms could potentially be explained purely – if not now, then in the future – by the medical model.

Functional

When the term *functional illness* was first described (Stearns 1946), it implied that despite the absence of obvious organic pathology there was some physiological process not yet clearly understood which could account for the symptoms (Trimble 1982). However, over the years the meaning has changed, and it is now often used to imply that patients are either exaggerating or feigning their symptoms or that the symptoms are psychological in nature. Interestingly, with the advent of new technology such as positron emission tomography, functional anatomy and physiological processes associated with medically unexplained somatic experiences are being elucidated (Marshall et al 1997, Vogt et al 1992). Research in this area is embryonic, but as methodologies are refined further, work of this kind should help to debunk the myth that patients are feigning symptoms. The term *functional overlay* is frequently used in neurological settings when the degree of disability associated with symptoms is in excess of what the health professionals would normally expect. Despite its original meaning, it now has a pejorative flavour.

Classification

Patients present with somatic symptoms without obvious organic pathology in every specialism within the health service. For example, in neurology, patients present with non-epileptic attacks, atypical facial pain or unexplained dizziness. In gastroenterology, patients experience abdominal pain associated with intermittent diarrhoea and constipation. This attracts the label of irritable bowel syndrome. In cardiology, patients are seen with non-cardiac chest pain. Other popular categories include CFS and fibromyalgia. All of these diagnoses have something in common. Patients are experiencing real physical symptoms without clear-cut organic pathology, are usually distressed at not being able to control the symptom and will have varying degrees of disability which stops them from carrying out everyday

activities. In addition, many of these patients believe they are physically ill.

Somatoform disorders

The International Classification of Disease (ICD-10) (World Health Organization 1993), defines *somatoform* disorders as 'repeated presentations of physical symptoms, together with persistent requests for medical investigations, in spite of repeated negative findings and reassurances by doctors that the symptoms do not have any physical basis'. For the sake of clarity ICD-I0 defines seven categories: somatisation disorder, undifferentiated somatoform disorder, hypochondriacal disorder, somatoform autonomic dysfunction, persistent somatoform pain disorder, other somatoform disorders and somatoform disorder, unspecified. All have overlapping criteria and, in clinical practice, it is often difficult to differentiate between them. Neurasthenia, which overlaps with CFS, is categorised under other neurotic disorders but has things in common with the somatoform disorders.

For each disorder, a description is provided of the main clinical features. In contrast to DSM-IV which is more specific, some degree of flexibility is apparent. The guidelines are general and should not be used as a straightjacket. They can provide a useful stimulus for teaching and can guide the clinician in deciding on suitable management options. Two of the more common somatising disorders will now be described.

Hypochondriasis is an example of a somatoform disorder that most people will be familiar with. It is a persistent preoccupation with the idea of having one or more serious physical disorders. Patients experience persistent somatic complaints and even though numerous investigations reveal no physical abnormality, the preoccupation persists. There is an inability to accept the advice and reassurance of doctors that there is no physical abnormality underlying the symptoms.

Somatisation disorder is characterised by multiple, recurrent and frequently changing physical symptoms which have been present for many years. Most patients will have a long and complicated history of contact with both primary and secondary care, during which time many negative investigations and, in severe cases, fruitless operations will have been carried out. Symptoms may occur in any system of the body but gastrointestinal sensations are common as are abnormal skin sensations. The course of the disorder is chronic and fluctuating and is associated with marked disability affecting all aspects of a person's life.

It is helpful to make a distinction between hypochondriasis and somatisation disorder while also highlighting the similarities. The hypochondriacal patient constantly presents to the doctor seeking reassurance in the form of requesting tests to determine the presence of a disease. This temporarily relieves the anxiety being experienced but in the longer term maintains the anxiety and worry. In somatisation disorder, the patient requests treatment to remove the symptom and does not feel temporarily relieved at being reassured that the disease is not present. Although the two disorders overlap in that both involve the experience of physical symptoms with no clear-cut organic pathology, the differences need to be taken into account when deciding on management.

Chronic fatigue syndrome

CFS is categorised in ICD-10 under neurasthenia. The illness has attracted a variety of other labels including myalgic encephalomyelitis (ME) and post-infectious fatigue syndrome. Given that the term CFS does not imply any specific aetiology, it is the preferred term. The condition is charac-

terised by physical and mental fatigue, provoked by minimal exertion, which results in marked disability and is associated with a myriad of other symptoms. As with the somatoform disorders there should be no obvious organic pathology to account for the symptoms (Schluederberg et al 1992, Sharpe et al 1991).

Illness behaviour

Illness behaviour is defined as 'the way in which individuals experience, perceive, evaluate and respond to their own health status' (Mechanic 1962, 1980). For example, one person who has a common cold may react by taking to bed for a few days where another may battle on and continue to work despite not feeling well. Clearly then, illness behaviour lies on a continuum. In other words, different people respond to illness and symptoms in different ways and with varying degrees of success. However, rather unhelpfully, the term has been defined categorically (i.e. in terms of what is normal and abnormal).

Normal illness behaviour is defined as being carried out by those who appear to behave in an adaptive way to illness. In other words, they acknowledge they are ill and take action which could be perceived by others as appropriate in the circumstances. For example, someone who finds a breast lump would visit the GP to have it investigated and treated medically should it be necessary.

Abnormal illness behaviour is a concept which has been defined as 'inappropriate or maladaptive mode of experiencing, evaluating or acting in relation to one's own state of health, which persists, despite the fact that a doctor has offered accurate and reasonable information concerning the person's health status, and the appropriate course of management, with provision of adequate time for discussion, clarification and negotiation, taking into account the individual's age, educational and socio-cultural background' (Pilowsky 1997). Clearly, there is some divergence in what is considered normal or abnormal. However, the difficulty with this concept is that on the whole it is pejorative and tends to blame the patient for behaving in a way which is in some ways understandable. The term 'abnormal doctor behaviour' has been used to criticise the doctor for acting in a way which is unhelpful to the patient (Singh et al 1981). Rather than blaming either doctor or patient for behaving in ways which are not helpful, it would seem more profitable to attempt to understand the interactive processes between doctor and patient.

In summary, then, a wide variety of labels have been used to describe the universal phenomenon of somatic symptoms without associated organic pathology. Terminology is confused and muddling. However, broadly speaking all are referring to the same thing: that is, real physical symptoms which cause great distress to the sufferer and frustration to the health professional. The next section of this chapter will focus on describing a model for understanding and treating this phenomenon.

AETIOLOGY AND MODEL FOR UNDERSTANDING SOMATIC SYNDROME

As is the case with the majority of illnesses, a combination of factors which interact determines who experiences somatic symptoms and how they develop them. This will involve predisposing, precipitating and perpetuating factors which affect the individual's physiological (symptoms), behavioural (actions) and cognitive (thoughts) responses. Box 13.1 lists the factors which may be contributing to an individual's becoming ill in the first place and then remaining ill long-term. Some of the literature examining the role of these factors is considered. However, most of the

---

Box 13.1 Factors which contribute to the development and maintenance of somatic symptoms

Predisposing factors
Family history of illness during childhood
Unhelpful core beliefs about illness, e.g. physical symptoms are dangerous
Introverted personality

Precipitating factors
Negative life events/chronic stress
Illness/disease
Psychiatric disorder
Lack of social support
Heightened physiological arousal

Perpetuating factors
Behavioural
Reduction of activities
Frequent visits to the doctor/hospital
Poor sleep routine
Avoidance of tasks/specific places
Reassurance-seeking
Checking for presence of signs of illness

Cognitive
Fear of making symptoms worse
Physical illness attributions
Symptom focusing
Influenced by memory of past aversive experiences
Feeling out of control

Affective
Demoralisation
Low mood
Frustration

Social and cultural
Mind–body dualism
Misinformation in the media
Unhelpful advice
Being disbelieved
Role of family and friends

---

research carried out in this field is preliminary and although there are some exceptions, much is cross-sectional in nature.

Predisposing factors

It has been suggested that early childhood experiences influence the development of somatic syndromes (Craig et al 1993, Mechanic 1979). More specifically, it appears to be the experience of physical illness in a parent which leads the individual to experience more somatic symptoms later on in life (Blumer & Heilbron 1981, Hartwig & Sterner 1985, Hotopf 1996). However, this does not hold for personal childhood experience of illness, suggesting that from a developmental perspective, modelling behaviour of others is the potent factor. Craig et al (1993) have extended their model further, by hypothesising that lack of care contributes to the development of emotional disorder in the face of adversity, while exposure to illness in a parent predisposes their children to interpret symptoms of emotional distress as indicative of physical illness.

There is some preliminary evidence that patients prone to introspection and anxiousness are more likely to somatise (Costa & McRae 1985). However, it seems likely that personality will to some extent be influenced by childhood learning, making it impossible to distinguish between the role of early life experiences and personality. The prevailing culture also has to be taken into account. As CFS, well known in the media as ME, is being promoted as a disease with an as yet, undiscovered physical cause, it is likely that this will influence individual beliefs about symptoms and illness.

Precipitating factors

Examining the role of life events in the development of illness is complicated and costly. A recent study carried out by the author examined the role of negative life events in the development of chronic fatigue in primary care. An increase in the number of negative life events and lack of social support independent of prior psychological distress all contributed to the development of fatigue (Chalder 1998). Mayou et al (1995a) recently suggested that a lowering of mood brought about by a negative event may exacerbate both attention to symptoms and checking of symptoms, which in turn lead to increased concern and then consultation with doctors. A major physical illness could be viewed as a negative event and there is some evidence that non-cardiac chest pain is likely after a myocardial infarction or cardiac surgery (Mayou 1989). However, pain is difficult to measure, making it impossible in this situation to make a distinction between non-cardiac and cardiac pain.

Lack of confiding, which is often connected to lack of social support, is associated with increased physiological arousal and somatic symptoms (Pennebaker & O'Heeron 1984). In one study, relatives of individuals who had died unexpectedly by suicide or car accident were healthier if they had talked to others about their distress (Pennebaker & Susman 1988).

As one would expect, there is an overlap between psychiatric disorder and somatic syndromes (Simon & VonKorff 1991). Not only is there a strong correlation between somatic symptoms and psychological distress, but the greater the number of symptoms, the stronger the association with psychological distress and level of disability (Gomez & Dally 1977, Wessely et al 1996).

Perpetuating factors

Once a particular physiological response has been triggered, the problem is maintained essentially by cognitive and behavioural factors such as fear and avoidance.

Behaviour

In chronic pain and CFS, the role of avoidance behaviour is central in sustaining the cycle of symptoms and disability. Chalder et al (1996b), Philips (1987) and Sharpe et al (1992) found that avoiding exercise predicted disability, while Ray et al (1995) found an association between functional impairment and accommodating to the illness in patients with CFS. In hypochondriasis, a variety of behaviours – reassurance-seeking, intended to check current health status; avoidance of health-related stimuli (e.g. watching *Casualty* on television); and checking of symptoms (e.g. repeatedly palpating a small cut) – actually serve to increase anxiety (Warwick & Salkovskis 1990), as they prevent habituation (anxiety reduction) and maintain preoccupation with illness.

Illness attributions and cognitions

Most patients with somatic complaints, regardless of the type, have a tendency to persistently misinterpret innocuous physical symptoms as evidence of something more serious. In CFS, patients are fearful of making the symptom of fatigue worse (Chalder et al 1996a); in chronic pain, patients worry about exacerbating the pain; in hypochondriasis, physical symptoms are interpreted as evidence of serious disease such as AIDS. Longitudinal studies have demonstrated that making physical illness attributions for fatigue predicts degree of disability in patients with CFS (Chalder et al 1996b, Sharpe et al 1992, Wilson et al 1994). In an effort to control and reduce symptoms, patients become hypervigilant and oversensitised to bodily sensations. This symptom-focusing may serve to exacerbate unpleasant sensations (Warwick & Salkovskis 1990) and has been shown to be associated with fatigue in patients with CFS (Ray et al 1995).

Summary

A variety of complex factors such as childhood experience of illness and stressful life events are associated with the onset of symptoms. Symptoms are then maintained and perpetuated by unhelpful cognitions and avoidant or maladaptive coping strategies. Patient behaviour is also influenced by the behaviour of health professionals. While the prevailing culture in the health service is dualistic, health professionals and patients will continue to misunderstand one another. A three systems model which incorporates physiological, cognitive and behavioural aspects of illness can be useful for both understanding and managing these difficult problems.

It is easy to become judgemental about how patients manage their symptoms, but it is important to remember that patients have striven to make sense of a poorly understood condition and will have probably received a plethora of contradictory advice from health professionals and the media about the nature of the problem and its management. As already stated, many patients will be depressed or anxious, but those who are not will undoubtedly feel very frustrated and demoralised at being stuck in an ever-increasing spiral of symptoms and disability.

COGNITIVE–BEHAVIOURAL TREATMENT

A cognitive–behavioural model enables a practitioner to carry out a comprehensive assessment and to make an individual formulation of the patient's problems, which then lead onto effective cognitive–behavioural management. Cognitive–behaviour therapy (CBT) is a pragmatic approach to managing symptoms which involves enabling patients to change aspects of their behaviour and the way in which they think in order to bring about change in symptoms. This model is widely used in the treatment of anxiety disorders and is referred to as Lang's three systems model (Lang 1970, Hugdahl 1981). Physiological, behavioural and cognitive processes operate largely in synchrony with one another. Changing one particular system such as the person's behaviour will bring about changes in the other two response systems.

Treatment is usually conducted on a one-to-one basis for between 5 and 20 sessions. Each treatment session is structured. At the start of every session, an agenda is agreed between patient and therapist. This is to ensure that all issues are addressed within the time available. Sessions usually last up to 1 hour. Homework, which takes the form of specific behavioural goals which have previously been agreed, is discussed. Success with homework and problems is discussed. New homework is negotiated and agreed upon by therapist and patient. At the end of each session, the key points of the discussion are summarised. The therapist always keeps in mind the end-of-treatment targets which have previously been agreed, as these are to be worked towards systematically.

Box 13.2   Treatment process

Phase 1 – the development of a therapeutic alliance
Phase 2 – generating the willingness to change
Phase 3 – behavioural analysis
Phase 4 – giving the patient a rationale for treatment
Phase 5 – conducting the treatment
Phase 6 – monitoring and evaluating progress
Phase 7 – generalising the progress and ending therapy

The process of treatment, from assessment to discharge, will be described. Kanfer & Schefft (1988) formulated a process model which described seven phases in the ideal course of treatment (see Box 13.2). This framework will be used to illustrate some of the ways in which patients can be enabled to manage their symptoms. The example of CFS will be used, because although approaches to the treatment of somatic problems are varied, the approach can easily be modified and adapted for use in a wide range of somatising illnesses. Salkovskis (1989) described a number of general principles that should be kept in mind when engaging and treating patients with somatic problems and these factors are incorporated into the following exposition.

Treatment process

Phase 1 – the development of a therapeutic alliance

Before health professionals begin the assessment of a patient with a somatic complaint, it is important for them to prepare themselves. It is helpful to have read some relevant literature on the nature of the complaint the patient is presenting with. In addition, a clear idea of what questions to ask during the first interview is essential. During the early phases of treatment, any communication that could be interpreted negatively should be avoided. There should be a value-free acceptance of the patient's world and no attempt should be made to try to dissuade patients from their point of view. Patients must feel they are being listened to. It is imperative to be explicit in conveying belief in the reality of the symptom. Patients may be hypervigilant in looking for signs that they are not believed. They should not be given any grounds for suspicion. In keeping with the model of somatic symptoms already described, any discussion about whether the problem is psychological or physical should be avoided. It is likely that the patient's views about what is wrong with them will be and will have been influenced by their interactions with health professionals. Usually, when a broad interactive model of the patient's symptoms is adopted, antagonistic responses are avoided. Even if the view of the health professional is markedly different from that of the patient, it is important that the patient's view is respected and not disagreed with. The focus of the discussion should shift from cause to symptom-management. This will inherently challenge the *therapeutic nihilism*, the feeling that nothing can be done, which surrounds these problems, and leads into the next phase.

Phase 2 – generating the willingness to change

The next phase involves persuading the patient that change is possible. Many patients feel demoralised when they present for treatment. They may already have seen a number of other professionals who have not offered any hope of recovery or improvement. Several studies have demonstrated that support is experienced positively by patients and helps to elicit behavioural change. It can be helpful to examine formally the advantages and disadvantages of change. Research carried out demonstrating the effectiveness of a particular intervention should be shared with the patient.

Phase 3 – behavioural analysis

During the first session, a behavioural analysis should be conducted using the three systems model as guidance. As well as information about the number and severity of symptoms, it is important to establish precisely what patients are *unable to do* as a *consequence* of their symptoms. In the case of CFS or chronic pain, the patient should be asked to describe a couple of typical days detailing social, work, private and home-related activities. It is important to get some idea, however vague at this stage, whether the patient has long-term plans regarding work and the extent to which the patient's social life has been disrupted. In hypochondriasis, many patients will spend a lot of time talking about their symptoms and seeking reassurance. It is essential that details regarding these behavioural excesses are elicited as these will be the focus of the intervention initially, regardless of what contributed to the onset.

Specific fears about the nature of symptoms and illness attributions should be enquired about. Future discussions will be directed to some extent by the patient's degree of psychological sophistication, and patient's perceptions about the illness will give some indication of how broad the patient's view is. It is helpful to have a longitudinal view of the illness. It is important therefore to establish what was happening in the patient's life prior to the onset of the illness. Enquiring about family illness in childhood may be helpful later on in treatment but may serve to irritate the patient if asked about these issues too early. It is important to check whether the patient is depressed or anxious. Finally, it can be revealing to ask how patients think their life might be in 5 years' time and whether they envisage any change.

Phase 4 – giving the patient a rationale for treatment

After an assessment has been completed, a preliminary formulation of the patient's problems can be decided upon. This should be integrated into a rationale for treatment. It is essential that the formulation and rationale for treatment are individualised, making them acceptable and plausible to the patient. It is impossible and foolish to include everything in the rationale for treatment at the beginning. At best, it would confuse the patient and at worst, it would antagonise them. It can be helpful to divide the rationale for treatment into two parts. The first part will involve some discussion about factors which triggered the problem off; the second part will include more detailed discussion about the factors which have kept the problem going and how any unhelpful patterns can be changed. The rationale will need to be repeated several times during the process of treatment and the patient should be asked to describe the rationale in order to check understanding of it. Lang's three systems model (i.e. the relationship between physiological, behavioural and cognitive responses) should be used to illustrate the approach (Lang 1970).

An example of a treatment rationale for someone with CFS follows:

'It sounds as though from what you've said that the problem started about 3 years ago when you developed the flu. You mentioned that you were particularly busy at work at the time and had been feeling under pressure. You had difficulty getting over the flu and in fact started to feel constantly fatigued. Am I right in thinking that it wasn't the sort of tiredness you used to feel when you were well? ... Um ... Gradually the fatigue got worse and in an attempt to make yourself better, you rested. Initially, resting worked but when you tried to go back to work the fatigue got worse again. So gradually over a long period of time your ability to do things has reduced and the symptoms have got worse. Does that seem like a fair description so far?'

At this point, there may be some discussion about the course of the illness and how resting, even though helpful in the short-term, can inadvertently make the symptoms worse in the long-term. This will lead automatically into the next phase of the rationale; that is, how to do things differently and what to expect.

'So, even though it is understandable that you rest when you feel fatigued, it does in fact help to keep the fatigue going in the long-term. I understand that you are worried about making the fatigue worse, but if you carry out activities consistently (i.e. spread activity throughout the day and intersperse activity with rest), you will slowly start to build up both your activity levels and your strength.'

More detailed discussion about the precise nature of activity scheduling is required and the patient should be told that the idea is to break the association between experiencing symptoms and stopping activity. The patient should continue with whatever activity is being done despite feeling tired. If the patient does this, then the fatigue

---

Box 13.3 Interventions for patients with somatic symptoms

1. Diary of behavioural avoidance or excess (activity scheduling in CFS/checking behaviour in hypochondriasis)
2. Graded, consistent approach to activity (CFS)
3. Establishing a sleep routine
4. Treatment of associated problems (exposure for phobias)
5. Attention to reinforcement (e.g. family member may be reinforcing unhelpful illness behaviour)
6. Ban on reassurance-seeking (hypochondriasis)
7. Cessation of investigations (all involved to agree to this)
8. Discuss advantages and disadvantages of changing
9. Role-play new behaviours in face-to-face session
10. Rationalise medication
11. Discuss how patient will explain improvement to others (face-saver important)

---

will improve gradually with time. The key to success in the beginning is consistency, starting off at a low enough level of activity to achieve success and gradually increasing activity as confidence grows.

It can help to state that if patients change what they do, then it will affect how they feel (i.e. their physical symptoms). This is in keeping with Lang's three systems model described earlier.

Phase 5 – conducting the treatment

Clearly the interventions used will depend entirely on the assessment and the nature of problem the patient presents with. The treatment for hypochondriasis, for example, is quite different from the treatment for CFS. (See Box 13.3 for a list of possible interventions.) At the outset of treatment, patients' relatives or significant others should be involved in the treatment process. This is essential when treating children and adolescents (Garralda 1995), but in adults the behaviour of others may shape the patient's illness behaviour, often dramatically. It is wise when planning treatment of any kind to start with the simplest solution. The patient is then more likely to comply with treatment and, if successful, will repeat the intervention more enthusiastically. This usually means focusing on perpetuating factors such as the behavioural avoidance in CFS.

In CFS, changing the pattern of activity takes time. Noticeable improvements in fatigue levels do not occur for several months. What is required is persistence and patience on the part of the therapist and the patient. In short, active treatment involves negotiating weekly targets of structured, planned activity and rest and establishing a sleep routine.

Examples of specific interventions used in chronic fatigue syndrome. *Activity scheduling.* Goals are initially negotiated using baseline diaries and typically involve a variety of specific tasks, a mixture of social, work and leisure-related activities. Short walks or tasks carried out in even chunks throughout the day are ideal, interspersed with rests. The emphasis is on consistency and breaking the association between experiencing symptoms and stopping activity. The goals are gradually built up as tolerance to symptoms increases, until the longer-term targets are reached. This usually takes several months. Fatigue levels do not decrease very much initially but between discharge and follow-up marked reductions in fatigue can be expected. Patients are warned that a worsening of symptoms may occur as activities are increased but are advised to press on with the programme; increases in fatigue, if any, are usually temporary. Tasks such as reading, which require concentration, can be included but mental functioning seems to improve in synchrony with physical functioning.

Care must be taken when setting goals to ensure that they fall within the tolerance level of the patient. It is far more rewarding for the patient to start off with small achievable goals than to be overly ambitious, which inevitably leads to failure to achieve goals. At times, it is necessary to give advice to patients. This does not mean that the collaborative style of the health professional is lost. Patients expect to be educated. That is why they have presented for treatment. Resistance to change will occur from time to time and a range of strategies can be used to overcome it (Casper & Grawe 1981, Zimmer 1983).

Establishing a sleep routine. Disturbed sleep is very common in patients with CFS. Some complain of hypersomnia (sleeping too much) while others wake up intermittently throughout the night. It is often associated with lack of activity and exercise, although sometimes it is related to worry. The quality of sleep will usually improve once the patient starts to do more. However, by tackling the sleep disturbance directly, a more rapid improvement is expected.

Early on in treatment, patients are asked to keep a diary of bed time, sleep time, wake up time and get up time. The total number of hours spent asleep is calculated. Bed restriction is then used to improve quality of sleep. A routine of going to bed and getting up at a pre-planned time, while simultaneously cutting out daytime catnaps, helps to prevent insomnia. Change in sleep routine can be done slowly depending on the severity of the problem (Morin 1993). For those patients who tend to worry when they get into bed, it can be useful to teach them problem-solving techniques which can be used prior to going to bed. Used in conjunction with stimulus control, where the patient is asked to get up, rather than to lie in bed tossing and turning, and then to return to bed 15 minutes later, the effect can be quite powerful.

Cognitive restructuring. Worry about health will involve misperceptions about the meaning of symptoms. Many patients with CFS will not only experience fatigue but will also notice other frightening symptoms which they will ascribe to the 'disease'. It is important to remember that symptoms are real, but they may not mean what the patient thinks they mean. Specific fears will include worry about the effects of increasing activities but these diminish quite quickly once treatment starts. However, any residual, unhelpful thoughts can be tackled using traditional, cognitive techniques (Burns 1980).

Negative automatic thoughts are referred to as such, because they tend to pop into people's heads almost unconsciously. They are difficult to control, particularly as they may be plausible. An example of a negative thought might be 'If I go shopping today, I am bound to pay for it tomorrow and will feel so exhausted that I'll have to rest for a couple of days to get over it.' For a patient with CFS that is in fact what has been happening. If patients carry out activity scheduling as described without any seriously adverse effects, then gradually their fear will subside along with symptoms. Change in symptoms, however, does take time. It is during this transition period that cognitive strategies can be usefully employed.

Patients are asked to write down negative thoughts like the example just given as precisely as possible. They are then taught to evaluate these thoughts in an objective way. Patients will usually have a bias in their thinking and will tend to ignore certain facts in favour of others which support their negative view. There are many ways of challenging unhelpful thoughts but essentially the main skill they are asked to master is that of a questioning solicitor. They should ask themselves a series of questions which will steer them away from taking a black-and-white view of the situation, to a more balanced view based on new information or evidence which has previously been ignored. A number of alternative explanations may be generated at any one time. The aim is to get away from viewing situations as positive or negative,

another unhelpful dichotomy, and to assist the patient to develop a more balanced view. For example, in response to the negative thought mentioned previously, a patient might challenge it by saying 'If I go for a short walk twice a day and shop for only 15 minutes at a time, then I will gradually build up my strength and confidence. It is important for me not to overdo it on a good day. Consistency is what is important.'

The same technique can be used for different types of thinking such as perfectionism, self-criticism and guilt. A good therapist will be flexible in the use of cognitive techniques. Some patients will find the approach useful at the start of therapy while others will need to develop more psychological sophistication before they will find it useful. The skill is in using the right technique at the right time.

Phase 6 – monitoring and evaluating progress

During the process of change, patients need to receive direct feedback about progress. This can be in the form of positive feedback (Barkham & Shapiro 1986) but, at times, patients may need to be confronted. Frank & Sweetland (1962) report an increase in insight after confrontation. It is likely that at the beginning of treatment patients feel elated at the rate of change but it is also usual for them to plateau. It is at this stage that it is important for the health professional to feedback to the patient that this is to be expected.

Phase 7 – generalising the progress and ending therapy

At the beginning of treatment, patients should be told roughly how many sessions they expect to receive. It can be quite motivating to know that therapy will not go on for ever. It also reinforces the idea that therapy should be both enabling and goal-directed. As time passes by, patients should be encouraged to take on more and more responsibility for their own treatment. It is likely that when therapy ends, there will still be much more to be achieved. It can be helpful therefore to help the patient to set goals which are to be worked towards after therapy has finished. Minor setbacks should be predicted and a plan of action identified to manage them.

EVIDENCE-BASED PRACTICE

There is a growing body of evidence suggesting that cognitive–behavioural approaches are effective in reducing disability and symptomatology in patients with somatic complaints (see Mayou et al 1995b for a review). A good example is a study conducted by Speckens et al (1995) in the Netherlands. They set out to examine the additional effect of CBT for patients with medically explained symptoms in comparison to optimised medical care. The intervention group received between 6 and 16 sessions of CBT. Techniques used included identification and modification of dysfunctional automatic thoughts and behavioural experiments aimed at breaking the vicious cycles of the symptoms and their consequences. At the 6-month, follow-up point, the frequency and intensity of symptoms had reduced and illness behaviour had changed for the better. These improvements were maintained to 1-year follow-up.

Similar impressive results have been demonstrated in chronic fatigue (Chalder et al 1997), chronic fatigue syndrome (Deale et al 1997, Sharpe et al 1996), chronic pain (Heinrich et al 1985, Nicholas et al 1992, Turner & Clancy 1988), non-cardiac chest pain (Klimes et al 1990) and hypochondriasis (Warwick et al 1996).

Sometimes it is hard to translate from research trials to clinical practice. Often treatment is carried out by highly trained and experienced therapists. However, with some training it is possible for less qualified and less experienced nursing staff to carry out psychological interventions. A study carried out by the author (Chalder et al 1997) evaluated the efficacy of a self-help book and specific advice compared with a no-treatment control in reducing chronic fatigue in a primary care population. Both groups were interviewed by a research nurse, using the Clinical Interview Schedule (CIS-R) (Lewis et al 1992), which is used for detecting psychiatric morbidity in primary care populations. The intervention group also received a self-help book. Both groups improved, while the self-help group showed greater improvements. This study demonstrates that effective interventions can be delivered by nurses, both general and psychiatric, with minimal extra training.

CONCLUSIONS

A variety of labels and ways of classifying somatic symptoms not explained by organicity have been used. What is important from a clinical perspective is that the health professional is aware of the various explicit and implicit meanings of these labels. Most of the labels in current use evolve from a world perspective which assumes mind and body are separate. It is difficult to escape this trap because our society and therefore our language are rooted in this philosophy. As far as the author is aware, certainly in the Western world, we do not have a word or phrase which describes the whole, that is body and mind. It is very difficult therefore to adopt a way of thinking and practising which allows us to understand and manage somatic syndromes in a way which is practically helpful. What is actually required is a personal philosophical shift. It has been suggested that a three systems cognitive–behavioural model of understanding illness and symptoms can offer the health professional a way of becoming more effective as a practitioner.

There have been a number of reasonably well-executed studies which demonstrate the usefulness of a cognitive–behavioural approach to somatic syndromes. All health professionals have a moral obligation to engage in evidence-based practice which ensures that patients receive the best care available at the time.

While it is acknowledged that training in pragmatic interventions such as CBT is required, vast sums of money are not necessarily needed to meet this need. Future nursing courses should focus on teaching specific skills including assessment, rationale-giving and problem-solving. In addition, it may be helpful to shift the emphasis away from a dichotomous view of health (i.e. psychological and physical, mind and body) and steer health professionals towards a more integrated view of health and illness. Nurses interested in developing skills in this area should consider undertaking post-registration training courses which emphasise both theory and practice.

Exercise

Think of a patient you are currently looking after who has physical symptoms without clear-cut organic pathology. Write down the patient's symptoms, the activities they are not able to do and the thoughts which are stopping them. What behavioural changes do you think the patient would benefit from? What rationale are you going to give the patient in order to help facilitate change?

KEY TEXTS FOR FURTHER READING

Deale A, Chalder T, Marks I, Wessely S 1997 A randomised controlled trial of cognitive behaviour versus relaxation therapy for chronic fatigue syndrome. American Journal of Psychiatry 154:408–414

Hugdahl K 1981 The three systems model of fear and emotion – a critical examination. Behaviour Research and Therapy 19:75–85

Mayou R, Bass C, Sharpe M 1995a Overview of epidemiology, classification and aetiology. In: Mayou R,

Bass C, Sharpe M (ed) Treatment of functional somatic symptoms. Oxford University Press, Oxford, p 42–65

Mechanic D 1962 The concept of illness behaviour. Journal of Chronic Diseases 15:184–189

Speckens A, van Hemert A, Spinhoven P, Hawton K, Bolk J, Rooijmans G 1995 Cognitive behavioural therapy for medically unexplained physical symptoms: a randomised controlled trial. British Medical Journal 311:1328–1332

REFERENCES

Andersen R, Anderson O, Smedby B 1968 Perception of and response to symptoms of illness in Sweden and the United States. Medical Care 6:18–30

Banks M, Beresford S, Morrell D, Waller J, Watkins C 1975 Factors influencing demand for primary medical care in women aged 20–44 years: a preliminary report. International Journal of Epidemiology 4:189–195

Barkham M, Shapiro D 1986 Counsellor verbal response modes and experience of empathy. Journal of Counselling Psychology 33:3–10

Blumer D, Heilbron M 1981 The pain prone disorder. A clinical and psychological profile. Psychosomatics 22:395–398

Bradlow J, Coulter A, Brookes P 1992 Patterns of referral. A study of referrals to out-patient clinics from general practices in the Oxford Region. Health Services Research Unit, Oxford

Breuer J, Freud S 1955 Studies in hysteria, student edn vol 2.

Hogarth Press, London

Bridges K, Goldberg D 1985 Somatic presentations of DSM-111 psychiatric disorders in primary care. Journal of Psychosomatic Research 29:563–569

Burns D 1980 Feeling good. The new mood therapy. William Morrow, New York

Casper F, Grawe K 1981 Resistance in behaviour therapy. In: Petzold H (ed) Resistance: A controversial concept in psychotherapy. Junfermann, Paderborn

Chalder T 1998 Factors contributing to the development and maintenance fatigue in primary care. Unpublished PhD thesis, London

Chalder T, Butler S, Wessely S 1996a In-patient treatment of chronic fatigue syndrome. Behavioural Psychotherapy 24:351–365

Chalder T, Power M, Wessely S 1996b Chronic fatigue in the community: 'a question of attribution'. Psychological Medicine 26:791–800

REFERENCES (*contd*)

Chalder T, Wallace P, Wessely S 1997 Self-help treatment of chronic fatigue in the community: a randomised controlled trial. British Journal of Health Psychology 2:189–197

Costa P, McRae R 1985 Hypochondriasis, neuroticism, and ageing. When are somatic complaints unfounded? American Psychologist 40:19–28

Craig T, Boardman A 1990 Somatisation in primary care settings. In Bass C (ed) Somatization: Physical symptoms and psychological illness. Blackwell, Oxford, p 73–103

Craig T, Boardman A, Mills K, Daly-Jones O, Drake H 1993 The South London somatization study: longitudinal course and the influence of early life experiences. British Journal of Psychiatry 163:579–588

Creed F, Mayou R, Hopkins A 1992 Medical symptoms not explained by organic disease. Royal College of Physicians and Royal College of Psychiatrists, London

de Gruy F, Crider J, Hashimi D 1987 Somatisation disorder in a university hospital. Journal of Family Practice 25:579–584

Deale A, Chalder T, Marks I, Wessely S 1997 A randomised controlled trial of cognitive behaviour versus relaxation therapy for chronic fatigue syndrome. American Journal of Psychiatry 154:408–414

Deighton C, Nichol A 1985 Abnormal illness behaviour in young women in a primary care setting: is Briquet's syndrome a useful category? Psychological Medicine 15:515–520

Escobar J, Canino G 1989 Unexplained physical complaints. Psychopathology and epidemiological correlates. British Journal of Psychiatry 154: supplement, 24–27

Frank G, Sweetland S 1962 A study of the process of psychotherapy: the verbal interaction. Journal of Consulting Psychology 26:135–138

Garralda E 1995 The management of functional somatic symptoms in children. In: Mayou R, Bass C, Sharpe M (eds), Treatment of functional somatic symptoms. Oxford University Press, Oxford p 353–370

Gomez J, Dally P 1977 Psychologically mediated abdominal pain in surgical and medical outpatient clinics. British Journal of Psychiatry 1:1451–1453

Hannay D 1978 Symptom prevalence in the community. Journal of the Royal College of General Practitioners 28:492–499

Hartwig P, Sterner G 1985 Childhood psychologic environmental exposure in women with diagnosed somatoform disorders. A case control study. Scandinavian Journal of Social Medicine 13:153–157

Heinrich R, Cohen M, Naliboff B, Collins G, Bonebakker A 1985 Comparing physical and behaviour therapy for chronic low back pain on physical abilities, psychological distress, and patient's perceptions. Journal of Behavioural Medicine 8:61–78

Hotopf M 1996 Psychiatric disorder and childhood experience of illness in the development of physical symptoms in adulthood: a prospective cohort study. London School of Hygiene and Tropical Medicine, London

Hugdahl K 1981 The three systems model of fear and emotion – a critical examination. Behaviour Research and Therapy 19:75–85

Kanfer F, Schefft B 1988 Guiding the process of therapeutic change. Campaign: Research Press,

Katon W, Von Korff M, Lin E, Lipscomb P, Wagner E, Polk E 1990 Distressed high utilisers of medical care DSMIII-R diagnoses and treatment needs. General Hospital Psychiatry 12:355–362

Kellner R 1990 Somatization:theories and research. Journal of Mental and Nervous Diseases 178:150–160

Kendell R 1972 A new look at hysteria. Medicine 30:1780

Klimes I, Mayou R, Pearce M, Coles L, Fagg J 1990 Psychological treatment for atypical non cardiac chest pain: a controlled evaluation. Psychological Medicine 20:605–611.

Lang P 1970 Stimulus control, response control and the desensitization of fear. In: Lewis D (ed) Learning approaches to therapeutic behaviour. Aldine Press, Chicago, p 148–173

Lewis G, Pelosi A, Araya R, Dunn G 1992 Measuring psychiatric disorder in the community: a standardised assessment for lay interviewer. Psychological Medicine 22:465–486

Lipowski ZL 1988 Somatization: the concept and its clinical application. American Journal of Psychiatry 145: 1358–1368

Marshall J, Halligan P, Fink G, Wade D, Frackowiak R 1997 The functional anatomy of a hysterical paralysis. Cognition 64:B1–B8

Mayou R 1989 Invited review : atypical chest pain. Journal of Psychosomatic Research 33:373–406

Mayou R, Bass C, Sharpe M 1995a Overview of epidemiology, classification and aetiology. In: Mayou R, Bass C, Sharpe M (eds) Treatment of functional somatic symptoms. Oxford University Press, Oxford

Mayou R, Bass C, Sharpe M 1995b (eds) The treatment of functional somatic systems. Oxford University Press, Oxford

Mechanic D 1962 The concept of illness behaviour. Journal of Chronic Diseases 15:184–189

Mechanic D 1979 Development of psychological distress among young adults. Archives of General Psychiatry 36:1233–1239

Mechanic D 1980 The experience and reporting of common physical complaints. Journal of Health and Social Behaviour 21:146–155

Morin C M 1993 Insomnia. Psychological assessment and management. Guilford Press, New York

Nicholas M, Wislon P, Goyen J 1992 Comparison of cognitive behavioural group treatment and an alternative non-psychological treatment for chronic low back pain. Pain 48:339–347

Pennebaker J, O'Heeron R 1984 Confiding in others and illness rate among spouses of suicide and accidental death victims. Journal of Abnormal Psychology 93:473–476

Pennebaker J W, Susman J R 1988 Disclosure of traumas and psychosomatic processes. Social Science and Medicine 26:327–332

Philips C 1987 Avoidance behaviour and its role in sustaining chronic pain. Behaviour Research and Therapy 25:273–279

Pilowsky I 1997 Abnormal illness behaviour. Wiley, Chichester

Ray C, Jeffries S, Weir W 1995 Coping with chronic fatigue syndrome: illness responses and their relationship with fatigue, functional impairment and emotional status. Psychological Medicine 25:937–945

REFERENCES (contd)

Reber A 1988 The Penguin dictionary of psychology. Penguin, Harmondsworth

Salkovskis P 1989 Somatic problems. In: Hawton K, Salkovskis P, Kirk J, Clark D (eds) Cognitive behaviour therapy for psychiatric problems: a practical guide. Oxford University Press, Oxford, p 235–276

Schluederberg A, Straus S, Peterson P et al 1992 Chronic fatigue syndrome research: definition and medical outcome assessment. Annals of Internal Medicine 117:325–331

Sharpe M, Archard L, Banatvala J et al 1991 Chronic fatigue syndrome: guidelines for research. Journal of the Royal Society of Medicine 84:118–121

Sharpe M, Hawton K, Seagroatt V, Pasvol G 1992 Follow-up of patients with fatigue presenting to an infectious diseases clinic. British Medical Journal 302:347–352

Sharpe M, Hawton K, Simkin S et al 1996 Cognitive behaviour therapy for chronic fatigue syndrome; a randomized controlled trial. British Medical Journal 312:22–26

Simon G, VonKorff M 1991 Somatization and psychiatric disorder in the NIMH epidemiologic Catchment Area Study. American Journal of Psychiatry 148:1494–1500

Singh B, Nunn J, Martin J, Yates J 1981 Abnormal treatment behaviour. British Journal of Medical Psychology 54:67–73

Smith G, Monson R, Ray D 1986 Patients with multiple unexplained symptoms. Archives of Internal Medicine 146:69–72

Speckens A, van Hemert A, Spinhoven P, Hawton K, Bolk J, Rooijmans G 1995 Cognitive behavioural therapy for medically unexplained physical symptoms: a randomised controlled trial. British Medical Journal 311:1328–1332

Stearns A 1946 A history of the development of the concept of functional nervous disease during the past twenty–five hundred years. American Journal of Psychiatry 103:471–473

Swartz M, Blazer D, George L, Landermann R 1986 Somatisation disorder in a community population. American Journal of Psychiatry 143:1403–1408

Trimble M 1982 Functional diseases. British Medical Journal 285:1768–1770

Turner J, Clancy S 1988 Comparison of operant behavioural and cognitive behavioural group treatment for chronic low back pain. Consulting and Clinical Psychology 56:261–266

Vogt B, Finch D, Olsen C 1992 Functional heterogeneity in cingulate cortex: the anterior executive and posterior evaluative regions. Cerebral Cortex 2:435–443

Warwick H, Salkovskis P 1990 Hypochondriasis. Behaviour Research and Therapy 28:105–117

Warwick H, Clark D, Cobb A, Salkovskis P 1996 A controlled trial of cognitive behavioural treatment of hypochondriasis. British Journal of Psychiatry 169:189–195

Wessely S, Chalder T, Hirsch S, Wallace P, Wright D 1996 Psychological symptoms, somatic symptoms and psychiatric disorder in chronic fatigue and chronic fatigue syndrome: a prospective study in the primary care setting. American Journal of Psychiatry 153:1050–1059

Wilson A, Hickie I, Lloyd A et al 1994 Longitudinal study of the outcome of chronic fatigue syndrome. British Medical Journal 308:756–760

World Health Organisation 1993 The ICD-10 classification of mental and behavioural disorders: clinical descriptions and diagnostic guidelines. The World Health Organisation, Geneva

Zimmer D 1983 The therapeutic relationship: Concepts and empirical findings regarding the therapist–client relationship and its formation. Edition Psychologie, Germany. Ed. Weinheim.

Key points   243

Introduction   244

Anorexia nervosa   244
Diagnosis and classification   244
Comorbidity   245
Aetiology   245
Clinical features   247
Behavioural assessment   248
Mental state assessment   249
Medical complications   249
Treatment   252
The environment of care   252
Current models of treatment   254
Prognosis   255
Measurement   256

Bulimia nervosa   256
Diagnosis and classification   256
Clinical features   256
Comorbidity   257
Aetiology   257
Sociocultural factors   258
Medical complications   259
Treatment   259
Prognosis   259

Summary and conclusions   260

Exercise   260

Key texts for further reading   260

References   260

14

Eating disorders

Janet Treasure   Gill Todd
Ulrike Schmidt

KEY POINTS

- Anorexia nervosa is a rare disorder. The incidence is probably not increasing although the prevalence may be because the illness has a more ominous course.

- Anorexia nervosa involves a problem in the definition of the self which is triggered by stress in the context of a genetic vulnerability. Family and wider cultural factors are important in maintenance.

- In-patient treatment is necessary for the most severe cases.

- Psychotherapy involving motivational aspects, and which addresses the core schema, is also necessary.

- Bulimia nervosa was described in 1979 and is rapidly increasing in incidence and prevalence.

- The aetiology involves developmental stress in the context of a culture that endorses dieting.

- Cognitive–behaviour therapy is effective in 50% of cases. In a proportion of cases, these skills can be given in a self-help format.

INTRODUCTION

Following the introduction of bulimia nervosa to the world in 1979 as 'an ominous variant of anorexia nervosa' by Professor Gerald Russell of the Maudsley Hospital, there has been a tendency to 'lump' the two conditions together and to think about them as 'eating disorders'. However, we know now that the majority of cases of bulimia nervosa do not have a history of anorexia nervosa. Moreover, recent research suggests that the aetiology, course and response to treatment of the two syndromes differ considerably. Therefore we have chosen to separate the two conditions in this chapter.

ANOREXIA NERVOSA

Anorexia nervosa has a long history and was described clearly in the Western medical texts of the last century (Gull 1874, Lasègue 1873, Marcé 1860). In earlier times, female self-starvation may have been explained as a form of zealous religiosity (the holy anorexia of Bell 1985) or as a scientific curiosity, miraculous maids who could survive without eating (Fowler 1871).

Anorexia nervosa remains a rather rare condition with the incidence of new cases of 7 per 100 000 population (Turnbull et al 1996). Approximately 4000 new cases arise in the UK per year. The average duration of the disorder is 6 years (Herzog et al 1997b) and so the prevalence is much higher (see Box 14.1). The prevalence in young women (the population at greatest risk) ranges from 0.1 to 1% (Gillberg et al 1994, Hoek 1993, Lucas et al 1991, Rastam et al 1989). This puts it amongst the three commonest chronic disorders in adolescence alongside asthma and obesity (Lucas et al 1991). Although earlier research suggested that anorexia nervosa might have increased in frequency, we now know this not to be the case (Fombonne 1995, Nielsen 1990,

Turnbull et al 1996). However, some evidence suggests that the prevalence of the illness may have increased as a result of the illness becoming more severe.

Box 14.1 Epidemiology of anorexia nervosa

- One of the top three chronic conditions of adolescence
- Incidence rate 7/100 000 of total population
- Prevalence 0.1–1% of young women
- Mean age of onset: mid-teens
- 90–96% of cases are female
- Median duration of illness: 6 years

Diagnosis and classification

There have been recent changes in the Diagnosis and Statistical Manual (DSM-IV, American Psychiatric Association 1994) criteria for anorexia nervosa, in that two sub-types have been defined. The classical form of anorexia nervosa is now termed 'restricting sub-type' which is distinguished from anorexia nervosa, binge–purge sub-type, in which in addition to the weight loss, the individual concerned regularly engages in binge-eating and/or purging behaviour (i.e. self-induced vomiting or the misuse of laxatives, diuretics or enemas). In the ICD-10 classification (World Health Organization 1992), there is no such sub-classification (see Table 14.1).

However, many authorities in the field (Lee 1995, Littlewood 1995, Russell 1995) have voiced disquiet about the diagnostic criteria regarding weight and shape concerns, because they are framed within contemporary Western culture and not generalisable to other times or cultures. Russell (1995) recommends attention to the core features which are 'that the patient avoids food and induces weight loss by virtue of a range of psychosocial conflicts whose resolution she perceives to be within her reach through the

Table 14.1 Criteria for the classification of anorexia nervosa

DSM-IV	ICD-10 F50
Refusal to maintain body weight over a minimal norm/leading to body weight 15% below expected	Significant weight loss (BMI < 17.5 kg/m^2) or failure of weight gain or growth
	Weight loss self-induced by avoiding fattening foods and one or more of the following: a. vomiting b. purging c. excessive exercise d. appetite suppressants f. diuretics
Intense fear of gaining weight or becoming fat	A dread of fatness as an intrusive, overvalued idea and the patient imposes a low weight threshold on herself
Disturbance in the way in which one's body weight, size or shape is experienced, e.g. 'feeling fat' {denial of seriousness of underweight or undue influence of body weight and shape on self-evaluation}	
Absence of three consecutive menstrual cycles	Widespread endocrine disorder: a. amenorrhoea b. raised growth hormone c. raised cortisol d. reduced T3
{Restricting type: Binge–purging type: binge-eating or vomiting/misuse laxatives diuretics}	

{ }, proposed addition to DSM-IV; BMI, body mass index.

achievement of thinness and or the avoidance of fatness.'

Comorbidity

Comorbidity with both axis I (other psychiatric problems) and axis II (personality disturbance) is common in anorexia nervosa. Some of the comorbid conditions are a consequence of starvation and these are ameliorated by weight gain

(Pollice et al 1997). Depression, obsessive–compulsive disorder and social phobia are particularly common (Halmi et al 1991, Laessle et al 1987). The binge–purge sub-type is associated with higher levels of depression and alcohol and substance misuse. Symptoms of post-traumatic stress disorder are common in mixed anorexia nervosa and bulimia nervosa (Turnbull et al 1998). A quarter of the group with restricting anorexia nervosa have avoidant, dependent or obsessive–compulsive personality types, whereas 40% of those with the binge–purge sub-type have a borderline or histrionic type of personality (Braun et al 1994, Herzog et al 1992).

Box 14.2 Comorbidity

- Some of the axis I comorbidity is a consequence of starvation
- 50% have major affective disorder
- 33% have social phobia
- 25% have obsessive–compulsive disorder

Binge–purge sub-type
- 80% have depression
- 10–20% have alcohol and substance abuse

Personality disturbance
- 25% of restricting anorexia nervosa disorder have avoidant, dependent or obsessional personalities
- 40% of binge–purge sub-type of anorexia nervosa have borderline or histrionic personality disorders.

Aetiology

Most explanations of causation are multidimensional and include genetic factors, other biological factors, psychological vulnerability and family and sociocultural setting conditions. However, one of the problems with such an all-encompassing model is that it is very difficult to prove or disprove and it makes any attempts at prevention very difficult as so many facets may be important.

Biological factors

Genetic. Anorexia nervosa is often linked to leanness within the family (Hebebrand & Remschmidt 1995). The risk of having a first degree relative with anorexia nervosa is increased sevenfold (Treasure & Holland 1995). Twin studies suggest that anorexic traits and the syndrome have a significant genetic component (Rutherford et al 1993, Treasure & Holland 1995). Female relatives have a 10-fold risk of developing the disorder (Strober et al 1990) and the incidence in relatives is 7%.

Other biological aspects. One possibility is that anorexia nervosa is caused by a dysfunction in the control of body composition which has a large (approximately 70%) heritable component (Owen 1992, Treasure & Owen 1997). One of the key components in the control of body composition, leptin, a hormone secreted by fat cells, has only recently been discovered. When the size of fat cells increases, more leptin is produced. Leptin is transported into the brain where it switches off the appetite system and activates metabolism and exercise. Preliminary research does not suggest that there is any abnormality in leptin function in anorexia nervosa (Grinspoon et al 1996); leptin levels are low when patients are underweight and are increased with weight gain (Casaneuva et al 1997) and in the normal range on recovery (Brown et al 1996).

Another possibility is that anorexia nervosa develops because of an abnormality in the hypothalamic pituitary adrenal (HPA) system which leads to a catabolic response to chronic stress (Connan & Treasure 1998). Several groups have suggested that the vulnerability to develop anorexia nervosa is related to abnormal 5HT function (Treasure & Campbell 1994, Study Group on Anorexia Nervosa 1995). A recent report suggests that an abnormality on one of the genes that controls one of the sub-types of sero-tonin receptors may be more common in women with anorexia nervosa (Collier et al 1997).

Social factors

Although sociocultural factors have shaped the presentation of the disorder, in that concerns about weight and fatness now predominate, it is probable that these features are not necessary. For example, there is no convincing evidence that there has been an increase in the incidence of anorexia nervosa associated with the increased prevalence of dieting (Fombonne 1995, Turnbull et al 1996). This contrasts with bulimia nervosa (see below). It is possible that a cultural focus on dieting serves to maintain the illness and may cause the course to be more severe, which can account for the trend for a higher mortality (Sullivan 1995) and increased re-admission rates (Nielsen 1990).

Many feminist writers have suggested that the changing roles of women shifting the assumptions of power and control may have led to the emergence of eating disorders. Such arguments are made about eating disorders in general and are probably more relevant to bulimia nervosa. (For a review of this area see Fallon et al 1994.) Katzman & Lee (1997) arguing from a feminist/transcultural perspective suggest that a phobia of control may be an appropriate definition of the psychopathology of anorexia nervosa which is free from cultural colouring.

Family factors

Although family factors are often included in the multidimensional, aetiological model of anorexia nervosa, there is little evidence to support any gross disturbance in family functioning (Schmidt et al 1993). The metaphors and explanations used in the family models are exciting and creative, which perhaps explains their widespread

Box 14.3 Aetiology
<ul><li>Twin studies suggest that genetic factors are important</li><li>A biological vulnerability involving 5HT or the HPA axis and stress at puberty may be relevant</li><li>Life events or difficulties occur in 70% of cases prior to onset</li><li>An obsessive–compulsive personality and perfectionism are possible vulnerability factors</li><li>No evidence of gross childhood adversity</li><li>Family risk factors include poor problem-solving</li><li>Sociocultural factors have shaped the form of the illness and probably increased the risk of developing anorexia nervosa, binge–purge sub-type</li><li>No evidence that sociocultural factors have increased incidence of anorexia nervosa</li></ul>

influence (Minuchin et al 1978, Selvini-Palazzoli 1974). Minuchin et al (1978) suggested that families of patients with anorexia nervosa showed specific traits: rigidity, lack of conflict resolution, enmeshment and overinvolvement. However, some of these features appear to be a consequence of having a sick child in the family. For example, enmeshment and overinvolvement are also seen in families caring for a child with cystic fibrosis (Blair et al 1995). In this study, the main difference between anorexia nervosa families and cystic fibrosis families was that families with a child with anorexia nervosa were less adept at problem-solving. This links with the finding that patients with anorexia nervosa react to stress both in childhood and adulthood (Troop & Treasure 1997) with a helpless style of coping and a tendency to use avoidance strategies intra- and inter-personally.

Psychological factors

The onset of anorexia nervosa usually (70% of cases) follows a severe life event or difficulty (Schmidt et al 1997). There is a tendency for these patients to have a maladaptive coping response to the triggering event exemplified by avoidance

and helplessness. This cognitive and emotional set is present from childhood (Troop 1996, Troop & Treasure 1997). Obsessional personality traits (Gillberg et al 1995), associated with self-disgust and a sensitivity to criticism, may lead to compensatory strategies such as perfectionism, and a tendency to please others and submit to their wishes.

Clinical features

The clinical descriptions of anorexia nervosa have been derived from both qualitative and quantitative approaches.

Who is involved?

The illness usually affects young women (male to female ratio 1:10) with the onset commonly occurring within a few years of menarche. The median age of onset is 17. Cases as young as 8 and as old as 60 have been described.

It used to be thought that the prevalence of anorexia nervosa was higher in women of high socio-economic class, but this link with social class has not been confirmed (Gard & Freeman 1996, Turnbull et al 1996). There is, however, an association with educational achievement.

What behaviours are seen?

There is avoidance of high calorie foods. Presently this takes the form of avoiding fat rather than carbohydrate. Overactivity, both mentally in terms of perfectionist detail to work and physically in the form of obsessional exercise routines, is common. The length of time sleeping is shortened. A sensitivity to the cold develops. This is usually compensated for by wearing layer upon layer of clothes. There is often an associated preoccupation with food (browsing through supermarkets or cookery books) and cooking for others. Rituals related to eating develop; for example, the individual will only use certain cooking or eating utensils, she may cut up her food a certain number of times and she may use excessive amounts of condiments.

What physical features occur?

One of the first physical indications of poor nutrition is the cessation of periods although this may be masked if the individual is on the contraceptive pill. The circulation is poor. This leads to cold, blue hands, feet and nose. At its extreme this results in chilblains and even gangrene, particularly in children. The blood pressure and heart rate are low and can lead to faints.

What is the mental state?

Despite severe weight loss, the person feels well and usually does not see any need to seek help. There are various gradations in this level of denial. Parents may describe a change in temperament, and that their previously 'good girl' has become 'difficult', emotional and excessively conscientious. Perfectionism and obsessional rituals, especially relating to order and symmetry are common. Anhedonia, lack of motivation and concentration, sadness, irritability, poor sleep and many other characteristic features of a major affective disorder may be present.

Box 14.4 Brief screen

1. Do you think you have problems with your weight and eating?
2. Are your doctors or any of your family and friends concerned about your weight and eating?
3. Do you ever have times when you feel that your eating is out of control and you quickly eat a large amount of food, much more than anyone else you know?

Behavioural assessment

At the simplest behavioural level the clinician wants to know the following by the end of the assessment interview:

a. Is undernutrition present and how severe is it? Is there a history of significant overweight?
b. Is there constant dietary restriction or are there episodes of overeating?
c. What are the weight control measures used?

These behavioural criteria are easy to define and elicit but they are also of clinical utility as they guide management.

a. Is undernutrition present and how severe is it? Is there a history of significant overweight?

This is addressed by measuring weight and height and is usually done at the end of the interview with the physical examination (see below).

A detailed lifetime weight and diet history is helpful. The patient should be asked when she first noticed a problem with her weight or when she first began to focus on weight as a topic of personal importance. Both the rate of weight loss and the absolute level of weight are markers of dangerousness. Marked fluctuations in weight suggest that there is self-induced vomiting or abuse of laxatives and diuretics.

The patient should be asked what her heaviest ever weight was, and when this occurred, and similarly about her lowest ever weight. The weight at which her periods began needs to be established, as does the weight at which her periods stopped (if relevant). This is important as the weight at which the patient's normal biological functions recover will generally be slightly above the former and so can give an indication of how much weight needs to be gained. It is also useful to get a family weight history. There may be a strong family history of obesity in bulimia nervosa or of leanness or eating disorder in anorexia nervosa. A corroborating eating and weight history obtained from the parents can be of help.

b. Is there constant dietary restriction or are there episodes of overeating?

It is often necessary to directly question the person about bulimic behaviour, as this may not be mentioned spontaneously, because of the shame attached. A suitable line of enquiry is: 'Do you have episodes when your eating seems excessive or out of control?' You need to probe gently to elicit whether the amount eaten is excessive (objective binge > 1000 kcalories) or not (subjective binge).

c. What are the weight control measures used?

In addition to dietary restriction, the commonly employed methods are self-induced vomiting, chewing and spitting of food, abuse of laxatives, diuretics, street drugs (e.g. amphetamines & ecstasy), caffeine, prescribed medication such as thyroxine, or health food preparations and excessive exercise.

Mental state assessment

Overvalued ideas about shape and weight, in which the assessment of self-worth is made exclusively in these terms, are considered primary features of bulimia nervosa. Not all patients with anorexia nervosa express such ideas.

Body image distortion (a statement that they are fat when they are underweight) is no longer regarded as one of the necessary criteria for anorexia nervosa. A less culturally bound description of this phenomenon is that the emaciated state is overvalued.

The patient should also be asked what weight she would ideally like to be. Often patients with

anorexia nervosa will try to please the therapist by giving a higher weight than they are aiming for. It may be helpful to probe this response in some detail: 'If you got to 7 stones, would you be happy there?' If the patient says 'No', it can be helpful to press her as this may help her realise that she has a problem: 'So if you were 7 stones, you might want to weigh $6\frac{1}{2}$, but what then?'

Box 14.5 Diagnostic features to look out for

- Body mass index less than 17.5 kg/m^2
- Use of weight control measures

Box 14.6 Spot diagnosis – physical signs

- Parotid or submandibular gland enlargement
- Eroded teeth
- 'Russell's sign' callus on back of hand
- Cold blue hands, feet and nose
- Lanugo hair

Medical complications

It is impossible to cover the medical complications of anorexia nervosa more than superficially and for more detailed information we would suggest the following resources: American Psychiatric Association 1993, Bhanji & Mattingly 1988, Kaplan & Garfinkel 1993, Sharpe & Freeman 1993, Treasure & Szmukler 1995.

Skin and hair changes

The skin is dry and fine downy hair, so-called lanugo hair, develops. There is often loss of head hair and this will appear thin and lifeless.

Musculoskeletal problems

Muscles. Individuals with severe anorexia nervosa have poor muscle strength and a decrease in stamina. Eventually, proximal myopathy develops with difficulty standing from a crouch or lifting the arms above the head to comb the hair. The poor muscle strength also leads to an impairment in respiratory function (Murciamo et al 1994).

Bones. Osteoporosis and pathological fractures are one of the commonest causes of pain and disability in anorexia nervosa (Treasure & Szmukler 1995). The annual incidence of non-spine fractures of 0.05 per person year in anorexia nervosa is sevenfold higher than the rate reported from a community sample of women aged between 15 and 34 (Rigotti et al 1991). Risk factors for this complication are a long duration and an increased severity of illness (Serpell & Treasure 1997). Refeeding alone produces a rapid rise in bone turnover (Stefanis et al 1999) and an increase in bone mineral content (Orphanidou et al 1997). Insulin growth factor also increases bone turnover (Grinspoon et al 1996). The value of hormone replacement therapy is uncertain; overall it produces no effect although it may protect against further bone loss in the sub-group who remain chronically unwell (Klibanski et al 1995). It is uncertain whether it is possible to restore bone mass to normal levels. Patients who have gained weight and have had a return of menses over many years had persistent osteopenia (Ward et al 1997). Duration of amenorrhoea/illness was the best predictor of osteopenia, but also an index of the duration of recovery was highly correlated with outcome.

Dental changes

The commonest stigma of persistent vomiting is erosion of dental enamel, in particular from the inner surfaces of the front teeth. Eventually dentine is exposed and the teeth become over-sensi-tive to temperature and caries develops. Dental complications such as abnormal tooth wear are not limited to the group which vomit (Robb et al 1995). The other causes of poor dental health are overconsumption of acidic foods such as fruit and carbonated drinks, grinding and loosening of the teeth caused by osteoporosis of the jaw.

Effects on the central nervous system

Brain substance decreases in anorexia nervosa and the ventricular spaces and the sulci increase in size (Dolan et al 1988, Katzman et al 1996, Krieg et al 1988). The increased resolution offered by magnetic resonance imaging has also shown that the pituitary is smaller (Dolan et al 1988, Katzman et al 1996). To a degree these structural abnormalities persist despite weight recovery for over a year which suggests that there may be a degree of irreversible destruction even in this group which had good prognostic features (Lambe et al 1997). The cause of the cerebral atrophy is uncertain. However, hormonal factors may be of relevance as oestrogen protects brain function whereas cortisol increases the vulnerability to toxic influences. It may be a general effect of starvation or may result from the high level of cortisol which is present in anorexia nervosa and which is known to be toxic to dendrites (Sapolsky 1992). A post-mortem study of a 13-year-old girl who died of anorexia found that the dendrites showed evidence both of stunting of growth and of neuronal repair (Schönheit et al 1996). In addition, women with anorexia nervosa may be at greater risk of Alzheimer's disease because of their prolonged state of oestrogen deficiency, if it is possible to extrapolate from the findings in post-menopausal women in whom it was found that oestrogen treatment appeared to delay the onset of dementia (Tang et al 1996).

Cognitive impairment can occur with deficits in memory tasks, flexibility and inhibitory tasks persisting despite weight recovery (Kingston et al 1996).

Cardiovascular problems

The heart becomes smaller and less powerful, because muscle is lost and the blood pressure and heart rate are lowered. This can lead to faints. There is poor circulation in the periphery and this leads to cold, blue hands, feet and nose. At its extreme, this results in chilblains and even gangrene, particularly in children.

There have been reports of cardiac valvular problems (Johnson et al 1986) although many of the murmurs that are heard are flow murmurs. Sudden death occurs in anorexia nervosa and may result from arrhythmias (Isner et al 1985). QT prolongation is common in anorexia nervosa (Cooke et al 1994). Low potassium which results from many of the methods of weight loss can exacerbate this problem.

Fertility and reproductive function

Fertility is reduced in women with anorexia nervosa. In part this is due to suboptimal physical recovery. In a follow-up of 12.5 years in Denmark, the fertility rate was a third of that expected and the perinatal mortality rate was six-fold higher (Brinch et al 1988). The birthweight of children born to anorexic mothers is lower than average (Treasure & Russell 1988). Women with anorexia nervosa may also have difficulties in feeding their children who may become malnourished and stunted in growth (Russell et al 1998).

Endocrine system

The hypothalamic–pituitary–gonadal axis regresses to that of a prepubertal child. The pituitary does not secrete follicle stimulating hormone and luteinising hormone and the ovaries decrease in size. The ovarian follicles remain small and do not produce oestrogens or progesterone (Treasure 1988). By contrast, the hypothalamic–pituitary–adrenal axis is overactive, probably driven by excess corticotrophin releasing factor CRF, with high levels of cortisol which are not constrained by any feedback (Gwirtsman et al 1989).

Gastrointestinal complications

Residual gastrointestinal problems such as irritable bowel syndrome are common after recovery from anorexia nervosa (Herzog et al 1992, Kreipe et al 1989). Functional abnormalities such as delayed gastric emptying and generalised poor motility are related to the degree of undernutrition (Szmukler et al 1990). Anatomical abnormalities as a result of the trauma of vomiting and overeating or loss of mesenteric fat occur. Structural abnormalities such as ulcers are common (Hall et al 1989). Finally, it is important not to overlook the effects of sorbitol present in sugar-free gums and sweets which can cause abdominal distension, cramps and diarrhoea (Orlich 1989).

Salivary glands hypertrophy and produce increased levels of amylase (Kinzl et al 1993). Pancreatitis is an extremely rare complication (Gavish et al 1987).

Liver

In cases of severe emaciation, fatty infiltration of the liver occurs and liver enzymes increase (Hall et al 1989).

Blood

All components of the bone marrow are diminished but the order in which this is discernible in the peripheral blood is white cells, red cells and finally platelets. The level of marrow dysfunction relates to the total body fat mass (Lambert et al 1997). The immune system is compromised with a decrease in CD8 T cells (Mustafa et al 1997).

Blood chemistry

In restricting anorexia nervosa the most common abnormality is a low urea level, which is a function of a low protein intake. Low potassium levels result from vomiting or laxative and diuretic abuse. Usually, this is associated with raised levels of bicarbonate but some laxatives can produce a metabolic acidosis. Many other salts and metabolites are reduced, for example magnesium, phosphate, calcium, sodium and glucose.

Treatment

Patients with anorexia nervosa are notoriously ambivalent about treatment (Bruch 1973, Vitousek et al 1997). Charles Lasègue in 1879 quoted one of his patients as saying: 'I do not suffer therefore I must be well.'

The transtheoretical model of Prochaska & Di Clemente (1992) has five stages of readiness to change:

- precontemplation (no recognition that there is a problem)
- contemplation (patient is ambivalent about costs and benefits of change)
- preparation
- action
- maintenance.

Patients with anorexia nervosa, when they come for an assessment, are usually in either the precontemplation or contemplation phase (Blake et al 1997, Ward et al 1996). Therefore, if the therapist begins to talk about active change, the therapist will be met with resistance and hostility as this produces a mismatch between the agendas of patient and therapist. It is therefore important to build a good therapeutic alliance by spending the first part of the interview eliciting the patient's concerns and her agenda. A key component of the assessment will be to elicit the patient's concerns about her condition: for example, physical and psychological side-effects, and effects on social life, family, career and education. Patients with anorexia nervosa are usually not concerned that they have anorexia nervosa, that they are not eating and that their weight is low. They may, however, be concerned about their poor concentration that affects their ability to study. In such a case, gentle feedback about the brain effects of anorexia nervosa may be of use.

Box 14.7 Essential facets of treatment for anorexia nervosa

1. Engender motivation
2. Find out what are the patient's beliefs about the illness
3. Develop a good therapeutic alliance
4. Formulation: links between behaviour and core schemata
5. Match therapeutic processes to stage of change
6. Balance move to change against degree of resistance

The environment of care

A theoretical model as a useful frame for treatment model is that anorexia nervosa occurs as a reaction to psychosocial stress and is a form of avoidance (see Russell's definition on p. 244). Anorexia nervosa serves to suppress awareness of the stress and the attendant negative emotions. For example, the developmental regression with loss of periods and sexual drive serves to help the patient avoid confronting and resolving any conflicts over adult sexual behaviour (avoidance of cognitive dissonance). Similarly, the overt physical ill-health and fragility mobilises parents to respond by increasing their care and protection (positive reinforcer of increased attention) so that the patient can avoid leaving home (avoidance of negative reinforcer, i.e. becoming independent).

Staff working with eating disorder patients need to understand that their expectation of change involves the patient giving up a cherished and valued state. This is a difficult task and can only take place in an atmosphere of warmth and empathy which fosters the patient's self-efficacy and a positive self-concept. This is no easy feat.

One of the core problems in anorexia nervosa is that it involves a disturbance in the development of the self. Rather than a sense of self which is good enough and reasonably stable, these patients have extreme core schemas which pertain to self as defective or as weak. These schema drive compensatory behaviours such as the striving for power or for specialness through perfectionism, and self-control. These lead to particular patterns of interactions with others such as despised and admiring or subordinate and dominant. Also, patients with anorexia nervosa can have insecure patterns of attachment. The core schemas underlying this are that close others may abandon you, or others need care or others are not to be trusted. These extreme constructions of others can oscillate to the opposite pole. For example, there may be compensatory yearnings for fused care, to be selfish and to be controlled. These intra- and interpersonal schemas will be triggered within the ward environment and play an important role in the ward management. They will colour relationships with other patients and with all members of the team.

The strength of the therapeutic alliance is of critical importance in working with patients with anorexia nervosa. The team and the key-nurse need to avoid resistance by working at the correct stage of change, by developing accurate empathy and by not entering into a dysfunctional role driven by the patient's core schema. Patients with anorexia nervosa can be drawn into the role of pleasing and giving the therapist what they think they want to hear rather than the truth. Issues of power and control, criticism and judgement can come to the fore when the team sets tasks, goals or rigid expectations about weight gain. Holidays and inconsistencies can trigger fears of abandonment. The avoidance of closeness can lead to silence and empty sessions.

In our practice we find it helpful to map the schema and the behaviours that they cause and their effects on others onto diagrams. This can be a helpful method to monitor the patterns and processes of interpersonal relationships. The development and exploration of the activity of the core schema throughout the patient's life history need to be explored. Schemas are either overt or appear as compensatory behaviours or as behaviours which allow them to be avoided.

The care environment has to be a judicious balance of control, trust, compromise and negotiation in the context of the reality, which is that people have to eat to live and there is no choice in this. The issue of control (a compensatory behaviour for self as weak) needs to be seen as providing both a positive and a negative experience. Care needs to be seen as a compromise of control, a letting-go of some rigidly held beliefs and embracing of untried and unthought ideas. The caring environment therefore provides calculated risks for the patient in the form of 1:1 meetings with professional strangers. Alternative therapies (dance therapy, drama therapy, art therapy, acupuncture, relaxation) group work, family/carer work, career guidance and occupational therapy, voluntary work, school work and regular meals are situations in which the schema and their attendant cognitions and emotions can be explored. The core environment needs to model a reasoning and flexible state of mind. It needs to be able to say no when some limits are transgressed and to say why. It needs to be able to say 'We have let you down' and 'We have failed you' which will enable the patient to see that mistakes can be useful. Perfectionism (the compensatory behaviour from self as defective) needs to be seen as an impossible state for man/woman/nurse/ward and that responsibility, blame and guilt can be acceptable and handled as part of everyday experience.

Patients with anorexia nervosa have extreme poles of ambivalence. So extreme are the ideas that they rarely reach consciousness at the same time. Furthermore, patients with anorexia nervosa find it difficult to tolerate more than one state of mind. As one patient said, 'I wish all of life could be put into little boxes and I could take them up and deal with them one at a time.'

Good communication skills are of critical importance in this patient group. Listening, hearing, explaining, rephrasing, repeating, checking out meaning, making a space for conversation and discussion have to be taught and practised by both staff and patients. Diagrams and letters may enable the patient to hold several ideas in the same place at the same time. In a time-pressured environment patients and staff have to be helped by structure, and have to use every available opportunity for communication. No type of communication can be assumed to be informal (i.e. not worth attending to). Denial has to be gently challenged with kindness.

Everyone's expectations have to be checked and rechecked. Staff must be given regular supervision both in groups and 1:1 to help them express their frustrations, prejudices, anger and hopes. Clinical supervision must always be available to extricate staff from experiencing

themselves as always right or always wrong or always supported or always ignored. The polarised thinking of the patient can be contagious to the staff. A ward group can function only as well as its weakest member. Help should always be available. Negative emotions such as fear and paranoia should not be seen as problems but as information which can be understood in terms of the interpersonal relationships that are evoked.

Change and choices are difficult because of the rigid thinking of the patients which is transmitted to the staff. Regular planning and evaluation meetings are important so that a degree of flexibility and readjustment in the light of feedback and re-evaluation is possible without the situation descending into the chaos of no plans or goals.

All members of the team will be affected by counter-transference. There may be a tendency for differences in the type of roles to be played out with different members of staff. Those with more power in the team will tend to evoke attachment patterns such as a parental type of relationship. More junior members will be drawn into peer types of relationship with competition or co-operation/alienation, in and out groups. None of these types of relationship is better or worse than any other, they are just different. They need to be recognised for what they are and what underlies them. After judicious reflection they can give a wealth of information that can be used to good effect.

Current models of treatment

The choice of treatment depends upon (1) the patient's age, (2) medical severity and (3) duration of the disorder. In patients under the age 17, it is helpful to have the family of the patient involved in treatment (Russell et al 1987, Eisler et al 1997). Also, if the onset of the illness was in early adolescence – no matter what the patient's chronological age is – it is usually helpful to involve the family in some capacity. Parental counselling (i.e. helping the family to understand the illness and to deal with the problems it causes) is as effective and more acceptable than a traditional form of family therapy (Le Grange et al 1992).

Out-patient psychotherapy or counselling can be effective if there has not been too much weight loss (i.e. less than 25%). Specialist psychotherapy such as cognitive analytic therapy (Treasure et al 1995, Treasure & Ward 1997) or modified dynamic therapy is more effective than supportive psychotherapy (Eisler et al 1997). New models of cognitive–behaviour therapy are being developed and are being tested as techniques to prevent relapse. Frequently, the therapy has to be continued long term. It is important that psychological treatment is supplemented by regular medical monitoring.

In-patient treatment is necessary for those with severe weight loss. An historical approach to the treatment of anorexia nervosa involved isolation. This was advocated in France by Charcot (Silverman 1997). The use of isolation and strict behavioural regimes should now be consigned to history as such coercive practices are deeply traumatic and reinforce the core features of the illness which are self-disgust and ineffectiveness. Furthermore, more lenient regimes use less staff time, provide less opportunity for patients to manipulate individual staff members and result in the patients being more motivated to change (Touyz et al 1984, Touyz & Beaumont 1997).

Staff with expertise in management of eating disorders can provide a judicious mixture of psychotherapy and nutritional support. This type of expertise is found in teams working in specialised units.

In extreme circumstances, an anorexic patient may need to be detained under the Mental Health Act. If at all possible, this should only be done within a specialised unit, where the treatment team have enough expertise to build up trust with the patient, so that their extreme avoidance strategies can be left behind and the problems clearly formulated and processed.

Prognosis

The median duration of the illness is 6 years (Herzog et al 1997b). A third of patients have a poor prognosis. The mortality is 0.06% per year after onset which means that anorexia nervosa has the highest mortality of any psychiatric illness (Patton 1988, Sullivan 1995). Approximately half of the deaths result from medical complications and the rest result from suicide (Herzog et al 1992). Treatment in specialised centres probably improves the outcome as the mortality rate in areas without a specialised service is higher (Crisp et al 1992). Also, the outcome appears to be better in cohorts who have been recruited from clinical centres than in the one centre which was able to detect cases from the schoolgirl population in one town (Gillberg et al 1994).

Outcome is usually defined using the Morgan & Russell scales (or an equivalent) which measure outcome in terms of physical status (weight and menstruation); psychological status (specific psychopathology: attitudes to shape, weight and eating; general psychiatric comorbidity, e.g. depression and obsessive–compulsive disorder); psychosexual adjustment, socio-economic ad-

---

Box 14.8   Prognosis of anorexia nervosa

1. Median duration is 6 years
2. 30% have a poor prognosis
3. Mortality is 1% per year
4. Treatment in specialised centres improves the outcome
5. Residual problems in good outcome group

justment and relationships with family. Even patients with a good outcome often have residual problems such as abnormal attitudes to food and eating.

Abnormally low serum albumin levels and a low weight (≤ 60% average body weight) predict a lethal course (Herzog et al 1997a).

Measurement

Many instruments have been designed to measure the psychopathology of eating disorders but we will mention only those which are in most use. The Eating Disorder Examination is a structured interview which assesses the relevant psychopathology (Cooper et al 1989). Several self-report questionnaires are also in common use. The Eating Attitudes Test (EAT) is a self-report questionnaire which has been validated in clinical samples but has poor sensitivity and specificity when used in the community (Garner & Garfinkel 1979). The Eating Disorder Inventory is also a self-report questionnaire produced later by the same group (Garner et al 1983) which incorporates factors from the EAT and, in addition, personality dimensions. The Bulimia Investigatory Test, Edinburgh (BITE; Henderson & Freeman 1987) is a self-report questionnaire which is widely used for bulimic features.

BULIMIA NERVOSA

The incidence of bulimia nervosa has rapidly increased and the disorder is now two or three times more common than anorexia nervosa – incidence 14 per 100 000 (Turnbull et al 1996). Approximately 2% of young women suffer from the illness (Kendler et al 1991). The demand for services is lower than the level suggested by the prevalence rates as less than a third of all cases present for treatment (Hoek 1993). Many suffer-

ers have mixed feelings about disclosing their condition and seeking help.

Diagnosis and classification

Bulimia nervosa was only recently included in the European classificatory system (ICD-10, World Health Organization 1992). DSM-IV (American Psychiatric Association 1994) defines two sub-types of bulimia nervosa, a purging and a non-purging sub-type. The main difference between the DSM and ICD definitions of bulimia nervosa is the absence of a frequency criterion in the ICD classification (see Table 14.2). Recent interest in obese binge eaters led to the suggestion that binge-eating disorder should be included in DSM-IV as a separate disorder (Spitzer et al 1992, 1993). However, this idea has been criticised (Fairburn et al 1993) on the basis of a community-based cluster analysis which failed to support it (Hay et al 1996) and the inclusion of binge-eating disorder in DSM has been put on hold until further clarification of its diagnostic usefulness.

Clinical features

The median age of onset of bulimia nervosa is 18, slightly later than that of anorexia nervosa. Females predominate (M:F ratio = 1:10) and all social classes are affected. Patients are usually of a normal body weight. Approximately a third have a past history of anorexia nervosa and another third a history of obesity.

A history of weight loss preceding onset is typical. There is usually an attempt to follow a strict diet with protracted periods of fasting. The content of binges varies from an array of 'forbidden' palatable foods to foodstuffs which would be normally treated with disgust such as leftovers or food from the dustbin. The usual precipitants for

Table 14.2 Criteria for the classification of bulimia nervosa

DSM-III-R Bulimia nervosa (307.51)	ICD-10 Bulimia nervosa (F50.1)	DSM-IV Binge-eating disorder
Recurrent episodes of binge-eating {(1) large amount of food (2) loss of control}	Episodes of overeating	{Recurrent episodes of binge-eating (1) large (2) no control}
Feeling of lack of control of eating during binge		*Binge-eating associated with at least three of the following:* *a. rapid eating* *b. uncomfortably full* *c. eat without hunger* *d. shameful, solitary eating* *e. disgust, guilt, depression after* *overeating*
Regular use of methods of weight control: a. vomiting b. laxatives c. diuretics d. fasting/strict diet e. vigorous exercise {DSM-IV Purging (vomiting, laxatives, diuretics) Non-purging}	Methods to counteract weight gain: a. vomiting b. laxatives c. fasting d. appetite suppressants e. metabolic stimulants f. diuretics	Marked distress after binge-eating
Minimum average of two binges a week in 3 months		Binge-eating on average at least 2 days a week for 6 months
Persistent overconcern with shape or weight {Self-evaluation is unduly influenced by body weight or shape}	Morbid fear of fatness with a sharply defined weight threshold	
{The disturbance does not occur exclusively during episodes of anorexia nervosa}	Often a history of anorexia nervosa	Disturbance not exclusively present with anorexia nervosa or bulimia nervosa

Italics, proposed deletion in DSM-IV; { }, proposed addition to DSM-IV.

binges are transgressions of self-imposed dietary rules or feelings of depression, anxiety, loneliness and boredom. A wide variety of weight control strategies are used. The most common are vomiting followed by laxatives and diuretics.

Comorbidity

Lifetime rates of major depression range from 35 to 70%. Major depression can precede, occur simultaneously with or start after the onset of bulimia nervosa (see Halmi 1995 for review). Many clinic-based samples of women with bulimia nervosa have high levels of alcoholism and drug abuse but this association was not seen in a community-based sample (Welch & Fairburn 1996b). Cases of bulimia nervosa did exhibit higher levels of self-harm (overdoses and cutting). Personality disorder is common (Levine & Hyler 1986, Wonderlich et al 1990), with a mixture of the borderline spectrum and anxious, avoidant personality problems occurring equally commonly (Braun et al 1994). 37% of cases of bulimia nervosa have a lifetime history of post-traumatic stress disorder (Dansky et al 1997).

Aetiology

Genetic

The estimated heritability for bulimia is between 30 and 35% (Kendler et al 1995). Some of the genetic liability to bulimia nervosa is non-specific and shared with the liability to phobia and panic disorder. The common, clinical manifestations of this genetic vulnerability are acute and short-lived.

Other biological factors

Early menarche is a risk factor for bulimia nervosa. The mechanism for this is uncertain, although Fairburn et al (1997) speculate that it may be linked to an earlier onset of dieting in these cases. Early menarche is also a feature of obesity which in itself is a strong risk factor for the development of bulimia, as is parental obesity. Plasma leptin levels are in the normal range in patients with bulimia nervosa and correlate with body mass index (Ferron et al 1997). Central 5HT is lowered (Jimerson et al 1997, Levitan et al 1997) and this is thought to be implicated in the aetiology or maintenance of the disorder (Halmi 1997).

Family developmental aspects

In general, three classes of family experiences have been described as being implicated in the aetiology of bulimia nervosa:

a. *The general quality of early social interactions and the inferences children draw about their acceptability.* These kind of experiences are often shared by siblings growing up in the same family. Bulimia nervosa differed from other psychiatric disorders examined in a large population study of twins in that the analysis suggested that common environmental factors played a significant part in the aetiology (Kendler et al 1995). Interestingly, Fairburn et al (1997) also found that in a community sample of women with bulimia nervosa difficulties such as low contact with the parents and high parental expectations and parental alcohol abuse were more common in

individuals with bulimia nervosa than in individuals with depression. This reflects the findings in clinical populations with bulimia nervosa which have found high levels of adversity within the family with discord and neglect (Schmidt et al 1993).

b. *Experiences related to childhood sexual and physical abuse.* Childhood sexual and physical abuse occur significantly more commonly in cases of bulimia nervosa ascertained from the community, than in well women in the community (Welch & Fairburn 1994). These risk factors are not specific to bulimia nervosa and are also found in other psychiatric groups, although repeated severe sexual abuse was more common in bulimia nervosa (Welch & Fairburn 1996a). Later, adverse, sexual experiences are more common in bulimia nervosa: rape 27% vs 13% comparison group; aggravated assault 27% (Dansky et al 1997).

c. *Factors in the family environment which increase the risk of dieting.* In comparison to families of psychiatric control patients in families of bulimic individuals more family members dieted and had eating disorders (Fairburn et al 1997). Also, in this study, there were higher levels of critical comments, made by family members of bulimics about weight, shape and eating.

Sociocultural factors

There has been a major increase in the incidence of bulimia nervosa in recent years (Kendler et al 1991, Turnbull et al 1996), which is likely to be the result of an increase of dieting in younger women. Bulimia nervosa is especially common in groups where weight and shape issues are of importance such as ballet dancers, models and actresses.

An interesting study examined the effects of childhood physical and sexual abuse on a community cohort of mothers and daughters

(Andrews et al 1995). While in the generation of the mothers those who had been abused in childhood had higher levels of depression but not eating disorder, the converse was found in the generation of the daughters. Thus age was a major factor which determined the psychopathology and in younger cohorts sexual and physical abuse is linked to bulimia nervosa.

Medical complications

These are usually either due to nutritional deficits and self-starvation (see anorexia nervosa p. 249) or to the after-effects of vomiting or laxative misuse (e.g. dental problems, electrolyte disturbance, see pp. 250, 252).

Treatment

The Royal College of Psychiatrists Report (1992) recommends a stepped approach to treatment. Low-intensity interventions such as self-help manuals, groups or guided self-care are useful in the first instance. Medium-term interventions such as cognitive–behavioural or interpersonal therapy require more specialist skills. Patients with personality difficulties, for example the multi-impulsive or borderline patient or those with additional physical morbidity such as diabetes mellitus, may need long-term psychotherapy or in-patient treatment (for review, see Schmidt 1998).

Group treatment has been widely used and better outcomes are associated with longer, more intensively scheduled groups and with the addition of other components such as individual work (Hartman et al 1992). However, in a quasi-experimental study, the addition of group psychotherapy (12 sessions) did not improve short-term outcome in comparison to five sessions of group psycho-education alone (Davis et al 1997). It may be helpful to match the charac-teristics of the client with the treatment to increase engagement and effectiveness and to decrease drop-out rates (McKisack & Waller 1997).

Antidepressants, especially SSRIs, are also widely used in the treatment of bulimia nervosa disorders, although their effect size is lower than that of psychotherapy (for review, see Schmidt 1998).

Box 14.9   Essential facets of treatment for bulimia nervosa

1. Engender motivation
2. Develop good motivation
3. Formulation: are there links between behaviour and core schemata? Is there a biological disposition to poor weight control?
4. Education/skills of nutritional balance
5. Education/skills of emotional balance

Prognosis

The median duration is between 3 and 6 years. Approximately 50% of patients remain symptomatic with short-term therapy (Wilson 1996). Keel & Mitchell (1997) recently reviewed 88 studies that conducted follow-up assessments of subjects with bulimia nervosa at least 6 months following presentation. Altogether these studies covered 2194 subjects. The crude mortality was 0.3%. In the short term, within 4 years after treatment, approximately one-third of cases relapse. The outcome 5 to 10 years after presentation was that 50% had no disorder and 20% met full criteria. There have been very few reliable markers of a poor prognosis although impulsivity may be linked to chronicity.

Box 14.10   Prognosis of bulimia nervosa

- Crude mortality 0.3%
- 5–10 years after presentation: 50% had no disorder, 20% met full criteria
- Impulsivity associated with a poor prognosis

SUMMARY AND CONCLUSIONS

Much progress has recently been made in delineating the differences between anorexia nervosa and bulimia nervosa. It is hoped that over the next few years this may translate into a better informed public opinion, moving away from, on the one hand, the trivialising notion that anorexia nervosa and bulimia nervosa are 'slimmers' diseases', affecting only fashion-conscious young women or, on the other hand, that sufferers from these conditions are totally untreatable 'freaks'.

Exercise

1. Think of something or someone that you might cherish, for example, your children, pet, or family. With a friend/colleague, carry out a role play exercise in which your colleague tries to get you to give up this cherished object or person.
2. Read the texts on motivational interviewing and practise the given exercises, then repeat the above, using the new approach.

KEY TEXTS FOR FURTHER READING

Garner D M, Garfinkel P E (eds) 1987 Handbook of treatment for eating disorders. Guilford Press, New York

Fallon P, Katzman M, Wooley S C 1994 Feminist perspectives on eating disorders. Guilford Press, New York

Hoek H, Treasure J L, Katzman M 1998 The integration of neurobiology in the treatment of eating disorders. Wiley, Chichester

Szmuckler G, Dare C, Treasure J 1995 Handbook of eating disorders. Wiley, Chichester

Brownell K D, Fairburn C G 1986 Eating disorders and obesity. Guilford Press, New York

---

REFERENCES

American Psychiatric Association 1993 Guidelines for the treatment of eating disorders. APA, Washington DC

American Psychiatric Association 1994 Diagnostic and statistical manual of mental disorders (DSM-III-R), 4th edn revised. APA, Washington DC

Andrews B, Valentine E R, Valentine J D 1995 Depression and eating disorders following abuse in childhood in two generations of women. British Journal of Clinical Psychology 34:37–52

Bell R 1985 Holy anorexia. Chicago University Press, Chicago

Blair C, Freeman C, Cull A 1995 The families of anorexia nervosa and cystic fibrosis patients. Psychological Medicine 25:985–993

Blake W, Turnbull S, Treasure J L 1997 Stages and processes of change in eating disorders: implications for therapy. Clinical Psychology and Psychotherapy 4:186–191

Bhanji S, Mattingly D 1988 Medical aspects of anorexia nervosa. Wright, London

Braun D L, Sunday S R, Halmi K A 1994 Psychiatric comorbidity in patients with eating disorders. Psychological Medicine 24:859–867

Brinch M, Isager T, Tolsrup K 1998 Anorexia nervosa and motherhood: reproductive pattern and mothering behaviours of 50 women. Acta Psychiatrica Scandinavica 77:611–617

Brown N, Ward A, Treasure J et al 1996 Leptin levels in anorexia nervosa (acute and long-term recovered). International Journal of Obesity 20:37

Bruch H 1973 Eating disorders: Obesity, anorexia nervosa and the person within. Routledge and Kegan Paul, London

Casanueva F F, Dieguez C, Popovic V, Peino R, Considine R V, Caro J F 1997 Serum immunoreactive leptin concentrations in patients with anorexia nervosa before and after partial recovery. Biochemistry and Molecular Medicine 60:116–120

Collier D A, Arranz M J, Li T, Mupita D, Brown N, Treasure J 1997 Association between a promotor polymorphism in the 5HT 2A gene and anorexia nervosa. Lancet 350:412

Connan F, Treasure J L 1998 Stress eating and neurobiology. In: Hoek K, Treasure J, Katzman M (eds) Neurobiology in the treatment of eating disorders. Wiley, Chichester, p 211–236

Cooke R A, Chambers J B, Singh R et al 1994 QT interval in anorexia nervosa. British Heart Journal 72:69–73

Cooper Z, Cooper P J, Fairburn C G 1989 The validity of the eating disorder examination and its subscales. British Journal of Psychiatry 154:807–812

Crisp A H, Callender J S, Halek C, Hsu L K G 1992 Long-term mortality in anorexia nervosa: a 20-year follow-up of the St George's and Aberdeen cohorts. British Medical Journal 161:104–107

Dansky B S, Brewerton T D, Kilpatrick D G, O'Neil P M 1997 The National Women's Study – Relation of victimisation and post-traumatic stress disorder to bulimia nervosa. International Journal of Eating Disorders 21:213–228

Davis R, Olmsted M, Rockert W, Marques T, Dolhanty J 1997 Group psychoeducation for bulimia nervosa with and

REFERENCES (*contd*)

without additional psychotherapy process sessions. International Journal of Eating Disorders 22:25–43

Dolan R J, Mitchell J, Wakeling A 1988 Structural brain changes in patients with anorexia nervosa. Psychological Medicine 18:349–353

Eisler I, Dare C, Russell G F M, Szmukler G, Le Grange D, Dodge E 1997 A five year follow-up of a controlled trial of family therapy in severe eating disorder. Archives of General Psychiatry 54:1025–1030

Fairburn C G, Welch S L, Doll H A, Davies B A, O'Connor M E 1997 Risk factors for bulimia nervosa: a community based case control study. Archives of General Psychiatry 54:509–517

Fairburn C G, Welch S L, Hay P J 1993 The classification of recurrent overeating: the 'binge eating disorder' proposal. International Journal of Eating Disorders 13:155–159

Fallon P, Katzman M A, Wooley S C 1994 Feminist perspectives on eating disorders. Guilford Press, New York

Ferron F, Considine R V, Peino R, Lado I G, Dieguez C, Casanueva F F 1997 Serum leptin concentrations in patients with anorexia nervosa, bulimia nervosa and non-specific eating disorders correlate with body mass index but are independent of the respective disease. Clinical Endocrinology 46:289–293

Fombonne E 1995 Anorexia nervosa. No evidence of an increase. British Journal of Psychiatry 166:462–471

Fowler R 1871 A complete history of the case of the Welch fasting girl (Sarah Jacob) with comments thereon, and observations on death from starvation. Henry Renshaw, London

Gard M C E, Freeman C P 1996 The dismantling of a myth: a review of eating disorders and socioeconomic status. International Journal of Eating Disorders 20:1–12

Garner D M, Garfinkel P E 1979 The Eating Attitudes Test: an index of the symptoms of anorexia nervosa. Psychological Medicine 9:273–279

Garner D M, Olmsted M P, Garfinkel P E 1983 Development and validation of a multidimensional eating disorder inventory for anorexia nervosa and bulimia. International Journal of Eating Disorders 48:173–178

Gavish D, Eisenberg S, Berry E M 1987 Bulimia an underlying behavioural disorder in hyperlipidaemic pancreatitis: a prospective multidisciplinary approach. Archives of Internal Medicine 147:705–708

Gillberg I C, Rastam M, Gillberg C 1994 Anorexia nervosa outcome: six-year controlled longitudinal study of 51 cases including a population cohort. Journal of the American Academy of Child and Adolescent Psychiatry 33:729–739

Gillberg I C, Rastam M, Gillberg C 1995 Anorexia nervosa 6 years after onset: Part I. Personality disorders. Comprehensive Psychiatry 36:61–69

Grinspoon S, Baum H, Lee K, Anderson E, Herzog D, Klibanski A 1996 Effects of short-term recombinant human insulin-like growth factor I administration on bone turnover in osteopenic women with anorexia nervosa. Journal of Clinical Endocrinology and Metabolics 81:3864–3870

Grinspoon S, Gulick T, Askari H et al 1996 Serum leptin levels in women with anorexia nervosa. Journal of Clinical Endocrinology and Metabolics 81:3861–3863

Gull W W 1874 Anorexia nervosa (apepsia hysterica, anorexia hysterica). Transactions of the Clinical Society of London 7:22–28

Gwirtsman H E, Jaye W H, George D T, Jimerson D C, Eberet M H, Gold P W 1989 Central and peripheral ACTH and cortisol levels in anorexia and bulimia. Archives of General Psychiatry 46:61–69

Hall R C W, Hoffman R S, Beresford T P, Wooley B, Hall A K, Kubasak L 1989 Physical illness encountered in patients with eating disorders. Psychosomatics 30:174–191

Halmi KA 1995 Current concepts and definitions. In: Szmukler G, Dare C, Treasure J (eds) Handbook of eating disorders: Theory, treatment and research. Wiley, Chichester

Halmi K A 1997 Models to conceptualize risk factors for bulimia nervosa. Archives of General Psychiatry 54:507–508

Halmi K A, Eckert E, Marchi P A, Samfpugnaro V, Apple R, Cohn J 1991 Comorbidity of psychiatric diagnosis in anorexia nervosa. Archives of General Psychiatry 48:712–718

Hartman A, Herzog T, Drinkmann A 1992 Psychotherapy of bulimia nervosa: what is effective? A meta-analysis. Journal of Psychosomatic Research 36:159–167

Hay P J, Fairburn C G, Doll H A 1996 The classification of bulimic eating disorders: a community-based cluster analysis study. Psychological Medicine 26:801–812

Hebebrand J, Remschmidt H 1995 Anorexia nervosa viewed as an extreme weight condition: genetic implications. Human Genetics 95:1–11

Henderson M, Freeman C P L 1987 A self-rating scale for bulimia: 'The Bite'. British Journal of Psychiatry 150: 18–24

Herzog W, Deter H C, Fiehn W, Petzold E 1997a Medical findings and predictors of long-term physical outcome in anorexia nervosa – a prospective 12 year follow-up study. Psychological Medicine 27:269–279

Herzog W, Schellberg D, Deter H C 1997b First recovery in anorexia nervosa patients in the long-term course: a discrete time survival analysis. Journal of Consulting and Clinical Psychology 65:169–177

Herzog D B, Keller M B, Lavori P W, Kenny G M, Sacks N R 1992 The prevalence of personality disorders in 210 women with eating disorders. Journal of Clinical Psychiatry 53:147–152

Hoek H W 1993 Review of the epidemiological studies of eating disorders. International Review of Psychiatry 5:61–74

Isner J M, Roberts W C, Heymsfield S B, Yager J 1985 Anorexia nervosa and sudden death. Archives of Internal Medicine 146:1525–1529

Jimerson D C, Wolfe B E, Metger E D, Finkelstein D M, Cooper T B, Levine J M 1997 Decreased serotonin function in bulimia nervosa. Archives of General Psychiatry 54:529–534

Johnson G L, Humphries L L, Shirley P B, Mazzoleni A, Noonan J A 1986 Mitral valve prolapse in patients with anorexia nervosa and bulimia. Archives of Internal Medicine 146:1525–1529

Kaplan A S, Garfinkel P E 1993 Medical issues and the eating disorders. Brunner, Mazel, New York

REFERENCES (*contd*)

Katzman M A, Lee S 1997 Beyond body image: the integration of feminist and transcultural theories in the understanding of self-starvation. International Journal of Eating Disorders 22:385–394

Katzman D K, Lambe E K, Mikulis D J, Ridgely J N, Goldbloom D S, Zipursky R B 1996 Cerebral grey matter and white matter volume deficits in adolescent females with anorexia nervosa. Journal of Paediatrics 129:794–803

Keel P K, Mitchell J E 1997 Outcome in bulimia nervosa. American Journal of Psychiatry 154:313–321

Kendler K S, MacLean C, Neale M, Kessler R, Heath A, Eaves L 1991 The genetic epidemiology of bulimia nervosa. American Journal of Psychiatry 148:1627–1637

Kendler K S, Walters E E, Neale M C, Kessler R C, Heath A C, Eaves L J 1995 The genetic and environmental risk factors for six major psychiatric disorders in women. Archives of General Psychiatry 52:374–383

Kingston K, Szmukler G, Andrews D, Tress B, Desmond P 1996 Neuropsychological and structural brain changes in anorexia nervosa before and after refeeding. Psychological Medicine 26:15–28

Kinzl J, Bieble W, Herold M 1993 Significance of vomiting for hypoamylasaemia and sialadenosis in patients with eating disorders. International Journal of Eating Disorders 13:117–124

Klibanski A, Biller B M K, Schoenfeld D A, Herzog D B, Saxe V C 1995 The effects of estrogen administration on trabecular bone loss in young women with anorexia nervosa. Journal of Clinical Endocrinology and Metabolism 80:898–904

Kreipe R E, Churchill B H, Strauss J 1989 Long-term outcome of adolescents with anorexia nervosa. AUDC 143:1322–1327

Krieg J C, Pirke K M, Lauer C, Backmund H 1988 Endocrine, metabolic and cranial computed tomographic findings in anorexia nervosa. Psychological Medicine 18:349–353

Laessle R G, Kittl S, Fichter M M, Wittchen H U, Pirke K M 1987 Major affective disorder in anorexia nervosa and bulimia. British Journal of Psychiatry 151:785–789

Lambe E K, Katzman D K, Mikulis D J, Kennedy S H, Zipursky R B 1997 Cerebral gray matter deficits after weight recovery from anorexia nervosa. Archives of General Psychiatry 54:537–542

Lambert M, Hubert C, Depresseux G et al 1997 Haematological changes in anorexia nervosa are correlated with total body fat mass depletion. International Journal of Eating Disorders 21:329–334

Lasègue, C 1873 On hysterical anorexia. Medical Times and Gazette ii:265–266, 367–369

Lee S 1995 Self starvation in context: towards a culturally sensitive understanding of anorexia nervosa. Social Science Medicine 41:25–36

Le Grange D, Eisler I, Dare C, Russell G F M 1992 Evaluation of family therapy in anorexia nervosa: a pilot study. International Journal of Eating Disorders 12:347–357

Levine A P, Hyler S E 1986 DSM-III personality diagnosis in bulimia. Comprehensive Psychiatry 27:47–53

Levitan R D, Kaplan A S, Joffe R T, Levitt A J, Brown G M 1997 Hormonal and subjective responses to intravenous meta-chlorophenylpiperazine in bulimia nervosa. Archives of General Psychiatry 54:521–527

Littlewood R 1995 Psychopathology and personal agency: modernity, culture change and eating disorders in south Asian societies. British Journal of Medical Psychology 68:45–63

Lucas A R, Beard C M, O'Fallon W M, Kurland L T 1991 50-year trends in the incidence of anorexia nervosa in Rochester, Minnesota: a population based study. American Journal of Psychiatry 148:917–922

Marcé L-V 1860 On a form of hypochondriacal delirium occurring during consecutive dyspepsia, and characterized by refusal of food. Journal of Psychological Medicine and Mental Pathology 13:264–266

McKisack C, Waller G 1997 Factors influencing outcome of group psychotherapy for bulimia nervosa. International Journal of Eating Disorder 22:1–13

Minuchin S, Rosman B L, Baker L 1978 Psychosomatic families. Harvard University Press, Cambridge, Massachusetts

Murciamo D, Rigaud D, Pinleton S, Armengaud M H, Melchior J C, Aubier M 1994 Diaphragmatic function in severely malnourished patients with anorexia nervosa. Effects of renutrition. American Journal of Respiratory Critical Care Medicine 150:1569–1574

Mustafa A, Ward A, Treasure J, Peakman M 1997 T-lymphocyte subpopulations in anorexia nervosa and refeeding. Clinical Immunology and Immunopathology 82:282–289

Nielsen S 1990 The epidemiology of anorexia nervosa in Denmark from 1973 to 1987: a nationwide register study of psychiatric admission. Acta Psychiatrica Scandinavica 81:507–514

Orlich E S, Aughey D R, Dixon R M 1989 Sorbital abuse among eating disorder patients. Academic Psychosomatic Medicine 30:295–298

Orphanidou C I, McCarger L J, Birmingham C L, Belzberg A S 1997 Changes in body composition and fat distribution after short term weight gain in patients with anorexia nervosa. American Journal of Clinical Nutrition 65:1034–1041

Owen J B 1992 Genetic aspects of appetite and feed choice in animals. Journal of Agricultural Science 119:151–155

Patton G C 1988 Mortality in eating disorders. Psychological Medicine 18:947–951

Pollice C, Kaye W H, Greeno C G, Weltzin T E 1997 Relationship of depression, anxiety and obsessionality to state of illness in anorexia nervosa. International Journal of Eating Disorders 21:357–376

Prochaska J O, Di Clemente C C 1992 The transtheoretical model of change. In: Norcross J C, Goldfried M R (eds) Handbook of psychotherapy integration. Basic Books, New York

Rastam M, Gillberg C, Garton M 1989 Anorexia nervosa in a Swedish urban region: a population based study. British Journal of Psychiatry 155:642–646

Rigotti N A, Neer R M, Skates S J, Herzog D B, Nussbaum S R 1991 The clinical course of osteoporosis in anorexia nervosa. Journal of the American Medical Association 265:1133–1137

Robb N D, Smith B G, Geidry S, Leeper E 1995 The distribution of erosion in the dentitions of patients with eating disorders. British Dental Journal 178:171–175

REFERENCES (*contd*)

Royal College of Psychiatrists 1992 Eating disorders. Council report. RCP, London

Russell G F M 1979 Bulimia nervosa an ominous variant of anorexia nervosa. Psychological Medicine 9:429–448

Russell G F M 1995 Anorexia nervosa through time. In: Szmukler G, Dare C, Treasure J (eds) Handbook of eating disorders: Theory, treatment, research. Wiley, Chichester

Russell G F, Szmukler G I, Dare C, Eisler I 1987 An evaluation of family therapy in anorexia nervosa and bulimia nervosa. Archives of General Psychiatry 44:1047–1056

Russell G F M, Treasure J L, Eisler I 1998 Children of mothers with anorexia nervosa. Psychological Medicine. 28:93–101

Rutherford J, McGuffin P, Katz R J, Murray R M 1993 Genetic influences on eating attitudes in a normal female twin population. Psychological Medicine 23:425–436

Sapolsky R M 1992 Stress and the ageing brain and the mechanisms of neuron death. MIT Press, Cambridge, Mass

Schmidt U 1998 Treatment of bulimia nervosa. In: Hoek H W, Treasure J L, Katzman M A (eds) The integration of neurobiology in the treatment of eating disorders. Wiley, Chichester, p331–362

Schmidt U, Tiller J, Treasure J 1993 Setting the scene for eating disorders: childhood care, classification and course of illness. Psychological Medicine 23:663–672

Schmidt U, Tiller J, Blanchard M, Andrews B, Treasure J 1997 Is there a specific trauma precipitating the onset of anorexia nervosa? Psychological Medicine 27:523–530

Schönheit B, Meyer U, Kuchinke J, Schulz E, Neumärker K J 1996 Morphometric investigations on lamina V pyramidal neurons in the frontal cortex of a case with anorexia nervosa. Journal of Brain Research 37:269–280

Selvini-Palazzoli M P 1974 Self-starvation. Chaucer, London

Serpell L, Treasure J L 1997 Osteoporosis – a serious health risk in chronic anorexia nervosa. European Eating Disorders Review 5:149–157

Sharpe C W, Freeman C P L 1993 The medical complications of anorexia nervosa. British Journal of Psychiatry 153:452–462

Silverman J A 1997 Charcot's comments on the therapeutic role of isolation in the treatment of anorexia nervosa. International Journal of Eating Disorders 21:295–298

Spitzer R L, Devlin M, Walsh B T et al 1992 Binge eating disorder. A multisite field trial of the diagnostic criteria. International Journal of Eating Disorders 11:191–203

Spitzer R L, Yanovski S, Wadden T et al 1993 Binge eating disorder: its further validation in an multisite study. International Journal of Eating Disorders 13:137–153

Stefanis N, Mackintosh, Abraham H, Treasure J, Moniz C 1999 Dissociation of bone turnover in anorexia nervosa. Clinical Biochemistry 35:709–716

Strober M, Lampert C, Morrell W, Burroughs J, Jacobs C 1990 A controlled family study of anorexia nervosa: evidence of familial aggregation and lack of shared transmission with affective disorders. International Journal of Eating Disorders 9:239–253

Study Group on Anorexia Nervosa 1995 Anorexia nervosa – directions for future research. International Journal of Eating Disorders 17:235–241

Sullivan P F 1995 Mortality in anorexia nervosa. American Journal of Psychiatry 152:1073–1074

Szmukler G I, Young G P, Lichtenstein M, Andrews D 1990 A serial study of gastric emptying in anorexia nervosa and bulimia nervosa. Australian and New Zealand Journal of Medicine 20:220–225

Tang M X, Jacobs D, Stern Y 1996 Effect of oestrogen during menopause on risk and age of onset of Alzheimer's disease. Lancet 348:429–432

Touyz S W, Beaumont P J V, Glaun D, Phillips T, Cowie I 1984 A comparison of lenient and strict operant conditioning programmes in refeeding patients with anorexia nervosa. British Journal of Psychiatry 144:517–520

Touyz S W, Beumont P J V 1997 Behavioural treatment to promote weight gain. In: Garner D M, Garfinkel P E (eds) Handbook of treatment of eating disorders. Guilford Press, New York

Treasure J L 1988 The ultrasonographic features in anorexia nervosa and bulimia nervosa: a simplified method of monitoring hormonal states during weight gain. Clinical Endocrinology 29:607–616

Treasure J L, Campbell I 1994 The case for biology in the aetiology of anorexia nervosa. Editorial. Psychological Medicine 24:3–8

Treasure J L, Holland A J 1995 Genetic factors in eating disorders. In: Szmukler G, Dare C, Treasure, J (eds) Handbook of eating disorders. Theory, treatment and research. Wiley, Chichester

Treasure J L, Owen J B 1997 Intriguing links between animal behaviour and anorexia nervosa. International Journal of Eating Disorders 21:307–311

Treasure J L, Russell G F M 1988 Intra-uterine growth and neonatal weight gain in anorexia nervosa. British Medical Journal 296:1038

Treasure J L, Szmukler G 1995 Medical complications. In: Szmukler G, Dare C, Treasure J (eds) Handbook of eating disorders. Wiley, Chichester

Treasure J L, Ward A 1997 Cognitive analytical therapy (CAT) in eating disorders. Clinical Psychology and Psychotherapy 4:62–71

Treasure J, Todd G, Brolly M, Tiller J, Nehmed A, Denman F 1995 A pilot study of a randomized trial of cognitive analytical therapy versus educational behavioural therapy for adult anorexia nervosa. Behaviour Research and Therapy 33:363–367

Troop N 1996 Coping and crisis support in eating disorders. Unpublished PhD thesis, Institute of Psychiatry, London

Troop N A, Treasure J L 1997 Setting the scene for eating disorders. II. Childhood helplessness and mastery. Psychological Medicine. 27:531–538

Turnbull S, Ward A, Treasure J, Jick H, Derby L 1996 The demand for eating disorder care: an epidemiological study using the general practice research data base. British Journal of Psychiatry 169:705–712

Turnbull S J, Troop N A, Treasure J L 1998 The prevalence of post-traumatic stress in eating disorder and its relation to childhood adversity. European Eating Disorders Review 5:270–277

Vitousek K, Watson S, Wilson G T 1997 Enhancing motivation in eating disorders. Clinical Psychology Review (in press)

Ward A, Brown N, Treasure J 1997 Persistent osteopenia after recovery from anorexia nervosa. International Journal of Eating Disorders 22:71–75

Ward A, Troop N, Todd G, Treasure J L 1996 To change or not

REFERENCES (*contd*)

to change. 'How' is the question. British Journal of Medical Psychology 69:139–146

Welch S L, Fairburn C G 1994 Sexual abuse and bulimia nervosa: three integrated case control comparisons. American Journal of Psychiatry 151:402–407

Welch S L, Fairburn C G 1996a Childhood sexual and physical abuse as risk factors for the development of bulimia nervosa: a community based case control study Child Abuse and Neglect 20:633–642

Welch S L, Fairburn C G 1996b Impulsivity or comorbidity in bulimia nervosa. A controlled study of deliberate self-harm and alcohol and drug misuse in a community sample. British Journal of Psychiatry 169:451–458

Wilson T G 1996 Treatment of bulimia nervosa: when CBT fails. Behaviour Research and Therapy 34:197–212

Wonderlich S A, Swift W J, Slotnick H B, Goodman S 1990 DSM-III-R personality disorders in eating-disorder sub-types. International Journal of Eating Disorders 9:607–616

World Health Organization 1992 ICD-10. Clinical descriptions and diagnostic guidelines. WHO, Geneva

15

Anger and impulse control

Tracey Swaffer   Clive R. Hollin

CHAPTER CONTENTS

Key points   265

Introduction   266

Anger   266

Impulse control   268

Anger and physical health   269
Physical ailments   269
Psychological constructs   269

Anger and mental health   270
Self-esteem   270
Depression   271

Anger and self-injury   271
Self-injury and mental illness   272
Self-injury and learning difficulty   272

Anger and violent behaviour   272
Understanding family violence   273
Violence towards care staff   273

The management of anger   273
Assessment   275
Cognitive preparation and assessment   276
Skill acquisition and rehearsal   277
Skill application   277
Evaluation   278

Case study Carl   279
Information obtained from the assessment period
279
Design of the anger-management package   280
Cognitive preparation and assessment   280
Skills acquisition and rehearsal   281
Absence   282
Skills application   283
Follow-up   283
Results   284
Summary   285

Concluding remarks   286

Exercise   286

Key texts for further reading   287

References   287

KEY POINTS

- Anger is a complex emotion, which can be conceived of in terms of an interplay between environmental events, thoughts, and physiological arousal.

- Impulse control disorders stem from a failure to resist a temptation to behave in ways that are harmful.

- Chronic anger is associated with a range of psychological and behavioural disorders and medical conditions.

- Anger management programmes have been used successfully with many different types of angry and impulsive people. These programmes typically consist of training in recognition of anger cues, development of self-control and social skills, and role-play practice of these skills.

INTRODUCTION

When unchecked, anger and poor impulse control can negatively impact upon people's lives, causing problems both for the individual concerned and for the individual's carers. This chapter explores what we mean by 'anger' and impulse control and their potential detrimental effects; how negative impacts can be rectified through the use of anger-management packages; and an example of how such a package can be implemented and evaluated.

ANGER

Anger is a particularly complex emotion as it can have a positive *or* negative impact (Novaco & Welsh 1989). This chapter will deal with the experience and expression of negative or dysfunctional anger. Anger is considered to be dysfunctional when the experience and expression of the emotion have an extremely negative impact upon the person experiencing emotion. Dysfunctional anger has been related to poor physical health (Blackburn 1993, Spielberger 1988), adverse mental health (Lester 1988), and self-injurious behaviour (Green 1967). Anger is also considered to be dysfunctional when the experience and expression of anger by an individual have a negative impact upon other people, such as violent behaviour that is directed at people who are caring for the angry individual (Gentry & Ostapiuk 1989, Haller & Deluty 1988). Each of the above relationships will be explored in more detail in this chapter. However, even with all this information about the maladaptive relationship between anger and other aspects of human functioning, it is important to define what is meant by the term anger. Anger is said to be an emotion. However, as Dodge & Garber (1991:3) state, 'Emotion is like pornography: the experts have great difficulty defining it, but we all know it when we see it'.

The most influential theory of anger, and related approach to its management, is provided by Novaco (1975, 1994). Novaco states that anger is a subjective emotional state which involves the presence of both physiological and cognitive components. Novaco particularly uses this model to give an account of aggressive and violent behaviour (see Fig. 15.1).

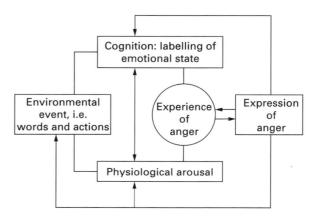

Figure 15.1 Determinants and consequences of anger (adapted from Novaco 1994).

To explain this model in more detail, it is important to explore how a person becomes angry.

According to Novaco, for a person to become angry, some environmental event triggers cognitive and physiological arousal. Most typically, this event is the words and actions of another person. When the event triggers cognitive and physiological arousal, the first step is that the individual labels the resultant, subjective, emotional state as 'anger'. A subjective emotional state is therefore the result of the interaction between physiological processes and cognitive structures and processes. Physiological processes that are typically associated with anger are increased body temperature, perspiration, muscular tension and increased cardiovascular activity.

Cognitive structures and processes are umbrella

terms for the cognitive labelling of the emotional state as 'angry', or something semantically similar such as 'annoyance'. Novaco & Welsh (1989) suggest that such labelling of the emotional state can be facilitated by the existence of schemas which are a 'pre-existing system of belief, knowledge and propositions' (Novaco & Welsh 1989:49). People use schemas to speed up the time that they take to process information, but this increase in speed can lead to potential bias in judgements. Dodge & Newman (1981) suggest that certain predispositions in the schemas and processes of some individuals can increase the possibility of anger experiences (Dodge & Newman 1981). Novaco & Welsh (1989) have identified five of these information-processing biases within the schemas of individuals prone to anger experiences and expression:

1. attentional cueing
2. perceptual matching
3. attributional error
4. false consensus
5. anchoring effects.

All of these five cognitive biases are concerned with the encoding of external and internal cues and the interpretation and mental representation of those cues.

Attentional cueing refers to the tendency of people who consistently become angry to see provocation everywhere. *Perceptual matching* implies that when people are exposed to a new situation, their reaction will depend upon what they have done before; that is, if people have found that an outward display of anger achieves their goal, they may be more likely to behave that way in the future. *Attributional error* refers to how individuals are more likely to perceive their own behaviour as being situationally determined, but the behaviour of other people is seen as a personal characteristic. This basic attributional error contributes to a higher chance of blaming the

other person not the circumstances. This process is linked to the fourth area which deals with *false consensus*.

Novaco & Welsh (1989) explain false consensus by suggesting that individuals who have problems with anger are predisposed to assume that more people agree with them than actually do. If an individual is unable to perceive another person's point of view, the individual may be more likely to make an attribution of blameworthiness to the other individual. Finally, there is the issue of the *anchoring of effects*. Once individuals have made their initial value judgement, they are unlikely to change this perspective even when presented with facts to the contrary.

However, at the same time as this cognitive labelling, which may or may not be influenced by the processing biases mentioned above, the individual is also more or less inclined to act in a confrontational manner towards the source of the provocation. Whether or not a person will react in an aggressive manner is based upon the disinhibition of internal and external controls which prevent outward displays of aggression. Disinhibition is achieved through the person-specific factors such as increased physiological arousal, previous experience of aggression, a low possibility of punishment, and the surrounding context of the event.

Novaco (1993) states that both the assessment and treatment of anger can be improved by using a contextual perspective. This perspective acknowledges that factors outside of the individual, such as the physical environment and time of day, impact upon a person's experience and expression of anger. Novaco (1993) points out that some hospitalised psychiatric patients are often seen as dangerous because their anger and aggressive behaviour are perceived by staff to be spontaneous. This perception occurs because both the individual experiencing the anger and the observer often view anger as having a proximity bias. In other words, the source of anger is typically identified as having just occurred, rather than being a consequence of more distal factors, and patients may well be labelled as dangerous because of the nature of their perceived unpredictable behaviour. Novaco (1993) suggests that therapists working with anger should focus upon three factors when using a contextually orientated perspective:

1. embeddedness
2. inter-relatedness
3. transformationality.

The notion of *embeddedness* refers to how anger should be understood within time and space, such as daily physical conditions of traffic congestion and social conditions such as work pressures and relative deprivation. *Inter-relatedness* refers to how people can be angry in different environments that are related, so that if someone is angry at work, it may be that following provocation at work they become angry at home. Finally, *transformationality* refers to how anger can be related to change, in that anger can create positive or negative change in personal and social circumstances. Therefore, as Haller & Deluty (1988) highlight, anger-precipitated assaults that occur within institutions are shaped by many factors such as environmental design, institutional philosophy, staff ratios and attitudes, and the effectiveness of treatment programmes, as well as the individual patient's perceptions and behaviour. Rather than focusing upon a notion that violence in psychotic people comes solely from their underlying pathology, it is important also to focus upon how environmental circumstances or staff might have precipitated the patient's anger and violence.

IMPULSE CONTROL

Unlike anger, disorders that are characterised by a lack of impulse control have a formal psychiatric diagnosis. According to the *Diagnostic and Statistical Manual*, 4th edition (DSM-IV):

> The essential feature of Impulse Control Disorders is the failure to resist an impulse, drive or temptation to perform an act that is harmful to the person or to others.
>
> American Psychiatric Association 1994:609

Of this group of disorders, one which is of particular interest here is intermittent explosive disorder (IED). An IED is characterised by three elements:

1. there are discrete events in which the individual fails to resist aggressive impulses which culminate in serious assaults against people and property;
2. the level of aggression displayed by the individual is out of proportion with the level of antecedents;
3. the aggressive episode cannot be better accounted for by another mental disorder, substance abuse, or another medical condition.

It has been suggested that IED could be seen as a formal diagnosis of anger, but, as DSM-IV highlights, unlike anger, IEDs are very rare (Novaco & Welsh 1989). DSM-IV suggests that it may be a more accurate conceptualisation, and of more clinical use, to perceive aggressive behaviour as being a product of anger.

Nevertheless, both anger and impulse control disorders recognise that an individual can react to a provoking stimulus in a manner that can be harmful to the individual or to other people. The impact of dysfunctional anger will now be considered in relation to four areas:

1. physical health
2. mental health
3. self-injury
4. and violent behaviour directed towards others.

ANGER AND PHYSICAL HEALTH

Although anger can be a consequence or reaction to illness (Burish & Bradley 1983), some research has focused on anger as a predictor of certain types of physical ill-health, and on anger in people suffering from ill-health. Anger has been associated with chronic heart disease (CHD) (Barefoot et al 1983), hypertension (Engebretson et al 1989), and carotid and coronary atherosclerosis (Dembroski et al 1985, Julkunen et al 1994). Researchers working within this field have looked at the personality of the individual experiencing the physical ill-health (Rosenman et al 1975), as well as the individual's style of expressing anger (Siegman 1993).

The research discussed in this section is divided into two sub-sections: the first focuses upon actual physical ailments directly associated with anger; the second focuses upon psychological constructs associated with anger and physical ill-health.

Physical ailments

Carotid atherosclerosis. The term carotid atherosclerosis refers to the disease in which deposits of fat cause the neck arteries to thicken. Julkunen et al (1994) found that poor anger control and high levels of cynical distrust, as measured on the Cynical Distrust Scale (Greenglass & Julkunen, 1989) and the Anger Expression Scale (Spielberger et al., 1985), to be risk factors for progression of carotid atherosclerosis over a 2-year period. Ultrasonographically assessed, common, carotid atherosclerosis has a strong association with the risk of CHD.

Coronary atherosclerosis. The term coronary atherosclerosis refers to the disease in which deposits of fat cause the arteries that supply the heart muscle to thicken. Barefoot et al (1983) concluded that not only do high scores on the

Minnesota Multiphasic Personality Inventory Cook and Medley Hostility Scale (Ho) contribute to progression of coronary atherosclerosis, but they may also be indicative of an individual's ability to survive other disorders. Dembroski et al (1985) argue that hostility in conjunction with acquired coping mechanisms such as anger suppression might be at the centre of coronary prone behaviour.

Hypertension. Engebretson et al (1989) identified anger instigation as the mechanism that connected negative interpersonal experiences with elevated blood pressure. Ewart & Kolodner (1994) suggest that high trait anger coupled with negative affect in one's youth are accompanied by elevated levels of ambulatory blood pressure, which is an early biological precursor of essential hypertension and has been related to cardiovascular diseases.

Psychological constructs

Type A personality

The search for psychological predispositions towards ill-health, especially CHD, has centred upon the Type A personality profile (Barefoot et al 1983). Friedman & Rosenman (1959) identified a coronary-prone behaviour pattern, which they labelled Type A. The classic profile of a Type A individual involves excessive competitiveness, drive, aggressiveness and hostility. Within this profile, anger and the closely related construct of hostility have been seen as the primary factors connecting a Type A behaviour pattern to heart problems. Evidence linking Type A behaviour pattern and CHD is provided by the Western Collaborative Group Study (Rosenman et al 1975). This study monitored over 3500 males in an attempt to ascertain what variables could be seen as predictive of CHD. At the onset of the study (in 1964), 113 males were known to be suffering from a form of CHD, and of these 80 were clinically judged to be Type A. At this point in the study, the findings were indicative of a likely relationship between Type A and CHD but not sufficiently substantive to be predictive of any causal link between the two factors. However by 1975, Rosenman et al could show that individuals who had been diagnosed as being Type A were twice as likely as non-Type A's to develop CHD. In addition, the Type A men who started the study with CHD were five times as likely to experience a second CHD problem, even when traditional risk factors were controlled (Barefoot et al 1983).

Anger suppression

The suppression of anger has long been seen within psycho-analytic theory as having a detrimental effect on an individual's health (Siegman 1993). Freud initially perceived the libido as a finite amount of internal energy that powers internal dynamic struggles. If energy became blocked, an emotional reservoir would form which must be released through catharsis (Tavris 1989). However, Freud never advocated the full-blown expression of anger, in all its expressive paraverbal intensity, as a desirable form of catharsis. Nevertheless, the cascading of psycho-analytic thought into numerous schools has fostered the general idea of the harmfulness of suppression of anger.

However, research conducted by Siegman (1993) showed that the full-blown expression of anger is actually associated with heightened cardiovascular reactivity (CVR) and is a risk factor for CHD, rather than the experience of or suppression of anger. Burns et al (1992) suggested that it was not the inwards or outwards direction of anger, but the *experience* of anger that caused the most cardiac reactivity.

It would appear that anger can and does have

an impact upon physical ill-health, both directly and through a personal style that is prone to anger.

ANGER AND MENTAL HEALTH

It has been hypothesised that the experience and expression of anger can have an effect upon psychological constructs such as anxiety (Wickless & Kirsch 1988), self-esteem (Kernis et al 1989), depression (Clay et al 1993), and one's general sense of well-being (Comunian 1994). However, given current space limitations, only self-esteem and depression will be explored here to illustrate the relationship between anger and mental health.

Self-esteem

The term self-esteem is used to describe an individual's perception of his or her own self-worth. Self-esteem can be thought of as a continuum, with low self-esteem implying that a person has a low self-opinion, contrasted with high self-esteem where a high opinion of one's self-worth is held. The interaction between levels of self-esteem and anger experience and expression is complex. This interaction is usually explored from one of three perspectives: (1) individuals with low self-esteem; (2) those with high self-esteem; (3) those in whom self-esteem is unstable.

Kernis et al (1989) suggested that individuals with stable, high self-esteem may be prone to more experiences of anger, as they perceive threats to their self-worth as being unjustified. It has also been suggested that individuals with stable, low self-esteem have high levels of anger experience and expression as they perceive a wide range of environmental stimuli as provoking (Averill 1982).

Baumeister et al (1996) state that the proposed link between low self-esteem and violence is based on an assumption that people who lack self-esteem hope to gain it by aggressively dominating others. Therefore, violence is seen as a vehicle for enhancing the self. However, Baumeister et al (1996) point out that people with low self-esteem are unlikely to place themselves in situations in which their vulnerable self-esteem would be highlighted. It is perhaps more likely that individuals with high self-esteem will believe that they would 'win' in a violent situation and therefore be more willing to engage in a violent transaction.

However, it has also been suggested that it is not the 'amount' of self-esteem individuals possess that causes an increase in their anger, but the *stability* of their self-esteem (Kernis et al 1989, Kugle et al 1983).

Kugle et al (1983) suggested that unstable self-esteem was likely to enhance individuals' sensitivity to feedback from their environment and lead to a heightened concern of how they are perceived by others. Such a level of self-awareness and attention could predispose the individual to perceive more events as provoking and therefore increase the likelihood of anger (Novaco & Welsh 1989). Comunian (1994) supports these opinions by reporting a negative correlation between scores on an anger scale and scores on a sense of well-being scale. Kernis et al (1989) also reported an association between unstable, high self-esteem and a tendency to experience substantially more anger, compared to those with stable levels of high self-esteem.

Low levels of self-esteem as well as unstable levels have also been related to depression (Kernis et al 1989).

Depression

Depression is:

> An emotional state marked by great sadness and apprehension, feelings of worthlessness and guilt, withdrawal from others, loss of sleep, appetite, and sexual desire, or interest and pleasure in usual activities; and either lethargy or agitation.
>
> Davidson & Neale 1986:G5

Some psycho-analytic theories take the view that depression is anger turned against oneself (Davidson & Neale 1986), and several studies have unearthed links between the direction of anger expression and depression (Clay et al 1993, Riley et al 1989).

For example, Clay et al (1993), using the State-Trait Anger Expression Inventory (STAXI, Spielberger 1988), reported that scores obtained on scales that indicated the preferred mode of anger expression as being outwards or controlled were not related to scores on a depression sub-scale. Yet scores that reflected a propensity to direct anger inwards were related to scores on a depression scale. These findings are substantiated by the work of Riley et al (1989) who found that depressed individuals reported higher levels of anger suppression.

ANGER AND SELF-INJURY

Deliberate self-injury is an exceptionally distressing behaviour both for individuals who cause themselves damage and for the people who care for those who self-damage (Fahmy & Jones 1990). Self-injury is defined as any non-accidental behaviour initiated by the individual which directly results in physical harm to that individual. Therefore, self-injury encompasses a broad range of behaviours such as self-cutting, swallowing sharp or dangerous objects, taking an overdose of drugs and self-strangulation. Fahmy & Jones (1990) report that deliberate self-injurious behaviour occurs in two broad populations: (a) people with a psychiatric diagnosis; (b) people who have learning difficulties.

Self-injury and mental illness

Within the psychiatric field, self-injurious behaviour is often seen as the maladaptive expression of aggression. Freud postulated that there is a need for the outlet of aggression and that when this is not possible, self-addressed aggression appears in the form of self-injury. Within the psychiatric field, self-addressed aggression has often been studied in young women, and has also been seen as being indicative of gender differences in the expression of anger.

Green (1967) looked at the prevalence of self-injury in 70 schizophrenic children. He concluded that the higher rate of self-injury found in females could be explained by social reinforcement of the non-expression of anger and aggression by women. Through a process of socialisation, young women are taught that the expression of anger is not acceptable and is, in fact, disapproved of and discouraged (Sharkin 1993). This unexpressed anger is seen as causing self-directed aggression in the form of self-injury.

Self-injury and learning difficulty

A common explanation of the occurrence of self-injury for people with learning difficulties (or autism) is that it arises from organic factors within the individual such as Lesch–Nyhan syndrome and Cornelia de Lange syndrome (Fahmy & Jones 1990). However, the most popular explanation for self-damage in people with learning difficulties is that the behaviour is maintained by both positive and negative reinforcement. Positive reinforcement contingencies arise through the social attention of carers that self-damage can produce. It has been suggested that restraints which are used to prevent self-injury can be negatively reinforcing as the process of restraint tends to involve the moving of the individual to another room, which may facilitate an escape from an aversive situation. The process of restraint may also be positively reinforcing as it provides individual attention.

ANGER AND VIOLENT BEHAVIOUR

It is important at this point to clarify what is meant by the terms aggression and violence, as these terms are often used interchangeably in the literature (McDougall & Boddis 1991). The term *violence* is understood to denote acts of strong physical force against another person (Blackburn 1993). *Aggression* is defined here as the 'intentional infliction of harm, including psychological discomfort as well as injury' (Blackburn 1993:211). Unlike violent acts, actions are deemed to be aggressive if they are *perceived* by an observer to be unjustified (Blackburn 1993): for example, acts of self-defence which involve the infliction of harm are rarely perceived as being aggressive. However, acts of aggression are also divided by the perceived underlying intent of the act. The distinction is made between hostile/angry aggression and instrumental/incentive aggression (Blackburn 1993). Angry aggression has received the most attention in clinical and forensic research (Browne & Howells 1996). It encompasses acts motivated by anger, 'in which harm or injury to the victims reduces an aversive emotional state' (Blackburn 1993:211). While incentive aggression incorporates acts that are incentive motivated, 'in which injury facilitates the attainment of non-aggressive goals' (Blackburn 1993:211). It is important to note that anger does not always precipitate aggression or violence (Blackburn 1993, Novaco & Welsh 1989). However, it has been suggested that anger tends to precipitate most instances of unplanned aggression and violence (Berkowitz 1986).

Hollin & Howells (1989) suggest that clinical intervention is best suited with angry acts of violence. However, before focusing upon the management of anger, it is important to consider how anger contributes to violent behaviours, such as serious assault. A serious assault may be defined as an attack which inflicts severe wounding and physical harm on the victim (Hollin & Howells 1989). The role of anger in family violence and assault on care staff will be considered to illustrate how anger can contribute to violence.

Understanding family violence

Violence and aggression between family members is not a new phenomenon, although it is only since the 1960s that physical abuse of children and women has been widely recognised (Blackburn 1993). Although family violence should be fully understood by taking a cultural and social approach (Browne 1989), in clinical practice it is important to focus on the personal characteristics of individuals committing acts of violence towards their partners. This focus is driven by the work of Deschner (1984) who suggested that anger and hostility serve as primary triggers of domestic violence.

Characteristics often associated with domestically violent men include low self-esteem, alcohol abuse, attitudes of power and control, and jealousy (Dobash & Dobash 1979, Maiuro et al 1988). However, Frude (1991) suggests that a principal determinant of the seriousness of an assault on a spouse is the degree of anger that precipitates the attack, with extreme anger being correlated with more serious attacks. This hypothesis gathers support from the work of Maiuro et al. (1988) who found that men who committed domestic violence had higher levels of anger and hostility than a non-violent control group.

Violence towards care staff

The prevalence of violence in institutions that provide services for psychiatrically disordered people is well documented (Haller & Deluty 1988). However, the nature of the link between mental disorder and violent behaviour is not well understood (Whittington & Wykes 1996). There is a tendency in the literature to view violence by psychotic people as being directly derived from an underlying pathology, rather than actually focusing upon all the circumstances surrounding a violent event (as recommended by Novaco's model). Whittington & Wykes (1996) looked at 63 instances of assault by patients on psychiatric care staff across 13 wards in a range of settings. The patient, the assaulted staff member and a staff witness were interviewed within 72 hours of the assault. It was found that 86% of assaults had been immediately preceded by the nurse delivering an aversive stimulus to the patient (such as an injection) which had angered the patient, rather than the assault being a spontaneous outcome of the patient's mental state. While this finding does not mean that all violence occurs because the patient has become angry, it does illustrate how a full assessment of an event would show the real nature of the relationship between anger and violence.

As discussed in the previous section, dysfunctional anger can negatively impact upon physical health, can affect mental health, and can lead to violent behaviour directed towards both the self and to others. It follows that there are advantages in providing assistance in anger management. The next section of this chapter focuses upon the design of an anger-management package based on Novaco's model of anger.

THE MANAGEMENT OF ANGER

Given the relationship between anger and violent behaviour, it has been suggested that anger management should form part of a 'clinical' orientation to the prevention of violent behaviour

(Howells 1989). This does *not* mean that anger-management programmes will prevent all forms of aggression and violence (Browne & Howells 1996), but may be helpful when aggression and violence are motivated by anger (Blackburn 1993).

Anger-management programmes do not teach the participants that anger is wrong, rather the purpose is to show that the control of anger is preferable to an unchecked expression of anger (McDougall et al 1990). LeCroy (1988) compared anger-*management* packages with anger-*expressive* interventions and found that participants in the anger-expressive group actually increased their aggressive behaviours when compared to the anger-management group. When working with violent people who are motivated by anger, the aim of intervention would not be to increase the amount of violent behaviour displayed; rather, control of such behaviour is the primary aim.

Anger-management packages have been effectively used with a range of groups including Vietnam veterans (Reilly et al 1994), people with learning difficulties (Black & Novaco 1993), adolescents (Feindler 1995), police officers (Novaco 1977), undergraduates (Deffenbacher et al 1988, 1990) and young offenders (McDougall et al 1990). Pharmacological therapies have been used successfully to manage anger in people who have met the DSM-IV classification for impulse control disorder (Campbell et al 1992).

When designing effective anger-management packages, it is important for participants to understand how anger can lead to unwanted violent or aggressive behaviour: packages that integrate conceptual issues with treatment outcome results are considered the most effective (Edmondson & Conger 1996).

Therefore, referring back to Novaco's model, individuals may have learnt that aggressive behaviour achieves their goal, and they will therefore be more likely to behave similarly when the setting conditions indicate that reinforcement may be forthcoming. Thus, by assessing the antecedents of the event, the behaviours that occur at the time of the event, as well as the consequences for the individual after the event, a functional analysis can be completed.

This analysis facilitates discussion between care-givers, clients and professional staff to establish why self-harm and other forms of violence are happening. This process allows effective use of anger-management techniques that can prevent the violence from initially occurring (Black & Novaco 1993).

The most influential theory of anger and related approach to its management was produced by Novaco (1975, 1994). Novaco states that there is a reciprocal relationship between anger, physiological arousal, behaviour and surrounding external events. Novaco's stress inoculation therapy for anger control was the first systematic psychological intervention for anger problems (Levey & Howells 1990). This intervention is comprised of three stages:

1. *cognitive preparation*, in which the treatment rationale and education about the function of anger and personal patterns of anger are established
2. *skills* acquisition and rehearsal, in which the participant models and rehearses cognitive, affective and behavioural techniques designed to manage anger
3. an *application* phase in which the participant practises the skills learnt in stage two through role-plays.

The model provides a step-by-step breakdown of both the components involved in becoming angry and the reciprocal relationship between these components, which makes this technique particularly appropriate for use with violent people (Browne & Howells 1996). This approach provides participants with a means by which they can understand and monitor their personal anger patterns, and provides them with skills for preventing their maladaptive anger expression. Packages based upon Novaco's principles have been shown to be successful in the reduction of anger (Browne & Howells 1996, Deffenbacher et al 1990, McDougall et al 1990). The next section of this chapter will focus upon issues that practitioners using a cognitive–behavioural approach will encounter. These practical considerations will be discussed in five sections that reflect the three stages of Novaco's programme of intervention, as well as the initial assessment stage and the evaluation of the package.

Assessment

Before any treatment rationale or education about the function of anger and personal anger patterns is established, the appropriateness of anger management for an individual needs to be established. To assess fully the relationship between an individual's anger and aggressive behaviour, it is necessary to focus on environmental, cognitive, physiological and behavioural factors (Black & Novaco 1993, Levey & Howells 1990).

Self-report questionnaires

The experience and expression of anger can be measured by questionnaires such as the STAXI (Spielberger 1988) and the Novaco Anger Scale (NAS, Novaco 1994). Currently, the STAXI has available a wide range of normative data, while the NAS provides normative data only for mentally disordered populations. Alongside standardised self-report questionnaires, the current level of anger is often assessed by the use of self-monitoring and direct behavioural observation.

Self-monitoring

Self-monitoring devices vary across several dimensions:

1. *structure* (whether they are highly structured or informal diary entries)
2. *level of analysis* (whether they look in detail at individual components of anger, or embrace a global perspective)
3. *frequency of completion*
4. what type of *reinforcement* a participant receives for their completion (Feindler & Ecton 1986).

Self-monitoring procedures can provide rich and detailed descriptions of the participants' experience and expression of anger. However, as there is no control over how the participant completes the assessment, it is usually better to use self-monitored evidence in conjunction with data gathered from other sources.

Direct behavioural observation

Direct behavioural observation refers to the process whereby specific behaviours are identified, observed and recorded as they occur, by someone other than the participant (Feindler & Ecton 1986). Observational data are extremely useful as they can be collected over a long period of time and can therefore serve as a baseline against which to measure the individual's future performance. However, the behaviours being observed may change if the individual is aware of being observed (Feindler & Ecton 1986).

Other sources

When working with individuals who are in institutions, it is often a statutory requirement to keep a daily log or record of their behaviour (e.g. as required by the Children Act 1989). This type of institutional data is recommended by researchers as a good source of archival data that can contribute to a comprehensive assessment (Feindler & Ecton 1986).

Thus, a multimodal approach to assessment, which includes different sources of information, various assessment methods, and an examination of functioning in different environments, is the key to effective treatment packages (Feindler 1995).

Therapeutic relationship

DiGiuseppe et al (1994) highlight several issues that practitioners have to be aware of when commencing any form of anger management. Primarily, the participant's attitudes towards change have to be established. Practitioners must establish the client's beliefs about anger; participants may view themselves as the aggrieved party (Howells 1989), so that they are totally justified in being angry; or believe that expressing anger is healthy; or that anger expression is an effective way of controlling others (DiGiuseppe et al 1994). Feindler (1995) emphasises the importance of understanding the role of hostile attribution styles and poor problem-solving abilities in maladaptive anger (Novaco & Welsh 1989). However, Feindler (1995) does suggest that this attributional style can be assessed through the use of structured interviews, and emphasises the use of individualised treatment programmes. The participant needs to appreciate that the aim is to control the anger, not to remove it, and the participant has to accept that anger is the treatment target.

Cognitive preparation and assessment

Feindler & Ecton (1986) suggest that the primary goal at this stage is to encourage participants to become experts in recognising their own personal anger patterns. This goal is achieved by presenting a model of anger, such as Novaco's, which demonstrates how the cognitive, physiological, behavioural and surrounding environment all interact to create an experience and expression of anger. Participants should be taught how to apply this conceptual model of anger to their own individual anger experience (information recorded through informal diaries or from structured interviews could be used at this point). Participants should become able to identify the positive and negative outcomes of their reactions to provocations (Feindler & Ecton 1986, McDougall et al 1990). Finally, Feindler & Ecton (1986), like DiGiuseppe et al (1994), emphasise the importance of establishing a therapeutic alliance with participants and their 'significant others' such as a member of their family, or another member of institutional staff.

Management of the environment

On a wider basis, it is essential that not only is the participant prepared during the cognitive and education stage, but also that other staff members are made aware of the anger-management package (Levey & Howells 1990). Schlichter & Horan (1981) found that some staff members in a residential establishment were actively working against an anger-management package. This resistance came in the form of inaccurate behavioural ratings, and in some cases actively encouraging participants to express their anger, thereby directly opposing other staff members who were working from an anger-control perspective. If staff are aware of the techniques and theories of the anger-management package, then there is an increased chance of generalising the skills the participants have acquired to naturally occurring, anger-provoking situations (Levey & Howells 1990).

Skill acquisition and rehearsal

The goal of this phase is to help participants acquire cognitive–behavioural techniques that they can use to cope more effectively with anger-provoking situations (Feindler & Ecton 1986). Feindler (1995) states that ideal anger-management packages should initially focus upon teaching participants to recognise physiological arousal (such as increased heart beat and sweating), and how accurately to label and manage their arousal in provoking situations. It is at this stage that techniques from relaxation training, such as deep breathing, should be introduced. Deffenbacher et al (1988) found anecdotal evidence that participants in anger-management groups with a relaxation component were less resistant in initial sessions and were more accepting when cognitive components of therapy were introduced, when compared to participants in an anger-management group that did not have a relaxation component. However, when working specifically with young offenders, McDougall et al (1990) recommended that the relaxation aspect of the course should be used towards the end of the sessional work, as the young offenders may not take the exercises seriously during the first stages of group work.

The next stage is to teach participants the techniques of self-instructional training. Self-instructional training has been used effectively to generate alternative verbal commands to control impulsive behaviour and guide appropriate social behaviour (Feindler 1995). This technique provides participants with the means to restructure their angry thoughts into something more positive, using, for example, *thought-stopping techniques* (Feindler & Ecton 1986).

When using thought-stopping techniques, the participant is encouraged to think of something negative, and is then taught how to break the thought pattern, using a 'stopping statement'.

Initially, the trainer should interrupt the participant's thought pattern. This goal is achieved by getting the participant to imagine a negative situation, and then shouting 'Stop'. For instance, the participant could be asked to think about being prevented from taking part in a pre-arranged trip, because of staffing shortages. As the participant ruminates on this scenario, the trainer should stop, to break the participant's thought pattern. Eventually the participant should be able to complete this process of monitoring and interrupting thought-patterns without help. McDougall et al (1990) suggest that this process can be facilitated by breaking down the participant's self-reported, angry incidents into what happened before, during and after the angry episode. This breakdown of each incident allows the participant to generate a range of positive self-statements at each stage that can replace earlier negative statements (McDougall et al 1990).

Finally, the behavioural skills training component of the package should include five components that address areas of co-operation, assertion, responsibility, empathy, and self-control. The participant is also taught non-verbal social skills such as eye contact, as well as verbal skills such as appropriate loudness of tone (Feindler 1995). These social skills are usually taught through the use of instructions, modelling, role-playing and performance feedback. Role-plays provide a safe environment in which the participant can model new behaviours and practice these new skills, without running the risk of retribution if the behaviour is not managed appropriately (Hughes 1996).

The final stage of the programme is the application of the newly acquired skills.

Skill application

The goal of this final stage is slowly to expose the participant to graduated, stressful anger-provoking situations to allow the participant to practise the newly acquired anger-management skills (Feindler & Ecton 1986). Achievement of this goal can be facilitated by discussing the participant's previous experiences and expressions of anger. McDougall et al (1990) found that for young people with a limited attention span, video-taped role-plays were a good way of maintaining attention, with the participants both commenting on and contributing to the video-taped role-plays. The part of provokers and provoked in the role-plays may be alternatively played by the participant and the practitioner.

Finally, the impact of these packages needs to be evaluated.

Evaluation

Evaluation of anger-management packages can be carried out by repeating the assessments originally completed during the initial assessment. This repetition can be carried out immediately after the anger-management package has been completed, and then again after longer intervals. Deffenbacher et al (1990) assessed the effectiveness of a cognitive, relaxation and behavioural coping skills package for reducing general anger: they found this type of combined programme was generally effective in impacting upon general anger. However, they noted that the inclusion of *all* these components would necessitate the extension of both the number of sessions and time of each sessional period. It is important to focus briefly upon the potential session structures that can be employed by practitioners.

Sessional structure

Sessions in anger management can either be run concurrently, requiring that the group all move at the same pace (Clark 1992), or can be run independently (Stermac 1986). Traditionally, anger-

control packages work on a 12-sessional basis, but the number and length of sessions can be altered to suit the needs of individual participants (Box 15.1).

Black & Novaco (1993), working with a man with learning difficulties, recommended that the

---

Box 15.1 A 12-session timetable for anger management

Cognitive preparation

Session 1 — Aims and objectives of the course
Conceptual model of anger to be used
Focus on the participant's personal experience of anger

Session 2 — Re-presentation of the model of understanding anger
Illustration of how the participant can use the model

Session 3 — Using the model of anger
Participant should describe and deconstruct a personal experience of anger, using the model of anger

Session 4 — Revision of work covered in Sessions 1, 2 and 3

Skills acquisition

Session 5 — Cognitive techniques
Self-instructional training

Session 6 — Behavioural skills training
Co-operation
Assertion
Responsibility
Empathy
Self-control
Extensive use of role-plays

Session 7 — Continual practice of skills learnt in Sessions 5 and 6

Session 8 — Continual practice of skills learnt in Sessions 5, 6 and 7

Skills application

Session 9 — Learning to use the taught skills in a variety of imagined and then real situations

Session 10 — Learning to use the taught skills in a variety of imagined and then real situations

Session 11 — Learning to use the taught skills in a variety of imagined and then real situations

Review

Session 12 — Re-appraisal of the aims and objectives of the course, and feedback from both the trainer and the participant standard 12 1-hour sessions were changed to 28 sessions and lasted for only 40 minutes. However, a 6-session format could also be used, whereby 4 sessions are devoted to stage one of the intervention, and the remaining sessions deal with stages two and three (Valliant et al 1995).

Returning to the issue of evaluation, Stermac (1986) emphasises the importance of collecting both psychometric and observational data at fol-low-up. This is especially important in the long-term evaluation of anger-management pro-grammes with offenders as it is often assumed that participation in an anger-management pro-gramme will have some impact on the likelihood of future criminal behaviour. Hughes (1996) found that recidivism of violent crime had fallen to 40% up to 4 years after offenders had partici-pated in an anger-management programme.

Case study 15.1 Carl

The final section of this chapter provides an illustrative case study of a successful anger-management package which was used with a young man who assaulted care staff within a secure institutional setting.

When Carl was initially admitted to the institution, his day-to-day behaviour was observed by the staff who worked closely with him. Over the assessment period, it became apparent through direct observation that Carl was experiencing and expressing anger towards members of staff, culminating in physical attacks and assaults.

Carl's suitability for an anger-management course was assessed by a wide range of methods, as well as the direct observation of his behaviour on the living unit. Carl completed a semi-structured interview (see Swaffer & Hollin 1997), his daily institutional records were analysed, and he completed two psychometric assessments – NAS (Novaco 1994) and *State-Trait Anger Expression Inventory*, STAXI (Spielberger 1988).

Carl's anger directed towards staff was divided into three separate categories: (1) anger-precipitated verbal assault; (2) anger-precipitated physical threats; (3) anger-precipitated physical assault. Whenever Carl displayed any of the above behaviours (which had been clearly defined, following Hartman (1984)), a full account would be noted within his daily record book. For example, staff were trained to record the antecedents to the event and the details of what occurred during the event. Staff reported that the operational definitions of each of the behaviours

were easy to use, and all instances of Carl's anger-precipitated behaviours were recorded. These 'incident logs' were then coded by a researcher into instances of verbal assault if intentional infliction of psychological discomfort had been Carl's aim. Instances of physical threat were recorded if Carl verbally stated his intent physically to harm the source of his provocation, while brandishing a weapon at the same time (a weapon was defined as anything from Carl shaking his fist to picking up a chair and threatening to throw it). Finally, Carl was deemed to have physically assaulted someone if he had intentionally inflicted physical harm on another person through the use of strong physical force. This wide range of assessment measures was used as reliance on self-report measures alone does not provide the detailed information that effective treatment planning requires (DiGiuseppe et al 1994).

Information obtained from the assessment period

First, the information gathered from Carl's detailed assessment was refined into meaningful data that would help to structure an individualised anger-management package. When asked to consider what anger meant to him, Carl primarily reported the physiological arousal that he associated with anger, such as an increased heart rate. The importance of physiological arousal to Carl's experience of anger was confirmed in his responses on the NAS, where he rated items within the arousal domain as being the most problematic. This assessment indicated that intervention required a focus upon the physiological arousal that Carl associated with anger, and ways in which such arousal could be reduced (see Table 15.1).

Table 15.1 Carl's self-reported scores on the NAS pre- and post-intervention

Sub-scale	Pre-intervention	Post-intervention
Cognitive domain	27	22
Attentional focus	8	7
Rumination	7	5
Hostile attitude	4	4
Suspicion	8	6
Arousal domain	30	18
Intensity	10	4
Duration	6	4
Tension	7	4
Irritability	7	6
Behavioural domain	29	19
Impulsive reaction	9	4
Verbal aggression	6	5
Physical confrontation	7	6
Indirect expression	7	4
Part B	65	38
Disrespectful treatment	13	6
Unfairness	17	10
Frustration	12	7
Annoying traits	13	6
Irritations	10	9

Carl reported that when he felt angry he would ruminate about the source of his provocation. Again these statements were supported by Carl's responses to items on the NAS. This part of the assessment indicated that the intervention should encompass a cognitive change to deflect his thoughts away from the source of his provocation.

Carl reported expressing his anger outwardly in a number of ways. This self-report was supported by his responses on the anger-out and anger expression scale of the STAXI, as well as through his scores on the behavioural domain of the NAS, and through direct observation of his behaviour. This section of the assessment indicated that the intervention should include a skills acquisition component that focused upon Carl's management and subsequent control over the expression of his

anger, diverting the anger away from aggressive and violent acts.

Finally, Carl stated that he became angry, aggressive and violent in order to show his power over another person. Therefore, the anger-control course would require a component which taught Carl socially acceptable ways in which he could assert himself, to achieve 'respect' from staff.

Design of the anger-management package

As noted in the previous section of this chapter, Novaco's intervention strategy involves three stages: (1) cognitive preparation; (2) skills acquisition and rehearsal; (3) an application phase. Each of the sessions ran for a period of 40 minutes to 1 hour, and was held away from the daily living units in an empty classroom to prevent interruption from staff or other young people. Initially, the sessions were conducted with two trainers; however, the last six sessions were conducted with only one trainer, as the other trainer left the institution. The sessions ran for a period of 6 months.

Cognitive preparation and assessment

The most important aspect of this phase is to enable clients to become expert at recognising their own anger patterns (Feindler & Ecton 1986).

Session 1

The aims of this session were (a) to make Carl aware that his anger should be managed, not stopped; (b) to present him with a conceptual model of anger; (c) to start Carl thinking particularly about physiological and behavioural components of anger (as he had reported an association between these two components in his own experience and expression of anger).

It was explained to Carl that the purpose of the sessions was not to prevent him from being angry, rather to help him to manage his anger. Carl was presented with a simplified version of Novaco's model of anger, and the principles of the model were explained to him. As Carl had reported the importance of physiological arousal in his own experience of anger, the trainer began a discussion concerning types of physiological arousal associated with anger. Carl was asked to think of all the different types of physiological responses a person might have while angry, such as muscle tightening and sweating.

During the second part of the session, Carl was asked to think of different ways people react when they are angry. To finish the session, Carl was asked to classify all of the behaviours he had thought of into verbal and non-verbal actions.

At this stage, Carl was asked to complete the homework task of keeping a diary of incidents of anger. The goal of this task was for Carl to generate episodes of anger that could be used as role-plays or discussion topics in the following sessions. However, it soon became apparent that Carl was not prepared to complete the diary as instances of Carl becoming angry had been observed on the unit, which Carl would acknowledge verbally but which he would not commit to paper. Therefore, examples of Carl's anger were mainly gathered from the continual direct observation of his behaviour.

Session 2
The aims of this session were (a) to familiarise Carl with three components of anger – cognition, physiological arousal, and behaviour; (b) to encourage Carl to use this model to deconstruct his own experience and expression of anger, so that he would eventually be aware of the different techniques he could use to control his anger more effectively.

```
┌─────────────────────────────┐
│                             │
│   Physical Sensations       │
│                             │
│                             │
│   HEART POUNDING            │
│                             │
└─────────────────────────────┘
```

Figure 15.2   A 'Physical Sensations' card.

At the beginning of the second session, Carl was again shown and talked through Novaco's model of anger. Carl was then presented with three sets of cards, grouped under the titles of 'Physical Sensations', 'Thoughts' and 'Acts'. Each group contained individual cards all of which had a different statement written on them which referred back to the broad group heading. For instance, 'Acts' cards had actions on them such as shouting, hitting, and throwing things, whereas 'Physical

Sensations' cards had words such as tense, heart pounding, and dry mouth written on them (Fig. 15.2).

The trainers and Carl discussed two incidents when Carl had become angry. Carl was presented with each incident in turn and asked to select cards from each pile to describe what he felt during each event.

Session 3
The aim of this session was to consolidate the information that had already been presented to Carl. To facilitate this process, he was encouraged to describe and deconstruct his own experience of anger, without assistance from the trainers. However, Carl was also encouraged to consider how the surrounding environment might impact upon his experience and expression of anger. This was achieved by asking Carl how his behaviour or thoughts might have differed if the angry incident had occurred outside secure conditions.

Finally, Carl was presented with a range of scenarios in which he was asked to state why he thought the people had become angry, and to identify the different components of their anger. This procedure aimed to reinforce the techniques of breaking down anger into the components that Carl had previously learnt.

Session 4
The aim of this session was to reinforce the learning from the previous three sessions and to focus in more detail upon how the surrounding environment might impact upon Carl's experience and expression of anger. As Carl appeared to be competent in identifying the cognitive, physiological and behavioural aspects of his anger, as well as the possible impact of the surrounding environment, it seemed appropriate that the sessional work should move onto the second stage of the intervention, skills acquisition and rehearsal.

Skills acquisition and rehearsal
The goal of this second stage is to help participants master the cognitive–behavioural techniques that they can use to cope effectively with anger-provoking situations (Feindler & Ecton 1986). Feindler (1995) recommends that the first skill to be acquired and rehearsed is that of

recognising physiological arousal and how to label and manage the arousal in provoking situations.

The accepted method of achieving this goal is to utilise techniques from relaxation training. Carl began a separate relaxation course at the same time as he started the anger-management programme. The relaxation training occurred three times a week, over a period of 2 months. Initially, Carl was instructed in basic relaxation techniques such as controlling his muscular movements and deep breathing. When he had mastered the basic skills of relaxation, he moved to the skills acquisition component of the anger-management programme. Carl began using self-instructional training in his relaxation sessions, whereby the identifiable physiological reactions that he associated with anger were paired using self-statements with relaxation techniques such as deep breathing.

Session 5
The aim of this session was to encourage Carl to consider how his cognitions could lead to angry arousal. Using the technique of pairing, that he had already mastered during relaxation training, it was anticipated that Carl would be able to pair his hostile attributions with calming statements. Therefore, the aim of the self-instructional training sessions was to focus upon the generation of alternative verbal commands to control his impulsive behaviour and guide appropriate social behaviour (Feindler 1995).

Following the recommendations of McDougall et al (1990), self-instructional training was facilitated by breaking Carl's self-reported angry incidents into stages of antecedents, behaviours and consequences. When focusing upon the antecedents to angry incidents, Carl was presented with a list of common cognitive distortions that can lead to angry thoughts and actions. Carl was then encouraged to consider the thoughts that he would have when angry, and was encouraged to try pairing these thoughts with statements such as 'Take a deep breath', and 'Ignore this'.

Session 6
Assessment had identified that Carl had a tendency to ruminate when he became angry. This implied that he would benefit from the ability to

restructure his angry thoughts using thought-stopping techniques (Feindler & Ecton 1986). The aim of this session was therefore to equip Carl with the basic skills to utilise thought stopping. The session was designed to build upon the work initiated in Session 5. During Session 6, Carl was asked to role-play a situation in which he had become angry. Carl was initially asked to state what was 'on his mind' at the points of antecedent, behaviour and consequence of the incident. The aim was to create an awareness that he may have misinterpreted the intention of the person who made him angry. Carl was encouraged to role-play the same situation again, talking through what he was thinking about. When Carl stated a negative belief about the situation, the trainer said 'Stop', and encouraged Carl to employ his relaxation skills, and use a thought-stopping statement such as 'Take a deep breath', or 'Chill out'.

Carl practised this technique for another two personal angry incidents; on the first occasion, he spoke the thought stoppers out loud, and on the second occasion, he began to internalise these statements.

Absence
Unfortunately, shortly after this session, Carl absconded from the institution and did not return for a period of 6 weeks. During this time, there was no contact between Carl and the institution. After a resettling period of 2 weeks, Carl returned to the anger-management course.

Session 7
Because of Carl's absence, this session served as a review of the content of the previous six sessions. Carl appeared to recall the basic content of all of the sessions, as well as the techniques he had been taught.

Sessions 8, 9 and 10
The final part of the skills acquisition stage is the behavioural skills training component of the programme. This should include the five components that address areas of co-operation, assertion, responsibility, empathy and self-control (Feindler 1995).

The overall aim of these three sessions was to equip Carl with a range of behavioural skills to help him manage his anger. The sessions are reported here in a block as the range of behavioural skills was taught concurrently, being explored, explained and practised for each episode of anger that was discussed. For instance, to encourage empathy, Carl was asked to recall an angry incident and then to participate in a role-play, where he played himself and the trainer played the person who was the source of provocation. Carl was then asked to repeat the exercise with the trainer playing Carl and Carl playing the other person. The point of this exercise was to encourage Carl to consider the other person's perception of the event and to take responsibility for angry incidents that he had instigated.

During these role-plays, Carl was also encouraged to modify some of his non-verbal skills. To achieve this, Carl was presented with a series of cards which had expressions such as direct eye contact, threatening posture, and 'angry' face/'happy' face written on them. Carl was asked to 'act' out each of the postures, and received feedback from the trainer. When Carl participated in subsequent role-plays, he was prompted to consider how his non-verbal behaviour might be interpreted by other people, and possibly be perceived as aggressive. Finally, for each role-play, an alternative ending was presented to Carl: this alternative ending entailed Carl being assertive rather than aggressive. He was taught how the techniques of broken record, empathic assertion, escalation assertion and fogging (Feindler & Ecton, 1986) could be used to divert and manage his anger.

At every stage of these role-plays, the emphasis and responsibility for the management of his anger were placed with Carl. It was continually repeated that he had to take responsibility for his actions and that although the trainer had helped him develop the necessary skills with which to control his anger, it was Carl's responsibility to use these skills.

It was then judged that Carl was ready to begin the final stage of the programme, actually applying the skills and techniques he had learnt in real situations.

Skills application

The final part of an anger-management programme requires participants to be exposed to graduated, stressful anger-provoking situations so they can practise their newly acquired anger-management skills.

Session 11
The aim of this session was gradually to introduce Carl to applying his skills. To begin with, it was appropriate for Carl to explain how and why he would use his skills using situations that were not directly and personally related. Therefore, Carl was asked to watch a video that contained 20 sequences of people becoming angry. For each sequence, Carl was asked to pinpoint the different components of anger being displayed, and the techniques that 'actors' could have used to manage their anger.

The second stage of this session was to engage Carl in a role-play of an imaginary provoking incident. Carl was encouraged to practise his newly acquired skills, and to explain why he had selected to use each specific technique to manage his anger.

Session 12
The aim of this final session was to build upon the work started in Session 11, as well as to bring the sessions to a close. Again, several role-play scenarios were carried out between the trainer and Carl, using both imaginal and his own personal experiences and expressions of anger. At all stages, Carl was encouraged to use his newly acquired skills.

The formal anger-management sessions were then drawn to a close. This was achieved by the trainer speaking broadly about what had been covered in the course, and asking Carl for his opinion about the framework of the course, and the usefulness of the skills he had acquired.

Follow-up

As Carl was concurrently completing a life-skills programme as well as the anger management, the application stage of the programme continued to occur in the outside community as Carl's access to mobility trips outside the secure institution was extended. When out in the community with a member of staff if he started to become angry, the member of staff was instructed to prompt Carl to use his anger-management skills. This strategy was continued until the end of the evaluation period. Carl was also re-tested using the STAXI and the NAS after the formal intervention stage had finished.

Results

Institutional data

Carl was officially separated from the other residents within the institution on three occasions during the course of intervention, and on one occasion after intervention had ceased. During intervention, on two occasions (following anger) he verbally assaulted and made physical threats towards members of staff, and on the other occasion he physically assaulted a member of staff after becoming angry. After the intervention, Carl was separated on one occasion for physically threatening a member of staff after a request had been denied.

Self-report questionnaires

Carl was assessed both pre-and post-intervention using the STAXI and the NAS.

Carl's responses on each of the STAXI sub-scales improved after intervention (except for state anger when the minimum score was achieved in both instances). People with high scores on the anger control scale are seen as investing a great deal of energy in monitoring and preventing the experience and expression of anger and would

therefore be less likely to express anger. Before intervention, Carl had been recording significantly higher responses for the scales of trait anger, angry temperament, anger-out and anger expression.

Although appropriate normative data are not supplied by Novaco (1994), visual inspection of Carl's scores reveals that he has reduced his scores on all of the sub-scales of the NAS except for hostile attitude in which he achieved the same low score both pre- and post-intervention.

Direct observation

Carl's anger-precipitated behaviour directed towards staff was observed both before, during and after intervention. The actual instances of each type of behaviour, verbal assault, physical threat, or physical assault, are displayed in Figs. 15.3, 15.4 and 15.5.

As Fig. 15.3 illustrates, Carl did not stop verbally assaulting staff; however, this behaviour had decreased to two incidents per month after the intervention period.

As Fig. 15.4 shows, Carl has reduced the frequency of his physical threatening behaviour directed towards staff over the intervention period.

As Fig. 15.5 illustrates, Carl has not assaulted a member of staff since the end of the intervention.

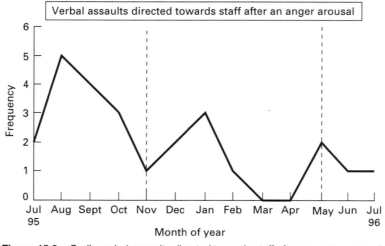

Figure 15.3 Carl's verbal assaults directed towards staff after an anger arousal.

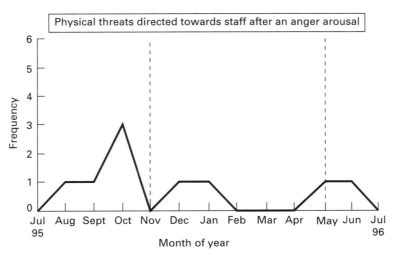

Figure 15.4   Carl's physical threats directed towards staff after an anger arousal.

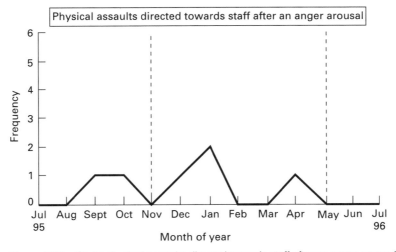

Figure 15.5   Carl's physical assaults directed towards staff after an anger arousal.

Summary

In summary, the young man who participated in this work has provided rich and detailed information about his own experience and expression of anger. Carl showed a dramatic decrease in both his expression of anger and his experience of anger, when comparing his pre- and post-intervention performance. Official records of Carl's expression of anger show that he reduced both the frequency and seriousness of his anger-precipitated acts of aggression and violence.

When all the assessment data were collated, it became apparent that Carl had a particular problems with physiological arousal and anger. After tailoring the anger-management course to address this issue, there was success as Carl reported a marked decrease in his scores on physiological aspects of anger. Similarly, Carl's tendency to ruminate while angry was identified during assessment as problematic and the training was again specifically tailored to address this issue. Its success in reducing rumination is reflected in Carl's responses on the NAS.

Finally, Carl had a problem with his frequent expressions of anger. Again, by taking detailed assessment information into account, Carl's anger-management course was specifically tailored to address these issues. His responses on both the STAXI and the NAS reflect a reduction in his inappropriate expression of anger-precipitated violent behaviour.

Therefore, the results from this section suggest that the person-specific tailored approach to anger management (Nugent 1991) has been successful in targeting and reducing the problematic aspects of Carl's anger.

Direct observation

The first point to highlight is that baselines can be problematic when the trend in the data is in the same direction as the expected treatment effect, as this makes it difficult to distinguish treatment effects from spontaneous change (Long & Hollin 1995). The frequency of the targeted behaviour of verbal assaults to staff reduced before the intervention had occurred, and therefore these findings will be discussed first.

When considering the targeted behaviour of Carl's verbal assaults directed towards staff, it becomes apparent that the frequency of such assaults has decreased across the intervention period. It is interesting to note that the greatest decline in verbal assaults occurred between January and March, which corresponds with the period of time when Carl was learning new skills to manage and express his anger. Visual inspection of the data regarding physical threats made towards staff shows that during intervention Carl's behaviour stabilised at a low rate and actually decreased to zero before he absconded. However, after Carl returned from absconding, his behaviour again increased in frequency, although it did not exceed the previously high level seen during the baseline period. When these data are seen alongside the psychometric measures and institutional data, it can be concluded that overall a positive treatment effect has occurred. As a general summary, it would seem prudent to conclude that the anger-management programme was mainly successful in changing Carl's problematic experience and expression of anger.

CONCLUDING REMARKS

This chapter has outlined a conceptual framework for understanding anger; it has shown how anger can impact upon an individual's health and cause violent behaviour; and the chapter has provided an example of how dysfunctional anger can be corrected. Anger is a very complex emotion, comprising cognitive, physiological and behavioural components that are all affected by the environment. To prevent the expression of dysfunctional anger, an anger-management package must address all three of these components, and acknowledge the impact of the surrounding environment.

Exercise

What makes you angry?
Many people, perhaps particularly those who tend towards an anger problem, are often unaware of the triggers for their anger. One way to assess triggers for anger is to keep an anger diary, or 'hassle log' as Americans might say. Simply record over a few days what happened when you felt angry: where were you? who else was there? what was said by whom? With a detailed picture, it is often possible to see patterns associated with feeling of anger: this might include particular places, or certain types of social situations, or occasions when you might feel badly done to, or when some personal slight has been made against you, or if someone has behaved in a way that you find objectionable. Keeping an anger diary is interesting personally, is often helpful for clients with anger problems, and can be illuminating for health care professionals.

KEY TEXTS FOR FURTHER READING

Feindler E L, Ecton R B 1986 Adolescent anger control: Cognitive–behavioural techniques. Pergamon Press, Elmsford, NY. *This book provides theoretical and practical advice for the running of anger-management packages with adolescents. It contains approaches that are designed for both individual participants and groups.*

Howells K, Hollin C R (eds) 1989 Clinical approaches to violence. Wiley, Chichester. *This edited book contains a selection of chapters that address the impact of anger and violence in a range of institutional settings.*

Novaco R W 1993 Clinicians ought to view anger contextually. Behaviour Change 10:208–218 *This article explains the surrounding context that may be important in causing an arousal of anger.*

Novaco R W 1994 Anger as a risk factor for violence among the mentally disordered. In: Monahan J, Steadman H (eds) Violence and mental disorder. University of Chicago Press, Chicago p. 21–59. *This book chapter describes the conceptual framework behind the design of the Novaco Anger Scale, as well as providing initial reliability and validity data.*

Kassinove H (ed) 1995 Anger disorders: Definition, diagnosis, and treatment. Taylor & Francis, Washington DC. *This edited book provides an overview of the different approaches to conceptualising and managing anger.*

REFERENCES

American Psychiatric Association 1994 Diagnostic and statistical manual of mental disorders, 4th edn. American Psychiatric Association, Washington DC.

Averill J R 1982 Anger and aggression: An essay on emotion. Springer-Verlag, New York

Barefoot J C, Dahlstrom W G, Williams R B 1983 Hostility, CHD incidence, and total mortality: A 25-year follow-up study of 255 physicians. Psychosomatic Medicine 45:59–63

Baumeister R F, Smart L, Boden J M 1996 Relation of threatened egotism to violence and aggression: The dark side of high self-esteem. Psychological Review 103:5–33

Berkowitz L 1986 Some varieties of human aggression: criminal violence as coercion, rule following, impression management, and impulsive behaviour. In: Campbell A, Gibbs J J (eds) Violent transactions: The limits of personality. Blackwell, Oxford, p 87–103

Black L, Novaco R W 1993 Treatment of anger with a developmentally handicapped man. In: Wells R A, Giannetti V J (eds) Casebook of brief psychotherapies. Plenum, New York, p 143–158

Blackburn R 1993 The psychology of criminal conduct: Theory, research and practice. Wiley, Chichester

Browne K D 1989 Family violence: spouse and elder. In: Howells K, Hollin C R (eds) Clinical approaches to violence. Wiley, Chichester, p 119–154

Browne K, Howells K 1996 Violent offenders. In: Hollin C R (ed) Working with offenders. Wiley, Chichester, p 188–210

Burish T G, Bradley L A (eds) 1983 Coping with chronic disease. Academic Press, New York

Burns J W, Freidman R, Katkin E S 1992 Anger expression, hostility, anxiety and patterns of cardiac reactivity to stress. Behavioral Medicine 18:71–78

Campbell M, Gonzalez M M, Silva R R 1992 The pharmacologic treatment of conduct disorders and rage outbursts. Psychiatric Clinics of North America 15:69–85

Clark D A 1992 Development of anger management module for sex offenders. Paper presented at the 2nd Annual Conference of the DCLP, International Conference Centre, Harrogate, March

Clay D L, Anderson W P, Dixon W A 1993 Relationship between anger expression and stress in predicting depression. Journal of Counseling and Development 72:91–94

Comunian A L 1994 Anger, curiosity, and optimism. Psychological Reports 75:1523–1528

Davidson G C, Neale J M 1986 Abnormal psychology: An experimental clinical approach. Wiley, New York

Deffenbacher J L, Story D A, Brandon A D, Hogg J A, Hazaleus S L 1988 Cognitive and cognitive-relaxation treatments of anger. Cognitive Therapy and Research 12:167–184

Deffenbacher J L, McNamara K, Stark R S, Sabadell P M 1990 A comparison of cognitive–behavioral and process-orientated group counseling for general anger reduction. Journal of Counseling and Development 69:167–172

Dembroski T M, MacDougall J M, Williams R B, Haney T L, Blumenthal J A 1985 Components of Type A, hostility, and anger-in: relationship to angiographic findings. Psychosomatic Medicine 247:210–233

Deschner J P 1984 The hitting habit: Anger control for battering couples. The Free Press, New York

DiGiuseppe R, Tafrate R, Eckhardt C 1994 Critical issues in the treatment of anger. Cognitive and Behavioral Practice 1:111–132

Dobash R E, Dobash R 1979 Violence against wives. The Free Press, New York

Dodge K A, Garber J 1991 Domains of emotion regulation. In: Garber J, Dodge K A (eds) The development of emotion regulation and dysregulation. Cambridge University Press, New York, p 3–11

Dodge K A, Newman J P 1981 Biased decision making processes in aggressive boys. Journal of Abnormal Psychology 90:375–379

Edmondson C B, Conger J C 1996 A review of treatment efficacy for individuals with anger problems: conceptual, assessment, and methodological issues. Clinical Psychology Review 16:251–275

Engebretson T D, Matthews K A, Scheer M F 1989 Relations between anger expression and cardiovascular reactivity: reconciling inconsistent findings through a matching hypothesis. Journal of Personality and Social Psychology, 57:513–521

Ewart C, Kolodner K B 1994 Negative affect, gender, and expressive style predict elevated ambulatory blood pressure in adolescents. Journal of Personality and Social Psychology 66:596–605

REFERENCES (*contd*)

Fahmy V, Jones R S P 1990 Theories of the etiology of self-injurious behaviour – a review. Irish Journal of Psychology 11:261–276

Feindler E L 1995 Ideal treatment package of children and adolescents with anger disorders. In: Kassinove H (ed) Anger disorders: Definition, diagnosis and treatment. Taylor and Francis, Washington, DC, p 173–196

Feindler E L, Ecton R B 1986 Adolescent anger control: Cognitive–behavioral techniques. Pergamon Press, Elmsford, NY

Friedman M, Rosenman R H 1959 Association of specific overt behaviour pattern with blood and cardiovascular findings. Journal of the American Medical Association 169:1286

Frude N 1991 Understanding family problems: A psychological approach. Wiley, Chichester

Gentry M R, Ostapiuk E B 1989 Violence in institutions for young adolescents. In: Howells K, Hollin C R (eds) Clinical approaches to violence. Wiley, Chichester, p 250–266

Green A M 1967 Self-mutilation in schizophrenic children. Archives of General Psychiatry 17:234–244

Greengrass E R, Julkunen J 1989 Construct validity and sex differences in Cook–Medlay hostility. Personality and Individual Differences 10:209–218

Haller R M, Deluty R H 1988 Assaults on staff by psychiatric in-patients: a critical review. British Journal of Psychiatry 152:174–179

Hartman D P 1984 Assessment strategies. In: Barlow D H, Hersen M (eds) Single case experimental designs: Strategies for studying behavior change, 2nd edn. Pergamon, Elmsford, NY, p 107–139

Hollin C R, Howells K 1989 An introduction to concepts, models and techniques. In: Howells K, Hollin C R (eds) Clinical approaches to violence. Wiley, Chichester p 3–24

Howells K 1989 Anger-management methods in relation to the prevention of violent behaviour. In: Archer J, Browne K (eds) Human aggression: Naturalistic approaches. Routledge, London, p 153–181

Hughes G V 1996 Short and long term outcomes for a cognitive–behavioral anger management package. In: Davies G, Lloyd-Bostock S, McMurran M, Wilson C (eds) Psychology, law, and criminal justice: International developments in research and practice. Walter de Gruyter, New York, p. 487–494

Julkunen J, Salonen R, Kaplan G A, Chesney M A, Salonen J T 1994 Hostility and the progression of carotid atherosclerosis. Psychosomatic Medicine 56:519–525

Kernis M H, Grannemann B D, Barclay L C 1989 Stability and level of self-esteem as predictors of anger arousal and hostility. Journal of Personality and Social Psychology 56:1013–1022

Kugle C L, Clements R O, Powell P M 1983 Level and stability of self-esteem in relation to academic behaviour of second graders. Journal of Personality and Social Psychology 44:201–207

LeCroy C W 1988 Anger management or anger expression: which is most effective? Residential Treatment for Children and Youth 5:29–39

Lester D 1988 Relationship between locus of control and depression mediated by anger toward others. Journal of Psychology 129:413–414

Levey S, Howells K 1990 Anger and its management. Journal of Forensic Psychiatry 1:305–327

Long C G, Hollin C R 1995 Single case design: a critique of methodology and analysis of recent trends. Clinical Psychology and Psychotherapy 2:177–191

McDougall C, Boddis S 1991 Discrimination between anger and aggression: implications for treatment. In: McMurran M, McDougall C (eds) Proceedings of the First DCLP Annual Conference: Issues in criminological and legal psychology. The British Psychological Society, Leicester, p 101–106

McDougall C, Boddis S, Dawson K, Hayes R 1990 Developments in anger control training. In: McMurran M (ed) Applying psychology to imprisonment: young offenders. Issues in Criminological and Legal Psychology 15: The British Psychological Society, Leicester, p 39–44

Maiuro R D, Cahn T S, Vitaliano P P, Wagner B C, Zegree J B 1988 Anger, hostility and depression in domestically violent versus generally assaultive men and non-violent control subjects. Journal of Consulting and Clinical Psychology 56:17–23

Novaco R W 1975 Anger control: The development and evaluation of an experimental treatment. D. C. Health, Lexington, MA

Novaco R W 1977 A stress inoculation approach to anger management in the training of law enforcement officers. American Journal of Community Psychology 5:327–346

Novaco R W 1993 Clinicians ought to view anger contextually. Behaviour Change 10:208–218

Novaco R W 1994 Anger as a risk factor for violence among the mentally disordered. In: Monahan J, Steadman H (eds) Violence and mental disorder. University of Chicago Press, Chicago, p 21–59

Novaco R W, Welsh W N 1989 Anger disturbances: cognitive mediation and clinical prescriptions. In: Howells K, Hollin C R (eds) Clinical approaches to violence. Wiley, Chichester, p 39–60

Nugent W R 1991 An experimental and qualitative analysis of a cognitive behavioral intervention for anger. Social Work Research and Abstract 27:3–8

Reilly P M, Clark H W, Shopshire M, Lewis E W, Sorensen D J 1994 Anger management and temper control: critical components of post-traumatic stress disorder and substance abuse treatment. Journal of Psychoactive Drugs 20:401–407

Riley W T, Treiber F A, Woods M G 1989 Anger and hostility in depression. Journal of Nervous and Mental Disease 177:668–674

Rosenman R H, Brand R J, Jenkins C D, Friedman M, Sraus R, Wurm M 1975 Coronary heart disease in the Western Collaborative Group Study: final follow up experience of $8^{1}/_{2}$ years. Journal of American Medical Association 233:872–877

Schlichter K J, Horan J J 1981 Effects of stress inoculation on the anger and aggression management skills of instutionalised juvenile delinquents. Cognitive Therapy and Research 5:359–365

Sharkin B S 1993 Anger and gender: theory, research and implications. Journal of Counseling and Development 71:386–389

REFERENCES (*contd*)

Siegman A W 1993 Cardiovascular consequences of expressing, experiencing, and repressing anger. Journal of Behavioral Medicine 16:539–569

Spielberger C D 1988 Manual for the State-Trait Anger Expression Inventory (STAXI). Psychological Assessment Resources, Odessa, FL

Spielberger C D, Johnson E H, Russell S F, Crane R S, Jacobs G A, Worden T J 1985 The experience and expression of anger: construction and validation of an anger expression scale. In: Chesney M A, Rosenman R H (eds) Anger and hostility in cardiovascular and behavioural disorders. Hemisphere/McGraw-Hill, New York, pp 5–30

Stermac L 1986 Anger control treatment for forensic patients. Journal of Interpersonal Violence 1:446–457

Swaffer T, Hollin C R 1997 Adolescents' experience and expression of anger within a residential setting. Journal of Adolescence 20:567–575

Tavris C 1989 Anger: The misunderstood emotion, 2nd edn. Simon & Schuster, New York

Valliant P M, Jensen B, Raven-Brook L 1995 Brief cognitive behavioural therapy with male adolescent offenders in open custody or on probation: an evaluation of management of anger. Psychological Reports 76:1056–1058

Whittington R, Wykes T 1996 Aversive stimulation by staff and violence by psychiatric patients. British Journal of Clinical Psychology 35:11–20

Wickless C, Kirsch I 1988 Cognitive correlates of anger, anxiety and sadness. Cognitive Therapy and Research 12:367–377

CHAPTER CONTENTS

Key points 291

Introduction 292

**Theoretical models of post-traumatic stress
    disorder 293**
    Behavioural model 293
    Cognitive and informational processing models
    294
    Biological models 295
    Psychodynamic models 296
    Psychosocial models 296

Assessment 297

Measurement 298

Treatment 298
    Psycho-analytical therapy 298
    Cognitive–behaviour therapy 299
    Exposure therapy 299
    Anxiety management 301
    Cognitive therapy 301
    Eye movement desensitisation and reprocessing
    302
    Pharmacology 303
    Summary 303

Process of treatment 304
    Therapeutic relationship 304
    Imaginal exposure 304
    The rationale 304
    Principles of imaginal exposure 305
    Live exposure 306
    Cognitive therapy 306
    Difficulties in treatment 307

Supervision 309

Conclusion 309

Exercise 309

Key texts for further reading 309

References 309

16

Post-traumatic disorders

Karina Lovell   Sheena Liness

KEY POINTS

- Post-traumatic stress disorder is characterised by three clusters of symptoms: (1) re-experiencing; (2) avoidance and numbing; and (3) increased arousal.

- Post-traumatic stress disorder affects between 1 and 9% of the general population and up to 50% of those exposed to a traumatic event.

- A comprehensive structured assessment using validated measures is an essential prerequisite of an effective treatment plan.

- Research studies have demonstrated the efficacy of behavioural and cognitive treatments.

- Difficulties which may arise in treatment include engagement, severe depression, numbing and detachment, guilt and disability.

- Effective, structured and regular supervision is required by therapists engaged in treating clients with the disorder.

INTRODUCTION

Following a severe trauma such as rape, physical assault, major disasters or witnessing such an event, a person can be expected to have some immediate psychological effects. These effects include feelings of vulnerability, hopelessness, numbness, despair and being overwhelmed. Such symptoms can be seen as a normal response to an abnormal event and for many people these symptoms will be severe and distressing but will subside within a month or so (Rothbaum et al 1992). Although some people will continue to have some mild symptoms they will not generally lead to impaired social or occupational functioning. However, for others, exposure to a severe stressor results in a persistence of a wide range of symptoms which is termed post-traumatic stress disorder (PTSD).

Historically, there have been many accounts of psychological disturbance following a traumatic event. Trimble (1981) provides a detailed description of psychological difficulties following traumatic incidents since the 17th century. Pepys writing in his diaries describes the emotional turmoil he felt following the Great Fire of London (Daly 1983). The history of the recognition of psychological disturbance after trauma is well documented in the literature (Kinzie & Goetz 1996). Historically, psychological disturbance from trauma has been described under numerous terms such as traumatophobia (Rado 1942), battle fatigue, war neurosis (Grinker & Spiegal 1943), shell shock (Myers 1940) and rape trauma syndrome (Burgess & Holstrom 1974).

However, despite many accounts of a picture close to PTSD as it is known today, it was not until 1980 that a diagnostic category finally emerged in the *Diagnostic Statistical Manual on Mental Diseases* (DSM) (American Psychiatric Association 1980). In the most recent classification DSM-IV (American Psychiatric Association 1994), PTSD is described as an extreme stressor where (a) a person experienced, witnessed, or was confronted with an event or events that involved actual or threatened death or serious injury, or a threat to the physical integrity of self or others and (b) the person's response involved intense fear, helplessness, or horror.

Three clusters of symptoms are found with PTSD: re-experiencing, avoidance and numbing, and increased arousal. Re-experiencing symptoms include flashbacks, intrusive thoughts and images, nightmares and physiological re-activity to reminders of the trauma. The second cluster of symptoms includes avoidance and numbing features and consists of avoidance of thoughts and feelings about the trauma, avoidance of activities of reminders of the trauma, psychogenic amnesia, diminished interest, detachment, restricted affect and a sense of foreshortened future. The third cluster comprises symptoms of increased arousal, including sleep disturbance, irritability or outbursts of anger, poor concentration, exaggerated startle response and hypervigilance. As well as these symptoms, there are several associated features not included in the diagnostic category but which often occur such as guilt, anger, disillusionment with authority, homicidiality, sadness and depression.

It is important to note that these reactions are normal responses to an abnormal event, but it is the persistence of such symptoms which results in PTSD.

The prevalence of PTSD has been studied across community samples and specific 'at risk' groups. Community studies have found the prevalence of PTSD to be between 1 and 9% (Davidson et al 1991, Kessler et al 1995). In specific 'at risk' groups, the most studied events have been rape and combat. In a prospective study of rape survivors (Rothbaum et al 1992), 94% of the sample had PTSD in the week following the rape, 64% at 1 month and 47% at 3 months following the assault. In a large study of Vietnam veterans (n = 1599), a PTSD lifetime prevalence of 30% was found (Kulka et al 1990). Gender differences have been investigated and one study reported that the traumas most commonly associated with women were sexual molestation, and among men, combat and witnessing a traumatic event (Kessler et al 1995). It is difficult to determine the exact prevalence of PTSD, because of the wide ranging different assessment tools and criteria used to define levels of PTSD in various studies. However, it is estimated that about 25% of those who are exposed to criterion (a) stressor develop PTSD (Green 1994).

There is a high level of comorbidity with PTSD. The most common co-existing diagnosis is major depression. Community studies show a remarkably consistent pattern of between 40 and 60% of individuals with PTSD having major depression (Kessler et al 1995). Other mental health disorders that commonly occur with PTSD are generalised anxiety disorder (GAD), personality disorders, obsessive–compulsive disorder and substance misuse (Green 1994). The rate of substance misuse tends to vary with different populations, being particularly high in war veterans (Keane & Wolfe 1990) and less so in other traumas such as major disasters (Green 1994).

Why is it that some people develop PTSD and others do not? Much research has gone into answering this question but as yet there are few clear answers. One of the strongest predictors of PTSD is the 'dose response' or severity of the trauma (Foy et al 1984, Green 1994) and strong evidence has been found that social support buffers PTSD (Jones & Barlow 1992). However, other variables such as personality type, previous psychiatric disorder and prior life events have been looked at, and have been supported in some studies but not in others; thus the evidence for these factors remains inconclusive.

THEORETICAL MODELS OF POST-TRAUMATIC STRESS DISORDER

Several theoretical models have been proposed to account for the acquisition and maintenance of PTSD.

Behavioural model

Behavioural conceptualisations of PTSD have used Mowrer's (1947, 1960) two-factor theory of learning fear and avoidance to account for the acquisition and maintenance of PTSD (Keane et al 1985). Thus, this theoretical model emphasises both classical and instrumental conditioning. Classical conditioning involves stimulus–stimulus learning, where a previously neutral stimulus is paired with an aversive stimulus (unconditioned stimulus – UCS). The UCS elicits an unconditional response (UCR), that is fear and anxiety, and after repeated pairings the neutral stimulus becomes the conditioned stimulus (CS) which elicits the now conditioned response (CR) in the absence of the UCS. The second element in two-factor learning is instrumental conditioning which suggests that an organism behaves in whatever way is necessary to avoid and escape from the CS and the UCS. Thus, avoidance and escape are learned behaviours which are reinforced and maintained by their reduction of arousal.

Keane et al (1985), using the above model, suggest that exposure to a traumatic event such as combat (UCS) elicits increased physiological arousal and psychological distress (UCR). Previously neutral external stimuli (sounds, smells and other environmental stimuli) and internal stimuli (thoughts) that were present at the time of the trauma become conditioned stimuli (CS) which produce high levels of physiological arousal and psychological distress. Further, such cues that were present at the time of the trauma elicit similar responses to those evoked by the trauma and in an effort to avoid fear and anxiety, the person escapes and avoids them. Thus avoidance behaviour is negatively reinforced, by anxiety reduction.

The behavioural model has been heavily criticised. Mowrer's two-factor learning theory model fails to account for all aspects of the maintenance of fear (Mineka 1979). The behavioural model is said to fail to explain the aetiology and maintenance of PTSD, and ignores symptoms such as nightmares, flashbacks, increased startle response and hypervigilance (Foa et al 1989). Further, this model only accounts for pathological, and not 'normal' responses.

Cognitive and informational processing models

Several cognitive (Creamer et al 1992, Janoff-Bulman 1992, Krietler & Krietler 1988) and informational processing models (Chemtob et al 1988, Foa et al 1989) have been developed to account for PTSD.

Cognitive processing models

Cognitive processing models of post-trauma reactions propose that people enter situations with pre-existing mental schema. These schema contain information about people's past experiences and their beliefs, assumptions, and expectations in regard to future events (Creamer et al 1992).

Janoff-Bulman (1992) argues that three core assumptions are shared by most people and are said to be particularly affected after a traumatic event:

1. the world as benevolent
2. the world as meaningful
3. the self as worthy.

She argues that most people see the world as good, safe, meaningful and comprehensive. Drawing on Lerner's (1980) 'just world hypothesis' (i.e. that people get what they deserve) she contends that people perceive that they have control over negative events and states:

> A meaningful world is one in which a self-outcome contingency is perceived; there is a relationship between a person and what happens to him or her.
>
> (Janoff-Bulman 1992:8)

The third assumption that the self is worthy is related to the view that people evaluate themselves in a positive light; that is good, worthy, benevolent and moral beings. From these assumptions comes a sense of invulnerability, and while people are aware that negative events can and do occur, they underestimate the likelihood of these events happening to themselves.

Janoff-Bulman argues that following an intensely traumatic event these assumptions become shattered and account for the psychological disequilibrium that follows. She states:

> survivors experience 'cornered horror', for internal and external worlds are suddenly unfamiliar and threatening. Their basic trust in their world is ruptured. Rather than feel safe, they feel intensely vulnerable.
>
> Janoff-Bulman 1992; 63

Survivors need to re-evaluate and rebuild these shattered assumptions and the individual needs to come to terms with the idea that the world is sometimes a bad place and that people are not entirely invulnerable. However, this view needs to be balanced; the victim needs to re-establish a view of the world which is benevolent and meaningful, and redevelop a positive self-image, including perceptions of worth, strength and autonomy.

Although Janoff-Bulman's theory has an immediate attractiveness in terms of its surface common sense and the ease with which clinicians can communicate the rationale to clients, it has an inherent weakness. Principally, it fails to account for PTSD symptoms. Shattered beliefs could equally well result in depression or other anxiety disorders.

Informational processing models

Foa et al (1989) have proposed the most influential informational processing model. Basically they argue that PTSD is acquired and maintained as a result of a failure to emotionally process a traumatic event. Based on Lang's (1979) work Foa & Kozak (1986) argue that fear structures are contained in memory as a network of 'propositional representations' and contain three types of information:

1. information about the feared stimulus situation
2. information about the verbal, physiological and behavioural responses
3. interpretative information about the meaning the stimuli has for sufferers and their responses.

They argue that this fear structure is seen as a programme for escaping and avoiding danger.

The fear structure is said to differ from other informational structures by its stimulus, response and especially its meaning elements. Further, PTSD is differentiated from other anxiety disorders because (1) the trauma is of monumental significance and violates previously held views of safety; (2) the intensity of the response elements; (3) the size of the fear structure; and (4) the fear structure is easily accessible.

To achieve or enhance satisfactory emotional processing and hence change the fear structure and resultant fear reduction requires two conditions: (1) fear-relevant information has to be accessed and (2) corrective information which is incompatible with that in that fear structure needs to be provided.

Although recent work has looked at aspects of informational processing (Joseph et al 1996, Thrasher et al 1993), further empirical work is necessary to substantiate information processing mechanisms (Litz & Keane 1989).

Biological models

Biological models have been conceptualised to account for PTSD, and comprehensive reviews are detailed by Davidson (1992), Charney et al (1993) and Pitman (1993). Distinct biological changes are associated with PTSD. Abnormalities found in individuals with PTSD are concerned with sympathetic arousal, hypothalmic–pituitary–adrenocortical function and physiology of sleep, of dreaming and of endogenous opioids (Friedman 1991). One model proposed is that of Van der Kolk (1987), who bases his model on learned helplessness theory. He argues that animal research has found that when animals are exposed to inescapable shock, there is a depletion of brain norepinephrine and dopamine.

Extending this model to humans, he argues that a similar depletion occurs in the development of PTSD. Further, he suggests that this depletion becomes a conditioned response, leading to greater norepinephrine receptor hypersensitivity. Adding to Van der Kolk's model, Krystal et al (1989) suggested that inescapable shock produces massive noradrenergic activation, which may lead to a learned traumatic response, thereby eliciting fear behaviours similar to some symptoms of PTSD. Kolb (1988) proposes a conditioned response model, where excessive and prolonged intense stimulation from trauma results in cortical neuronal and synaptic changes in chronic PTSD. He argues that this leads to an inability to discriminate between threatening and non-threatening stimuli, impaired concentration, repetitive dreams, hyperactivity and aggression.

Others such as Friedman (1991) have suggested that repeated exposure to traumas can result in biological changes within limbic structures which leave the victim open to the development of PTSD. Such sensitisation has been called *kindling*. Related to this is the view that exposure to one or more traumas may sensitise the person to other stressors of lower intensity (Antelman 1988).

Biological models do not explain the entire constellation of PTSD symptoms, or why only some people develop PTSD and not others, nor do they account for other variables such as social support that mediate the development of PTSD (Jones & Barlow 1990).

Psychodynamic models

The main psychodynamic model for PTSD is Horowitz's (1986) 'stress response syndrome' defined as 'all personal reactions when a sudden, serious life event triggers internal responses with characteristic symptomatic patterns' (Horowitz & Kaltreider 1980:163).

Horowitz's model (1986), although psychodynamic in orientation, emphasises information processing and cognitive theories. He argues that people have several schema or cognitive maps of the self and world as established by experience. Such schema allow the individual to process information unconsciously and automatically. In the event of a trauma, there is a mismatch of information received during the event and existing schema. For example, the death of a loved one is at odds with that individual's world.

This mismatch of information leads the person to become overwhelmed, and cognitive processes thereafter try to incorporate this 'contrary' information into previously stable schema experience. Horowitz argues that two opposing internal

processes 'intrusion' and 'denial' are at work to try to assimilate such information.

Thus the trauma survivor oscillates between these two opposing internal processes: thinking about the trauma (*intrusion*) and avoiding thinking about the trauma (*denial*). Denial is seen as a defence against intrusion. It manifests as emotional numbness, avoidance of thoughts and of activities, and stimuli that resemble the trauma. In contrast, intrusion manifests as re-experiencing phenomena. These processes of intrusion and denial progress to a stage where the individual integrates this new and revised information (known as 'working through') into their cognitive schema. Horowitz posits that when old and new information are matched and revised this is termed the 'completion tendency'. He states:

> Inner models or schemata are now relatively congruent with the new information about the self and the world, and with the actual external situation to the extent that it is represented accurately in that new information.
>
> Horowitz 1986:96

Horowitz argues that the above is a predictable and normal stress response syndrome after a serious life event, and that psychopathology occurs if this process is 'blocked' or 'prolonged' or becomes intolerably intense (Horowitz & Kaltreider 1980). Horowitz's model fails to account for delayed PTSD, and is said to ignore the behavioural and social effects of trauma (Kleber & Brom 1992).

Psychosocial models

Psychosocial models incorporate many of the above perspectives and try to account for why only some individuals develop PTSD. Green et al (1985) suggest that PTSD develops and is maintained by the interaction of the traumatic event, individual characteristics and the social/cultural environment. Jones & Barlow (1990, 1992) propose a biopsychosocial model, and suggest that PTSD shares a number of features with other anxiety disorders, particularly panic disorder, and develops from a complex interaction between biological and psychological vulnerability, the development of anxiety, the occurrence of stressful life events and alarms, and the adequacy of coping strategies and social support.

In sum, diverse theoretical perspectives for PTSD have helped us to understand some of the processes that may account for the acquisition and maintenance of PTSD. Further research is necessary to account for all symptoms of PTSD, the maintenance of the disorder and why it occurs in some people and not others.

ASSESSMENT

A clear, comprehensive and structured assessment is a prerequisite for the development of an effective treatment plan. In essence, an effective assessment includes gaining an accurate view of the presenting complaints, understanding the impact these complaints have on the individual's life, an overview of the individual's life history, developing a therapeutic alliance, assessing mental state and developing a collaborative treatment plan. Good assessment skills require advanced interviewing and interpersonal skills. It is not the aim of this chapter to describe a full cognitive–behavioural assessment (Hawton et al 1989), although specific factors pertaining to assessing an individual with PTSD are detailed.

Although it is necessary to obtain a detailed account of the traumatic event, the initial interview should focus on the symptoms and the impact such symptoms are having on the individual's life. The assessor needs to identify the frequency, intensity, and when, where and with whom these symptoms occur. As well as PTSD symptoms, the assessor needs to determine any other associated features that may be present.

When assessing the traumatic event, it is important to assess the facts of the event and the client's thoughts, feelings and events at the time of the trauma. It is also important to ask clients what the trauma meant for them. This question often elicits thoughts of guilt, self-blame and anger which may not have been accessed on questioning of specific symptoms. This question often highlights changes in pre-existing and current beliefs and assumptions about themselves, the world or the future. For example, a rape survivor, raped by an acquaintance might express that she believes that the rape meant she was a bad person. This may relate to her pre-existing belief and current belief that women cannot be raped by someone they know.

As important as the traumatic event is the aftermath of the trauma, which can be as traumatic as the event itself. For example, eliciting views from clients on how they were treated by the emergency services, employers, court and family may highlight to the assessor that these issues need to be addressed as part of the treatment plan. Other factors that may affect treatment such as compensation and litigation issues also need to be included. Such issues often lead to much anger and bitterness by clients because of the length and time taken for many cases to go through the legal process.

As mentioned above, other disorders often coexist with PTSD and thus it is necessary to determine any other comorbid diagnosis. Clearly, where severe depression and suicidal ideas or intent are present, these need to be managed and treated prior to treatment of the PTSD.

Further, as with any assessment, details of past psychiatric treatment, past and current medical history, family and personal history, the use of prescribed medication and illicit drugs, alcohol and a full mental state examination are essential for a comprehensive assessment.

MEASUREMENT

A prerequisite of any assessment is the use of a range of valid and reliable clinical process and outcome measures. Clinical measurement not only provides the clinician with valuable information regarding the clinical interventions but also allows the clinician information which might lead to changes in the treatment plan; it also provides clients with valuable feedback. Specific measures that are used in assessing PTSD are the Impact of Events Scale (IES, Horowitz et al 1979), the Post-traumatic stress disorder Symptom Scale (PSS, Foa et al 1993) and the Clinician Administered PTSD Scale (CAPS, Blake et al 1990). Another useful measure given the frequent co-existence of depression is the Beck Depression Inventory (BDI, Beck et al 1974). A measure often used by cognitive–behaviour therapy (CBT) clinicians is a problem and targets rating (Marks 1986). This is where clients are asked to describe their problem in a sentence and to rate on a 0 to 8 scale how much it upsets them or interferes with their life (0 denoting not at all to 8 continuously). Clients are also asked to identify four goals which they would wish to achieve at the end of treatment and again rate them on a 0 to 8 scale (0 denoting complete success to 8 no success). In addition, it is important to use a measure that assesses impairment of work and social functioning; a user-friendly measure that can be assessor or client rated is the Work and Social Adjustment Scale (Marks 1986).

TREATMENT

Despite the increasing volume of research being carried out on PTSD, there is still a lot to learn about the most suitable treatment for the multitudinal symptoms which result from trauma. Since its inception as a psychiatric disorder in 1980, a variety of treatments have been implemented with varying degrees of success. These include psycho-analytical therapy (Brom et al 1989, Lindy et al 1983), CBT (Foa et al 1991, Resick & Schnicke 1992), eye movement desensitisation and reprocessing (Shapiro 1989a, Vaughn et al 1994) and pharmacology (Frank et al 1988, Van der Kolk et al 1994).

Psycho-analytical therapy

There have been many case reports but few controlled trials evaluating the effectiveness of psychodynamic therapy with PTSD. The most used and developed theory is that of Horowitz (1986) who developed a brief psychodynamic therapy for stress response syndromes. Using this model, Brom et al (1989) carried out a large scale study of 112 people suffering serious disorders following traumatic events and compared trauma desensitisation, hypnotherapy and brief psychodynamic therapy. All three treatments reduced trauma-related symptoms. However, only 23 patients had experienced a traumatic event while the rest had bereavement as their main problem and treatment methods used were not fully explained. Lindy et al (1983) have shown psychoanalytical treatment to have some effect in treating PTSD. 30 survivors of a club fire entered 6 to 12 sessions of short-term psychodynamic psychotherapy 6 months to 1 year after the fire. Treatment completers showed considerable improvement on measures at 3-month follow-up. However, initial diagnosis varied from PTSD, anxiety, complicated bereavement to major depression alone and limited measures were used. The Horowitz model was used in group psychotherapy (Roth et al 1988) for 13 women survivors of sexual assault which involved weekly, $2\frac{1}{2}$-hour group sessions over 1 year facilitated by two therapists. Participants also had concurrent individual psychotherapy. While there was no improvement in PTSD symptoms by week 8, there was improvement by week 20. Despite the lack of controlled trials, there is therefore some evidence to suggest that focused psychodynamic therapy may be of benefit to PTSD sufferers.

Cognitive–behaviour therapy

Although there is as yet no definitive treatment of choice, undoubtedly the most extensive and effective work to date has been carried out in the field of CBT with a number of randomised controlled trials proving its efficacy. These have focused particularly on the techniques of exposure, anxiety management and cognitive restructuring, alone and in combination.

Exposure therapy

Exposure therapy has its foundations in learning theory, classical conditioning and instrumental learning in particular (see models of treatment pp 293–297) and is now widely recognised as the treatment of choice for a variety of anxiety disorders such as specific phobias, agoraphobia and obsessive–compulsive disorder (Marks 1987). Exposure involves the gradual and repeated confrontation of a feared stimulus, memory or situation without escape or avoidance in order to facilitate habituation, that is the gradual reduction of a response such as anxiety. The two principal methods of exposure are imaginal and live. More recently, Foa & Kozak (1986) have posited an emotional processing theory to explain fear reduction in exposure. Exposure therefore not only reduces anxiety to feared stimuli and memories, it also accesses and changes the meaning of the event so that it can be incorporated and resolved.

Efficacy of exposure

Exposure therapy has been used to treat PTSD, though it has been given a variety of different descriptions including flooding (Cooper & Clum 1989, Keane & Kaloupek 1982), implosive therapy (Keane et al 1989), direct therapeutic exposure (Boudewyns & Hyer 1990), and prolonged exposure (Foa et al 1991).

Cooper & Clum (1989) compared their standard treatment for veterans which involved individual and group sessions to standard treatment plus flooding. Overall, imaginal flooding led to increased improvement in nightmares and anxiety but seemed to have had little effect on depression. Keane et al (1989) randomised 24 veterans to 14 sessions of implosive therapy or waiting list control. Treatment involved an introduction and conclusion of relaxation with flooding to traumatic memories in between. Treatment reduced anxiety, startle response, depression and re-experiencing but did not improve numbing or avoidance symptoms.

Boudewyns & Hyer (1990) randomly assigned in-patient Vietnam veterans to direct therapeutic exposure or a control of one-to-one counselling. However, both groups also had standard in-patient treatment specifically designed for PTSD which included an element of exposure and it is not clear what the control counselling included or excluded. The exposure group had less anxiety post-treatment compared to standard treatment alone and by 3-month follow-up had improved significantly on some measures. However, specific PTSD symptoms were not measured which leaves the results unclear. Foa et al (1991) randomly assigned 45 women survivors of assault to 1 hour of prolonged exposure (PE) imaginal and live and stress inoculation training (SIT), involving education, coping skills, cognitive restructuring, self-dialogue, modelling and role-play, supportive counselling or waiting list control. PE and SIT improved on all PTSD symptoms. PE further improved in follow-up. Supportive counselling and waiting list control improved on arousal but not avoidance or re-experiencing. A second study (Foa & Meadows 1997) compared PE, SIT, combination SIT and PE, and waiting list control with all three active treatments, significantly improving PTSD symptoms.

Richards et al (1994) treated 14 patients with mixed trauma to four sessions of imaginal exposure followed by four sessions of live exposure or vice versa. Both groups significantly improved with a very high symptom improvement of 65 to 80% which continued to 1-year follow-up. However, there were no control or blind evaluations. Thompson et al (1995) gave 23 patients eight weekly sessions of imaginal and live exposure. Although all improved on a variety of measures, treatment also included elements of debriefing and cognitive interventions.

It also has to be pointed out that most studies to date have been carried out in the USA on combat and sexual assault victims although later studies are emerging in a mixed trauma population. Lovell et al (1996) attempted to separate the key components of CBT by using pure behavioural (exposure) and cognitive techniques (cognitive restructuring) with a view to assessing if particular interventions targeted specific symptoms as hypothesised in the literature (Hacker-Hughes & Thompson 1994, Solomon et al 1992). In a controlled trial, 87 patients with PTSD according to DSM-III(R) criteria of at least 6 months duration were randomly assigned to 10 sessions of either prolonged exposure (imaginal and live) alone, cognitive restructuring alone, a combination of prolonged exposure and cognitive restructuring or a control group of relaxation. They used blind assessors and standardised measures and 77 patients completed treatment. Results showed that exposure and cognitive restructuring individually or combined significantly improved PTSD symptoms when compared to the control relaxation, and that improvement covered the wide range of PTSD

symptoms, irrespective of the treatment delivered. Another interesting angle on the treatment of PTSD is the issue of self-help programmes, and although very much in its infancy Frueh (1995) reported a Vietnam veteran using self-exposure with good results.

Foy et al (1996) questioned why so few trauma therapists use exposure as a treatment technique given its extensive validation in the literature. They also concluded that the findings of Shipley & Boudewyns (1980) that exposure might drive patients into crisis because of intolerable levels of stress were unfounded. They found that in a survey on patients' reasons for terminating treatment, exposure was mentioned by only 8%. They suggest some refusal to use exposure may be due to inexperience and fear of distress and that training in this technique may be necessary. While complications have been reported (Pitman et al 1991), these have mainly been reported in chronic, combat-related PTSD which is commonly recognised as complex PTSD and generally difficult to treat. Of course, as with all forms of treatment, exposure does not work for everyone. Jaycox & Foa (1996) identified three obstacles that can interfere with the successful implementation of exposure: intense anger, emotional numbing and overwhelming anxiety, and in such cases, exposure may need to be modified, or other techniques implemented concurrently.

There is, however, enough evidence in the literature to date supporting exposure as an effective treatment for PTSD. One key question arising is whether exposure targets and improves symptoms such as avoidance and re-experiencing while cognitive therapy may better target other common symptoms of guilt, shame and anger (Soloman et al 1992). While Foa et al (1989) propose that exposure leads to fear reduction and thereby alters perceptions of danger, Resick & Schnicke (1992) argue that other emotional reactions such as conflicts, misattributions or expectations may also need to be addressed. However, this argument has not so far been borne out in the literature with two major studies (Foa et al 1991, Lovell et al 1996) finding no significant difference between exposure and SIT, or exposure and cognitive restructuring, and no difference in specific symptoms improved by the different treatments. There was also no significant difference in outcome with combined techniques. Jaycox & Foa (1996) suggest that exposure is easier to implement compared to SIT or cognitive interventions and should therefore be favoured as the treatment of choice, and that future research should focus on identifying which client group benefits from exposure alone and which requires other techniques.

Anxiety management

A second type of behavioural intervention commonly used to treat PTSD is anxiety management, usually based on the stress inoculation training of Meichenbaum (1975). While exposure aims to activate fear and promote habituation or anxiety reduction, anxiety management aims to provide coping skills to manage anxiety. This involves education in a variety of coping strategies to deal with anxiety, such as relaxation, controlled breathing, problem-solving and cognitive restructuring. Kilpatrick & Veronen (1983) developed an anxiety-management package for rape survivors using relaxation, role-play, thought stopping and self-guided dialogue with positive effect. In a controlled study, Foa et al (1991) found anxiety management to be as effective as prolonged exposure although it was less effective in follow-up; they concluded by hypothesising that clients were less likely to carry on strategies taught outside formal treatment. All studies so far have therefore been limited to women survivors of sexual assault. A generally reported difficulty with anxiety management, however, is

that it is difficult to administer and carry out because of the variety of strategies used and that it is also unclear what the effective components of the treatment really are.

Cognitive therapy

Many studies have found cognitive therapy to be effective with depression (Dobson 1989) and panic (Clark et al 1994), which are comorbid diagnoses of PTSD, and a limited number of studies have found cognitive therapy to be effective with PTSD (Forman 1980, Thrasher et al 1996). Most cognitive therapy has used a Beckian-style, cognitive restructuring, involving education on the relationship between thoughts, feelings and behaviour, and identification and challenging of negative or unhelpful thoughts. The effect of cognitive restructuring in Forman's (1980) case study of a rape victim is however confounded by the use of thought stopping. In Foa, et al's (1991) controlled trial mentioned earlier, cognitive restructuring was included as a component of SIT but differential effects of the variety of techniques incorporated in SIT need evaluation.

Cognitive processing therapy (CPT) was used by Resick & Schnicke (1992) to treat victims of sexual assault. Based on the information-processing theory of PTSD, it includes education, exposure and cognitive components. Although the term 'cognitive' is in the title, it also incorporates a variety of techniques. 19 sexual assault victims received 12 weekly group sessions of CPT and were compared to a waiting list group. CPT subjects improved significantly with treatment which was maintained at 6-month follow-up. CPT also emphasises the five main areas of beliefs disrupted by trauma, which are intimacy, trust, power, safety and esteem, and it targets these in treatment. Resick & Schnicke also hypothesised that people who deny the possibility they might experience a traumatic event are more likely to develop PTSD if it does happen.

Thrasher et al (1996) found cognitive restructuring alone with PTSD to be effective in two case studies but the most sophisticated trial to date using a pure Beckian cognitive restructuring model with PTSD in a mixed trauma population (Lovell et al 1996) showed cognitive restructuring to be as effective as exposure. Patients in the cognitive restructuring group were taught to identify negative automatic thoughts and elicit rational alternative thoughts by using Socratic questioning and probabilistic reasoning. The aim was to change their view of their role in the trauma and distorted beliefs in the world post-trauma. Exposure instructions were excluded. Added to the recent controlled trials, there have been excellent accounts of different cognitive techniques and their appliance to PTSD sufferers. Carroll & Foy (1992) applied cognitive techniques to combat-related PTSD and Kubany (1994) gives an account of combat-related guilt and provides a comprehensive conceptual base and treatment outline for trauma-related guilt which includes guilt associated with perceived wrong doing, responsibility and hindsight bias.

Eye movement desensitisation and reprocessing

Eye movement desensitisation and reprocessing (EMDR) has been at the centre of controversy since its appearance as a technique in 1989 for treating PTSD (Acierno et al 1994; Herbert & Mueser 1992). Criticisms include the fact that it has no clearly accepted theoretical base, that the initial claims by therapists of single session success were exaggerated and because of the monopoly on the training and dissemination of the technique by the Shapiro Foundation, and, more importantly because of the serious methodological flaws in the initial research carried out.

Shapiro (1989b) describes EMDR as an accelerated form of information processing which uses the same mechanisms now acknowledged in rapid eye movement sleep. It therefore acts on a physiological level and links neural networks. In EMDR, the patient is asked to focus on a disturbing image or memory from the traumatic event along with the accompanying thoughts and feelings, while carrying out saccadic eye movements created by tracking the therapist's finger from side to side. The belief in the thought is rated using a validity of cognition (VOC) scale, and a subjective units of discomfort (SUDS) level then rates the distress of feeling. The goal of the session is then to reduce the distress associated with the image or memory and to replace a negative thought with a positive one, increasing the validity of the positive thought.

One of the main difficulties with the literature to date is that despite an abundance of studies, the majority have major methodological flaws in that they lack clear diagnoses and fail to use or report on standardised objective measures for outcome, relying on the self-rated VOC and SUDS ratings to measure improvement (Marquis 1991, Shapiro 1989a, Wolpe & Abrams 1991). More sophisticated studies have recently been completed. Wilson et al (1995) randomised 80 subjects to either EMDR or a waiting list control. EMDR significantly improved on PTSD measures compared to the waiting list. However, there was no information on diagnoses and no treatment control. Vaughn et al (1994) compared EMDR with image habituation training (exposure to verbal descriptions of trauma) or applied muscle relaxation. They included standardised measures and independent assessment. All three groups improved equally.

Recent studies have also compared EMDR with and without eye movement (Renfrey & Spates 1994, Sanderson & Carpenter 1992) with simple phobics and found no significant difference between the two techniques. Shapiro (1995) has now relegated the importance of the eye movement in the treatment. An extensive study is currently being carried out with combat veterans (Boudewyns & Hyer 1996) with PTSD diagnoses (DSM-III(R)), comparing EMDR with an exposure control (eyes fixed) and a second control of standard treatment using standardised measures. Standard treatment excludes exposure instructions but does include discussion of the traumatic experiences. To date, results have indicated no significant differences between EMDR and the exposure control.

Clearly, EMDR may have a role to play in the treatment of PTSD with evidence emerging that it does improve PTSD symptoms compared to a control and is equal to other more extensively researched treatments. However, conclusive evidence awaits the outcome of randomised controlled trials using recognised standardised measures and comparing it to other evidence-based effective treatments such as exposure. It has been claimed (Boudewyns & Hyer 1996) that EMDR is equal rather than superior to clinically evaluated techniques such as exposure but that it can be carried out using fewer sessions, and that patients and therapists prefer it. The claims need to be tested in a systematic manner. The exposure control used in the EMDR studies are also EMDR with eyes fixed rather than exposure as carried out in other studies.

Pharmacology

Pharmacological treatment has focused mainly on antidepressants with controlled trials (Davidson et al 1990, Frank et al 1988, Van der Kolk et al 1994) comparing antidepressants to a control placebo. Overall, antidepressants improved PTSD symptoms, although improvement was modest. Difficulties with the trials were that no long-term follow-up was carried out when the medication was stopped and sample sizes are small. Overall, medication for PTSD may be useful in reducing distress, depression, increased arousal and irritability and can be used as an adjunct to psychological treatment (Friedman 1988).

Summary

In summary, despite the increasing sophistication of treatment trials for PTSD, we are no closer to finding the definitive treatment of choice. It appears that several psychological treatments are equally effective. Comparison is difficult with many of the major studies focusing on particular trauma populations such as exposure for combat veterans and cognitive therapy or SIT for rape victims. The criticisms of exposure alone that negative emotions such as guilt, shame and depression do not extinguish are not supported in recent trials, while cognitive restructuring equally reduced anxiety and fear (Lovell et al 1996). Similar results were also found with an obsessive–compulsive population (Van Oppen et al 1995) in that there was no significant difference in outcome of treatment between pure exposure and cognitive restructuring.

Marks et al (personal communication) talk of a paradigm shift towards viewing emotions as being linked by a physiological, behavioural and cognitive network so that by focusing on the symptoms from any one angle would gradually alter the connecting network. In our view, this has comparisons to Lang's three systems (verbal, behavioural, physiological) model of fear (1979). As such, any psychological treatment focusing directly on the trauma in a systematic and structured way should be beneficial. It may be that the key part of treating PTSD is focused work on the traumatic event to enable the processing of unresolved emotions and that this can be accessed by various channels, cognitive, behavioural, or focused psychodynamic psychotherapy. Undoubtedly, most research shows CBT to be the most consistently effective treatment for PTSD with treatment outcome improving in this field over the last 5 years (Richards & Lovell 1997). Another remaining question is the key timing of treatment. There have been a number of recent pilot studies (Foa et al 1995) investigating early intervention following assault to assess prevention of PTSD symptoms which have promising outcome. There do, however, remain many questions in treating this multifaceted syndrome.

PROCESS OF TREATMENT

Therapeutic relationship

Establishing and maintaining a therapeutic relationship is a key prerequisite to any form of treatment. Sufferers of PTSD are particularly vulnerable, entering treatment with common fears that they are losing control or going crazy because they have not been able to get over this event in their life. It is therefore paramount with this client group that therapists are particularly attentive to the basic therapist skills in order to provide a therapeutic context to facilitate the processing and understanding of what has happened to their clients in a productive and supportive fashion.

A key component of the therapeutic process is the giving of a clear and valid treatment rationale in order to gain the clients' agreement and co-operation in what might be at times a very difficult, anxiety-provoking treatment. Each stage of treatment needs to be clearly explained and understood, and feedback should be sought from clients regarding their awareness and understanding of the next step. A core symptom of PTSD is poor concentration and memory; therefore, it is also good practice to provide clients with a written or typed handout explaining the key points of the session and particularly the rationale for the type of treatment offered to take away and read in their own time.

Imaginal exposure

Imaginal exposure involves direct exposure to the memories of the traumatic incident until a reduction in fear and distress is experienced by the client (a process called habituation). PTSD sufferers attending for treatment have often avoided or been unable to talk in detail to anyone about what happened. Their memories of the event are often fragmented and confused and involve high levels of anxiety and distress and while this avoidance is understandable as a short-term coping mechanism, in the long run avoidance prevents adequate processing of the event and maintains fear. Imaginal exposure involves going over the trauma in a systematic, focused way so that memories and feelings can be explored to enable distressing emotions to be processed and their impact reduced. It is important to convey to clients that the aim is not that they accept what happened but that they are able to come to terms with the incident. It is also often important to look at what happened in the aftermath of the trauma as sometimes the way people were treated or reacted to worsened the effects of the trauma.

The rationale

The giving of a treatment rationale is probably one of the most important aspects of starting treatment. It is paramount both for ethical and collaborative reasons that clients understand the principles of the treatment they are agreeing to undertake and that informed consent is gained. When outlining the treatment approach, details from the client's own experience should be used as much as possible to encourage client participation and check understanding. It is essential that adequate time is spent explaining the principles of treatment and that feedback is sought for any doubts or uncertainties. This may well prove a key factor in engaging and motivating the client into treatment. Outlined in Box 16.1 is an example of the type of rationale used to explain imaginal exposure in PTSD.

Principles of imaginal exposure

Having explained the treatment rationale, clients now need a clear and comprehensive explanation of their role and how imaginal exposure is facilitated by the therapist. The key principles of imaginal exposure are that it is carried out:

1. in the first person, present tense
2. using as much detailed information as possible
3. using all sense modalities (what they saw, heard, smelt, touched)
4. using audio-tapes of sessions for homework
5. and that imaginal exposure is prolonged (at least 45 to 60 minutes).

We therefore ask them to go over the event as if they are re-living it, using the first person, present tense, all sense modalities, focusing in detail on what happened, their response, and, if possible, what it meant to them. They are encouraged to include as much detail as they can and to try to stay with the feelings this evokes. Each session is audio-taped and clients then take the tape away with them to listen to daily as homework. At each recounting of the event, clients rate their level of distress/anxiety on the following 0 to 8 scale, identifying also the worst parts.

0	2	4	6	8
No distress/ anxiety				Severe distress/ anxiety

As anxiety and distress reduce during the recounting of the incident overall, these worst parts then become the focus of the exposure using a 'rewind and hold' technique (Richards & Rose 1991) when clients are asked to focus on a particular image, thought or feelings, again to enable processing of these particular points. The greatest amount of reduction in distress and anxiety generally occurs between sessions, but sometimes also occurs in-session. As therapists, we are present to facilitate the processing of the trauma which may involve several clinical choice points during the recounting of the event. Generally, while the event is being recounted,

---

Box 16.1   Rationale for imaginal exposure

When you think about the traumatic experience, or are reminded of it, what do you experience [client may express extreme anxiety or distress] and what do you do [client usually tries to avoid or push it away]? The trauma was a very frightening and distressing experience. It causes fear and anxiety now and so pushing it away is an understandable way of coping. You may wish you could just forget about it. What has happened when you have pushed it away or tried to distract yourself? [Client has found this unsuccessful as it continues to intrude in the form of thoughts, images or nightmares.] As you already know, no matter how hard you try to push away thoughts about the trauma, the experience keeps coming back. These symptoms indicate that what happened is unfinished and that the event has somehow remained unprocessed. In this treatment, our goal is to help you by systematically confronting the feared memories connected with the incident until your anxiety and distress reduce.

Initially reliving your memory will be distressing but we will support you through this. By focusing on these memories over a period of time, the fear, anxiety and distress should reduce. [It is often helpful at this point to use an analogy to reinforce the explanation, for example what happens when a person experiences a bereavement (as long as there is no unresolved grief in the presentation).] Have you ever lost someone you loved as a result of death or break-up? How did you react then and what happened? [Immediately after the loss, the client may have felt numb, sad and upset, and may have kept thinking about the loved one when the client did not want to, but over time the thoughts and feelings settled down until the client felt able to carry on. This is what we want to happen with the traumatic experience.]

our input is minimal, particularly if it is producing affect in the client. However, there may be times when we have to prompt, encourage further details or ask clients to focus on a key point. We also have to ensure that the client does not leave the session in a high state of distress by allowing time at the end to explore the session, de-role and debrief and gain clear feedback that homework is clearly understood. We may also need to make ourselves more available to clients for support, particularly for the first few sessions either by telephone, or with the offer of more frequent sessions. Foa & Kosak (1986) found three types of responses during exposure treatment correlate with good improvement: (a) the degree of initial response, that is, activation; (b) habituation within the exposure session; and (c) habituation across sessions.

Box 16.2 Key components of imaginal exposure

The following guidelines are essential in the setting up and carrying out of imaginal exposure:
- a treatment rationale is given with clear feedback of the client's understanding
- an explanation of the procedure and client's role is given
- distress ratings are used
- therapist involvement is fully explained
- continual feedback is gained from the client
- homework setting and closure are essential

Live exposure

As well as being fearful and anxious when remembering the traumatic incident, PTSD sufferers also come to fear and avoid associated reminders and environmental cues. Live exposure involves the confrontation of feared and avoided situations or objects related to the trauma which may now restrict the clients' general level of functioning. In chronic PTSD, avoidances have often become extensive and generalised to non-trauma-related cues and situations. For example,

someone involved in a train disaster may start by avoiding images of trains, which may then progress to being unable to travel on public transport and avoiding crowds. The survivor of an assault may avoid going out alone. Indeed, phobic avoidance versus realistic precautions is a key point in the case of sexual assault victims. While again this avoidance is an understandable reaction and brings short-term relief, in the long run the avoidance maintains the fear and anxiety and often this then begins to spread (generalisation of fear, Keane et al 1985) to other areas until the client's life is severely restricted. With live exposure, the client would gradually face these phobic avoidances in a graded and repeated way until the client has experienced a reduction in anxiety over time ('habituation'). We have to be very clear from the outset that it is the avoidance of realistically safe situations we will be working on. In treatment, clients would be asked to draw up a hierarchy of feared objects or situations and to face them in a graded, systematic way and for a prolonged length of time, starting with the least anxiety-provoking first. Again, they would be asked to continue tasks as homework on a daily basis.

Cognitive therapy

People's perceptions of themselves and the world can drastically change following a traumatic event. For example, victims of an assault may blame themselves for not taking preventative action to have avoided the assault. At the same time, they may now view the world as a violent dangerous place where no-one can be trusted. Although this is an understandable reaction to a severe trauma, such thoughts maintain feelings of anxiety, depression and guilt and affect behaviour. Cognitive therapy is therefore based on the theory that an individual's emotional disturbance is maintained as a result of this type of negative thinking and aims to elicit and modify maladaptive or unhelpful thoughts and beliefs that emerge. Initially, the person is educated about the connection between thinking, feelings and actions and the maintenance of a vicious circle. Using daily thought diaries clients are taught to identify and challenge any unhelpful thoughts which may be maintaining feelings of anxiety, guilt or hopelessness and to focus on interpretations and distorted assumptions about their traumatic experience. A variety of cognitive techniques may be used such as looking for evidence for and against the thought, probabilistic reasoning, identifying thinking errors, testing out beliefs and looking for alternative viewpoints in the sessions. They are then asked to continue the work as homework by keeping daily diaries. The process is therefore structured, collaborative and focused with the therapist using a Socratic style of questioning wherever possible to help patients elicit and analyse their own thoughts. The overall aim is to reduce distress, and enable them to develop a view of themselves and the world which is more balanced but one which takes into account the traumatic experience.

Difficulties in treatment

There are many difficulties that can arise in the treatment of PTSD. In the following we will outline and discuss some of the more common difficulties, some of which are recognised in the literature relating to specific symptoms.

Engagement

Engaging clients in treatment is a particular problem. General attendance for initial assessment can be low. In Foa et al's study of rape victims (1991), approximately half of the women did not attend for initial assessment which they sug-

gest may be due to their reluctance to deal with the rape memory. Another difficulty is high drop-out rates with many studies having a fairly high attrition level (Solomon et al 1992). Epstein (1989) states that non-compliance is an issue in this client group with high drop-out and refusal rates making analysis difficult as it is unclear if those who stay in treatment are representational. It has also been suggested that PTSD sufferers who may have been functioning well prior to trauma are reluctant to seek help from psychiatric services (Schwarz & Kolowalski 1992). It is therefore important to be aware of the client's vulnerability at assessment and to be aware that we are asking them to divulge details that they have tried to forget and so to probe lightly. As discussed earlier, a clear and viable rationale for treatment is also of vital importance. It may be beneficial to pre-empt their reluctance to start treatment, to acknowledge it as a common feeling of PTSD sufferers and to problem solve the advantages and disadvantages of seeking help and engaging in treatment. It may also be helpful to use outside social support where appropriate, and if possible the involvement of patients who have benefited from treatment in the past.

Depression

As discussed on page 293, depression is widely recognised as a comorbid diagnosis of PTSD (Green 1994, Kessler et al 1995). Any assessment must involve a thorough mental state examination, including a risk assessment for suicidal ideation and intent and an agreed management plan with ongoing re-assessment as required. In a community study, Davidson et al (1991) found PTSD sufferers eight times more likely to have attempted suicide. As with any other type of treatment, the safety of the client is paramount and needs the application of a clear treatment plan. In some cases, active treatment may be delayed until severe depression has been effectively treated by medication and the input of other health professionals.

Anger

Anger and irritability are recognised symptoms of PTSD and in many cases are an understandable result of the patient's experiences. A traumatic event may have involved the violation of someone by another person, group of people or a negligent employer. Survivors may have been left with physical injuries or suffered a bereavement. They may also now find themselves involved in lengthy complicated legal and compensation procedures in which they are having to prove their psychological and physical disabilities which does little to aid their recovery. In the majority of cases, anger reduces with appropriate treatment and in the recent trial with a mixed trauma population (Lovell et al 1996), anger did not affect outcome of treatment. There is however some indication (Foa et al 1995) that overwhelming anger is a poor predictor of outcome in treatment and it has been suggested that this level of anger may impede emotional processing during exposure (Jaycox & Foa 1996). Indeed, treatment of intense anger often requires a variety of cognitive–behavioural techniques. The anger may need to be broken down to identify the sources of the different areas of focus, such as anger towards the perpetrator and towards the legal system, and may need to be worked on using different techniques. In these cases, it can be useful to focus on the adverse impact the anger is having on the person's life. Impulsive anger may also require anger management, particularly in cases where the need for revenge or homicidal tendencies are being expressed.

Numbing and detachment

Emotional numbing is another recognised symptom of PTSD which can lead to difficulties in treatment. Jaycox & Foa (1996) suggest that numbing equally affects emotional processing and provides an obstacle to effective exposure therapy. An added difficulty can be differentiating between emotional numbing, avoidance of engaging in treatment and clinical depression which can have similar clinical presentations. In our experience, numbing and detachment often present in more complex cases, where a variety of treatment techniques need to be applied.

Guilt

Guilt is a symptom which is not officially recognised in DSM-IV criteria for PTSD but is generally accepted as a common associated feature. In the recent Lovell (1997) study, 50% of participants experienced feelings of guilt. Survivors may experience guilt over things they did or did not do. They may have guilt from surviving an event where others died, and some might blame themselves, often irrationally, for what happened. In our experience, guilt is most easily addressed using cognitive techniques to help clients to challenge any irrational thinking over the event and their actions. Another effective technique is the guilt cake of Kubany (1994) where clients are asked to apportion blame amongst the various people or factors involved to aid them to see the event and their role in it more objectively.

Disability and loss

By the time clients present for treatment, many have lost their previous employment, relationships and social life and some are left with permanent physical injury, disfigurement and chronic pain. Treatment of such cases needs to address the loss of their previous functioning and to work with coping strategies to help clients adjust to their current level of functioning. There has been some indication of treatment improving post-traumatic chronic pain (Hekmat et al 1994, Muse 1986) although both are case studies and are limited in design and measures used. Some clients may also benefit from referral to a specialist pain clinic.

SUPERVISION

Undoubtedly, working with survivors of trauma is demanding and emotional work. As therapists, we are at risk of vicarious traumatisation in hearing detailed accounts of traumatic events, both in terms of distressing content and becoming more aware of the risks and pitfalls of daily living. It is therefore of the utmost importance to have appropriate and regular supervision to express concerns and deal with any difficult issues. It is also important that we are aware of our own limitations and vulnerabilities and feel able to refer clients to other agencies where appropriate.

CONCLUSION

Overall, the response and recovery of PTSD sufferers are determined by a complexity of personal and environmental factors and any treatment plan has to take into account the variety of difficulties faced in such cases. With the variety of symptoms presented by PTSD, it may mean that the search for any definitive treatment of choice will continue to elude us and that future research should focus more on effective treatment strategies for differing PTSD protocols.

Exercise

Using some of your own clinical material, role-play with a partner the assessment process of a client with PTSD. Discuss which CBT intervention you would use and why. Role-play the delivery of the treatment rationale and discuss the overall treatment plan and difficulties that may arise.

KEY TEXTS FOR FURTHER READING

Saigh P 1992 Post traumatic stress disorder: A behavioural approach to assessment and treatment. Macmillan, New York. *An excellent book that details the history, epidemiology, assessment and behavioural treatment of PTSD.*
Foy D W 1992 Treating PTSD: cognitive behavioural strategies. Guilford Press, New York. *A comprehensive text for the practising therapist, detailing various CBT interventions with different trauma types.*
Green B L 1994 Psychosocial research in traumatic stress disorder: an update. Journal of Traumatic Stress 7:341–362.

A well written and readable article, highlighting much of the research into PTSD and also detailing the methodological problems of such research.
Black D, Newman M, Harris-Hendricks J, Mezey G 1997 Psychological trauma: a developmental approach. Gaskell, London. *An up-to-date text with contributions from many experts in the field, covering human response to stress, the impact of many of the recent disasters, diagnosis and treatment and legal aspects.*

REFERENCES

Acierno R, Hesen M, Van Husselt V B, Tremont G 1994 Review of the validation and dissemination of eye movement desensitisation and reprocessing: a scientific and ethical dilemma. Clinical Psychology Review 14(4):287–299
American Psychiatric Association 1980 Diagnostic and statistical manual of mental disorders, 3rd edn. APA, Washington DC
American Psychiatric Association 1994 Diagnostic and statistical manual of mental disorders, 4th edn. APA, Washington DC
Antelman S M 1988 Time-dependent sensitisation as the cornerstone for a new approach to pharmocotherapy: drugs as foreign/stressful stimuli. Drug Development Research 14:1–30
Beck A T, Rial W Y, Rickels R 1974 Short form of depression inventory: cross validation. Psychological Reports 34:1184–1186

REFERENCES (*contd*)

Blake D D, Weathers F W, Nagy L M et al 1990 A clinician rating scale for assessing current and lifetime PTSD: the CAPS-1. The Behaviour Therapist: 18:187–188

Boudewyns P A, Hyer L 1990 Physiological response to combat memories and preliminary treatment outcome in Vietnam veteran PTSD patients with direct therapeutic exposure. Behaviour Therapy 21:63–87

Boudewyns P A, Hyer L A 1996 Eye movement desensitisation and reprocessing (EMDR) as treatment for post traumatic stress disorder (PTSD). Clinical Psychology and Psychotherapy 3(3):185–195

Brom D, Kleber R J, Defares P B 1989 Brief psychotherapy for posttraumatic stress disorder. Journal of Consulting and Clinical Psychology 57:607–612

Burgess A W, Holstrom L L 1974 Rape trauma syndrome. American Journal of Psychiatry 131:981–986

Carroll E M, Foy D W 1992 Assessment and treatment of combat-related post-traumatic stress disorder in a medical centre setting. In: Foy D W (ed) Treating PTSD: cognitive and behavioural strategies. Guilford Press, New York Press, p 39–68

Charney D S, Deutch A Y, Krystal J H, Southwick S M, Davies M 1993 Psychobiologic mechanisms of posttraumatic stress disorder. Archives of General Psychiatry 50: 294–304

Chemtob L, Roitblat H L, Hamada R S, Carlson J G, Twentyman C T 1988 A cognitive action theory of post-traumatic stress disorder. Journal of Anxiety Disorders 2:253–275

Clark D M, Salkovskis P M, Hackman A, Middelton H, Anastasiades P, Gelder M 1994 A comparison of cognitive therapy, applied relaxation and imipramine in the treatment of panic disorder. British Journal of Psychiatry 164:759–769

Cooper N A, Clum G A 1989 Imaginal flooding as a supplementary treatment for PTSD in combat veterans. A controlled study. Behaviour Therapy 20:381–391

Creamer M, Burgess P, Pattison P 1992 Reaction to trauma: a cognitive processing model. Journal of Abnormal Psychology 101:452–459

Daly R J 1983 Samuel Pepys and post-traumatic stress disorder. British Journal of Psychiatry 143:64–68

Davidson J 1992 Drug therapy for post-traumatic stress disorder. British Journal of Psychiatry 160:309–314

Davidson J R T, Hughes D, Blazer D, George L 1991 Post-traumatic stress disorder in the community: an epidemiological study. Psychological Medicine 21:713–721

Davidson J R T, Kudler H, Smith R et al 1990 Treatment of posttraumatic stress disorder with amitryptiline and placebo. Archives of General Psychiatry 47:259–266

Dobson K 1989 A meta-analysis of the efficacy of cognitive therapy for depression. Journal of Consulting and Clinical Psychology 57:414–419

Epstein R S 1989 Posttraumatic stress disorder: A review of diagnostic issues. Psychiatric Annals 19:556–563

Foa E B, Kozak M J 1986 Emotional processing of fear: exposure to corrective information. Psychological Bulletin 99:20–35

Foa E B, Meadows E A 1997 Psychosocial treatments for post traumatic stress disorder: A critical review. In: Spence J (ed) Annual review of psychology. Annual Review, Palo Alto, CA

Foa E B, Hearst-Ikeda L, Perry K J 1995 The evaluation of a brief cognitive–behavioural programme for the prevention of chronic PTSD in recent assault victims. Journal of Consulting and Clinical Psychology 63(6):948–955

Foa E B, Riggs D S, Dancu C V, Rothbaum B O 1993 Reliability and validity of a brief instrument for assessing post-traumatic stress disorder. Journal of Traumatic Stress 6:459–473

Foa E B, Rothbaum B O, Riggs D S, Murdock T B 1991 Treatment of posttraumatic stress disorder in rape victims. A comparison between cognitive and behavioural procedures and counselling. Journal of Clinical and Consulting Psychology 59:715–723

Foa E B, Steketee G, Rothbaum B O 1989 Behavioural/cognitive conceptualisations of post-traumatic stress disorder. Behaviour Therapy 20:113–120

Forman B D 1980 Cognitive modification of obsessive thinking in a rape victim: a preliminary study. Psychological Reports 47:819–822

Foy D W, Kagan B, McDermott C, Leskin G, Sipprelle R C, Paz G 1996 Practical parameters in the use of flooding for treating chronic PTSD. Clinical Psychology and Psychotherapy 3(3):169–175

Foy D W, Sipprelle R C, Rueger D B, Carroll E M 1984 Etiology of posttraumatic stress disorder in Vietnam veterans: analysis of premilitary, military, and combat exposure influences. Journal of Consulting and Clinical Psychology 52:70–87

Frank J B, Kosten T R, Giller E L, Dan E 1988 A randomised clinical trial of phenelzine and imipramine for post-traumatic stress disorder. American Journal of Psychiatry 145:1289–1291

Friedman M J 1988 Towards rational pharmacotherapy for post-traumatic stress disorder: an interim report. American Journal of Psychiatry 145:281–284.

Friedman M J 1991 Towards rational pharmocotherapy for post traumatic stress disorder. An interim report. American Journal of Psychiatry 145:281–284

Frueh C B 1995 Self administered exposure therapy by a Vietnam veteran with PTSD. Letters to the editor. American Journal of Psychiatry 152:1831–1832

Green B L 1994 Psychosocial research in traumatic stress: an update. Journal of Traumatic Stress 7:341–362

Green B L, Wilson T, Lindy J D 1985 Conceptualising post-traumatic stress disorder: a psychosocial framework. In: Figley C R (ed) Trauma and its wake. Brunner/Mazel, New York: p 53–69

Grinker R R, Spiegal J P 1943 War neurosis in North Africa, the Tunisian Campaign, January to May 1943. Josiah Macy Foundation, New York

Hacker-Hughes J G H, Thompson J 1994 Post-traumatic stress disorder: an evaluation of behavioural and cognitive behavioural interventions and treatment. Clinical Psychology and Psychotherapy 1:125–142

Hawton K, Salkovskis P, Kirk J, Clark D 1989 Cognitive behaviour therapy for psychiatric problems: a practical guide. Oxford University Press, Oxford

Hekmat H, Croth S, Rogers D 1994 Pain ameliorating effect of eye movement desensitisation. Journal of Behaviour Therapy and Experimental Psychiatry 25(2):121–129

Herbert J D, Mueser K T 1992 Eye movement desensitisation:

REFERENCES (*contd*)

a critique of the evidence. Journal of Behaviour Therapy and Experimental Psychiatry 123(3):169–174

Horowitz M J 1986 Stress response syndromes, 2nd edn. Aronson, New York

Horowitz M J, Kaltreider N B 1980 Brief psychotherapy of stress response. In: Karsau T, Bellack L (eds) Specialised techniques in individual psychotherapy. Brunner/Mazel, New York

Horowitz M J, Wilner N, Alverez W 1979 Impact of event scale: a measure of subjective distress. Psychosomatic Medicine 41:207–218

Janoff-Bulman R 1992 Shattered assumptions. Free Press, New York

Jaycox L H, Foa E B 1996 Obstacles in implementing exposure therapy for PTSD: case discussions and practical solutions. Clinical Psychology and Psychotherapy 3(3):176–184

Jones J C, Barlow D H 1990 The etiology of posttraumatic stress disorder. Clinical Psychology Review 10:299–328

Jones J C, Barlow D H 1992 A new model of posttraumatic stress disorder: implications for the future. In: Saigh P A (ed) Posttraumatic stress disorder: A behavioural approach to assessment and treatment. McMillan, New York: p 147–165

Joseph S, Dalgleish T, Thrasher S, Yule W, Williams R, Hodgkinson P 1996 Chronic emotional processing in survivours of the Herald of Free Enterprise disaster: the relationship of intrusion and avoidance at 3 years to distress at 5 years. Behaviour Research and Therapy 34:357–360

Keane T M, Kaloupek D 1982 Imaginal flooding in the treatment of a posttraumatic stress disorder. Journal of Consulting and Clinical Psychology 50:138–140

Keane T M, Wolfe J 1990 Comorbidity in post traumatic stress disorder: an analysis of community and clinical studies. Journal of Applied Social Psychology 20:1776–1788

Keane T M, Fairbank J A, Caddell J M, Zimmering R T 1989 Implosive (flooding) therapy reduces symptoms of PTSD in Vietnam combat veterans. Behaviour Therapy 20:149–153

Keane T M, Fairbank J A, Caddell J M, Zimmering R T, Bender M E 1985 A behavioural approach to assessing and treating post-traumatic stress disorder in Vietnam veterans. In: Figely C R (ed) Trauma and its wake: The study and treatment of posttraumatic stress disorder. Brunner/Mazel, New York, p 254–294

Kessler R C, Sonnega A, Bromet E, Hughs M, Nelson C B 1995 Posttraumatic stress disorder in the national comorbidity survey. Archives of General Psychiatry 52:1048–1060

Kilpatrick D G, Veronen L J 1983 Treatment for rape related problems: crisis intervention is not enough. In: Cohen L H, Claiborn W L, Spector C A (eds) Crises intervention. Human Sciences Press, New York, p 85–103

Kinzie J D, Goetz R R 1996 A century of controversy surrounding posttraumatic stress-spectrum syndromes: the impact on DSM-III and DSM-IV. Journal of Traumatic Stress 9:159–179

Kleber R J, Brom D 1992 Coping with trauma: Theory, prevention and treatment. Swets and Zeitlinger, Amsterdam

Kolb L C 1988 A critical survey of hypotheses regarding post-traumatic stress disorder in light of recent findings. Journal of Traumatic Stress 1:291–304

Krietler S, Krietler H 1988 Trauma and anxiety: the cognitive approach. Journal of Traumatic Stress 1:35–56

Krystal J H, Kosten T R, Southwick S, Mason J W, Perry B D, Giller E L 1989 Neurobiological aspects of PTSD: review of clinical and preclinical studies. Behaviour Therapy 20:177–198

Kubany E S 1994 A cognitive model of guilt typology in combat-related PTSD. Journal of Traumatic Stress 7:3–19

Kulka R A, Schenger W E, Fairbank J A et al 1990 Trauma and the Vietnam generation. Report of the findings from National Vietnam Veterans Readjustment Study. Brunner/Mazel, New York

Lang P J 1979 A bio-information theory of emotional imagery. Psychophysiology 16:495–512

Lerner M J 1980 The belief in a just world. Plenum, New York

Lindy J D, Green B L, Grace M, Titchener J 1983 Psychotherapy with survivors of the Beverley Hills Supper Club fire. American Journal of Psychotherapy 37:593–610

Litz B T, Keane T M 1989 Information processing in anxiety disorders: application to the understanding of post traumatic stress disorder. Clinical Psychology Review 9:243–257

Lovell K 1997 Outcome of exposure therapy and of cognitive restructuring in post-traumatic stress disorder. PhD thesis, University of London

Lovell K, Marks I, Noshirvani H, Thrasher S, Livanou M 1996 Final results of a RCT in PTSD. Paper presented at BABCP Annual Conference, Southport, England

Marks I M 1986 Behavioural psychotherapy: Maudsley pocket book of clinical management. Wright, Bristol

Marks I M 1987 Fears, phobias and rituals: panic, anxiety, and their disorders. Oxford University Press, Oxford

Marquis J N 1991 A report on 78 cases treated by eye movement desensitisation. Journal of Behaviour Therapy and Experimental Psychiatry 22:187–192

Meichenbaum D A 1975 A self-instructional approach to stress management: a proposal for stress inoculation training. In: Speilberger C, Sarason I (eds) Stress and anxiety, vol 2. Wiley, New York, p 12–35

Mineka S M 1979 The role of fear in theories of avoidance learning, flooding and extinction. Psychological Bulletin 86:985–1010

Mowrer O H 1947 On the dual nature of learning: a reinterpretation of 'conditioning' and 'problem-solving.' Havard Educational Review 17:102–148

Mowrer O H 1960 Learning theory and behaviour. Wiley, New York

Muse M 1986 Stress-related post-traumatic chronic pain syndrome: behavioural treatment approach. Pain 25:384–394

Myers C S 1940 Shell shock in France 1914–18. Cambridge University Press, Cambridge

Pitman R K 1993 Biological findings in posttraumatic stress disorder: implications for DSM-IV classification. In: Davidson J R T, Foa E B (eds) Posttraumatic stress disorder: DSM-IV and beyond. American Psychiatric Press, Washington DC, p 173–190

Pitman R K, Altman B, Greenwald E et al 1991 Psychiatric

REFERENCES (*contd*)

complications during flooding therapy for posttraumatic stress disorder. Journal of Clinical Psychiatry 52:17–20

Rado S 1942 Psychodynamics and treatment of traumatic war neurosis (traumatophobia). Psychosomatic Medicine 42:363–368

Renfrey G, Spates C R 1994 Eye movement desensitisation and reprocessing: a partial dismantling procedure. Journal of Behaviour Therapy and Experimental Psychiatry 25:231–239

Resick P A, Schnicke M K 1992 Cognitive processing therapy for sexual assault victims. Journal of Consulting and Clinical Psychology 60:748–756

Richards D A, Lovell K 1997 Treatment of adults: behavioural and cognitive approaches. In: Black D, Newman M, Harris-Hendricks J, Mezey G (eds) Psychological trauma: A developmental approach. Gaskell, London, p 264–273

Richards D A, Rose J S 1991 Exposure therapy for post-traumatic stress disorder. British Journal of Psychiatry 58:836–840

Richards D A, Lovell K, Marks I M 1994 Post-traumatic stress disorder: evaluation of a behavioural treatment program. Journal of Traumatic Stress 7:669–680

Roth S, Dye E, Lebowitz L 1988 Group therapy for sexual assault victims. Psychotherapy 25:82–93

Rothbaum B O, Foa E B, Riggs D S, Murdock T, Walsh W 1992 A prospective examination of post-traumatic stress disorder in rape victims. Journal of Traumatic Stress 5:455–475

Sanderson A, Carpenter R 1992 Eye movement desensitisation versus image confrontation: a single-session crossover study of 58 phobic subjects. Journal of Behaviour Therapy and Experimental Psychiatry 23:269–275

Schwalrz E D, Kowalski J M 1992 Malignant memories. Journal of Nervous and Mental Disease 180 (12):767–772

Shapiro F 1989a Eye movement desensitisation: a new treatment for post-traumatic stress disorder. Journal of Behaviour Therapy and Experimental Psychiatry 20:211–217

Shapiro F 1989b Efficacy of the eye movement desensitisation procedure in the treatment of traumatic memories. Journal of Traumatic Stress 2:199–223

Shapiro F 1995 Eye movement desensitisation and reprocessing. Guilford Press, New York

Shipley R H, Boudewyns P A 1980 Flooding and implosive therapy: are they harmful? Behaviour Therapy 11:303–308

Solomon S D, Gerrity E T, Muff A M 1992 Efficacy of treatments for posttraumtic disorder: an empirical review. Journal of the American Medical Association 268:633–638

Thrasher S M, Dalgeish T, Yule W 1993 Information processing in post traumatic stress disorder. Behaviour Research and Therapy 32:245–247

Thrasher S M, Lovell K, Noshirvani H, Livanou M 1996 Cognitive restructuring in the treatment of post-traumatic stress disorder: two single cases. Clinical Psychology and Psychotherapy 3:137–148

Thompson J A, Charlton P F C, Kerry R, Lee D, Turner S W 1995 An open trial of exposure therapy based on deconditioning for post-traumatic stress disorder. British Journal of Clinical Psychology 34:407–416

Trimble M 1981 Post-traumatic neurosis. Wiley, New York

Van Oppen P, De Hann E, Van Balkrom A J, Spinhoven P, Hoogduin K, Van Dyke R 1995 Cognitive therapy and exposure *in vivo* in the treatment of obsessive–compulsive disorder. Behaviour Research and Therapy 33:379–393

Vaughn K, Armstrong M S, Gold R, O'Conner N, Jenneke S, Tarrier N 1994 A trial of eye movement desensitisation compared to image habituation training and applied muscle relaxation in post-traumatic stress disorder. Journal of Behaviour Therapy and Experimental Psychiatry 25:283–291

Van der Kolk B A 1987 Psychological trauma. American Psychiatric Press, Washington DC

Van der Kolk B A, Dreyfuss D, Michaels M et al 1994 Fluoxetine in posttraumatic stress disorder. Journal of Clinical Psychiatry 55:517–522

Wilson S A, Becker L A, Tinker R H 1995 Eye movement desensitisation and reprocessing (EMDR) treatment for psychologically traumatised individuals. Journal of Consulting and Clinical Psychology 63:928–937

Wolpe J, Abrams J 1991 Post-traumatic stress disorder outcome of eye movement desensitisation: a case report. Journal of Behaviour Therapy and Experimental Psychiatry 22:39–43

CHAPTER CONTENTS

Key points   313

Introduction   314
Disorders, problems and difficulties   314
Historical overview of child and adolescent mental
   health nursing   314

**Epidemiology of child and adolescent mental
   health problems and disorders   315**

**Characteristic mental health disorders of young
   life   316**
Anxiety disorders   316
Depression   317
Behavioural problems   318
Attention-deficit–hyperactivity disorders   319
Autism   320

**Assessment and detection of child mental health
   problems and disorders   320**
History from parent(s) or main carer   321
Interview with the child   322
Formulation   322

**Aetiology and underlying theoretical models
   323**
Psychological theories of development   323
Biological factors   324
Social factors   325
Resilience–protective factors   328

Treatment interventions   328
Psychological therapies   328
Cognitive–behaviour therapy   329
Psychotherapy   331
Family therapy   332
Residential settings   333
Biological treatment   333

Conclusions – the future   334
Child mental health services and disciplines   334
Nursing skills and roles within child and adolescent
   mental health services   336
Future directions for research, training and service
   development   337

Exercise   338

Key texts for further reading   338

References   338

17

Children's and adolescents' difficulties

Richard Soppitt   Panos Vostanis

KEY POINTS

- At any time, between 15 and 20% of children and adolescents have significant mental health problems and disorders.

- Characteristic mental health disorders of young life include anxiety, depression, oppositional and conduct disorders, attention-deficit–hyperactivity disorder, somatising disorders, autism and eating disorders.

- Aetiology is often multifactorial, involving interaction between developmental, psychological, biological and social factors.

- Treatment interventions include psychological therapies (psychotherapy, behaviour, cognitive and family therapies), pharmacological and residential treatment.

- Child mental health services are currently being developed on a four-tier model, which includes the full range of services from primary care to specialist settings. Links with primary health, education, social services and hospital child services are essential.

KEY POINTS (*contd*)

- Nursing staff are involved in the assessment and treatment of child mental health problems across all four tiers; for example, health visitors, school nurses, community psychiatric nurses, hospital paediatric and psychiatric nurses.

INTRODUCTION

Disorders, problems and difficulties

Mental health difficulties in childhood and early adolescence are best conceptualised as emotions or behaviour which are outside the normal range for age and sex, either linked with an impairment of development/functioning and/or where the child suffers as a result. Unlike the adult mental health field, it is often not the child who complains of problems but one of the many adults involved, either parents or one of the agencies with statutory responsibilities for education or child protection.

The term disorder is used in this chapter to imply the presence of a clinically recognisable set of symptoms or behaviours linked with distress and interference with personal functions for at least 2 weeks' duration. It should not imply stigmatisation, but rather help to organise helpful interventions and resources for children. Neither should it indicate the problem is entirely within the child, for many disorders may be largely resolved through a change in external circumstances. Indeed, this responsiveness to environmental factors marks another significant difference between childhood and adult mental health problems.

Unlike most adult mental health disorders, most symptoms in childhood are quantitative shifts from normality within a developmental framework. For example, the behaviours appropriate for a 3-year-old and his or her parents would not be apposite if demonstrated by a 15-year-old and his or her parents. Hence, it is not so much medical diagnosis but an individual appreciation of the whole child and the child's environment and development that is important to target interventions.

Historical overview of child and adolescent mental health nursing

The history of child and adolescent mental health nursing in the UK dates back to the Maudsley Residential Unit of 1947, which emphasised nurturing and containment and the basic needs of Maslow's hierarchy. Paplau in the 1950s distilled the importance of the therapeutic relationship as distinct from being in loco parentis. In 1975, the Joint Board of Clinical Nursing Studies was established, and with it the specialism of child and adolescent psychiatric nursing began to fight for recognition. In the UK, Teresa Wilkinson published *Child and Adolescent Psychiatric Nursing* in 1983; her American counterpart, Clunn, published a similar volume in 1991. In 1983, the English National Board took over nurses' training and the ENB 603 course was born, specifically for child and adolescent mental health. Approximately 630 nurses have trained in the discipline since 1975, and recent UK service development guidelines (Health Advisory Service 1995) have highlighted the great need for expansion in numbers, particularly in community mental health nursing.

This chapter aims to address the broad issues surrounding child and adolescent mental health disorders, covering the epidemiology of problems and disorders; characteristic mental health disorders of young life; the assessment and detection of problems and disorders; key aetiological/theoretical models; the main treatment modalities to which nurses will be exposed; and a forward look at the direction of child mental health services, disciplines and research, with particular emphasis on the nursing skills and role within the multidisciplinary team.

EPIDEMIOLOGY OF CHILD AND ADOLESCENT MENTAL HEALTH PROBLEMS AND DISORDERS

Interpretation of epidemiological research must take into account several methodological aspects. This applies to studies on the prevalence of child and adolescent mental health disorders, and explains the variation of the findings. The selection of the sample may not necessarily represent the general population, as it may be associated with mediating factors, such as socio-economic deprivation, which could account for the high rates of mental health problems. The definition of symptoms, behaviours, problems or disorders measured by the study is essential, as highlighted in the previous section. For example, many studies claim to have measured rates of *disorders* by using screening questionnaires or rating scales, rather than diagnostic interviews, when in fact these have established *general* rates of possible child psychopathology. These methodological problems also apply to research in adult mental health and other social sciences.

Research with children and adolescents faces additional difficulties, such as the reliance on multi-informant ratings. Because of continuous changes in cognitive development, different instruments are used for different age groups. There are several self-report measures (for depression, anxiety and general mental health problems – Kent et al 1997) for adolescents (12 to 16 years), although even in this age group corroborative information from parents and teachers is important. In the last few years, research

instruments have been developed for children of primary school age (6 to 11 years). In pre-school children, data collection is almost exclusively based on adult reports and direct observation. Discrepancies in multi-informant ratings may be related to informant characteristics, or to the presentation of certain behaviours (specifically related to the school or family environment). Surveys based on questionnaires are reliable in estimating general rates of mental health problems. In contrast, two-stage designs, with questionnaire screening at the first stage and interviewing at the second stage, are superior in estimating the prevalence of specific mental health disorders, but obviously costly and time consuming.

Another difficulty concerns the varying nature and presentation of phenomenology (symptoms) and their frequency according to developmental stage and sex (Richman & Lansdown 1988). For example, depressive disorders present equally in boys and girls until adolescence, but are more frequent in female than male teenagers; also, their overall rate increases with age. Such differences may be related to the aetiology of the disorders. Finally, the comorbidity (concurrent presentation) of disorders is not unusual in this age group. Depression may present together with either anxiety or conduct disorders, or both. Child mental health disorders are often comorbid with learning difficulties or developmental disorders.

Advances in the classification systems, methods of diagnosis and research measures have been reflected in epidemiological surveys during the last three decades (Rutter 1989). Epidemiological research has been strongly influenced by the Isle of Wight studies between 1964 and 1974 (Rutter et al 1976). These consisted of neuropsychiatric assessment of different age cohorts from the entire child population of the island. In the main survey with 10-year-old children, a prevalence rate of about 10.6% of psychiatric disorder was established. Because of the social characteristics of this population, this was compared with children from an inner city (London), where the deviance rate was almost double (19.1%, Rutter 1973). The substantial difference was attributed to different family and social indexes of deprivation.

Subsequent major epidemiological studies from North America, Western Europe and New Zealand established rates between 12% and 20% (e.g. 13.2% in pre-school children, Thompson et al 1996; 12.4% in 8 to 11-year-olds, Fombonne 1994; 18.1% in children and adolescents, Offord et al 1987). Recent evidence suggests a real increase of mental health problems among children and adolescents in Western societies. These are mainly accounted for by pre-school behaviour problems, and adolescent depression, substance abuse, self-harm and conduct disorders (Prosser & McArdle 1996).

In order to highlight the characteristics of child and adolescent mental health disorders, and their differences from disorders of adult life, five types of disorders with onset in childhood are briefly described in this chapter (anxiety, depression, behavioural problems, hyperactivity and autism). Other problems and disorders include bedwetting/enuresis, soiling/encopresis, adjustment disorders, child post-traumatic stress disorders, tics, Tourette's syndrome, somatising disorders and specific or general learning difficulties. Disorders with onset usually in adolescence or early adult life, such as anorexia and bulimia nervosa, schizophrenia and bi-polar affective disorders, resemble the adult-like conditions discussed in other chapters.

CHARACTERISTIC MENTAL HEALTH DISORDERS OF YOUNG LIFE

Anxiety disorders

The general term of *emotional disorders* is still often used by clinicians to describe a range of anxiety and depressive disorders, mainly because of their comorbidity in young life. In childhood (6 to 11 years), the prevalence of anxiety disorders varies between 5 and 10% in both sexes, while in adolescence there is higher prevalence in females (about 13%) than males (about 5%).

Causes involved include stressors, that is acute or chronic life events (such as bereavement, accidents or other traumas), personal predisposition (vulnerability) or a combination of these factors. Symptoms of anxiety are irritability, inability to relax, tension in muscles, poor sleep, nightmares, fear of death or loss (of child or parents), physical complaints (nausea, abdominal pain, sickness, headaches, sweating, heartbeats) and panic attacks (sudden onset, extreme fear, physical symptoms, faintness).

As in adult life, *phobic disorders* are characterised by persistent and irrational fear of specific objects, activities or situations, which leads to their avoidance. They include (a) simple phobias (dogs, insects, heights, dark), which are common in early childhood, and usually subside; (b) fear of public places, mainly in adolescence; and (c) social phobias (e.g. speaking, eating in front of others, also predominantly in adolescence). *Obsessive–compulsive disorders* also resemble those adult-like states, as they include intrusive and persistent obsessional thoughts (e.g. thoughts of counting, urge to wash hands or touch wood a certain number of times) and compulsive actions related to the thoughts. The young person is aware that these phenomena are unreasonable and tries to resist them, but often gives in.

Separation anxiety is manifest upon separation or threat of separation from attachment persons, usually the mother, and is a normal reaction between 18 months and 3 years. Its aim is to attract the care-giver's attention to the child. In a secure, mother–child relationship, this reaction gradually weakens as the child grows up and develops peer and alternative attachment relationships. In certain cases, usually in insecure attachment relationships, separation anxiety may persist into later childhood and even into adolescence. It may present with physical complaints (sickness, headaches, abdominal pain), nightmares with separation themes and school refusal.

Treatment of anxiety disorders includes behavioural therapy, consisting of gradual and increased exposure to the object or situation that brings anxiety, relaxation techniques, psychotherapy (brief or longer term) in order to gain understanding into the causes of anxiety, and medication. Antidepressants may be indicated, either because of a comorbid depressive condition or because of their anxiolytic effect, while minor tranquillisers are only indicated for acute anxiety, for a brief period and under medical supervision. Milder cases of anxiety disorder have good outcome, while chronic and severe cases are at risk of persisting or recurring in adult life.

School refusal is not a mental health condition, but is often associated with anxiety and depressive disorders. It is defined as an irrational fear of school attendance. This may be partly or fully based on fear of separation from one or both parents, and may be specific to school attendance (school phobia). It should be distinguished from truancy, which is disguised absence from school, linked to behavioural problems but without an accompanying fear of the school situation. School refusal often starts at a time of school change or after absence for other reason (minor illness), and usually has gradual onset and a history of previous absences. Children may present with physical symptoms of tension or anxiety linked to attendance (abdominal pain, headache, nausea, sickness, heartbeats), which tend to remit at weekends and holidays. They may maintain some peer relationships, although they usually have social difficulties. School refusal is not generally associated with learning difficulties. The child is often behind with school work because of prolonged absence. One or both parents may be 'worriers' and overtly close to the child, and there may be stressful factors at school, such as bullying or exam-related anxiety. Although minor forms of school refusal are common and difficult to measure, this has been found to occur in about 1 to 2% of the school population. There is no social class trend, and it presents equally in both sexes. It is important to exclude an underlying physical illness, treat comorbid anxiety or depressive disorders, and aim for a quick return to school, before the development of entrenched social difficulties and anticipatory anxiety. This should be gradual, but with clear, graded tasks. Joint work with teachers and education welfare officers, and family work are essential in the management of school refusers. With this approach, the majority of mild cases and many severe cases of acute onset will be resolved.

Depression

The presence of depression in childhood and adolescence has only been recognised in the last decade. During this period, there has been a substantial volume of research on its prevalence, phenomenology and aetiology. However, current classification systems (ICD-10, World Health Organization 1992 and DSM-IV, American Psychiatric Association 1994) still adopt criteria from adult depressed people, and there is little research on treatment for young people. In children, depression occurs in 0.5 to 2% of the general population (males = females), which rises to 3% in adolescence (higher in females). Children have non-specific symptoms, such as physical complaints, irritability and withdrawal. Adolescents present with adult-like symptoms and develop negative cognitions and attributions.

Such symptoms include depressed mood (persistent for at least 2 weeks), insomnia or excessive sleeping, change in appetite (usually decrease), weight changes (usually loss), suicidal thoughts or deliberate self-harm (DSH) behaviour, poor concentration, loss of interest for previously enjoyable activities, fatigue and negative cognitions (feeling useless, inadequate, ugly, guilty, hopeless). Young people with depression often have other mental health problems, such as anxiety, behavioural problems or eating disorders. Established causes are life events (trauma/loss), personal predisposition (genetic) and physical illness. Treatment includes management of underlying family, school or social problems, cognitive–behaviour therapy (aiming at changing maladaptive and negative ways of thinking – Vostanis & Harrington 1994, brief psychotherapy, antidepressant medication and social skills training (improving self-esteem and interpersonal relationships). The depressive episode usually remits, but there is a high risk of relapse (in at least one-third of young people over 2 to 3 years – Vostanis et al 1996). In a small proportion of young people, depressive symptoms may become chronic, and there is a risk of depression persisting in adult life.

Deliberate self-harm and suicide

Vague suicidal thoughts can occur in up to one-third of teenagers, with an annual prevalence of DSH (hospital-treated) of about 0.2% in the general population. The lifetime prevalence of DSH in adolescence has been found between 2 and 3.5% in studies from Europe and much higher in the USA (about 9%). DSH increases with age, is more common in females (3:1) and low socio-economic groups, and is often precipitated by arguments with family, friends or partner. The method is usually either by overdose of analgesics, antidepressants or other medication, or by inflicting lacerations. There are often associated mental health problems such as depression, behavioural problems, alcohol/drug misuse, but not necessarily severe mental health disorders. There is a high risk of eventual suicide (in up to 10% of the young people who self-harm).

Suicide in young life is rare, although it is possibly an underestimate, because of often being defined as accidental death – in less than one child of 5 to 14 years per 100 000 general population, and about 7 to 13 adolescents/young adults per 100 000 general population (or 14% of all deaths). There is an increasing trend in male teenagers. In contrast with DSH, suicide is more frequent in males, often there has been a history of previous attempts (in 25 to 50% of young people), and there is no association with social class. Methods tend to be more violent in males, while overdoses are more frequent in females. An important finding for nursing staff and other clinicians is that about 50% of young people who committed suicide had talked about their intent during the previous week, and that there has usually been an underlying mental health disorder, such as depression, substance abuse or conduct disorder.

Behavioural problems

Behavioural problems are classified as psychiatric disorders in both the ICD-10 and the DSM-IV. They are broadly divided into *oppositional disorders* (usually of milder severity and in younger children) and the more severe *conduct disorders* (in older children and adolescents, and often associated with delinquency, i.e. committing offences). The prevalence of behavioural problems that require assessment and treatment is about 6% in boys of 4 to 11 years and 2% in girls of the same age. In adolescence, the rates rise to 10% and 4%, respectively. There is a higher frequency in urban and socially deprived areas, which is almost double that in rural areas. Well-established, associated characteristics and risk factors are chronic marital conflict, family dysfunction and family breakdown, parenting (lack of affection and discipline/consistency), overcrowding, criminality of the father, exposure to violence (at home or among peers), and alcohol abuse in the family (Vostanis & Nicholls 1995).

A child with an oppositional disorder may present with temper tantrums, as being argumentative, defiant, annoying, blaming others, touchy, angry, resentful, or spiteful/vindictive. Severe symptoms (conduct disorder) include lying, initiating fights, cruelty to animals or people, destructiveness, fire-setting, stealing, truanting, running away, robbery and violence. At least one-third of children with behavioural problems also have learning difficulties. Other comorbid disorders are hyperactivity, depression and substance misuse. It is important to consider whether the behavioural problems are secondary to a developmental disorder such as autism or learning disability, because of impaired communication and social skills, as these children will need a different treatment approach.

Treatment and management include behaviour modification, parental counselling, family work or family therapy, social problem-solving, group therapy (for children and/or parents) and school-based interventions. There are continuities with antisocial behaviour in late adolescence and adult life, particularly if the onset was early (under 12 years) and several risk factors are present (cumulative risk), but many children escape from this cycle of adversity. In other words, there are also discontinuities from further psychosocial problems, usually in the presence of protective factors such as parental warmth, school achievement, high self-esteem and friendships.

Attention-deficit–hyperactivity disorders

Attention-deficit–hyperactivity disorder (ADHD) has attracted publicity in the media in the last few years, and is a good example of how changes in the diagnostic and classification systems affect clinical practice. ADHD has an onset before the age of 5 years, and is characterized by continuous (pervasive) motor hyperactivity, restlessness, poor attention and concentration, distractibility and impulsivity. The DSM classification system has always adopted a lower threshold; that is, these problems only need to occur for certain periods in the child's life, rather than continuously, for the diagnosis to be made. The ICD classification system has used a relatively 'narrow' definition, for which reason the estimated prevalence rates have been much lower in the UK (in about 1.5% of the general population) than in the USA. There has been greater convergence between the recently revised diagnostic systems (DSM-IV and ICD-10).

The condition is more common in boys (3:1). Between 30 and 50% of children with hyperactivity also have behavioural problems (this combination is more difficult to treat). No single cause has been found, but there is some evidence that biological/neurodevelopmental factors are involved. Family factors, such as parental attitudes, are only involved in the presence of behavioural problems. Treatment includes behavioural modification (to improve concentration and adverse behaviour), school intervention (these children benefit from structured teaching in a small size class, if possible) and medication (usually centrally acting stimulants such as methylphenidate). Medication may have a positive effect on attention, concentration and activity, but not directly on behavioural problems. However, if a child improves in some of the symptoms, this allows additional interventions to target the comorbid behavioural problems. There is limited research on long-term outcome. Hyperactivity, restlessness, attention-deficit and impulsivity improve with age, but other problems, such as poor school performance, impaired social skills and relationships, low self-esteem, behavioural problems, may persist.

Autism

This condition is characterised by onset in the first 3 years of life, delay and deviation in the development of social relationships and communication, and resistance to change. There is association with learning disability (mental retardation) and a range of neurological diseases, particularly epilepsy. The child may show little interest in other people and show preference for his own company, be preoccupied with objects, avoid going to parents for comfort, and have little or no understanding of other people's emotions (lack of empathy). Both comprehension and expression are usually markedly delayed. Children with autism develop no or limited pretend or imaginative play. When behavioural problems occur, these are usually secondary (i.e. a result of impaired communication). The child may have special abilities involving mechanical tasks (e.g. numbers) and memory, but difficulties in abstract thinking.

Typical autistic disorders occur in 3 to 4 per 10 000 children. If one includes cases of milder severity (high functioning), the prevalence rises to 10 per 10 000 children. It is as yet unclear whether there is a spectrum (or continuum) of autistic disorders according to severity, or groups of disorders with different aetiology and presentation. The diagnosis *Asperger's syndrome* is characterised by the same abnormalities of reciprocal social interaction as autism, together with a restricted and repetitive repertoire of interests and activities, but without the general delay in language or cognitive development of autism. These social difficulties are likely to continue in later life. The broad diagnostic term *pervasive developmental disorders* is used to describe all autism-like conditions. Autistic disorders are four times more common in boys than in girls. There is a genetic predisposition, with 2 to 3% of siblings being affected, and a higher proportion has non-specific language delay. In addition to comorbid neurological conditions, autism is also associated with a number of chromosomal abnormalities, particularly Fragile-X syndrome.

Management starts with a comprehensive assessment and explanation/reassurance to the parents. Support to the family should be long term. Appropriate educational placement is essential, depending on the nature and severity of the problems. Speech therapy or a behavioural programme can help maximise the child's communication skills. Behaviour modification also targets aggression and social difficulties, the latter through graded steps of social stimulation and interaction. The prognosis depends on the number and severity of problems and impairments. In severe disorders, a high proportion of individuals will require continuing care and support. In nearly all cases, there is continuing improvement throughout childhood and adolescence, so that each year the child gains some new skills.

ASSESSMENT AND DETECTION OF CHILD MENTAL HEALTH PROBLEMS AND DISORDERS

The assessment and diagnostic procedure, as well as the formulation and establishment of a management plan, are briefly discussed, in order to highlight issues specific to interviewing children and families. Our aim is to stress the general principles that apply to a variety of out-patient and in-patient settings, rather than only to child mental health services. Nursing staff are in contact with children, to a lesser or greater degree, throughout their training and career. Although the clinical circumstances (school nurse assessment, home visit by health visitor, accident and emergency department, paediatric ward, child development centre, out-patient clinic) obviously affect the nature, purpose and duration of contact with young patients, awareness of child mental health issues and ways of detecting them are essential for the appropriate diagnosis and treatment, whatever the primary reason for referral.

Even within the physical and time constraints of a busy clinic or hospital, a child should preferably be interviewed alone. Children are often inhibited or frightened to answer questions on their emotional state in front of parents or known adults. Children as young as 4 to 5 years are aware of adults' emotions and views, and this can limit their account of their own thoughts and feelings. Parents of pre-adolescents (i.e. younger than 12 years) should preferably be seen first, to give a more comprehensive history on their development and other related information. Adolescents may be more difficult to engage, particularly if they have been unclear about or opposed to the referral. In all cases, the young person should be reassured about the purpose of the interview. Family (joint) interviews are useful in establishing interaction of family members, as well as a means of initiating change in family relationships, but should not replace the initial, individual contact with young people.

History from parent(s) or main carer

The *reason for referral and the presenting complaints* (nature, context, duration) are explored first. Also, what kind of help or treatment has been previously received, why the family are seeking help at this particular time, and who initiated the referral. For example, parents may not share teachers' concerns on the child's behaviour, but feel obliged to attend, and their lack of motivation to change will be counter-productive in future treatment. Obviously, not all of the following items of children's potential problems will need to be explored in depth. At the same time of eliciting information on symptoms, the clinician can also assess parents' attitudes towards the child, the rest of the family and the described difficulties. Important areas of children's functioning include eating habits, somatic complaints (e.g. sickness, nausea, stomach aches, other kinds of pain), habits of elimination (soiling, wetting clothes at daytime, bed wetting), sleep pattern and habits, restlessness or overactivity, tics, speech, emotional state (depressive and anxiety symptoms), response to separation from main carer, attention and concentration, behaviour (accounts may be vague or critical of the child, particularly at the first assessment, for which reason it is useful to seek specific examples of reported behaviour: 'Could you give me an example of A being naughty? What happens when you ask him to go to bed? What does he actually do?').

The child's early *development* (motor skills, language, social functioning, toilet training, personal skills) and *temperament* (easy baby, placid, irritable) need to be explored, particularly the areas of parental concern. Knowledge of child development and normal milestones is important for the interpretation of the developmental history so that the clinician can decide what constitutes deviance or delay from the general population. *School history* includes exploration of learning capacity and social functioning. History or presence of *physical illness* and of medical/nursing treatment could be relevant.

Parents may be sensitive to questions on *family history* of mental illness or *family relationships*. An introductory statement/explanation can put them at ease ('I would like to get a picture of A's life at home by asking a few questions about the family.'). Use of genograms can be helpful. The child's *social functioning* and ability to make and maintain peer relationships is a good predictor of outcome, and is therefore a routine part of the assessment. Psychosexual and forensic history (offences, convictions) may be applicable to adolescents.

Interview with the child

Engaging the child should be the priority at the start of the assessment interview. This is achieved by clarifying the child's understanding of the referral, explaining the assessment procedure, and alleviating any fears of stigma attached to mental illness or attending a mental health service. Questions on hobbies, friends and interests enable an anxious child to relax, and to gain rapport with the interviewer. Some children will initiate a discussion on the presenting problems with very little prompting. Younger children often communicate through non-verbal means such as play and drawing. What is important is that the clinician remains sensitive and sympathetic, uses the child's clues or material in asking relevant questions, while remaining in control, and maintaining the structure and plan of the assessment interview. The child's perceptions of the family and school, as well as the child's self-perceptions are constantly being assessed. Important observations and information also include the child's appearance and behaviour during the interview, ability to make rapport and attitude to future treatment.

The structure of the mental state examination depends on the age of the child, particularly the child's cognitive development. Open and closed questions are asked on anxieties (about themselves, parents, past events or anticipation of the future) and related symptoms, mood and depressive symptoms, thoughts of self-harm, fears, obsessions, sleep, eating, and perception of behavioural problems, and also, in relation to abnormal (psychotic) experiences, such as delusions and hallucinations.

Formulation

Diagnosis comprises five categories (axes), according to recent *multi-axial* classification (World Health Organization 1996): presence of psychiatric disorder, developmental disorder, intellectual capacity (IQ), physical illness and psychosocial abnormalities (e.g. life events and family dysfunction). Such a comprehensive assessment enables the clinician to address three major questions:

- Which are the problems/disorders of this child in all areas of the child's development? (Rather than 'this is a child with behavioural problems'.)
- Why have these problems/disorders arisen and why are they presenting at this particular time? The understanding of the underlying aetiology, which is often multifactorial is enhanced by distinguishing between:
  a. *predisposing (risk) factors*, which made this child vulnerable to the development of mental health problems (e.g. early deprivation, abuse, chronic physical illness)
  b. *precipitating factors*, which happened before the onset of the current episode, such as a bereavement or a road traffic accident
  c. *maintaining factors*, that is risk factors that are still present and are likely to affect the child in the future, even if the child's current symptoms respond to treatment, such as ongoing domestic violence or parental mental illness.
- What types of treatment should one consider

for this episode and in order to prevent similar problems in the future? The *management/care plan* must be clear and focused, and discussed with the family. Its aims should be to reduce or alleviate presenting symptoms and distress, minimise future risk, and foster protective factors such as parental warmth, supportive peer relationships, school achievement, and positive self-esteem. Different treatment modalities, most of which are not exclusive of each other, are briefly described in this chapter.

AETIOLOGY AND UNDERLYING THEORETICAL MODELS

The aetiology of mental health disorders in childhood is multifactorial and may be conceptualised under three broad headings: psychological development, biological factors and social factors. However, aetiological factors are rarely discrete but often involve a complex interaction.

Psychological theories of development

Attachment and bonding

Bowlby stated that selective clinging behaviour, which starts at around 6 months, is an outward demonstration of a normal and biologically determined psychological process that deals with personal relationships with those who have a primary play and comforting role (usually the mother) for the infant. This will govern the quality of subsequent close relationships. The mother's presence calms the child; her actual or threatened absence induces separation anxiety which subsides over the pre-school years, depending on the temperament of the child, the parental handling, experiences of actual or threatened separations and the child's perception as to whether his or her mother will return or not.

The acute separation reaction in children between 6 and 24 months is shown by protest, despair and detachment. On return to the care of the attachment figure, clinging will reappear but will be prolonged and demanding, and hence an insecure attachment will be seen. However, previous brief and manageable separations, as well as good, previous relationships, are protective. Poor attachments are described as either insecure (chronically clingy and ambivalent) or avoidant (self-sufficient). Insecure attachments are associated with anxiety disorders (e.g. school refusal), while avoidant attachment is held to be a precursor of aggression and poor social functioning later. Multiple attachments are possible, however, as are successful adoptions in early to middle childhood.

Piaget: cognitive development

Jean Piaget (1896–1980) was a Swiss psychologist who viewed the child as an active organism that worked to overcome difficulties through problem-solving. He demonstrated that children do not think any less than adults; they think differently (Orr 1991). Piaget proposed that children progress through four stages of cognitive development:

- sensorimotor stage (0 to 2 years)
- pre-operational stage (2 to 7 years)
- stage of concrete operations (7 to 12 years)
- formal operations (12 years onward)

Learning theory

Learning theory as developed by Skinner and other behaviourists posits that all human behaviour is learned by conditioning, either classical Pavlovian or operant conditioning. Behavioural difficulties are attributed to faulty conditioning or problems with learning owing to learning disability or attention problems. This view has been challenged by studies of child development, which occur without specific instruction.

Learning theory aids the understanding of certain childhood mental health disorders, such as phobias, encopresis (soiling) and conduct disorders. Such theory is based on observed behaviour and ignores complex internal mental processes such as attachment and those involved in emotional disorders. However, these theories are useful for changing maladaptive behaviours, forming the foundation of behaviour therapy.

Cognitive–behaviour therapy

Extending learning theory, proponents of cognitive–behaviour therapy (CBT) propose that patients' negative emotions are linked to distorted cognitions. Beck suggested that negative thinking in depression has its origins in attitudes and assumptions arising from early life experiences and consequent cognitive schema or assumptions about themselves and the world, which are then used to organise perception and to govern and evaluate behaviour (Beck 1972).

Problems arise when critical incidents occur that reactivate negative core assumptions, for example, 'My worth depends on everybody liking me.' These can lead to spontaneous negative automatic thoughts, such as 'Nobody loves me.' Such thoughts lower mood and encourage further negative automatic thoughts congruent with that mood. A negative view of one's self, current experience and the future, termed a cognitive triad, can overtake a person's thinking, leading to biased processing. Behavioural factors will impinge on the depression, leading to reduced exercise or social withdrawal, hence reinforcing the low mood.

Psychodynamic theories

Sigmund Freud, the father of psycho-analysis, reported on Little Hans in 1909 and observed his own grandchildren. His daughter Anna and his pupil Melanie Klein developed new ways of observing and interpreting children's non-verbal communications which later became play therapy. Psychodynamic psychotherapy and play therapy blossomed in the child guidance clinics in the UK and North America in the 1930s and 1940s. Psychodynamic psychotherapy is influenced largely by Freudian psycho-analysis, adapted in the UK by object relations theorists such as Winnicot, Bion and Klein and attachment theorists such as Bowlby and Ainsworth. Other core ideas propose that children develop through initial imitation and subsequently internalise their parents by identifying with them. Such theories attempt to describe and explain all the internal mental processes experienced by patients as well as their behaviour. However, it has been difficult to verify treatment efficacy empirically.

Biological factors

Temperament

This can be regarded as the child's individual style of doing things, held to be genetically determined and therefore reasonably stable over time, which may be altered by experience and environmental influences. The New York Longitudinal Study (Thomas & Chess 1977) distinguished three temperamental constellations of functional significance:

- difficult temperament in 10% (i.e. irregularity, withdrawal, slow adaptability, high intensity and relatively negative mood)
- easy temperament in 40% (i.e. the opposite)
- slow to warm up in 15% (i.e. negative

responses to change with slow adaptability, and mild intensity of emotional reactions).

These findings are group trends, and not necessarily able to help predict development for individual children. Temperament is an interactional concept where the child is an active participant in its own development, shaping the reactions of others. Thomas & Chess found that difficult temperament is a risk factor by a factor two to three for subsequent behaviour disorder if it interacts with a discordant family. Temperament alone is not a good predictor of adult clinical outcome.

Genetics

There is a genetic contribution to most childhood disorders, although this is not due to single gene effects with Mendelian patterns of inheritance (for a review, see Bolton 1996). Childhood autism probably has a strong genetic component, transmitted by several genes, although there may be non-specific heritability of elements such as language delay. Other disorders with a significant genetic component include Tourette's syndrome (TS), schizophrenia, and severe learning disability (e.g. Fragile X) and to a less extent anorexia nervosa, ADHD and affective disorders.

Interestingly, research points to a TS/chronic tics/obsessive–compulsive disorder phenotype, inherited in a simple, autosomal dominant fashion. Harrington et al (1993) found that the lifetime prevalence of depressive disorder in the relatives of depressed children was double that of the relatives of matched non-depressed controls. Familial aggregation could be explained by familial adversity, rather than genes per se.

Neurodevelopmental

Mediation of mental health disorders may lie in early environmental factors *in utero* not determined genetically (Goodman 1990). For example, individuals exposed to obstetric complications are twice as likely as controls subsequently to develop schizophrenia. Other pointers to a neurodevelopmental basis in schizophrenia include an association with midline structural defects (Edelstyn et al 1997), as association with winter births and neuropathological studies which indicate faulty second trimester fetal development (Roberts 1991).

Learning disability. Prenatal environmental factors influencing development of learning disability, although uncommon, include infections (e.g. HIV), as well as toxins such as alcohol in fetal alcohol syndrome, and also serious systemic maternal disease. Perinatal factors are seen usually as markers of learning disability which reflect pre-existing causes. However, severe birth asphyxia may lead to later cerebral palsy.

Social factors

The last sub-section will examine the role of environmental social factors within the immediate family, highlighting protective and vulnerability factors to adversity. Stressors may be divided into acute and chronic.

Acute stressors

These events or circumstances imply sudden or rapid onset, marked by intense fearfulness. It is now well established that young people can demonstrate post-traumatic stress disorder symptoms after major life-threatening stressors, with prognosis dependent on the level of trauma, its meaning, and the support networks following the trauma. Where children believe they could have died during the disaster, they show increased psychopathology later. It is not clear if young pre-school children are protected by their cognitive immaturity.

Chronic adversity

Investigators have identified a set of six variables, reflecting chronic familial adversities, which are significantly associated with mental health disorder in children: severe marital discord; low social status; overcrowding/larger family size; paternal criminality; maternal psychiatric disorder; and the accommodation of a child with a local authority. These risk factors are additive. Thus a child with one risk factor did almost as well as those with none. Two risk factors increase the probability of disorder by a factor of four (Rutter 1985). Six similar risk factors were isolated by Kolvin et al (1988) in the longitudinal Newcastle Thousand Family Study of the development of criminality. A single deprivation was linked with a 29% rate of later criminality, with two criteria raising the rate to 69%.

Parental mental disorder

There is an association between parental and childhood mental health problems (Quinton et al 1990). It is clear from research on parental mental illness that the nature and severity of that illness is of less importance than how it directly impinges upon the child. Protective factors include a mentally healthy partner, restoration of family harmony and a good relationship with one parent. Gender issues are germane in that boys may be more at risk than girls, while sharing the ill parent's gender may also be a risk factor. A difficult temperament attracts parental hostility, whereas an easy temperament protects and deflects criticism.

Research on children of depressed parents shows raised levels of general problems in adjustment, with social and academic difficulties. Children are themselves prone to depression, especially with mothers suffering unipolar depression. Other work in the offspring of schizophrenic mothers suggests that the continuity of

a negative family and social environment pattern was mirrored in a dearth of support, restricted parenting and reduced opportunities for the child's development by an accumulation of 10 familial risk factors (Garmezy & Masten 1994).

Early parental loss

Longitudinal studies indicate that children who experience parental divorce, death or permanent separation in early childhood are significantly more likely to develop mental health problems and delinquency in early adult life. If the early loss leads to inadequate care of the children and to lack of emotional stability, then it is likely to auger depression (Birtchnell 1980). A person's cognitive set, that is, the person's sense of self-esteem and self-efficacy, facilitates coping. Parental death or institutionalisation may predispose to poor marriages. Early bereavement itself may be harder to cope with because of cognitive immaturity.

Divorce and interpersonal conflict

Divorce is now one of the most common life events impacting upon children. It is a complex and fluid process with cumulative stressors. Remarriage and subsequent divorce in a third of these marriages subject children to chronic adversity, with children often being used as ammunition in hostile disputes. Hence, like parental mental disorders, there is an association with childhood disorder and the disruption and hostility associated with the quality of the divorce rather than divorce per se.

Longitudinal studies demonstrate that boys have more problems than girls. The Virginia Longitudinal Study of Divorce and Remarriage (Hetherington et al 1985) found that for children living with their mother, re-marriage aided re-adjustment for boys, while disturbing girls on measures of emotional symptoms and social competence. Particular challenges surrounding mother–son relationships include coercive cycles arising from poor discipline, leading to non-compliance and escalating aggression.

Pre-school children, although initially very distressed, may be buffered by their cognitive immaturity and inability to remember negative aspects of divorce (Wallerstein 1991). Reported protective factors include an exceptionally good relationship with the mother, sibling support, grandparents living in the home, friends of older children and a structured, positive school environment.

Parenting characteristics

Parenting characteristics which have been empirically linked with mental health disorders appear to impact negatively on children's self-esteem, locus of control and self-reliance. Parental hostility, marital discord and illness, both physical and mental, can all impact on children as acute or chronic stressors. This may be through continuity of care, and the disruption of essential parenting functions such as stability, consistency and emotional warmth; facilitation of development, fostering of self-esteem, and the provision of rules and structure; finally, the experience of 'good-enough' attachments upon which to build successful relationships in later life. Power-assertive punishment techniques, such as screaming, are risk factors for behavioural problems.

Abuse

Methodological problems in research arise from lack of agreement on what constitutes abuse. It is generally agreed that abuse can be delineated into emotional, physical and sexual types, while there is overlap in definitions and often more than one type occurs concurrently. Emotional abuse describes the severe impairment of social and emotional development arising from repeated criticism, lack of affection, rejection and verbal insults shown by the primary care-givers to the child over a period of time. Physical abuse or non-accidental injury is akin to the original concept of child abuse which described the 'battered baby syndrome', and extends to include any chronic or dangerous subjection to physical insult or assault at any age in childhood. Sexual abuse may be defined as 'the involvement of dependent children and adolescents in sexual activities they do not truly comprehend, to which they are unable to give informed consent, or which violates social taboos of family roles.' Neglect includes a combination of adverse circumstances and poor parenting which leads to a serious failure of the care-giver to provide the basic essentials needed for healthy development.

Prevalence rates relating to sexual abuse would indicate 3 to 6% of women in the general population have suffered major, long-term psychological disturbance following sexual abuse. The rate for men is about half this (Glaser 1991). In 1988, 3.5 per 1000 children in the UK were on the Child Protection Register, and about 25% of these had suffered physical abuse, and about 1 in 8 neglect (Skuse & Bentovim 1994). It should be noted that although the different types of abuse are linked with a high risk of developing mental disorders, not all children will suffer them. The outcome of physical and emotional maltreatment is likely to be influenced by the nature and severity of the abuse or neglect, by the characteristics of the perpetrator, by the age of the children when the abuse occurred, and child characteristics including level of intelligence and the abused child's perception of his or her experiences as a victim.

Consequences of emotional abuse include the following: (1) impaired psychological development; (2) impaired physical development, for example, 'psychosocial dwarfism', which improves when a child is placed in a more nurturing milieu; (3) psychiatric disorder, including depression and reactive attachment disorder of infancy (Thompson & Kaplan 1996). Sequelae of sexual abuse include (1) psychosexual problems; (2) psychiatric disorders; (3) impaired psychological development. Greater long-term harm appears to be associated with abuse involving a father or a step-father and abuse involving penetration, long duration and accompanied by force or threat of force (Cosentino et al 1995).

Physical illness and disability

Ongoing childhood physical illness is a strong risk factor for mental health difficulties. If chronic illness affects the central nervous system, the rate of mental health disorders in children soars by a factor of five, even with normal intelligence. Children with chronic illness and disability show increased rates by a factor of two to three. The Isle of Wight Study discovered that nearly 6% of 10- to 12-year-olds suffered a chronic physical disorder. Risk factors may involve the additive risk of multiple hospitalisations, especially between the ages of 6 months and 2 years, with separations being especially hard in the second to fourth years of life. Other factors could include illness-specific neurobiological elements (e.g. with severe asthma comorbid depression is common).

Frustration, social restrictions and learned helplessness may lead to an external locus of control, demoralisation and low mood. Indeed, the effects can be bi-directional. Emotional stressors can exacerbate physical symptoms, such as asthma, as well. Related to this is somatisation or the manifestation of psychological difficulty through somatic symptoms such as abdominal pain, chronic fatigue syndrome or conversion disorders (Garralda 1996). Recurrent abdominal pain is common; 25% of 5- to 6-year-old children

had at least three episodes of pain over at least 3 months, leading to the child missing normal activities (Faull & Nicol 1986).

Resilience–protective factors

To conclude, not all children exposed to risk factors develop mental health problems. There is indeed hope for even 'high risk' children (Werner 1996). Disorders themselves mediate maladaptive coping strategies, and children can promote their own environmental difficulties. However, resilience–protective factors have been uncovered and include individual cognitive capacities; styles of acting rather than reacting; cognitive set or self-efficacy and problem-solving; positive experiences of secure relationships, success and temperament; qualities which engender a positive response from others, and competency through overcoming stress successfully (Rutter 1985).

TREATMENT INTERVENTIONS

Since the early days of mental health nursing within the Maudsley residential units, emphasis on containment and nurturing has evolved through understanding of the therapeutic relationship and the movement in part of nursing from the residential to the community setting. This in turn has opened up a wide range of therapeutic options to child and adolescent psychiatric nurses as they have become practitioners in their own right, alongside the former child guidance tripartite of social worker, psychologist and doctor.

Psychological therapies

Behaviour therapy

Based on learning theory, this is a problem-solving approach rooted in the understanding that behaviour is learnt and maintained and therefore interventions can impact to make it more or less likely to re-occur. Different sub-groups exist:

- stimulus–response theories, which include exposure to an avoided stimulus either gradually by systematic desensitisation, or flooding
- operant conditioning techniques use positive and negative reinforcement to modify behaviour
- social learning theory uses modelling, role-play and social skills to improve social problem-solving, assertiveness and self-esteem.

Key elements to a behavioural formulation are that of 'ABC': antecedents or triggers of the unwanted behaviour need to be identified. Parental diaries are useful in this respect. A clear description of the behaviour, its timing, interactions and meaning for the family should be elicited. The consequences which may reinforce the behaviour need to be established.

Procedures to increase deficits of behaviour include positive reinforcement, shaping (a steady approximation towards a desired behaviour) and modelling (imitation). Parents and teachers often see reinforcers as bribes, but an objective view of any adult behaviour will see the importance of positive feedback, social praise and material gain. It is important to choose attainable goals so that children succeed early on, before moving onto the next stage.

Procedures to reduce unwanted behaviour include:

- *differential reinforcement of other behaviour* by rewarding the child for set periods, say, without fighting
- *time out (from positive reinforcement)* requires removing the child from a situation where the adverse behaviour is being reinforced; consistency and clarity are vital and need to be used with positive reinforcers to encourage desired behaviours
- *desensitisation* is a treatment for simple phobias – children are gradually exposed to a graded hierarchy of anxiety provocation until they can cope with phobic stimulus (e.g. the treatment of school refusal)
- *relaxation training* – children tense and relax muscle groups and use positive mental imagery to reduce anxiety states and gain an internal locus of control.

Punishment, which is effective in the short-term, can risk escalation through habituation, particularly if more attention is gained as a result.

Case study 17.1 Helen

Helen, aged 11, was referred because of school refusal at the start of secondary education. She complained of being bullied at primary school and had recently been threatened at knife point in her neighbourhood by a teenage girl. She lived with her disabled mother, her father and two younger siblings. Helen was very reluctant to return to school. Liaison with the educational social worker and the head of year at school led to a re-integration plan, whereby Helen was accompanied to school by a relative who initially stayed in the school office to reassure her. Gradually, the time at school was extended, taking into account subject preferences, and each successful increment was rewarded with praise and a small present. After three terms, Helen was attending full time and asked to be discharged.

Cognitive–behaviour therapy

Cognitive deficiencies and distortions lead to clinical difficulties as discussed before (p. 324). In clinical practice, CBT theories are useful in the understanding and treating of a number of conditions such as anger and aggression, attention-deficit disorder with hyperactivity, anxiety disorders and depression. However, issues regarding long-term outcome remain to be answered (Reinecke et al 1996).

Anger and aggression

Aggressive children are overly sensitive and have a low threshold for perceiving aggression in others; they have poor, social problem-solving skills. They tend to have automatic responses which are aggressive, underestimating their own aggression and not empathising with their victims, believing that rewards will follow violence. Treatment involves self-monitoring and self-instruction, perspective-taking, social problem-solving, affect-labelling and relaxation. Outcome research documents positive results from interventions across school and home settings up to 3 years post-treatment.

Depression

Studies have found distortions in attributions, self-evaluation and perceptions of present and past in depressed young people. There are low levels of self-esteem relating to academic and social performance. Cognitive errors include over-generalisation, catastrophisation, inappropriate self-blame and selectively attending to the negative. Generally, depressed children have poor, social problem-solving skills. Treatment strategies include the recognition and labelling of emotions, the change of negative cognitive attributions and the enhancement of social skills (Vostanis & Harrington 1994). There is emerging evidence from school-based trials for specific effects of individual or group CBT in depression, although these need to be replicated with referred young people (i.e. with more severe cases).

Anxiety

Childhood anxiety is a multidimensional amalgam of the physiological (e.g. butterflies in the stomach), behavioural (e.g. avoidance) and cognitive ('I think I'm going to fail.'). Techniques focus on identifying physiological arousal and teaching methods to reduce this in the child, such as relaxation training. This can be used effectively with phobic children, by pairing fear and relaxation. Work shows that combinations of relaxation, problem-solving, calm imagery and positive self-talk can reduce anxiety.

Attention-deficit–hyperactivity disorder

ADHD involves the display of above-average levels of inattention, impulsivity and overactivity. Next to stimulant medication, behaviour modification is a most effective adjunct, as it allows the children to learn adaptive ways of behaving. The goals of treatment are to help the child internalise the components needed in problem-solving, to reduce impulsivity and to promote organisational behaviour by breaking

---

Case study 17.2 Fiona

Fiona was a 9-year-old girl referred with a 4-month history of abdominal pain, depressed mood and reluctance to attend school. She was described as outgoing, although she appeared to have low self-esteem and poor self-image prior to the described episode. At the time, her parents were considering divorce and were arguing regularly. Fiona fulfilled diagnostic criteria for a major depressive episode, and undertook a CBT programme to treat her depression.

sequences down into manageable steps. Parental and school co-operation with reinforced self-evaluation is essential in treatment programmes.

Fiona appeared surprised when she was asked to describe different emotional states. She was articulate but found it difficult to understand the concept of thoughts and to describe recent examples of mood–events–thoughts. During her first session, it was much easier for her to think of such examples related to an imaginary friend of hers (e.g. following the therapist's questions: 'Your friend is feeling very sad. What may be happening at that time? What is she thinking?'). She was subsequently capable of monitoring her mood and thoughts and she completed her diary in between sessions.

Fiona liked the idea of rewarding herself. Her mother was asked to reinforce her positive mood, her school attendance and the absence of physical symptoms. Despite her improved mood, Fiona was still concerned about her appearance and had difficulties in her peer relationships. She recalled examples of falling out with her friends, was able to generate solutions to social problems and practise them at school. She then attended for cognitive restructuring and was symptom-free 6 months after discharge.

Psychotherapy

Psychodynamic psychotherapy is based on a working relationship with the patient in the 'here and now', within the context of past history and external relationships. It employs concepts such as unconscious processes, defence mechanisms, and transference, which is the way by which patients transfer on to their therapist and recapitulate previous disturbed or dysfunctional relationships.

Many questions, including efficacy, remain untested in child and adolescent psychotherapy in contrast to the adult counterparts. For example, Barnett et al (1991) considered outcome and efficacy of individual child psychotherapy over 26 years. Individual psychotherapy was found to be equivalent to other therapies in more than half of the studies; in about a third, other forms of therapy were superior.

Other modes of therapy include:

- *Interpersonal psychotherapy* (developed by Harry Stack Sullivan) which focuses on the child's current life situation, symptoms and interpersonal relationships. It can be used to address developmental issues, e.g. adolescent maturational tasks.
- *Gestalt therapy*, developed by Perls, is largely a training in self-awareness, emphasising mind and body, and personal responsibility. Difficulties are dealt with in the present tense and externalised for ease of access by the patient (see Oaklander 1988).
- *Creative art therapies* include art, music and drama media. Children are encouraged to explore and express their inner conflicts non-verbally; and as these therapies can be less threatening for the patient, they foster self-awareness and personal growth. Drama therapy attempts to encourage the acting-out of feelings through script, role-play or improvisation. Psychodrama is based on the work of Moreno, who believed problems stemmed from the need to retain social roles. The principal actor acts out his or her conflict, involving other group members. As the experiences can be very powerful, they need careful handling and resolution.
- *Group therapies* can be divided into (a) *experiential groups*, based on the work of Bion, incorporating projection and transference with dependence, pairing and fight or flight processes, commented upon by the leader; therapy can be either open or closed; (b) *educative groups* include CBT and

psychotherapy approaches. Examples include social skills groups, child sexual abuse survivors, disaster groups and those with chronic illness or siblings of life-limited children.

Family therapy

Family therapy is an approach to psychological treatment where the family group, couple or part of a family is the basic family unit (Bloch et al 1995). It focuses on interpersonal processes, relationships and communication, while assuming that one person's behaviour impacts and is influenced by another family member. Key concepts derive from cybernetics and general systems theory. Types of family therapy include:

- *structural family therapy* (founded by Minuchin), which emphasises the need for clear boundaries, hierarchy and flexibility
- *strategic* (after Haley), which uses the presenting problem as a metaphor, and works with dysfunctional hierarchies
- *systemic or Milan*, which highlights the need for a circular rather than linear perspective, using hypothesising, circular questioning and neutrality to facilitate this.

Other categories include psychodynamic, behavioural and psycho-educational. Family work has been utilised effectively in schizophrenia, lowering expressed emotion (i.e. carers' negative emo-

---

Case study 17.3 Sarah

Sarah was a 16-year-old adolescent who had been referred for psychotherapy having been raped. She had self-destructive behaviours, putting herself at risk by walking alone at night, drinking excessive alcohol and mixing with violent young men. Sessions were contracted for the same time and venue each week. A working relationship was fostered using transference, counter-transference and interpretation to deal with difficult issues around a male/female therapeutic alliance. Sarah was able to understand that a part of her was keeping her hostage and putting herself at risk. At times, she would project great anxieties about keeping herself safe and alive onto the therapist. The intensity of emotions and feelings in the room required close and supportive supervision to ensure boundaries were kept safe and appropriate, to allow Sarah the experience of a non-abusive relationship. Sarah became more careful in her external world, but found it hard to come in touch with the pain inside her and defaulted appointments.

Case study 17.4 Nicholas

Nicholas was an 11-year-old boy who had been referred for soiling. He lost his mother aged 7 months and was brought up by his grandmother until the age of 5 when his father remarried. Inadequate bowel control stemmed from the time of the remarriage. There was no organic basis found by the paediatricians. Work was undertaken to explore relationships within the reconstituted and extended families. Circular questioning enabled greater communication, and use of a genogram elucidated family scripts, a need for the step-mother to be accepted as part of the wider family and not to be compared with the deceased mother, and for clearer boundaries between the three families and the married couple. Although it was difficult for the parents to come to terms with the pain they were feeling, they understood that Nicholas' difficulties had allowed them to receive help. Nicholas' bowel control improved significantly with a simultaneous behavioural programme and novel coping strategies generated by the family that allowed a redistribution of household chores, facilitating family time together at weekends.

tional attitudes), and in adolescents with anorexia nervosa.

Residential settings

In-patient treatment

In-patient units cater for a small minority of patients where the mental health problems of children are too severe to be managed in the community setting (e.g. severe anorexia nervosa). Following the 1950s epoch of custodial care, psychiatric nursing moved towards a one-to-one nurse–patient relationship as advanced by Peplau (1952). She believed that the interpersonal process within the nurse–patient therapeutic relationship promotes healthy adjustment and reduces anxiety, depression and insecurity. Environmental treatment components have developed, including physical restructuring to facilitate adjunct therapies; encouraging key attitudes and behaviours in staff, patient and families; and the use of planned activities that are ego-strengthening across work, recreation and education. The creation and management of a therapeutic milieu has been largely adopted by nurses. Specific in-patient nursing roles have been described (Critchley 1991), which include the provision of clinical supervision to other staff, treatment planning, programme planning, being a role model in a milieu team, and conducting clinical nursing research. The school facility attached to in-patient units allows detailed assessments of educational and social functioning.

Day units

These provide a treatment facility that shares the burden with the parents in a multidisciplinary framework. They are useful when children are too young to be separated from their parents, and allow supervision and parental guidance for families.

Therapeutic community schools

Therapeutic communities such as the Cotswold and Peper Harrow, originated in the 1930s. Here meaningful personal relationships are established that enable children to develop self-control through partaking in their own social control. Therapeutic community schools were aimed at helping severely damaged children with commitment and consistency and understanding of the profound roots of a child's very disruptive and frequently violent behaviour. Work focuses on building a secure emotional base and is intensive (Winkley 1996).

Biological treatment

Drug treatments in childhood have been controversial for a number of reasons, including the potential for side-effects, ideological stances precluding physical treatments and the issue of social control. Nevertheless, there is an important place for pharmacotherapy within a holistic, and individualised framework (Campbell & Cueva 1995). Specific issues encompassing the drug treatment in specific childhood disorders will be discussed below.

Obsessive–compulsive disorder

Obsessive–compulsive disorder (OCD) and/or TS benefit from medication. For OCD, the mainstays are the tricyclic agent clomipramine and some of the specific serotonin re-uptake inhibitors (SSRIs), combined with CBT. For TS, the best-known agents are the dopamine-blocking neuroleptics (pimozide, haloperidol and sulpiride), tetrabenazine and clonidine. Individual, family and social factors are important in treatment. There is a sub-group of patients with primary neurological or other psychiatric disorders who present with full or partial 'secondary OCD' or TS. Others argue that hair-pulling, nail biting and body dysmorphic disorder should be included under an OCD spectrum.

Depressive disorders

Antidepressant medication in childhood and adolescence is indicated in cases of severe depressive symptomatology which is unresponsive to psychotherapeutic treatments, shows risk of suicidal behaviour, or is linked with serious impairment in school, social or family arenas. Despite the response of adults to these agents, studies do not demonstrate superiority over placebo in children. However, children appear to respond more to environmental factors and placebo than adults, hence further work needs to be done.

Attention-deficit–hyperactivity disorder

The stimulant drugs available in the UK and Ireland include methylphenidate, dexamphetamine and pemoline. They are well proven to decrease the core features of ADHD. Their effects are seen in normal children; response therefore does not confirm diagnosis. It is not clear whether the response to increased doses increases behavioural control at the expense of cognitive benefit. Adverse effects can occur, therefore caution and close supervision are essential. It is vital to use stimulants as an element of a broad treatment plan, incorporating psycho-educational and social perspectives, particularly in the absence of studies showing long-term benefits from medication alone.

Schizophrenia

Schizophrenia with onset in childhood has been shown to be a discrete entity, but rare in young life. There is now evidence that antipsychotics are effective in its treatment, but there is a dearth of information on long-term efficacy and safety. Older age at onset and higher IQ appear to be predictors of drug response.

Case study 17.5 Christopher

Christopher, aged 6, was referred because of disruptive behaviour, and pervasive aggression. His parents were going through a turbulent separation and he witnessed domestic violence. He had been taken out of one school and his mother was poised to repeat this when the school felt it could no longer contain his behaviour. It became obvious that Christopher was unable to concentrate, and had been restless and inattentive since infancy. He was diagnosed as being hyperkinetic or having ADHD, and after careful assessment and failure of a behavioural programme, he was begun on methylphenidate (Ritalin). Within the behavioural programme, social support and assessment of special educational needs, the medication allowed Christopher to co-operate with the treatment plan, prevented permanent exclusion, and engendered learning of appropriate behaviours. Indeed, he began to help others with their school work in the class for the first time.

CONCLUSIONS – THE FUTURE

Child mental health services and disciplines

Research on mental health problems and disorders in young life indicates a high level of need among children and adolescents (between 15 and 20%), multifactorial aetiology and complex conditions of varying severity. Their recognition and treatment require different clinical skills, according to the presentation and complexity of the problems. For this reason, a four-tier (level) model of child and adolescent mental health services has been proposed by the Health Advisory Service in the UK (1995), and this is being widely adopted as the way forward for at least the next decade. It is apparent that existing staff resources are well below those required to meet population needs, particularly in inner-city deprived areas. A co-ordinated type of service, from primary care to tertiary/specialist units would help maximise clinical efficacy, as many primary health care workers are involved in the ongoing care of young people with mental health problems, but are often unsupported and work in isolation from child and adolescent mental health services (Kurtz et al 1994). The four proposed tiers (levels) of services are discussed below.

Tier 1 is usually the first point of health care contact for children with mental health problems and their families. It consists of health professionals such as school nurses, health visitors, general practitioners, school medical officers, speech therapists, and also teachers and social workers. The implications for nursing are substantial, as school nurses and health visitors come across the whole range of child mental health problems and disorders. Aims of Tier 1 services are the recognition of mental health problems and, either (a) management by Tier 1 staff of less complex cases, for example, oppositional problems such as temper tantrums, or sleep problems in young children; (b) treatment in liaison (consultation) with local child mental health services, for example, school refusal without significant anxiety/depressive symptoms or school-related behaviour problems; or (c) referral to local child mental health services of more complex mental health problems and disorders, such as eating disorders, self-harm and depression. The latter obviously requires regular links and direct access to child mental health services, joint

strategy planning and commissioning of services.

Tier 2 includes individual child and adolescent mental health professionals. They may also be members of a local mental health service, but working at schools or health centres (e.g. psychologists, community psychiatric nurses). Designated mental health social workers, educational psychologists and 'behaviour support' teachers are professionals working for the local authority. Within child health care, Tier 2 is provided by hospital and community paediatric nursing staff and paediatricians. As they are involved in the treatment of children with somatising disorders, eating disorders, self-harm, autism and hyperactivity, regular links and formal arrangements with the local child mental health service are essential (e.g. liaison work with paediatric wards, or assessment of young people following DSH).

Tier 3 consists of specialised out-patient multidisciplinary teams for a locality (geographical area) of 100 000 to 200 000 general population. The composition of these teams varies. A comprehensive Tier 3 service consists of community psychiatric nurses, child and adolescent psychiatrists (consultants and staff grade doctors), psychologists and social workers. In many settings, there are designated child psychotherapists, while some teams include family therapists. Specialist child mental health services should be well resourced, accessible to the previous two tiers, provide the whole range of treatment rather than work on a particular model, and initiate training for Tiers 1 and 2 staff.

Tier 4 services provide treatment for specific, complex and severe disorders. They include day and in-patient units (usually 20 to 30 beds per general population of at least 1 to 2 million, i.e. a considerably lower number than in adult psychiatric hospitals) for psychotic disorders, severe eating disorders, depression not responding to out-patient treatment and neuropsychiatric disorders. More specialised services (supra-regional or national) include units for deaf children and forensic (secure) provisions for young offenders.

Nursing skills and roles within child and adolescent mental health services

General mental health nursing skills are essential for nursing staff working in child and adolescent mental health services, which emphasises the need for continuing training within the specialism. However, the differences between adult and child mental health nursing also need to be stressed. Nurses within the specialty need to be able to communicate effectively with children of all ages in a variety of ways, and then act as an advocate for the child with parents, teachers or other professionals involved. It is important to acquire knowledge and understanding of theories related to child development (from infancy to adolescence), parenting, family functioning and a variety of treatment modalities. A broad range of training and experience enables one to adopt a holistic approach within the assessment, planning, implementation and evaluation (Clunn 1991).

Specialist clinical skills include:

1. establishment of a therapeutic relationship with young people and their families
2. assessment of needs and ongoing monitoring of children, adolescents and families
3. child-centred communication and relationships
4. detection of early signs of mental health problems
5. risk assessment (mainly for adolescents with self-harm behaviour, psychosis or repeated offending)
6. development, implementation and evaluation of a care programme
7. organisation and provision of a specialist service
8. teaching
9. research.

In addition to the collaboration with members of the multidisciplinary team, there are close links with primary health care professionals, schools, social services and hospital services. Specialist treatment skills appropriate to meeting the specific needs of children, teenagers and their families include behaviour therapy, child-centred counselling, play therapy and psychodynamic psychotherapy, family therapy, cognitive therapy, psychodrama and art therapy.

Community psychiatric nurses (CPNs) are responsible for their own caseload, function as members of the multidisciplinary team, liaise with referring and other agencies (e.g. outreach clinics in general practice, education or other local authority establishments), participate in family therapy teams, assess young people who self-harm, undertake risk assessment, provide inter-agency support, and supervise ENB and RMN nursing trainees. Many CPNs are now being recognised as expert witnesses in child protection and other complex cases, although this component has received little attention so far by training programmes. McMorrow (1995) suggested that CPNs should operate essentially as eclectic therapists, but with the training and clinical supervision that ensures this is an informed eclecticism and allows 'flexibility to the client's needs'.

Nursing staff working at *child and adolescent in-patient psychiatric units* have multiple roles in providing general nursing care, support and therapeutic work to young people (behaviour therapy, psychotherapy, group therapy, cognitive therapy, psychodrama) (Wilkinson 1983). They also offer support, advice to parents and family therapy. These roles can be conflicting. For example, a member of nursing staff may be the therapist for an adolescent with anorexia nervosa, and at the same time supervise the eating programme (calorific intake), which is obviously unpopular and distressing for the young person.

Future directions for research, training and service development

The last few years have seen a rise in the national and international profile of child mental health issues within the health service, local authorities and the general public. This is likely to continue in the foreseeable future. Child and adolescent mental health has been established as a specialty in its own right, despite its historical origins in paediatrics and adult psychiatry. Advances in the understanding of mental illness, as well as in children's rights and their position in society, have alleviated many fears on the concept of mental health in young life. This has been a catalyst for the rapid development of child and adolescent mental health services.

This expansion has also highlighted weaknesses in a field influenced by diverse theoretical models, which have not always been supported by research evidence. Population needs and broader changes in health care provision require better co-ordinated and more accessible child and adolescent mental health services, with comprehensive treatment provision and multiskilled staff. These requirements will be reflected in future research and development of training programmes.

Research in child mental health will include the evaluation of (a) diagnostic and outcome measures, (b) specific treatment modalities for different mental health disorders and (c) service models, particularly in relation to the described four-tier system. Advances in molecular biology, genetics and biochemistry are likely to have an impact on the understanding of the aetiology of autism and other pervasive developmental disorders, attention-deficit–hyperactivity disorders and depression in young life. There will also be increasing research in transcultural aspects of child psychopathology and treatment.

The importance of recognising and treating mental health problems in early life will have an effect on undergraduate and postgraduate training of health care professionals working with children, particularly nursing staff. There should be minimum teaching requirements for child development and child mental health in undergraduate nursing curriculums, with the parallel development of academic nursing posts in this field. Nationally recognised training necessary for nurses who wish to specialise in child mental health (currently ENB603 in the UK) will be complemented by post-ENB603 training on specific therapeutic approaches (e.g. individual psychotherapy, family therapy, CBT). Postgraduate training should be adapted to clinical needs of paediatric nurses, health visitors and school nurses, with increasing opportunities for different level (Diploma, Masters) courses in child and adolescent mental health. Community psychiatric nursing for children and families will continue to be the single most rapidly expanding discipline within the child mental health team, and will be critical for the successful establishment of links between traditional child mental health services, primary health care, schools and other local authority agencies.

Acknowledgement

We are grateful to Mrs Sandy Fitzgibbon for her advice and information.

Exercise

Consider a child from your existing caseload:
- What kind of mental health problems does this child have?
- Why have these problems developed?
- Consider the question 'Why now?'
- What risk and resilience factors are relevant to their presentation?
- What is the necessary treatment or management?

KEY TEXTS FOR FURTHER READING

Barker P 1995 Basic child psychiatry, 6th edn. Blackwell, Oxford

Graham P 1994 Child psychiatry: a developmental approach, 2nd edn. Oxford University Press, Oxford

Johnson B H 1995 Child, adolescent and family psychiatric nursing. Lippincott, Philadelphia

Rutter M, Taylor E, Hersov L (eds) 1994 Child and adolescent psychiatry: modern approaches, 4th edn. Blackwell Scientific, Oxford

Wilkinson T R 1983 Child and adolescent psychiatric nursing. Blackwell, Oxford

---

REFERENCES

American Psychiatric Association 1994 Diagnostic and statistical manual of mental disorders, 4th edn. American Psychiatric Association, Washington DC

Barnett R J, Docherty J, Frommelt G 1991 A review of child psychotherapy research since 1963. Journal of the American Academy of Child and Adolescent Psychiatry 30:1–14

Beck A 1972 Depression: causes and treatment. University of Pennsylvania Press, Philadelphia

Birtchnell J 1980 Women whose mothers die in childhood: an outcome study. Psychological Medicine 10:699–713

Bloch S, Hafner J, Harari E, Szmuckler G 1995 The family in clinical psychiatry. Oxford University Press, Oxford

Bolton P 1996 Genetic advances and their implications for child psychiatry. Child Psychology and Psychiatry Review 1(3):82

Campbell M, Cueva J 1995 Psychopharmacology in child and adolescent psychiatry: a review of the past seven years. Parts I and II. Journal of the American Academy of Child and Adolescent Psychiatry 34(9):1124–1132; 10:1262–1272

Clunn P (ed) 1991 Child psychiatric nursing. Mosby Year Book, St Louis

Cosentino C, Meyer-Bahlburg H, Alpert J, Weinberg S, Gaines R 1995 Sexual behaviour, problems and psychopathology: symptoms in sexually abused girls. Journal of the American Academy of Child and Adolescent Psychiatry 34:1033

Critchley D 1991 Nursing's contributions to a psychiatric in-patient treatment milieu for children and adolescents. In: Hendren R, Berlin I (eds) Psychiatric in-patient care of children and adolescents: A multicultural approach. Wiley-Interscience, New York, ch 15

Edelstyn N, Oyebode F, Riddoch M, Soppitt R, Moselhy H, George M 1997 A neuropsychological perspective on three schizophrenic patients with midline structural defects.

British Journal of Psychiatry 170:416–421

Faull C, Nicol A 1986 Abdominal pain in six year olds: an epidemiological study in a new town. Journal of Child Psychology and Psychiatry 27:251–260

Fombonne E 1994 The Chartres study: I. Prevalence of psychiatric disorders among French school-aged children. British Journal of Psychiatry 164:69–79

Garmezy N, Masten A 1994 Chronic adversities. In: Rutter M, Taylor E, Hersov L (eds) Child and adolescent psychiatry: modern approaches, 4th edn. Blackwell Scientific, Oxford, ch 12, p 192

Garralda M 1996 Somatisation in children. Journal of Child Psychology and Psychiatry 37:13–33

Glaser D 1991 Treatment issues in child sexual abuse. British Journal of Psychiatry 159:769–782

Goodman R 1990 Technical note: are perinatal complications causes or consequences of autism? Journal of Child Psychology and Psychiatry 31:809–812

Harrington R, Fudge H, Rutter M, Bredenkamp D, Groothues C, Pridham J 1993 Child and adult depression: a test of continuities with data from a family study. British Journal of Psychiatry 162:627–633

Health Advisory Service 1995 Child and adolescent mental health services: together we stand. HMSO, London

Hetherington E M, Cox M, Cox R 1985 Long-term effects of divorce and remarriage on the adjustment of children. Journal of the American Academy of Child and Adolescent Psychiatry 24(5):518–530

Kent L, Vostanis P, Feehan C 1997 Detection of major and minor depression in children and adolescents. Journal of Child Psychology and Psychiatry 38:565–573

Kolvin I, Miller F, Fleeting M, Kolvin P (1988) Social and parenting factors affecting criminal offence rates (findings from the Newcastle Thousand Families Study, 1947–1980). British Journal of Psychiatry 152:80–90

REFERENCES (*contd*)

Kurtz Z, Thornes R, Wolkind S 1994 Services for the mental health of children and young people in England: a national review. South Thames RHA, London

McMorrow R 1995 An eclectic model of care. Child Health 3:95–98

Oaklander V 1988 Windows to our children: a Gestalt therapy approach to children and adolescents. The Gestalt Journal Press, New York

Offord D, Boyle M, Szatmari P et al 1987 Ontario child health study: six-month prevalence of disorder and rates of service utilization. Archives of General Psychiatry 44:832–836

Orr J 1991 Piaget's theory of cognitive development may be useful in deciding what to teach and how to teach it. Nurse Education Today 11:65–69

Peplau H 1952 Interpersonal relations in nursing. Putnam, New York

Prosser J, McArdle P 1996 The changing mental health of children and adolescents: evidence for a deterioration? Psychological Medicine 26:715–725

Quinton D, Rutter M, Gulliver L 1990 Continuities in psychiatric disorders from childhood to adulthood in the children of psychiatric patients. In: Robins L, Rutter M (eds) Straight and devious pathways from childhood to adulthood. Cambridge University Press, Cambridge, ch 14, p 259–278

Reinecke M, Dattilio F, Freeman A 1996 Cognitive therapy with children and adolescents: a casebook for clinical practice. Guilford Press, New York

Richman N, Lansdown R 1988 Problems of preschool children. Wiley, Chichester

Roberts C 1991 Schizophrenia: a neuropathological perspective. British Journal of Psychiatry 158:8–17

Rutter M 1973 Why are London children so disturbed? Proceedings of the Royal Society of Medicine 66:1221–1225

Rutter M 1985 Resilience in the face of adversity: protective factors and resistance to psychiatric disorder. British Journal of Psychiatry 147:598–611

Rutter M 1989 Isle of Wight revisited: twenty-five years of child psychiatric epidemiology. Journal of the American Academy of Child and Adolescent Psychiatry 28:633–653

Rutter M, Tizard J, Yule W, Graham P, Whitmore K 1976 Isle of Wight studies, 1964–1974. Psychological Medicine 6:313–332

Skuse D, Bentovim A 1994 In: Rutter M, Taylor E, Hersov L (eds) Child and adolescent psychiatry: modern approaches, 4th edn. Blackwell Scientific, Oxford, ch 13

Thomas A, Chess S 1977 Temperament and development. Brunner/Mazel, New York

Thompson A, Kaplan C 1996 Childhood emotional abuse. British Journal of Psychiatry 168:143–148

Thompson M, Stevenson J, Sonuga-Barke E et al 1996 Mental health of preschool children and their mothers: I. Prevalence and ecological factors. British Journal of Psychiatry 168:16–20

Vostanis P, Harrington R 1994 Cognitive–behavioural treatment of depressive disorder in child psychiatric patients: rationale and description of a treatment package. European Child and Adolescent Psychiatry 3:111–123

Vostanis P, Nicholls J 1995 Nine-month changes of maternal expressed emotion in conduct and emotional disorders of childhood. Journal of Child Psychology and Psychiatry 36:833–846

Vostanis P, Feehan C, Grattan E, Bickerton W L 1996 A randomised controlled out-patient trial of cognitive–behavioural treatment for children and adolescents with depression. Journal of Affective Disorders 40:105–116

Wallerstein J 1991 The long-term effects of divorce on children: a review. Journal of the American Academy of Child and Adolescent Psychiatry 30:349–360

Werner E 1996 Vulnerable but invincible: high risk children from birth to adulthood. European Child and Adolescent Psychiatry 5(Suppl 1):47–51

Wilkinson T R 1983 Child and adolescent psychiatric nursing. Blackwell, Oxford

Winkley L 1996 Emotional problems in children and young people. Cassell, London, ch 1, p 21

World Health Organization 1992 The ICD-10 classification of mental and behavioural disorders. World Health Organization, Geneva

World Health Organization 1996 Multi axial classification of child and adolescent psychiatric disorders. Cambridge University Press, Cambridge

18

Mental disorders of older people

Peter Ashton   John Keady

CHAPTER CONTENTS

Key points   341

Introduction   342

Depression   342
Characteristics and prevalence   342
Assessment and interventions   344

Anxiety disorders   346
Characteristics and prevalence   346
Assessment and interventions   348

**Schizophrenia, paraphrenia and paranoia in old
age   349**
Characteristics and prevalence   349
Assessment and interventions   350

Alcohol misuse   351
Characteristics and prevalence   351
Assessment and interventions   352

Dementia   354
Historical and contemporary context   354
Prevalence of dementia   356
Policy and practice considerations   357
Dementia – impact on families   359
Family care – supportive interventions   361
The person with dementia   361
A basis for practice   363
Dementia care nursing – reflections and directions
363

Conclusion   364

Exercise   364

Key texts for further reading   365

References   365

KEY POINTS

- While mental health problems may be complicated by age-related factors, age in itself should not be seen as a barrier to the treatment of older people.

- Depression is the most commonly occurring mental health problem in old age.

- The risk of suicide increases with age, with men aged 75 and over being particularly vulnerable.

- Carers of people with dementia are more likely than other care-giving groups to experience emotional health problems such as stress, tiredness and depression.

- People with the early signs of dementia are able to verbalise and communicate their experiences.

- The nursing role in the assessment and treatment of older people with mental health problems needs to be more fully developed.

INTRODUCTION

The aim of this chapter is to provide an insight and understanding into five of the most common mental health needs experienced in old age. The chapter, therefore, will provide an overview of depression, anxiety disorders, psychosis in later-life, alcohol misuse and dementia, with attention being targeted primarily upon the twin towers of depression and dementia. Evidence will be reviewed relating to the nature and prevalence of each condition, as will approaches to intervention. However, it needs to be emphasised at this point that this is not a 'how to' chapter, rather it is a critical appraisal of the challenges and opportunities that exist in working with older people with mental health needs and their families. A separate reading list at the end of the chapter points the reader towards a more skills-based approach to a selection of the therapies mentioned in the text.

As we have already identified, the aim of this chapter is to provide an insight and understanding into five of the most common mental health needs experienced in old age. However, making a firm distinction between being an adult and being an older person is fraught with difficulties. At what age does a person become old? If, following a socially constructed approach to ageing, society considers old to be in receipt of the state pension (presently 60 years for women and 65 years for men, but subject to equality in the near future), then there is the possibility of a spread of some 30 years between these ages and old-old age when a person enters the ninth decade of life. Within this time-span, different generations will be encountered who will have quite distinct, and separate, views on what constitutes health and illness. Indeed, many older people in their 60s provide daily care not only for their partner, but also for their frail, older parent(s) (Wenger 1994).

Moreover, there is an urgent need to avoid the trap of adopting negative attitudes towards older people, and upholding a belief that social withdrawal and loneliness are inevitable consequences of ageing. While mental health problems may be complicated by age-related factors, age itself should not be seen as a barrier to the treatment of older people (Emery 1981). Indeed, the very existence of a separate chapter on mental health and old age within this text could, in itself, be a reinforcement of the segregation of older people within the general context of mental health practice and service delivery. In our opinion this would be an unfortunate outcome, as older people have the same underlying mental health needs as the remainder of the population; they are, we believe, simply expressed differently.

We will now turn our attention to an overview of five of the most common mental health problems in old age.

DEPRESSION

Characteristics and prevalence

While most people successfully adapt to the shifting circumstances of old age, a significant proportion experiences the signs and symptoms of depression. In fact, depression is now the most common mental health problem experienced by older people (Banerjee et 1996) with Murphy & Grundy (1984) reporting that as many as 40% of all new referrals to their psychiatric service for older people were found to have depression. Moreover, of those aged 65 to 75 years who present to psychiatrists, depression has long been reported as the most common diagnosis (Post 1982). For instance, in a community survey by Lindesay et (1989) of approximately 1000 older people in an urban area, 4.3% were identified as suffering from severe depression, with a further

13.5% experiencing depression to a mild to moderate degree.

Intuition may lead us to believe that dementia is by far the most common mental health problem in old age, but four extensive community surveys on the prevalence of mental illness within older people have shown that depression outranks dementia by a factor of three to one (Copeland et al 1987, Livingstone et al 1990). However, accurate estimates of the prevalence of depression can be problematic as different instruments and criteria are used to screen, measure and classify its existence. Despite these complications, estimates of the prevalence of depression in an older population are seen to range from 1 to 3% (Newmann 1989) to 45% (Koenig et al 1988). However, accepting these figures at face value is a little misleading as they represent studies which have used either different diagnostic criteria, or looked at subjects in different settings. For example, Newmann's (1989) figures refer to older people suffering from major depressive disorder, whereas Koenig et al (1988) refer to the frequency of depressive disorder in medical patients. Alongside these studies there have been a number of others which have produced quite different estimates of prevalence, for example:

- Banerjee (1993) found evidence of depression in 26% of people receiving home care services from a local authority social services department
- MacDonald (1986) identified the existence of depression in 31% of all older people attending their general practitioner
- Pitt (1991) reported a prevalence rate of depression of between 5 and 40% in 'geriatric' in-patient populations
- Ames (1991) identified a figure of 40% in a UK study of older people living in residential homes

- Copeland et al (1987) suggested that between 10 and 20% of all people aged 65 and over suffer from clinically significant depression, and that this figure is substantially higher for women.

Furthermore, depression has also been found to be very common among people diagnosed with Alzheimer's disease (AD), and it has been suggested that as many as 30% of people with AD have a co-existing major depressive disorder (Teri & Wagner 1991, Wragg & Jeste 1989).

Depression can be classified in a number of ways. Generally, the diagnosis of clinical depression is based on either the International Statistical Classification of Diseases and Related Health Problems (ICD-10) (World Health Organization (WHO) 1993a) or the Diagnostic and Statistical

---

Box 18.1   Main characteristics of depression

- The person reports or is observed having depressed mood most of the day, nearly every day.
- Generally, the person describes feeling sad, empty or 'down in the dumps'.
- Loss of interest and pleasure in normal everyday and social activities. The person starts to withdraw from participating in activities, stating that there is no longer any enjoyment from the activities, or it is too much effort to participate.
- The person reports having disturbed sleep which can include waking in the night, difficulty getting off to sleep or early morning rising.
- Reduced energy, resulting in complaints of fatigue and reduced levels of activity.
- Appetite can also be affected. Some people state that they are not as hungry or can no longer be bothered to cook their normal meals. Prolonged disturbance of appetite can lead to weight loss and a further loss of energy.
- Loss of concentration and attention, leading to lower levels of awareness and impaired judgement.
- Pessimistic views of self and the future. People may express distorted beliefs about themselves, often blaming themselves for negative aspects of their lives. Ideas of guilt and worthlessness are often expressed, as are beliefs that there is no future or prospects of things improving.

Sources: ICD-10 (WHO 1993a) and DSM-IV (American Psychiatric Association 1994)

Manual of Mental Disorders (DSM-IV) (American Psychiatric Association 1994). As Box 18.1 reveals within both these texts, evidence of depression is confirmed by the persistent existence of a number of core characteristics.

The intensity and combination of these beliefs can have serious consequences in terms of suicidal ideation, with people experiencing a strong sense of helplessness and hopelessness and being more at risk of self-harm and suicide. Set against the remainder of the population, suicide rates are higher amongst older people, particularly males aged 75 years and over (Clarke & Fawcett 1992, Murphy 1988). Indeed, in 1990, the suicide rate for those aged 65 and over was 50% higher than the average for the population as a whole (Millar 1992). While not all people who commit suicide are clinically depressed, an earlier study by Barraclough et al (1974) found that there was a diagnosis of depressive illness in 87% of suicides they examined. In a more recent study, in which Cattell & Jolley (1995) examined 100 cases of suicide in Manchester, they found that 61% of successful suicides had a clinically recognisable depressive illness.

In addition to these core characteristics, depression in older people has been found to include:

- increased levels of anxiety, agitation and hypochondriasis (Gurland 1976)
- delusions (Meyers & Greenberg 1986)
- the existence of physical disease (Murphy 1982).

There also seems to be a strong association with loss events, poverty and social isolation (Katona 1994), with depression being more common in women (Copeland et al 1987). Moreover, depression appears to have a poorer prognosis than in younger people, a finding that is reflected within the high rates of persistence and recurrence (Cole 1990). For example, Musetti et al (1989) found that previous episodes of depression in older people were as high as 67%, while mortality rates have also been found to be higher (Murphy 1983). However, as Benbow (1992) pointed out, these issues may well have been influenced by inappropriate, or non-existent, treatment and management regimens.

Assessment and interventions

These characteristics highlight that depression is a multidimensional condition which impacts upon the physical, psychological and social aspects of a person's life. Furthermore, the symptoms can have a detrimental effect upon family support systems, such as spouses, relatives and friends. It is also important to recognise that these symptoms exist within a continuum which ranges from mild to severe intensity. While a person would need to be at the severe end to be diagnosed as suffering from a clinical depression, people not reaching this level still experience significant difficulties in their lives. Unfortunately, many older people with depression, both severe and less severe, are not diagnosed (Blanchard & Mann 1994) or not identified (Iliffe et al 1993). This is of particular concern given the higher risk of suicide within the older population (Diekstra 1989).

Accurate and comprehensive assessment is the essential foundation for the effective treatment of depression, and an act which sits at the heart of the professional nursing response (Keady & Ford 1997). Furthermore, its importance has further significance given the higher risk of suicide in the older population. While the ideal place to conduct an assessment may be the person's own home (Warner 1996), assessments carried out elsewhere can be equally effective if they take into account the different dimensions of depression and the person's biographical history. A comprehensive assessment should also consider physical, psychological and social factors. When conducting an assessment it is also important to identify the personal impact and meaning that the reported symptoms have for the person concerned, and the efficacy of the coping strategies being used.

This approach to assessment can be achieved in a number of ways. For example, there are a number of different self-report assessment tools which can be used. The Beck Depression Inventory (BDI) and the Schwab–Gilleard Depression Scale have been shown to provide a valid and reliable measure of depressive symptoms in older people (Gallagher et al 1982, Richardson & Hammond 1996). Furthermore, the BDI is easy to use and can be re-used during the course of treatment to evaluate its effectiveness. Information should also be sought through the use of interviews with the person and, wherever practicable, with the person's spouse or relative(s). The skilful use of interviews not only provides an important insight into the person's world, but also helps to establish a therapeutic relationship which has a pivotal role in the intervention phase. Interviews with relatives or significant others provide an additional source of information which helps to establish an accurate picture of the older person and the person's biographical history. Observational information can also be sought as it makes a vital contribution to the assessment process.

For interventions to be effective, they need to be targeted at the specific symptoms and identified problems within the physical, psychological and social domains. Given that depression usually affects all three domains, interventions need to reflect this position. Generally speaking, interventions are most likely to be successful when a combination of approaches are used, such as pharmacotherapy, psychotherapy and social support. The combined use of these different approaches should not only enhance intervention effectiveness, but also help to prevent relapse. We will now review the efficacy of each of these different approaches to intervention.

Pharmacotherapy

Traditionally, the treatment of depression in older people has been via the use of pharmacotherapy (Larson et al 1991, Shepherd et al 1981) although the use of medication has produced mixed results. On the one hand, Georgotas et al (1986) found that between 30 and 40% of individuals with major depressive disorder did not achieve a satisfactory improvement from initial treatment with antidepressants. On the other hand, these findings suggest that up to 60% of people suffering from moderate to severe depression experience a significant improvement in their mental state with the use of antidepressants (see also Benbow 1992, Menon & Jacoby 1993).

Whichever way these figures are taken, considerable room for improvement remains. For instance, there is some evidence to suggest that antidepressants could be more effective if adequate doses were prescribed, or the medication was taken for a longer duration (Keller et al 1986). Richter et al (1983) also suggested that many older people are prescribed sub-therapeutic doses of antidepressants because of the increased risk of side-effects. Moreover, because older people are more vulnerable to side-effects, there is a heightened risk of non-compliance. In both situations, mental health nurses have a key role to play. Older people taking antidepressant medication need to be educated about their possible side-effects, and that the benefits of this treatment can often arise after the side-effects have subsided. Mental health nurses also need to be vigilant in their observation of possible side-effects, and in helping older people with depression to maintain their physical health status. Some older people with depression may require prompting, support and advice in areas such as diet, exercise, sleep and personal care. Indeed, neglect of these important aspects of everyday life may cause further complications and impede any recovery.

Physical treatments

While the use of electroconvulsive therapy (ECT) is now less common, recovery rates from its use appear encouraging, particularly in cases of endogenous depression (Benbow 1987, Fraser & Glass 1980). In a review of the use of ECT in the treatment of depression in old age, Benbow (1989) concluded that older people respond to ECT at least as well as younger people, if not better. Furthermore, Kendell (1981) suggested that old age should not be seen as a contra-indication to ECT because frail people in their 80s and 90s can tolerate ECT very well. It would appear that age on its own is not a barrier to the use of ECT, but rather, on moral as well as medical grounds, whether its use is more appropriate than other forms of intervention.

Psychosocial interventions

Although physical treatments have their place in the treatment of depression in older people, existing medical conditions, increased risk of side-effects and/or concurrent drug therapy may limit their use (Cohen-Cole & Stoudemire 1987). Consequently, medication can play only a limited role in reversing the psychological and social dysfunction that features in depression. Indeed, dysfunctional cognitions, bereavement reactions, social isolation and self-care difficulties need more than medication to effect a positive change.

In a meta-analysis of 17 controlled psychosocial treatment studies involving older people with depression, such interventions were shown to be highly effective (Scogin & McElreath 1994).

Hinrichsen (1992) also suggested that the successful resolution of family and interpersonal factors was the best longitudinal predictor of recovery and relapse from depression. In a comparative study of behavioural, cognitive and brief psychodynamic psychotherapy, Thompson et al (1987) found that all three therapies produced positive outcomes for older people. Moreover, these forms of psychotherapy have been reported to be effective for both endogenous and non-endogenous depressions (Gallagher & Thompson 1983). In studies examining the efficacy of cognitive–behaviour therapy (CBT), both individual and group approaches have been shown to be effective (Leung & Orrell 1993, Thompson & Gallagher 1984), with the literature indicating that CBT produces better long-term effects (Thompson et al 1987). We would contend that this outcome is probably due to the psycho-educational components of this type of therapy, with Yost et al (1986) further suggesting that the high degree of structure in CBT appeals to the compliance of older people to a specified treatment regimen.

In addition to the use of more structured psychotherapy, many older people with depression may benefit from help with their home and social situations. Loss of significant others, social isolation and deteriorating physical health can play a major role in the development and maintenance of depression. In these circumstances it is imperative that mental health nurses carefully assess the impact of these factors upon the older person, and seek ways of helping individuals to adjust to their circumstances.

ANXIETY DISORDERS

Characteristics and prevalence

Anxiety can be seen as a normal reaction to life's uncertainties and dangers, such as ill-health and crime. However, as in adult life, excessive anxiety in old age can cause significant distress and dysfunction for some people, in which the quality of life is diminished and the ability to function normally severely affected. Research into the existence and characteristics of anxiety in old age has, however, been problematic. For instance, at the turn of this decade, Hersen & Van Hasselt (1992) suggested that existing research in this area had a significant number of weaknesses, including:

- absence of structured diagnostic procedures
- use of assessment instruments with unknown psychometric properties
- use of community and medical populations in lieu of samples receiving clinical diagnosis.

Furthermore, a review of the literature indicates that there are, at present, too few studies examining the specific characteristics and treatment of anxiety disorders in old age. As with the younger population, anxiety in older people can manifest itself in a variety of ways, although for the purpose of this text we will focus upon the two disorders which have been identified as being the most common, namely:

1. generalised anxiety disorder (GAD)
2. phobic disorders.

Generalised anxiety disorder

This is characterised by excessive and persistent generalised anxiety and worry, accompanied by autonomic symptoms, apprehension, tension, hypervigilance and often depression. The presentation of GAD in later life appears similar to that identified in younger people (Beck et al 1996), with sufferers presenting with elevated anxiety, worry, social fears and depression. The focus of these symptoms is the existence of danger-related thoughts from which those experiencing the condition make an overestimation of the danger(s), and underestimate their ability to cope with them. Once the threat appraisals (cognitions) are activated, a vicious cycle of anxiety begins with danger-related thoughts leading to the development of unpleasant physical symptoms, and the subsequent use of behaviours to minimise the anxiety. These behaviours, however, often produce dysfunctional consequences, resulting in further problems and fears. For example, people with excessive worries about health may make frequent visits to their GP and end up with unnecessary investigations and medication.

Phobic disorders

Phobic disorders are characterised by the persistent and irrational fear of a situation, activity or object which results in a compelling desire to avoid the phobic stimulus. There are generally considered to be three main types of phobias:

1. Agoraphobia. The essential feature of agoraphobia is a marked fear of being alone, or being in a public place from which escape may be difficult, or help not available in the case of sudden incapacitation.

2. Social phobia. In social phobia, the individual experiences significant anticipatory anxiety in response to a fear of being humiliated, criticised or embarrassed in public situations. Frequently, people experiencing phobic disorders utilise avoidance as a coping strategy.

3. Specific phobias. Specific phobias refer to excessive anxiety in response to a specific object or situation, such as those presented by spiders or heights.

Whatever the type of phobia, the fear is recurrent, intense and perceived as beyond the person's control. Furthermore, people experiencing phobia frequently attempt to control and cope with their anxiety through the use of dysfunctional behaviours. For older people, this phenomenon was illustrated in a study by Lindesay (1991a) who demonstrated that as many of 30% of the people in their sample developed their fears after the age of 65, with agoraphobia, accompanied by severe social impairment, being the most common. In this instance it was found that the majority of older people developed their fear following a physical illness, or similar traumatic event. Of more concern, only a minority of the older people in the study who experienced a phobic disorder were receiving any form of appropriate psychological help.

While the presentation of anxiety disorders appears to fall with increasing age (Office of Population Census and Surveys (OPCS) 1983, 1986), there is evidence to suggest that they still affect a significant number of older people. For example, in a community survey carried out by Manela et al (1996) which involved 700 people aged 65 years and over, a total of 105 (15%) of the sample fulfilled the ICD-10 (WHO 1993a) diagnostic criteria for anxiety disorders. More specifically, 12% were found to have a phobic disorder and 4.7% to have GAD; of those with phobic disorders, 7.9% had agoraphobia and 5.9% had a specific phobia. These figures appear consistent with the findings of a much earlier study by Watts et al (1964) who identified a 10% overall level of anxiety within the older population. This study also reported that 91% of the subjects who had GAD also had a diagnosis of depression, which emphasises the high rate of comorbidity with depression. Furthermore, Ballard et al (1996) have also reported that anxiety is often present in people with dementia.

Assessment and interventions

Generally speaking, the assessment procedures and interventions used for anxiety disorders in older people are the same as those provided for younger adults. Assessment needs to identify the nature of the problem(s), what appears to be their cause, what maintains them and what outcomes are desired. The assessment process provides the opportunity and framework for both the mental health nurse and the older person to mutually explore the reality of the situation, and to develop an insight into current difficulties. To facilitate this process, the mental health nurse needs to develop a therapeutic relationship, and make good use of observational and interviewing skills. Additional information can also be obtained from significant others, and through the use of psychometric assessment instruments. In this capacity, a study by Stanley et al (1996b) found that the Spielberger State-Trait Anxiety Inventory, Worry Scale, Fear Questionnaire and the Padua Inventory were instruments that had good utility. Furthermore, the Beck Anxiety Inventory is an easy-to-use, self-report assessment tool which could be simply incorporated into the practice setting.

Interventions for older people experiencing an anxiety disorder usually consist of pharmacotherapy, anxiety-management techniques and psychotherapy, or a combination of all three approaches. However, as older people seeking help for a reduction in their levels of anxiety are initially assessed by their GP, it is, perhaps, no surprise to learn that the prescription of benzodiazepines is the first treatment of choice. Indeed, Salzman (1990) reported that between 17 and 50% of all older people who attended for consultancy have received prescriptions for minor tranquillisers, and it is only when the older person is referred to a specialist service that psychotherapy becomes available. Not surprisingly, Lindesay (1991b) suggested that this is not an ideal situation since psychological treatment approaches can be safer and provide more durable, long-term benefits.

From a psychological perspective, anxiety-management techniques can make a useful contribution (Woods & Britton 1985) and be safely carried out by mental health nurses. The use of relaxation tapes, breathing exercises, distraction and education on anxiety can help anxious older people to reduce and control their levels of anxiety. Rickard et al (1994) demonstrated that relaxation training had a considerable impact on reducing the level of subjective anxiety experienced by 25 older people who completed a set relaxation programme. These effects could have been further enhanced through the use of CBT. King & Barrowclough (1991) have provided some encouraging results from the use of CBT with older anxious people. In this study, the authors used CBT with 10 older people who had a diagnosis of either GAD (two); panic disorder (five); or a combination of both conditions (three). Following the commencement and evaluation of the efficacy of CBT with this client group, all but one older person in the study showed a reduction in symptoms, and these improvements were generally maintained at 3- and 6-month follow-up. Furthermore, eight of the study sample reported no recurrence of symptoms after a period of 6 months after completion of the study. These encouraging findings from individual CBT therapy are complemented by some equally positive results from the use of group CBT (Stanley et al 1996a).

It would appear that the use of CBT has particular merit in helping anxious older people to become more aware of their dysfunctional thinking, keep their anxieties in perspective and develop compensatory coping strategies. Moreover, increasing the availability of social support may also help to improve the older person's ability to manage the anxiety. A relatively straightforward intervention of promoting social contact with a close friend or neighbour may help an older person with high levels of anxiety to keep current worries in perspective, and reduce some uncertainty over the future.

SCHIZOPHRENIA, PARAPHRENIA AND PARANOIA IN OLD AGE

Characteristics and prevalence

Functional psychosis in old age can be seen to fall into two main categories. The first refers to people who have suffered from schizophrenia during adulthood and into old age. The second consists of older people whose first experience of functional psychosis occurs in old age. However, the classification and diagnosis of functional psychosis developed in old age appear to be the subject of much debate. For instance, do late-onset schizophrenia, paraphrenia and paranoia exist as separate entities, or are they versions of the same phenomenon? (For a discussion, see Flint et al 1991.)

Almeida et al (1994) state that the term 'paraphrenia' was first used by Emil Kraepelin in 1919 to describe a group of 'paranoid patients' with marked delusions and hallucinations in whom affect, will and personality continued to be preserved. During the middle part of this century, both Roth & Morrissey (1952) and Kay & Roth (1961) have suggested that this descriptor should be changed to 'late paraphrenia'; this, they contended, more appropriately described the situation of older people who presented with a well-organised system of paranoid delusions and hallucinations, and who had well-preserved personality and affect. However, Grahame (1984) takes an opposing viewpoint, suggesting that 'late paraphrenia' is simply a form of late-onset schizophrenia and that 'paraphrenic older patients' eventually develop clinical features similar to those of schizophrenia; in this scenario, paraphrenia is considered a manifestation of schizophrenia occurring in old age. Confusingly, there is also some uncertainty over the use of the terms 'paranoia' and 'paranoid'. These terms have been used interchangeably as a diagnostic label, a description for symptoms and as an illustration of personality type. Moreover, the classification of functional psychosis has been complicated by the exclusion of 'paraphrenia' from the ICD-10 diagnostic criteria for research (WHO 1993a).

Given the ongoing debate over the inclusiveness of diagnostic criteria, estimates of prevalence are, inevitably, problematic. The lack of social support and experience of isolation that is often a feature of older people with a functional psychosis, further complicate the picture. Nevertheless, in studies using the diagnosis 'paraphrenia', Howard (1993) suggested a prevalence rate of between 1 and 2%, whereas Holden (1987) estimated the annual incidence of paraphrenia to involve 17 to 26 older people per 100 000 of the population. These figures, of course, do not take into account the number of older people who developed schizophrenia at a younger age. Gurland & Cross (1982) suggested that 90% of the estimated 300 000 older people in the USA with schizophrenia developed the disorder before the age of 45. Conversely, this also suggests that a significant number of older people with enduring functional psychosis are present within the population, with the profile of this group increasing given future demographic trends (Coleman et al 1993).

While this suggests there are significant numbers of older people who have had schizophrenia from early adulthood, the characteristics, treatment and management can, again, be seen as being very similar to that provided for younger people. Most older people with younger onset schizophrenia will already be known to the service, and receiving an ongoing package of care. Consequently, the remainder of this section will consider those older people who have developed a functional disorder *for the first time* in old age.

Despite the previously outlined problems of classification, a study by Almeida et al (1995) sug-gested that 'late paraphrenia' presents with the following characteristics:

- a well-organised, paranoid, delusional system in which the most frequent delusions involved ideas of persecution and reference – complaints of neighbours being implicated in plots to harm or interfere with the person were frequently cited occurrences; the beliefs can also have a sexual nature
- the existence of hallucinations, which are often of an auditory and visual type
- an absence of thought disorder
- gender bias – 'late paraphrenia' appears to be more common in women, particularly amongst single women living alone
- negative symptoms such as apathy, inappropriate affect, withdrawn behaviour, poor motivation, decreased activity and reduced interests were not usually observed; where there are reports of reduced social activity, this can be seen as a natural response to the existence of persecutory beliefs.

Assessment and interventions

Once a diagnosis has been established, the purpose of the assessment is to identify the specific problems and difficulties the older person is experiencing. Problems often relate to how the person reacts to the delusions and hallucinations, and it is not uncommon to discover that the older person has problems relating to other people, such as neighbours, friends or relatives. People with 'late paraphrenia' may well be abusive to others in their attempt to deal with their dysfunctional beliefs and perceptions, and be so anxious about the nature of their persecutory beliefs that it interferes with their ability to carry out everyday living activities. Moreover, the older person may become more withdrawn and solitary and find contact with people difficult. The combination of these factors may well result in distress and a diminished quality of life and requires careful and skilled handling.

Interventions need to be targeted at both the disorder itself and its consequences. However, progress with interventions will largely be influenced by the nature of the therapeutic relationship. The tendency to be suspicious or even hostile towards other people makes the development of a trusting relationship a significant challenge. It is, therefore, important for mental health nurses to invest heavily in developing a good relationship with the person in their care, as the relationship will play a pivotal role in encouraging the older person to engage in any agreed intervention programme.

Older people suffering from paraphrenia also appear to respond well to both oral and depot medication. To this end, Howard & Levy (1992) suggested that the use of depot injections administered by a mental health nurse appears to be the most effective strategy for reducing symptoms. Furthermore, in such a situation, it is not hard to imagine that the mental health nurse working in the community becomes one of the most significant people in the older person's life. There is also a need for close monitoring and frequent communication with the GP so that the optimal dose of medication can be achieved with minimal side-effects. Generally, medication should be introduced at lower doses and gradually increased once tolerance is established. Although the efficacy of psychosocial interventions with older people with functional psychosis has yet to be established, interventions based upon these techniques should be considered, where appropriate. The psycho-educational element of this therapy may prove extremely useful, particularly with relatives or carers.

Carstensen & Fremouw (1981) have also noted that behavioural interventions can be successfully deployed to reduce the level of paranoid speech. Moreover, the re-integration of the older person back into the social environment can be progressed further once the medication starts to have an impact upon the psychotic symptoms. The use of community facilities and day centres can be helpful here, as can the support of close friends, relatives and support workers.

ALCOHOL MISUSE

Characteristics and prevalence

While alcohol misuse has long been recognised as a health problem within society, relatively little consideration has been given to its presence and treatment in older people. Until recently, little has been known about the extent and nature of alcohol misuse in older people. Recent research would indicate that alcohol misuse in older people constitutes a health problem of moderate proportions (Atkinson 1990), and although older people are less affected by alcohol misuse than younger people, it has been reported that 17% of men and 7% of women over 65 drink more than the recommended limits (OPCS 1996). Moreover, when researching the drinking behaviour of people aged 75 years and over, Iliffe et al (1991) found that 3.6% of men and 3% of women consume more than recommended limits. Further, in a study by Bridgewater et al (1987) which involved 101 adults aged 60 years and over in Newcastle upon Tyne, it was found that 27% of men and 9% of women were assessed as being 'at risk' drinkers. While these figures suggest a significant number of older 'problem drinkers', precise estimates of prevalence can be difficult to achieve for a number of reasons, including:

- many older people and their relatives may be reluctant to report alcohol misuse owing to fear of stigma and shame
- symptoms of alcohol misuse may be confused with other medical and psychiatric disorders

- assessment and identification methods which focus on consumption levels may not be sensitive enough to identify older drinkers who generally consume less than younger people
- accessing large representative community samples of older people can be problematic
- prevalence studies do not recognise the different types of older 'problem drinkers'.

Further to this last point, Zimberg (1978) suggests that there are three types of older 'problem drinkers':

1. people who start to misuse alcohol for the first time in old age (late-onset misuse)
2. people who have intermittently experienced alcohol misuse, but have not developed significant misuse until later in life
3. people who have misused alcohol throughout their life and into old age.

The significance of these categories is that late-onset alcohol misuse appears to have different characteristics than that presented by adults who have experienced alcohol misuse for most of their lives. For example, Ward & Goodman (1995) suggested that late-onset drinkers may drink excessively because of bereavement, to ease pain, to help induce sleep or to deal with boredom and loneliness. Women were also found to be more prone to late-onset alcohol misuse, particularly those who lived on their own (Gomberg 1994). However, Widner & Zeichner (1991) suggested that late-onset alcohol misusers had fewer behavioural and social problems and had a better prognosis for treatment. These authors also reported that late-onset alcohol misuse accounted for approximately one-third of all older alcohol misusers, with these numbers likely to increase in the future. Moreover, Widner & Zeichner (1991) contend that even if the number of 'younger alcoholics' remained at its present level, the absolute numbers will increase because of the expected growth of the older population. This observation would appear to challenge the assumption that younger people who seriously abuse alcohol would either be cured, or die, from its effects before reaching old age.

Despite methodological and epidemiological limitations in the available data, there does appear to be an urgent need to accept that a significant number of older people misuse alcohol, resulting in a diminished quality of life. Furthermore, it is important to recognise that older people who abuse alcohol may benefit from interventions which acknowledge their specific needs, beliefs and circumstances. We will now consider how this could be approached.

Assessment and interventions

As with any other serious condition, the interventions for alcohol misuse require careful and accurate assessment. Assessment needs to be both detailed and comprehensive, but should also be carried out in a sensitive manner. Many older people may be reluctant, or find it difficult, to discuss their alcohol misuse. As highlighted earlier, shame, guilt and stigma may serve to inhibit an older person from disclosing the reality of their situation. Also, for some older people, cognitive impairment may make it difficult to remember or describe fully their difficulties.

With these issues in mind, it is often helpful for the mental health nurse to validate the information presented by the older person against accounts provided by a spouse, relative or close friend. These significant others can often provide a different perspective on events which may help to enhance an understanding of the situation, and their early involvement can also prove to be very helpful in laying the foundation for future intervention. It is also important not to rush the assessment and bombard the older person with a series of questions which they may perceive as an interrogation. This is particularly important in home assessments, where older people may simply terminate the interview and refuse further contact should they feel uncomfortable at any time. To help avoid this situation, it is often useful to elicit the information through a more informal discussion which also aims to develop the therapeutic relationship. Many older people will only disclose sensitive information when a trusting relationship has been developed. Furthermore, the development of a trusting relationship will cement the foundations for effective collaboration within the intervention phase.

The main aim of the assessment should be to obtain an accurate picture of the older person's alcohol misuse. This should include details of the present drinking behaviour, and possible antecedents and consequences of alcohol misuse. Attention also needs to be given to the physical, psychological and social perspectives of misuse, and their possible interrelationships. Finney & Moos (1984) have suggested that chronic illness, social isolation and depression appear to co-exist with alcohol misuse, and attention to these in the assessment will build a suitable base for interventions.

The assessment should also provide the necessary information to ensure that treatment and management are responsive to the individual's needs and circumstances. While the treatment and management of alcohol misuse in older people share many of the characteristics described for younger people (see Ch. 17), Blake (1990) suggests that a broader range of treatment strategies may be needed for older people who misuse alcohol. In reviewing the available evidence, successful treatment of older people who misuse alcohol is more likely to occur if the following are considered:

- Both Glatt (1961) and Atkinson et al (1993) found that older people with alcoholism who were treated in age-specific groups responded better than those treated in mixed age groups.
- Schonfeld & Dupree (1995) commented that because older alcohol misusers have fewer social resources, more problems in everyday functioning and more life stresses, treatment should build upon increasing the available social support systems and utilising all possible services. This support would include involvement from health and social services, voluntary organisations and family, relatives and friends.
- Schonfeld & Dupree (1994) recommend that treatment approaches should be conducted at a slower pace, avoiding confrontation and placing emphasis on treatment for isolation and depression.
- Dupree et al (1984) reported good success for older people completing a behavioural treatment programme. This programme included analysis of drinking behaviour, development of drink management skills, alcohol information and education and the development of problem-solving skills. Similar to Schonfeld & Dupree (1995), the authors also noted that successful outcome was associated with the expansion of the older person's social network.
- Moos et al (1991) found that many late-onset problem drinkers responded well to education and informal social pressure and did not require formal treatment. This highlighted the value of relative involvement and the use of education on alcohol misuse.
- Wessen (1992) suggested that there is a general ignorance of what constitutes 'sensible' drinking levels for older people. Thus, the success of the joint health education initiative and literature provided by Alcohol Concern and Age Concern at the end of the last decade (Alcohol Concern 1988) would appear to have good utility.

Although older people who misuse alcohol are less likely to be detected (Curtis et al 1989), once identified, they respond as well as, or even better than, younger people in treatment (Atkinson 1994). These findings would suggest that more effort needs to be made to target potential older problem drinkers at the primary health care level. Improved surveillance and screening for alcohol misuse, coupled to improved health education and treatment availability, may well improve the situation for many older people.

DEMENTIA

In an attempt to provide a flavour of possibilities for dementia care practice, this section will now give a broad overview of the literature on the experience of dementia, and it will include a review of the main types of intervention which have proved to be clinically effective. This will be undertaken by following eight separate headings which are seen to link the experience of dementia from an individual and societal perspective.

Historical and contemporary context

A historical context for the present understanding of dementia can be attributed to Binswanger in 1898 and his description of 'presenile dementia' (Binswanger cited in Allison 1962). At the end of the last century, Binswanger used the term 'presenile' to refer to symptoms developing in a person between the ages of 40 to 60 years and 'dementia' to imply impairment of memory and intellect. As such the initial focus of medical research into the syndrome of 'dementia' was concerned with the link between younger people with impaired memory and intellect and the (as yet unknown) role-played by atheroma and arteriosclerosis in this process. Arnold Pick's writings between 1892 and 1908 exemplify this point fully when he described a rare and particular presenile 'cortical atrophy' in the frontal and temporal lobes of the brain; the reported syndrome (Pick's disease) continues to bears his name to this day and remains recognised as one of the 'early onset' dementias.

However, it was the seminal neurological and observational research on cognitive functioning and memory decline undertaken by Alzheimer in 1907 that was to change the course of medical and social understanding of dementia. Alzheimer's detailed case study was undertaken on Auguste D, a 51-year-old woman from the Frankfurt am Main insane asylum in Germany (see Maurer et al 1997). An English translation of this work by Stelzmann et al (1995) revealed that during her time in the asylum, Auguste was completely disorientated in time and place, suffered from auditory hallucinations and expressed paranoid ideas. What made Alzheimer's work so innovative was that, for the first time, he successfully managed to link diffuse cortical atrophy in the brain to the function and axonal spread of senile plaques and neurofibrillary tangles within the higher and dominant areas of the brain structure. Providing a complete understanding of the biology of dementia is a complex process and beyond the scope of this chapter, although if further information is required the authors would suggest reference to Jacques (1992) and Delieu & Keady (1996 a,b, 1997).

For the remainder of this century, the medical profession have attempted to systematically define the characteristics of dementia and place them within a medical context under the umbrella term of mental illness. However, it was not until the turn of the 1970s that the ICD-10 (WHO 1993a) and DSM-IV (American Psychiatric Association 1994) converged and set agreed diagnostic criteria for dementia; even then discrepancies in category formation still existed; for example, in the reference to multi-infarct dementia (American Psychiatric Association

1994) and vascular dementia (WHO 1993a) to broadly define the same set of signs and symptoms.

While there have been many attempts to provide a comprehensive definition of dementia, the following is now widely accepted:

> Dementia is the global impairment of higher cortical functions, including memory, the capacity to solve problems of day to day living, the performance of learned perceptuo-motor skills, the correct use of social skills and control of emotional reactions in the absence of gross clouding of consciousness. The condition is often irreversible and progressive.
>
> WHO 1986, cited in Jones & Miesen 1992:9

In keeping with its historical roots, both the ICD-10 and DSM-IV criteria divided the syndrome of dementia into two on the basis of age of onset, with 65 years and under being referred to as 'early-onset' dementia and 65 years and over being referred to as 'late-onset' dementia. The range of 'early-onset' dementias encompasses a diverse number of syndromes including Alzheimer's disease (AD), vascular dementia, Pick's disease, Creutzfeldt–Jakob disease, Huntington's disease, AIDS dementia complex and alcohol-related dementia. Although rare, dementia may also occur in children and young adolescents as a result of general medical conditions which include head injury, brain tumours, HIV infection, strokes and adrenoleuko-dystrophies (American Psychiatric Association 1994:137). Moreover, as stated in the WHO definition, there are also potentially treatable causes of dementia, examples of which include:

- deficiencies of vitamin B12, folate, niacin (pellegra), thiamine (Wernicke–Korsakoff syndrome)
- zinc and/or copper deficiencies
- endocrine disorders (hypo- or hyperthyroidism)
- normal pressure hydrocephalus

- drug- or medication-induced disturbances
- subdural haematoma
- toxin exposure
- cerebral tumour.

It is also important to recognise that dementia has many different causes (see Tables 18.1 and 18.2) and risk factors, and a correct diagnosis of dementia can only be made with about 80% certainty in any one instance (Alzheimer's Disease Society (ADS) 1995a). It is a sobering thought that as we approach the 21st century the only absolute means of confirming a diagnosis and type of dementia is in the performance of an autopsy (Jacques 1992).

Table 18.1 Causes of dementia with relatively rapid onset and course (from Byrne 1994:62, reproduced by kind permission of the publisher)

Degenerative	Diffuse Lewy body disease, Alzheimer's disease (rare)
Vascular	Cerebral infarction and embolus, cerebral aneurysm, cerebral vasculitis
Transmissible dementias	Creutzfeldt–Jakob disease, Gerstmann–Sträussler syndrome
Infection	Encephalitis (especially herpes simplex), Whipple's disease
Miscellaneous	Severe cerebral trauma (course may be prolonged), neuropsychiatric systemic lupus, rheumatoid, sarcoid, temporal arteritis

As Keady (1996) noted in a recent review of the literature, assessment is complicated further by the necessity to exclude other symptomatology which may further mimic the signs and symptoms of dementia, such as benign senescent forgetfulness; age-associated memory impairment and depressive pseudodementia. With these pressures in mind, it is, perhaps, not too surprising that GPs in primary health care settings have great difficulty in correctly identifying and diagnosing dementia, although recent evidence suggests that the history provided by close family members can play an important part in this process (Morris & Fulling 1988). Furthermore, both the ICD-10 and DSM-IV clinical criteria track the progression of dementia through three stages: mild, moderate and severe. These stages are able to be identified owing to the gradual nature of most dementias, in particular AD (see Table 18.2). This staging of dementia and its assigned clinical severity rating (see Hughes et al 1982) has come under increasing criticism as the stages from healthy–questionable–mild–moderate–severe dementia are seen as taking the 'personhood' out of the experience of dementia, and stop professional workers seeing the person behind the cluster of signs and symptoms (see Bell & McGregor 1995, Carr & Marshall 1993). We will return to the concept of 'personhood' later in this part of the chapter.

Table 18.2 Causes of dementia with gradual onset and prolonged course (from Byrne 1994:66, reproduced by kind permission of the publisher)

Degenerative	Alzheimer's disease, Pick's disease, Wilson's disease, Huntington's chorea, Diffuse Lewy body disease, dementia of the frontal type, corticobasal degeneration, multisystem atrophies, multiple sclerosis, motor neurone disease, thalamic dementia
Vascular	Binswanger's disease (subcortical arteriosclerotic encephalopathy)
Infections	Neurosyphilis
Space-occupying lesions	Primary intracranial tumours: meningioma, astrocytoma, chronic subdural haematoma
Metabolic and endocrine	Uraemia, chronic hepatic encephalopathy, carcinomatosis, hypothyroidism, hypopituitarism
Miscellaneous	Communicating hydrocephalus, alcoholic dementia

While there is no reliable pharmacological 'cure' for the vast majority of the dementias, including AD, there has been some recent advances. In March 1997, donepezil hydrochloride (Aricept) was the first drug licensed in the UK specifically to treat AD. According to an information sheet provided by the Alzheimer's Disease Society in April 1997 (ADS 1997a), donepezil works by reducing the breakdown of acetylcholine (a chemical involved in nerve cell communication which affects memory) in the brain by inhibiting the production of acetylcholinesterase (a chemical which controls the timing of the transmission of acetylcholine, its amount and concentration); thus more acetylcholine is able to be retained in the nerve cell, improving memory performance. The drug has been evaluated as being especially effective for people during the mild to moderate stage in improving their cognitive function (Harvey & Fairey 1997), but it is important to emphasise that donepezil is not a cure for AD and, according to the Alzheimer's Disease Society, does not appear to stop or slow down the progression of the disease (ADS 1997a). It is likely that many other similar compounds will be available in the near future which will focus the role of the mental health nurse within primary care upon earlier case identification, family assessment and support.

Prevalence of dementia

By the year 2000, the number of people aged 65 and over living in the world is expected to be about 423 million with nearly 50% of this total situated in developing countries (WHO 1993b). Commenting on these figures, Prince (1997) has suggested that by the year 2025 there will be 34.1 million people in the world with some form of dementia, 9.9 million situated in the developed world and 24.2 million in the developing countries. Against this backcloth, the Alzheimer's Disease Society (ADS 1996a) has estimated that there are presently 636 000 people with dementia living in the UK of whom nearly 500 000 have AD; this includes approximately 17 000 younger people with dementia or about 100 to 150 per district health authority (ADS 1995b, 1996b). In the UK, the prevalence of dementia is expected to rise to 894 000 by the year 2021 (ADS 1996a) and, within this overall figure, prevalence varies widely, being 0.1% (1 in 1000) in the age group 40 to 65 years; 2.0% (1 in 50) in the age group 65 to 70; 5.0% (1 in 20) in the age group 70 to 80 and 20% (1 in 5) in the age group 80 and over. Moreover, the acquisition of cognitive impairment and dementia in both old and young age has been significantly correlated to a reduction in life expectancy (Eagles et al 1990) and Magnússon & Helgason (1993) have placed an upper age limit of 75 years on this correlation. There is also emerging evidence of the genetic inheritance of 'early-onset' AD (Li et al 1995), a finding which has tremendous implications for mental health nursing in the conduction of genetic screening and family-centred counselling.

In the mid 1980s, Gilhooly (1986) found that the majority of people with dementia lived in the community (5 out of 6), but recent studies have found that this may be an overestimate. For instance, in the Bangor Dementia Studies (Wenger 1994), which drew on a large sample of older people living in Liverpool (n = 4500+), it was found that 43% of those with dementia lived in residential care, with the risk of earlier admission being heightened for the parent(s) of adult child carers. Moreover, the support networks of older people with dementia were more likely to be centred around the family system with less contact provided by friends, neighbours and community groups. It would appear, therefore, that a diagnosis of dementia is itself an indicator of increased risk into residential care. As suggested by Keady (1997a:21–22) studies would indicate that the family carers' decision to admit a person with dementia to residential care is influenced by a number of factors which include:

- perceived nature and quality of the emotional relationship between the carer and person with dementia
- carer's use of and access to services
- carer's age
- carer's reactions to the exhibited behaviours and ways of managing memory problems
- persistence of troublesome behaviours, including aggression and incontinence
- omission of satisfactions from the care-giving relationship
- availability and contact with friends and satisfaction from such help
- existence of another dependent relative
- employment situation of the carer.

However, as the prevalence of dementia increases exponentially with age, not all people with dementia living in the community do so with the support of a surviving spouse/partner or, because of social mobility, close to (any) existing family members, for example a son or daughter. As such in the UK, the Alzheimer's Disease Society has estimated there to be about 154 000 people with dementia living on their own (ADS 1994) with half this total aged 85 years and over. More alarmingly, this population was seen as being exposed to increased risks such as undetected self-neglect, financial exploitation and falls. This finding echoes the concern expressed in a recent joint Social Services Inspectorate (SSI) and Department of Health (DoH 1997) report where home support workers were seen as providing 'the most significant relationship' in the support of older people with mental health needs who live alone.

Policy and practice considerations

The social and economic impact of the increased prevalence of dementia has been recognised in the UK for some considerable time, with two reports issued at the beginning of the 1980s being particularly influential – Organic Mental Impairment in the Elderly (Royal College of Physicians 1981) and The Rising Tide (Health Advisory Service 1982). Both these reports embraced the importance of people with dementia and highlighted the need for well-staffed resources in both community and residential settings. The prominence of nursing, in particular that of mental health nurses, to meet these needs figured high upon their respective agendas and was allied to the drive towards more effective multi-agency working. At this time, the NHS was seen as steering the policy and service direction of dementia care practice, and this was witnessed in its full-scale commitment to the provision of continuing care facilities, even though they were usually located, and locked, within the totally inappropriate setting of the mental hospitals. However, propelled by the division of health and social care needs contained within the NHS and Community Care Act (Department of Health 1990), this full-scale commitment to meeting the community and residential care needs of people with dementia has altered significantly during recent years. Indeed, the 1997–1998 awareness campaign and report by the Alzheimer's Disease Society (ADS 1997b) have found a lack of planning by health services for people with dementia, and a significant reduction in the provision of continuing care facilities.

In the face of this changing and uncertain climate, the need to define precisely the role of mental health practice in dementia care in both residential and community care settings is vital, yet few clinical outcome studies exist to propagate its effectiveness in either of these settings. Fortunately, at present, the same can be said of most other professions (excluding, arguably, clinical psychology), and where clinical outcome studies in dementia care exist, most have focused

upon meeting the needs of family carers. This has usually been expressed in the measurement of structured interventions with family carers in support groups, especially in the teaching of coping strategies and education about dementia (for a review, see Miller & Morris 1993). Arguably, the challenge for mental health nursing is to embrace this role and advance its practice while operating firmly within a family systems approach to dementia care practice (Cotter & Miceli 1993).

One way of promoting this position is to clarify the underlying mental health role in assessment and intervention approaches. Unfortunately, the methods of conducting assessment and co-ordinating community care for people with dementia and their carers have, over the years, received relatively little policy attention. For instance, a joint SSI and DoH report (SSI/DoH 1996) was issued which based its substantial recommendations and suggestions for practice improvements following 1-day visits to five local authorities in England in the summer of 1995. In the report, the interface between GPs/primary health care teams and other agencies, such as social services and secondary health services, was seen as crucial in fostering assessment and care planning arrangements for people with dementia and their carers. However, as we have seen earlier, there is a major concern that GPs do not possess all the skills and interest necessary to perform the vital role of 'focal point' for joint assessment. As the report identified, GPs may be reluctant to refer people with dementia, and presumably their carers, to social services and other agencies when they experience delays in assessment and little feedback on its outcome. As with the findings of an earlier report (ADS 1995c), this report included a discussion on the 'vital' need for the early identification of dementia, although the resource implications and training necessary to create a more proactive response to dementia care were not addressed. This creates both a tension and a paradox as in the report early identification of dementia was not a common occurrence with older people with dementia not identified in the community until their problems became too severe, thus limiting the potential range of services and support that could be offered (SSI/DoH 1996); a finding all to a familiar to those practising in the field.

Dementia – impact on families

Without doubt the greatest weight of social research into dementia care has been conducted by clinicians and social scientists into interpreting the stress and coping behaviours of community-dwelling family carers (see carer-centred literature reviews by Kuhlman et al 1991, Morris et al 1988, Woods 1995). Indeed, it is hard to imagine that it is over 30 years since Grad & Sainsbury (1965) first measured the burden placed upon carers caused by the discharge home of older psychiatric patients from the institutional setting. In this important study, Grad & Sainsbury (1965) distinguished between *objective burden*, which described the behavioural dysfunctions and practical problems that were encountered by the carer, and *subjective burden* which referred to the carers' emotional adjustment in terms of increased stress and lowered morale. This division of burden and search for 'the truth' in interpreting the dynamics of family stress continued in the development of an immense social research agenda into dementia care-giving.

One of the earliest and most frequently cited papers in this context was provided by Sanford (1975). In this study, Sanford reviewed the tolerance of family carers to providing home care for people with dementia, and found that carers reported lack of time for themselves, immobility, faecal incontinence and sleep disturbances as the most stressful aspects of providing home care. As

highlighted by both Woods (1995) and Keady (1996), establishing the nature of burden in dementia care-giving is a complex issue and there is little unanimity in the field. However, from these reviews, the main features salient to establishing the nature of stress and burden in family care were found to relate to:

- those personnel visiting the home of people with dementia and their carers requiring adequate training and support
- the level of informal support available in home care not being seen as a significant factor to establishing the amount and degree of stress
- older carers being generally perceived as experiencing less care-giving stress
- the greatest care-giving strain attributed to the 'apathetic inactivity' on the part of the person with dementia
- the closer bond between care-giver and care-receiver, the more stressful the caring role
- the least well-tolerated behaviours included demands for attention, noisiness, falls and personality clashes
- the carer's ability to draw on a range of coping strategies was crucial for successful adaptation and management of the care-giving process
- establishing the nature and quality of the care-giving relationship was central to interpreting the outcome of family-based home care.

As the 1980s progressed, Keady (1996) also noted that social research in dementia care began to extend its boundaries from appraising stress and the care-giving burden to investigating such concepts as care-givers' gender and coping styles; access to information and services; participation in and effectiveness of support groups; adjustment and circumstances surrounding admission into care; perception of their own health needs and their expressions of anticipatory grief (see also Sweeting & Gilhooly 1997). Building upon the transactional model of stress outlined by Lazarus (1966), the studies described by Pearlin et al (1990) were particularly effective in starting a new research agenda for the 1990s built around identifying carers' coping patterns and styles, and their role in mediating patterns of stress. This new direction was also augmented by studies exploring positive dimensions in providing home care to people with dementia, such as the carers' experiences of warmth, comfort and pleasure (Cohen et al 1994, Motenko 1989), and that the amount and degree of satisfactions themselves helped to predict the physical and emotional health of carers (Nolan et al 1996).

However, despite these encouraging findings there is little doubt that caring at home for a person with dementia is a stressful and self-injurious process. In a survey of 1303 carers in the UK, the Alzheimer's Disease Society found that 97% of carers were suffering from some form of emotional health problem, such as stress, tiredness or depression, and that 36% had a physical complaint (e.g. back pain) as a direct result of being a carer (ADS 1993). In the same report, the Society found that 34% of carers had not been offered a full assessment and 59% complained that the person they cared for did not receive regular check ups by a doctor or nurse. These are disturbing findings, but ones which are, unfortunately, not unusual when considering access and availability of service provision to carers of people with dementia (for a comprehensive review and study, see Levin et al 1989).

Qualitative studies by nurse researchers also began to make a significant contribution to understanding the motivating factors involved in providing home care to people with dementia, and to explore its associated meaning for the care-giver and care-receiver (see Adams 1994,

Bowers 1987, 1988, Clarke 1995, Hirschfield 1983, Keady & Nolan 1995a). Following interviews with 30 care-givers, Hirschfield (1983) developed the concept of 'mutuality' as a critical variable to explain the social relationship between families and the person with dementia. Hirschfield suggested that 'positive mutuality' grew out of the carers' ability to find meaning, gratification and reciprocity in their care-giving role. Accordingly, feelings of 'low mutuality' were synonymous with poor adjustment within the family and negative feelings towards the person with dementia which, in turn, led the family to consider admission into care. This finding highlighted the importance of establishing both the *nature and quality* of the relationship during any professional assessment of need. Moreover, following interviews with 32 adult child carers caring for their parent with varying degrees of dementia, Bowers (1987) developed a five-stage temporal model of care-giving which consisted of the following stages: anticipatory care-giving; preventive care-giving; supervisory care-giving; instrumental care-giving; and protective care-giving. From the analysis of her data, Bowers suggested that 'protective care-giving' (i.e. protecting the self-image of the parent) was, for adult child carers, the most stressful experience in providing home care for a parent with dementia.

This necessity for services to be more sensitive to the needs of carers has also been noted by several authors (see, e.g., Badger et al 1990a,b, Harris 1993) and they have repeatedly urged service providers to be more aware of carers' information needs and gender. For instance, Badger et al (1990a,b) found that wives caring for husbands were much less likely than male carers to receive community nursing services, or home helps. In addition, providing information to carers of people with dementia appeared essential in helping both carers and people with dementia adjust to their new roles, with information providing the basis of a model for stress reduction and the identification of appropriate coping strategies (see Coyne 1991, Fortinsky & Hathaway 1990, Keady & Nolan, 1994a, Watkins 1988, Zarit et al 1985). However, studies have constantly found that a structured, personalised and systematic approach to the provision of information to carers is not forthcoming (ADS 1993, 1994, Collins et al 1994, Keady & Nolan 1995a, McWalter et al 1994) and that younger people with dementia have even less opportunity to access such important age-sensitive information (ADS 1996b).

Family care – supportive interventions

From this review, it can be seen that mental health nurses have a tremendous scope and role in working with family carers of people with dementia. Interventions may include:

- establishing the nature and quality of the carer–care-receiver relationship
- systematically building a relationship based upon mutual trust and support
- working within a family systems model, where the perspectives and beliefs of all family members are respected
- conducting stress management techniques
- introducing age-based and sensitive information to encourage autonomy
- eliciting carers' hopes and expectations for the future
- being sensitive to the carer's ethnicity, gender and coping patterns
- implementing counselling approaches and skills
- facilitating carer support groups in the community, ranging from teaching coping skills to facilitating group discussion
- providing innovative systems of support, such as a telephone support group

- liaison and networking with other agencies and voluntary organisations, such as the local Alzheimer's Disease Society branch to provide information and (where practicable) instigate financial support for family carers
- teaching new carers caring and coping techniques
- being open to and learning from more experienced carers
- teasing out the personal satisfactions in the care-giving and family relationship.

At all times, these interventions need to be carefully constructed and tailored to individual needs. Each family care-giving situation and biographical context will be different, and it must be remembered that family carers have a right not to care at any time in the process of dementia. Moreover, it is important to recognise that, at times, the expressed needs of the family carer and that of the person with dementia will conflict. Brokering a path through these two perspectives requires immense skill and experience.

The person with dementia

It is crucial that people with dementia are not seen as passive recipients in their dementia. As we have seen the majority of research in the 1980s and early part of this decade has been centred upon the needs of family carers. However, there is an increasing recognition of the need for people with dementia to have their voice heard (Goldsmith 1996) with this campaign for greater recognition being led by Tom Kitwood and his colleagues at the Bradford Dementia Group. Kitwood has built a persuasive argument for discovering the 'personhood' and 'well-being' of people with dementia (Kitwood 1997). In a direct challenge to the medical approach to dementia, where people are labelled and measured in terms of their cognitive and behavioural deficits,

Kitwood and his colleagues look to discover the personhood and well-being of people with dementia (Kitwood 1997, Kitwood & Benson 1995). Indeed, Kitwood believes that discovering personhood and well-being is a responsibility which involves both professional worker and the person with dementia. Following this paradigm, professional workers need to understand the social world as experienced by people with dementia, and interpret their efforts at communication through this, at times, opaque window. Adoption of this viewpoint results in a change of emphasis from the divisive view of 'us' (professional workers) and 'them' (people with dementia)' to, simply, 'us'. Kitwood & Bredin (1992) also view people with dementia as going through a growth experience (this has been named 'rementia') and that dementia care mapping can help in the identification of personhood and well-being within a residential care environment (Kitwood 1992).

The emergence of this philosophy has coincided with the publication of a few books written by people with AD about this experience (Davis 1989, McGowin 1993). Moreover, despite methodological and ethical difficulties, a small but growing number of qualitative researchers have interviewed people with dementia at symptom onset in an attempt to interpret this experience (see Goldsmith 1996, Gubrium 1987, Keady 1997b, Keady & Gilliard 1999, Keady & Nolan 1994b, 1995b,c, LeNavenec 1995, Sabat & Harré 1992, Wuest et al 1994). The Index for Managing Memory Loss (IMMEL) (Keady & Nolan 1995b), which lists 42 coping statements developed directly from the voices of people with the early signs of dementia against a likert scale, has been evaluated as a useful tool for helping people with dementia identify their range of coping behaviours, particularly during their adaptation to the diagnosis and prognosis (Kakemoto 1997, personal correspondence).

In a similar vein, a process model on the experience of AD was reported in an informative paper by Wuest et al (1994). In developing this grounded theory model, 11 people with AD (age range: 51 to 90 years) were interviewed together with their family carers (n = 15; age range: 28 to 83 years). The authors found that an overriding dimension of 'becoming strangers' described the full experience of AD and that the person with dementia and the carer 'moved together' towards an understanding of the dementia. To date this finding has not been replicated in other studies, or within the previously outlined individual accounts, with Keady & Gilliard (1999) describing the individual transition into dementia as being a fraught and secretive process with a need to continually 'cover your tracks' in order to avoid the experience of loss being discovered.

Recently there have been descriptions of individual accounts of suicide by people with AD who have awareness and knowledge of their diagnosis and prognosis (Rohde et al 1995), with a key feature of these accounts being the calculated preparation for the act itself and dissatisfaction with their performance in memory-enhancing drug trials. At present, no official statistics are kept on people with dementia who commit suicide, but we would suggest that this act is likely to increase substantially in the future, especially with the present drive towards earlier diagnosis and more openness in its communication (ADS 1995c, SSI/DoH 1996). Again, mental health nurses would appear to have a vital part to play at the time of the diagnosis, conducting health education programmes and carrying out intervention programmes that encourage the person with dementia and their family supporters to adapt to their new-found situation.

One way of working with dementia at this time is by the setting up and provision of a support group for people with the early experience of dementia, similar in design to that of carer support groups but with a more focused agenda. As studies have shown (Duff & Peach 1994, Gatz 1995, Gibson & Moniz-Cook 1996, LaBarge & Trtanj 1995, Yale 1995) such a group may involve the teaching of adaptive coping skills, sharing of information and providing markers about how to live within the shifting realities of the diagnosis. Support groups for people with the early experience of dementia are still in their infancy within the UK, as in other countries, but there is little doubt in our mind that this type of support will prove to be a major source of mental health intervention as pace is gathered towards the new millennium.

A basis for practice

The following interventions with people with the early experience of dementia may all be considered a basis for mental health nursing practice:

- help towards case identification and early assessment
- provision of memory training, life review and reminiscence approaches (see Haight 1992, Scogin 1992)
- facilitating and teaching adaptive coping skills at the onset and adjustment in dementia (see IMMEL as an example of operationalising this approach (Keady & Nolan 1995b))
- adoption and use of counselling skills and approaches
- move towards genetic counselling
- role of advocate
- role of independent confidante to act as a buffer between the person with dementia and the family supporter.

In themselves we would see the broad range of interventions as eclectic in nature with the personal and human qualities of the mental health nurse being just as important as any adopted intervention technique.

Dementia care nursing: reflections and directions

Working with people with dementia has traditionally been seen as an unattractive option in mental health practice, especially amongst nursing students (Åström 1986), and viewed as one where little could be done other than in the provision of 'tender loving care'. This is an unfortunate stereotype and, as we have seen, dementia care nursing is a dynamic field which embraces all the recognised skills of the mental health nurse (see Department of Health 1994:17–18). Indeed, we would visualise the practice of dementia care nursing on a continuum which extends from the contribution to case identification and diagnosis at the onset of dementia, to the personal and intimate acts of care provided at the end of human life. The care and support provided to families and their support networks will be evident throughout, and beyond, this continuum. The set of challenges this framework presents requires the mental health nurse to have a broad range of interpersonal and therapeutic skills, including a depth of subject-related knowledge, assessment skills and an ability to work both individually and collectively as part of a residential and/or community-based team. Successfully fulfilling this agenda may, at present, be considered a bridge too far, as the most recent review of mental health nursing (Department of Health 1994:34) found evidence of:

> …an under-investment in training, support and supervision for nursing staff in relation to the very complex and demanding needs of those suffering from dementia.

To begin to address this 'under-investment' it would appear vital that managerial and supervisory structures in dementia care practice are formalised, and specialist educational opportunities are made available to all nurses practising in the field. However, this is a position not reflected in the composition and teaching content of most pre- and post-registration programmes in mental health and social care (Nolan & Keady 1996), and the vexed question of 'What is to be done with dementia?' presently sits uncomfortably upon the shoulders of mental health nursing.

This is unfortunate as there is so much still to learn about dementia care practice within both residential and community settings. For instance, there is a need for residential services to provide more locally based living environments, such as those seen in Sweden under the philosophy of the Group Living Homes (Keady & Lundh 1997, Malmberg & Zarit 1993) and for the staff to operate in more person-centred ways. Moreover, there is an urgent need for more outcome studies in dementia care where the mental health nursing is not just seen as being valued (ADS 1995c, Furst & Sperlinger 1992) but evaluated. Meeting and subscribing to this challenge is, perhaps, the greatest of all those facing dementia care nursing and people considering entry into this work.

CONCLUSION

While it is contrary to the title and ethos of the book, perhaps the overriding feature we encountered in preparing this chapter has been the relative paucity of published accounts of evidence-based nursing practice applicable to older people with mental health needs and their families. Where evidence did exist, it was inevitably from other professions, or overseas, with the USA and Canada leading the way. Speaking from a purely UK perspective, this must change and older people must be moved from the margins to the mainstream of mental health education, practice, research design and service delivery. As we have seen repeatedly during this review, working with older people with mental health needs, and their families, draws consistently upon the expert skills of the mental health nurse, and pro-

vides a framework of opportunity for multi-agency practice in primary, secondary and tertiary care. Grasping this particular nettle is the responsibility of all the profession, with, we hope, students undertaking mental health nurse training, agitating for change and providing an effective voice for older people with mental health needs.

Exercise

After reading through the chapter, profile how mental health services for older people are constructed in your area. As a start consider the following questions:

- Is there a published strategy for providing mental health services for older people in your locality? If so, find a copy and discover what it contains.
- Is a separate mental health service for older people provided in your locality, or is this service integrated into adult services? How do staff working in the field feel about this system? Is there any scope for improvement/clarification?
- How are services for people with dementia provided and what appears to be the nursing role in this field? Are services for younger people with dementia integrated into older services?
- How effective are the mechanisms for the identification, assessment and treatment of older people with mental health problems in the community?

After conducting your profile, reflect upon the following question: to what extent does current practice reflect the evidence provided within this chapter ?

KEY TEXTS FOR FURTHER READING

Chiu E, Ames D (eds) 1994 Functional psychiatric disorders of the elderly. Cambridge University Press, Cambridge

Kitwood T 1997 Dementia reconsidered: the person comes first. Open University Press, Milton Keynes

Lindesay J (ed) 1995 Neurotic disorders in the elderly. Oxford University Press, Oxford

Miesen B M L, Jones G 1997 Care-giving in dementia: research and applications, vol 2. Routledge, London

Norman I J, Redfern S J (eds) 1997 Mental health care for elderly people. Churchill Livingstone, New York

Skills-Based texts

Beck A T, Emery G, Greenberg R L 1985 Anxiety disorders and phobias: A cognitive perspective. Basic Books, New York

Beck A T, Rush A J, Shaw B F, Emery G 1979 Cognitive therapy of depression. Guilford Press, Surrey

Haddock G, Slade P D 1996 Cognitive–behavioural interventions with psychotic disorders. Routledge, London

Hawton K, Salkovskis P M, Kirk J, Clark D M (eds) 1994 Cognitive behavioural therapy for psychiatric problems. Oxford Medical, Oxford

Jones G, Miesen B M L (eds) 1992 Care-giving in dementia: Research and applications. Routledge, London

Knight B G 1996 Psychotherapy with older adults. Sage, London

Myers W A (ed) 1991 New techniques in the psychotherapy of older patients. American Psychiatric Press, Washington DC

Stokes G, Goudie F 1990 Working with dementia. Winslow Press, Bicester

Wells A 1997 Cognitive therapy of anxiety disorders. Wiley, London

Yale R 1995 Developing support groups for individuals with early-stage Alzheimer's disease: Planning, implementation and evaluation. Health Professions Press, London

Yost E D, Beutler L E, Corbishley M A, Allender J R 1986 Group cognitive therapy: A treatment approach for depressed older adults. Pergamon Press, London

REFERENCES

Adams T 1994 The emotional experience of caregivers to relatives who are chronically confused – implications for community mental health nursing. International Journal of Nursing Studies 31(6):545–553

Alcohol Concern 1988 Alcohol and older people: Safer drinking for the over 60s. Series of three leaflets: (1) A DIY guide for older people; (2) A guide for family, relatives and friends; (3) A guide for health and social services and voluntary group workers. Alcohol Concern, London

Allison R S 1962 The senile brain: A clinical study. Edward Arnold, London

Almeida O P, Howard R J, Forstl H, Levy R 1994 Late onset paranoid disorders: Part 1: Coming to terms with late paraphrenia. In: Chiu E, Ames D (eds) Functional psychiatric disorders of the elderly. Cambridge University Press, Cambridge ch 18, p 303–315

Almeida O P, Howard R J, Levy R, David A S 1995 Psychotic states arising in late life. British Journal of Psychiatry 166:205–214

Alzheimer's Disease Society 1993 Deprivation and dementia. Report by Alzheimer's Disease Society, London

Alzheimer's Disease Society 1994 Home alone: Living alone with dementia. Report by Alzheimer's Disease Society, London

Alzheimer's Disease Society 1995a Dementia in the community: Management strategies for general practice. Report by the Alzheimer's Disease Society, London

Alzheimer's Disease Society 1995b Services for younger people with dementia. Report by the Alzheimer's Disease Society. Alzheimer's Disease Society, London

Alzheimer's Disease Society 1995c Right from the start: Primary health care and dementia. Report by Alzheimer's Disease Society, London

Alzheimer's Disease Society 1996a Opening the mind. Report by Alzheimer's Disease Society, London

Alzheimer's Disease Society 1996b Younger person with dementia: a review and strategy. Report by Alzheimer's Disease Society, London

Alzheimer's Disease Society 1997a New treatments for Alzheimer's disease. Information sheet 11. Alzheimer's Disease Society, London

Alzheimer's Disease Society 1997b No accounting for health. Report by Alzheimer's Disease Society, London

American Psychiatric Association 1994 DSM-IV: Diagnostic and statistical manual of mental disorders, 4th edn. American Psychiatric Association, Washington DC

Ames D 1991 Epidemiological studies of depression among the elderly in residential and nursing homes. International Journal of Geriatric Psychiatry 6:347–354

Åström S 1986 Health care students' attitude towards, and intention to work with, patients suffering form senile dementia. Journal of Advanced Nursing 11:651–659

Atkinson R M 1990 Aging and alcoholic use disorders: diagnostic issues in the elderly. International Psychogeriatrics 2:55–72

Atkinson R M 1994 Late onset problem drinking in older adults. International Journal of Geriatric Psychiatry 9:321–326

Atkinson R M, Tolson R L, Turner J A 1993 Factors affecting outpatient treatment compliance of older male problem drinkers. Journal of Studies on Alcohol 54:102–106

Badger F, Cameron E, Evers H 1990a Waiting to be served. The Health Service Journal 100(5183):54–55

Badger F, Cameron E, Evers H 1990b Slipping through the net. The Health Service Journal 100(5184):86–87

Ballard C, Boyle A, Bowler C, Lindesay J 1996 Anxiety disorders in dementia sufferers. International Journal of Geriatric Psychiatry 11:987–990

Banerjee S 1993 Prevalence and recognition rates of psychiatric disorder in the elderly clients of a community care service. International Journal of Geriatric Psychiatry 8:125–131

REFERENCES (*contd*)

Banerjee S, Sharmash K, Macdonald A J D 1996 Randomised controlled trial of effect of intervention by psychogeriatric team on depression in frail elderly people at home. British Medical Journal 313:1058–1061

Barraclough B M, Bunch J, Nelson B 1974 A hundred cases of suicide: clinical aspects. British Journal of Psychiatry 125:355–373

Beck G J, Stanley M A, Zebb B J 1996 Characteristics of generalized anxiety disorder in older adults: a descriptive study. Behaviour Research Therapy 34(3):225–234

Bell J, McGregor I 1995 A challenge to stage theories of dementia. In: Kitwood T, Benson S (eds) The new culture of dementia care. Hawker, London, ch 2, p 12–14

Benbow S M 1987 The use of electroconvulsive therapy in old age psychiatry. International Journal of Geriatric Psychiatry 2:25–30

Benbow S M 1989 The role of electroconvulsive therapy in the treatment of depressive illness in old age. British Journal of Psychiatry 155:147–152

Benbow S M 1992 Management of depression in the elderly. British Journal of Hospital Medicine 48(11):726–731

Blake R 1990 Techniques for counselling older persons. Journal of Mental Health Counselling 12(3):354–367

Blanchard M, Mann A 1994 Depression in primary care settings. In: Chiu E, Ames D (eds) Functional psychiatric disorders of the elderly. Cambridge University Press, Cambridge, ch 11, p 163–176

Bowers B J 1987 Inter-generational caregiving: adult care-givers and their ageing parents. Advances in Nursing Science 9(2):20–31

Bowers B J 1988 Family perceptions of care in a nursing home. Gerontologist 28(3):361–367

Bridgewater R, Lee S, James O F W, Potter J F 1987 Alcohol consumption and dependence in elderly patients in an urban community. British Medical Journal 295:884–885

Byrne E J 1994 Confusional states in older people. Edward Arnold, London

Carr J S, Marshall M 1993 Innovations in long-stay care for people with dementia. Reviews in Clinical Gerontology 3(2):157–167

Carstensen L L, Fremouw W J 1981 The demonstration of a behavioural intervention for late-life paranoia. Gerontologist 21:329–333

Cattell H, Jolley D J 1995 One hundred cases of suicide of elderly people. British Journal of Psychiatry 166:451–457

Clarke C L 1995 Care of elderly people suffering from dementia and their co-resident informal carers. In: Heyman B (ed) Researching user perspectives on community health care. Chapman and Hall, London, ch 8, p 135–149

Clarke D C, Fawcett J 1992 Review of empirical risk factors for evaluation of the suicidal patient. In: Bongar B (ed) Suicide: Guidelines for assessment, management and treatment. Oxford University Press, New York

Cohen C A, Pushkar-Gold D, Shulman, K I, Zucchero C A 1994 Positive aspects in caregiving: an overlooked variable in research. Canadian Journal of Aging 13(3):378–391

Cohen-Cole S A, Stoudemire A 1987 Major depression and physical illness: special considerations in diagnosis and biological treatment. Psychiatry Clinics of North America 10:1–17

Cole M G 1990 The prognosis of depression in the elderly. Canadian Medical Association Journal 142:633–639

Coleman P, Bond J, Peace S (1993) Ageing in the twentieth century. In: Bond J, Coleman P, Peace S (eds) Ageing in society: an introduction to social gerontology, 2nd edn. Sage, London, ch 1, p 1–18

Collins C E, Given B A, Given C W 1994 Interventions with family caregivers of persons with Alzheimer's disease. Nursing Clinics of North America 29(1):195–207

Copeland J R M, Dewey M E, Wood N, Searle R, Davidson I A, McWilliam C 1987 Range of mental illness among the elderly in the community. British Journal of Psychiatry 150:815–823

Cotter V T, Miceli D G 1993 Dementia and the family. In: Fawcett C S (ed) Family psychiatric nursing. Mosby, London, ch 21, p 356–375

Coyne A C 1991 Information and referral service usage among caregivers for dementia patients. Gerontologist 31(3):384–388

Curtis J R, Geller G, Stokes E J, Levine D M, Moore R D 1989 Characteristics, diagnosis and treatment of alcoholism in elderly patients. Journal of American Geriatric Society 37:310–316

Davis R 1989 My journey into Alzheimer's disease. Scripture Press, Buckinghamshire

Delieu J, Keady J 1996a The biology of Alzheimer's disease: 1. British Journal of Nursing 5(3):162–168

Delieu J, Keady J 1996b The biology of Alzheimer's disease: 2. British Journal of Nursing 5(4):216–220

Delieu J, Keady J 1997 The biology of dementia due to Parkinson's disease. British Journal of Nursing 6(14):806–810

Department of Health 1990 NHS and Community Care Act. HMSO, London

Department of Health 1994 Working in partnership; a collaborative approach to care. HMSO, London

Diekstra R F W 1989 Suicide and attempted suicide: An international perspective. Acta Psychiatrica Scandinavica 80:1–24

Duff G, Peach E 1994 Mutual support groups: A response to the early and often forgotten stage of dementia. Report, Dementia Services Development Centre, University of Stirling, Stirling

Dupree L W, Broskowski H, Schonfeld L 1984 The gerontology alcohol project: a behavioural treatment programme for elderly alcohol abusers. The Gerontologist 24(5):510–516

Eagles J M, Beattie J A G, Restall D B, Rawlinson F, Hagen S, Ashcroft G W 1990 Relation between cognitive impairment and early death in the elderly. British Medical Journal 300:239–240

Emery G 1981 Cognitive therapy with the elderly. In: Hollon S D, Bedrosian R C (eds) New directions in cognitive therapy. Guilford Press, New York

Finney J W, Moos R H 1984 Life stressors and problem drinking among older persons. In: Glanter M (ed) Recent developments in alcoholism, vol 2. Plenum Press, New York, p 267–288

Flint A J, Rifat S L, Eastwood R M 1991 Late-onset paranoia: distinct from paraphrenia? International Journal of Geriatric Psychiatry 6:103–109

REFERENCES (*contd*)

Fortinsky R H, Hathaway T J 1990 Information and service needs amongst active and former family care-givers of persons with Alzheimer's disease. Gerontologist 30(5):604–609

Fraser R M, Glass I B 1980 Unilateral and bilateral ECT in elderly patients: a comparative study. Acta Psychiatrica Scandinavica 62:13–31

Furst M, Sperlinger D 1992 Hour to hour, day to day: the service experiences of carers of people with pre-senile dementia in the London Borough of Sutton. Report for St Helier NHS Trust, Surrey

Gallagher D, Thompson L W 1983 Effectiveness of psychotherapy for both endogenous and non-endogenous depression in older adults. Journal of Gerontology 38:307–312

Gallagher D, Nies G, Thompson L W 1982 Reliability of the Beck Depression Inventory with older adults. Journal of Consulting and Clinical Psychology 50:152–153

Gatz I 1995 Early stage Alzheimer's patients find comfort in their own support group. Alzheimer's Disease International Global Perspective, Newsletter 6(1):6–7

Georgotas A, McCue R E, Hapworth W et al 1986 Comparative efficacy and safety of MAOIs versus TCAs in treating depression in the elderly. Biological Psychiatry 21:1155–1166

Gibson G, Moniz-Cook E 1996 It's good to talk – man to man. Journal of Dementia Care 4(5):20–22

Gilhooly M L M 1986 Senile dementia: factors associated with care-giver's preference for institutional care. British Journal of Medical Psychology 57:34–44

Glatt M M 1961 Treatment results in an English mental hospital alcoholic unit. Acta Psychiatrica Scandinavica 37:143

Goldsmith M 1996 Hearing the voice of people with dementia: Opportunities and obstacles. Jessica Kingsley, London

Gomberg E S L 1994 Risk factors for drinking over a women's life span. Alcohol Health and Research World 18(3):220–227

Grad J, Sainsbury P 1965 An evaluation of the effects of caring for the aged at home. In: Psychiatric disorders in the aged. WPA Symposium, Geigy, Manchester

Grahame P S 1984 Schizophrenia in old age (late paraphrenia). British Journal of Psychiatry 145:493–495

Gubrium J F 1987 Structuring and destructuring the course of illness: the Alzheimer's disease experience. Sociology of Health and Illness 9(1):1–24

Gurland B J 1976 The comparative frequency of depression in various adult age groups. Journal of Gerontology 31:283–292

Gurland B J, Cross P S 1982 Epidemiology of psychopathology in old age. Psychiatric Clinics of North America 5(1):11–26

Haight B 1992 The structured life-review process: a community approach to the aging client. In: Jones G, Miesen B M L (eds) Care-giving in dementia: Research and applications. Routledge, London, ch 16, p 272–292

Harris P B 1993 The misunderstood caregiver? A qualitative study of the male caregiver of Alzheimer's disease victims. Gerontologist 33(4):551–556

Harvey R, Fairey A 1997 Drug treatments on the way.

Alzheimer's Disease Society Newsletter, March, p 6

Health Advisory Service 1982 The rising tide. Report, NHS, Sutton, Surrey

Hersen M, Van Hasselt V B 1992 Behavioural assessment and treatment of anxiety in the elderly. Clinical Psychology Review 12:619–640

Hinrichsen G A 1992 Recovery and relapse from major depressive disorder in the elderly. American Journal of Psychiatry 149:1575–1579

Hirschfield M J 1983 Home care versus institutionalization: family caregiving and senile brain disease. International Journal of Nursing Studies 20(1):23–32

Holden N 1987 Late paraphrenia or the paraphrenias? British Journal of Psychiatry 150:635–639

Howard R 1993 Late paraphrenia. International Review of Psychiatry 5:455–460

Howard R, Levy R 1992 Which factors affect treatment response in late paraphrenia? International Journal of Geriatric Psychiatry 7:667–672

Hughes C P, Berg L, Danziger W L, Coben L A, Martin R L 1982 A new clinical scale for the staging of dementia. British Journal of Psychiatry 140:566–572

Iliffe S, Haines A, Booroff A, Goldenberg E, Morgan P, Gallivan S 1991 Alcohol consumption by elderly people: a general practice survey. Age and Ageing 20:120–123

Iliffe S, Tai S S, Haines A et al 1993 Assessment of elderly people in general practice: depression, functional ability and contact with services. British Journal of General Practice 43:371–374

Jacques A 1992 Understanding dementia, 2nd edn. Churchill Livingstone, Edinburgh

Jones G, Miesen B M L 1992 Care-giving in dementia: Research and applications. Routledge, New York

Katona C L E 1994 Depression in old age. Wiley, Chichester

Kay D W K, Roth M 1961 Environmental and hereditary factors in the schizophrenias of old age (late paraphrenia) and their bearing on the general problem of causation in schizophrenia. Journal of Mental Science 107:649–686

Keady J 1996 The experience of dementia: a review of the literature and implications for nursing practice. Journal of Clinical Nursing (Review Section) 5(5):275–288

Keady J 1997a Dementia: identification, assessment and support. Primary Health Care 7(6):17–22

Keady J 1997b Maintaining involvement: a meta concept to describe the dynamics of dementia. In: Marshall M (ed) The state of the art in dementia care. Centre for Policy on Ageing, London, ch 6, p 25–31

Keady J, Ford P 1997 Assessment of older people with mental health needs. Elderly Care 9(2):12–17

Keady J, Gilliard J 1999 The early experience of Alzheimer's disease: implications for partnership and practice. In: Adams T, Clarke C (eds) Dementia care: Developing partnerships in practice. Baillière Tindall, London, p 227–256

Keady J, Lundh U 1997 Living together: group homes in Sweden. The Journal of Dementia Care 5(3):26–28

Keady J, Nolan M R 1994a The carer-led assessment process (CLASP): a framework for the assessment of need in dementia caregivers. Journal of Clinical Nursing 3(2):103–108

Keady J, Nolan M R 1994b Younger-onset dementia:

REFERENCES (*contd*)

developing a longitudinal model as the basis for a research agenda and as a guide to interventions with sufferers and carers. Journal of Advanced Nursing 19:659–669

Keady J, Nolan M 1995a A stitch in time: facilitating proactive interventions with dementia caregivers: the role of community practitioners. Journal of Psychiatric and Mental Health Nursing 2(1):33–40

Keady J, Nolan M R 1995b IMMEL: assessing coping responses in the early stages of dementia. British Journal of Nursing 4(6):309–314

Keady J, Nolan M R 1995c IMMEL 2: working to augment coping responses in early dementia. British Journal of Nursing 4(7):377–380

Keller M B, Lavori P W, Klerman G L et al 1986 Low levels and lack of predictors of somatotherapy and psychotherapy received by depressed patients. Archives of General Psychiatry 43:458–466

Kendell R E 1981 The present status of electroconvulsive therapy. British Journal Psychiatry 139:265–283

King P, Barrowclough C 1991 Clinical pilot study of cognitive–behavioural therapy for anxiety disorders in the elderly. Behavioural Psychotherapy 19:337–345

Kitwood T 1992 Quality assurance in dementia care. Geriatric Medicine 22(9):34–38

Kitwood T 1997 Dementia reconsidered: the person comes first. Open University Press, Milton Keynes

Kitwood T, Benson S 1995 The new culture of dementia care. Hawker, London

Kitwood T, Bredin K 1992 Towards a theory of dementia care: personhood and well-being. Ageing and Society 12:269–287

Koenig H G, Meador K D, Cohen H J 1988 Detection and treatment of major depression in older medically ill hospitalised patients. International Journal Psychiatric Medicine 18(1):17–31

Kuhlman G J, Wilson H S, Hutchinson S A, Wallhagen M 1991 Alzheimer's disease and family caregiving: critical synthesis of the literature and research agenda. Nursing Research 40(6):331–337

LaBarge E, Trtanj F 1995 A support group for people in the early stages of dementia of the Alzheimer type. Journal of Applied Gerontology 14(3):289–301

Larson D B, Lyons J S, Hohmann A A, Beardsley R S, Hidalgo J 1991 Psychotropics prescribed to the US elderly in early to mid 1980s: prescribing patterns of primary care practitioners, psychiatrists and other physicians. International Journal of Geriatric Psychiatry 6:63–70

Lazarus R S 1966 Psychological stress and the coping process. McGraw Hill, New York

LeNavenec C 1995 Understanding the social context of families experiencing dementia: a qualitative approach. Paper presented at the 3rd European Conference of Gerontology, Amsterdam, September

Levin E, Sinclair I, Gorbach P 1989 Families, services and confusion in old age. Avebury, Aldershot

Leung M N S, Orrell M W 1993 A brief CBT group for the elderly: who benefits? International Journal of Geriatric Psychiatry 8:593–598

Li G, Silverman J M, Smith C J et al 1995 Age at onset and familial risk in Alzheimer's disease. American Journal of Psychiatry 152(3):424–430

Lindesay J 1991a Phobic disorders in the elderly. British Journal of Psychiatry 159:531–541

Lindesay J 1991b Anxiety disorders in the elderly. In: Jacoby R, Oppenheimer C (eds) Psychiatry in the elderly. Oxford University Press, Oxford, ch 20, p 735–757

Lindesay J, Briggs K, Murphy E 1989 The Guys/Age Concern survey prevalence rates of cognitive impairment, depression and anxiety in an urban elderly community. British Journal of Psychiatry 155:317–329

Livingstone G, Hawkins A, Graham N, Blizard B, Mann A 1990 The Gospel Oak study: prevalence rates of dementia, depression and activity limitation among elderly residents in inner London. Psychological Medicine 20:137–146

MacDonald A J D 1986 Do GPs miss depression in elderly patients? British Medical Journal 292:1365–1368

McGowin D F 1993 Living in the labyrinth: a personal journey through the maze of Alzheimer's disease. Mainsail Press, Cambridge

McWalter S, Toser H, Corser A, Eastwood J, Marshall M, Turvey T 1994 Needs and needs assessment: their components and definitions with reference to dementia. Health and Social Care in the Community 2(4):213–219

Magnússon H, Helgason T 1993 The course of mild dementia in a birth cohort. International Journal of Geriatric Psychiatry 8:639–647

Malmberg B, Zarit S H 1993 Group homes for people with dementia: a Swedish example. Gerontologist 33(5): 682–686

Manela C, Katona C, Livingston G 1996 How common are the anxiety disorders in old age? International Journal of Geriatric Psychiatry 11:65–70

Maurer K, Volk S, Gerbaldo H 1997 Auguste D and Alzheimer's disease. The Lancet 349:1546–1549

Menon R R, Jacoby R J 1993 Physical management of depression in the elderly. International Review of Psychiatry 5:417–426

Meyers B S, Greenberg R 1986 Late-life delusional depression. Journal of Affective Disorders 11:133–137

Millar B 1992 Threescore years and then? Health Service Journal Sept 3:10

Miller E, Morris R 1993 The psychology of dementia. Wiley, Chichester

Moos R H, Brennan P L, Moos B S 1991 Short-term process of remission and non-remission amongst late-life problem drinkers. Alcoholism: Clinical and Experimental Research 15:948–955

Morris J C, Fulling K 1988 Early Alzheimer's disease: diagnostic considerations. Archives of Neurology 45:345–349

Morris R G, Morris L W, Britton P G 1988 Factors affecting the emotional well-being of the caregivers of dementia sufferers. British Journal of Psychiatry 153:147–156

Motenko A K 1989 The frustrations, gratifications and well-being of dementia caregivers. Gerontologist 29(2):166–172

Murphy E 1982 Social origins of depression in old age. British Journal of Psychiatry 141:135–142

Murphy E 1983 The prognosis of depression in old age. British Journal of Psychiatry 142:111–119

Murphy E 1988 Prevention of depression and suicide. In: Gearing B, Johnson M, Heller T (eds) Mental health problems in old age. Wiley, Chichester, ch 8, p 67–73

REFERENCES (*contd*)

Murphy E, Grundy E 1984 A comparative study of bed usage by younger and older depressed patients. Psychological Medicine 14:445–450

Musetti L, Perugi G, Soriani A et al 1989 Depression before and after age 65:a re-examination. British Journal of Psychiatry 155:330–336

Newmann J P 1989 Aging and depression. Psychology and Aging 4(2):150–165

Nolan M, Keady J 1996 Training together: a challenge for the future. Journal of Dementia Care 4(5):10–13

Nolan M, Grant G, Keady J 1996 Understanding family care: A multidimensional model of caring and coping. Open University Press, Milton Keynes

Office of Population Census and Surveys 1983 Mortality statistics from general practice: third national study 1981–1982. HMSO, London

Office of Population Census and Surveys 1986 General household survey. HMSO, London

Office of Population Census and Surveys 1996 General household survey 1994. HMSO, London

Pearlin L I, Mullan J T, Semple S J, Scaff M M 1990 Caregiving and the stress process: an overview of concepts and their measures. Gerontologist 30(5):583–594

Pitt B 1991 Depression in the general hospital setting. International Journal of Geriatric Psychiatry 6:363–370

Post F 1982 Functional disorders : I. Description, incidence and recognition. In: Levey R, Post F (eds) The psychiatry of later-life. Blackwell Scientific, Oxford, p 176–221

Prince M 1997 The number of people with dementia is rising quickly. Alzheimer's Disease International Bulletin, 21 Sept 1997. Alzheimer's Disease International, London

Richardson C A, Hammond S M 1996 A psychometric analysis of a short device for assessing depression in elderly people. British Journal of Clinical Psychology 35:543–551

Richter J, Barsky A J, Hupp J A 1983 The treatment of depression in elderly patients. Journal of Family Practice 17:43–47

Rickard H C, Scogin F, Keith S 1994 A one-year follow-up of relaxation training for elders with subjective anxiety. The Gerontologist 34(1):121–122

Rohde K, Peskind E R, Raskind M A 1995 Suicide in two patients with Alzheimer's disease. Journal of the American Geriatrics Society 43:187–189

Roth M, Morrissey J 1952 Problems in the diagnosis and classification of mental disorders in old age. Journal of Mental Science 98:66–80

Royal College of Physicians 1981 Organic mental impairment in the elderly: A report by the Royal College of Physicians. College Committee on Geriatrics, Royal College of Physicians, London

Sabat S R, Harré R 1992 The construction and deconstruction of self in Alzheimer's disease. Ageing and Society 12(4):443–461

Salzman C 1990 Anxiety in the elderly: treatment strategies. Journal of Clinical Psychiatry 51:18–21

Sanford J R A 1975 Tolerance of debility in elderly dependents by supporters at home: its significance for hospital practice. British Medical Journal 3:375–376

Schonfeld L, Dupree L W 1994 Alcohol abuse among older adults. Reviews in Clinical Gerontology 4(3):217–225

Schonfeld L, Dupree L W 1995 Treatment approaches for older problem drinkers. Special issue: Drugs and the elderly: use and misuse of drugs, medicines, alcohol and tobacco. International Journal of Addictions 30(13–14):1819–1842

Scogin F 1992 Memory training for older adults. In: Jones G, Miesen B M L (eds) Caregiving in dementia: research and applications. Routledge, London, ch 17, p 260–271

Scogin F, McElreath L 1994 Efficacy of psychosocial treatments for geriatric depression: a quantitative review. Journal of Consulting Clinical Psychology 62:69–74

Shepherd M, Cooper B, Brown, Kalton G 1981 Psychiatric illness in general practice. Oxford University Press, Oxford

Social Services Inspectorate/Department of Health 1996 Assessing older people with dementia in the community: Practice issues for social and health services. HMSO, Wetherby

Social Services Inspectorate/Department of Health 1997 Older people with mental health problems living alone: anybody's priority? HMSO, Wetherby

Stanley M A, Beck G J, Glassco J D 1996a Treatment of generalized anxiety in older adults: a preliminary comparison of cognitive–behavioural and supportive approaches. Behaviour Therapy 27:565–581

Stanley M A, Beck G J, Zebb B J 1996b Psychometric properties of four anxiety measures in older adults. Behaviour Research Therapy 34(10):827–838

Stelzmann R A, Schnitzlein N, Murtagh F R 1995 An English translation of Alzheimer's 1907 paper, 'Uber eine eigenartige Erkrankung der Hirnrindle'. Clinical Anatomy 8:429–431

Sweeting H, Gilhooly M 1997 Dementia and the phenomenon of social death. Sociology of Health and Illness 19(1):93–117

Teri L, Wagner A 1991 Assessment of depression in patients with Alzheimer's disease: concordance between informants. Psychology and Aging 6:280–285

Thompson L W, Gallagher D 1984 Efficacy of psychotherapy in the treatment of late-life depression. Advanced Behaviour Research Therapy 6:127–139

Thompson L W, Gallagher D, Breckenridge J S 1987 Comparative effectiveness of psychotherapies for depressed elders. Journal of Consulting Clinical Psychology 53:385–390

Ward M, Goodman C 1995 Alcohol problems in old age, 2nd edn. Staccato, London

Warner J P 1996 Depression in older people: what does the future hold? International Journal of Geriatric Psychiatry 11:831–835

Watkins M 1988 Lifting the burden. Geriatric Nursing and Home Care 3(10):18–20

Watts C A H, Cawte E C, Kuenssberg E V 1964 Survey of mental illness in general practice. British Medical Journal 2:1351–1359

Wenger G C 1994 Support networks and dementia. International Journal of Geriatric Psychiatry 9:181–194

Wessen J 1992 The vintage years: Older people and alcohol. Aquarius, Birmingham

Widner S, Zeichner A 1991 Alcohol abuse in the elderly: review of epidemiology research and treatment. Clinical Gerontologist 11(1):3–18

REFERENCES (*contd*)

Woods B 1995 Dementia care: progress and prospects. Journal of Mental Health 4(2):115–124

Woods R T and Britton P G 1985 Clinical psychology with the elderly. Croom Helm, London

World Health Organization 1993a The ICD-10 classification of mental and behavioural disorders: Diagnostic criteria for research. World Health Organization, Geneva

World Health Organization 1993b Implementation of the global strategy for health for all by the year 2000, second evaluation: and eighth report on the world health situation. World Health Organization, Geneva

Wragg R E, Jeste D V 1989 Overview of depression and psychosis in Alzheimer's disease. American Journal of Psychiatry 146:577–587

Wuest J, Ericson P K, Stern P N 1994 Becoming strangers: the changing family caregiving relationship in Alzheimer's disease. Journal of Advanced Nursing 20:437–443

Yale R 1995 Developing support groups for individuals with early-stage Alzheimer's disease: Planning, implementation and evaluation. Health Professions Press, London

Yost E B, Beutler L E, Corbishley M A, Allender J R 1986 Group cognitive therapy: A treatment approach for depressed older adults. Pergamon, London

Zarit S, Orr N, Zarit M 1985 The hidden victims of Alzheimer's disease. New York University Press, New York

Zimberg S 1978 Diagnosis and treatment of the elderly alcoholic. Alcoholism: Clinical and Experimental Research 2:27–29

Mental health initiatives: new directions in mental health care

SECTION CONTENTS

19. Advocacy   373

20. Self-help initiatives   391

21. Alternatives to traditional mental
    health treatments   405

CHAPTER CONTENTS

Key points   373

Introduction   374

Advocacy – its meaning and manifestations   374

Different types of advocacy   376
   Legal advocacy   376
   Self-advocacy   377
   Peer advocacy   377
   Citizen advocacy   378
   Class or collective advocacy   378

Advocacy in mental health nursing – the literature and research   379

Advocacy schemes in mental health   382
   Clientbond   382
   Nottingham Advocacy Group   383
   Whitby Advocacy Project   384
   Barnsley Hospital Advocacy Service   385

Conclusions   385

Exercise   388

Useful addresses   388

Key texts for further reading   388

References   388

19

Advocacy

Bob Gates

KEY POINTS

● Advocates aim to represent, empower and advise clients.

● Advocacy has a high profile in mental health nursing.

● Empirical research supporting advocacy is limited, but clients report benefit.

● The roles of nurse and advocate may be mutually exclusive.

● Nurses are a potential force for the support of advocates and the advocacy movement.

INTRODUCTION

This chapter will explore a range of literature about, and report on, a number of advocacy schemes relevant to the specialism of mental health nursing. The chapter also explores the evidence, scant as it is, concerning the efficacy of advocacy in mental health nursing. This evidence will be undertaken from two perspectives: first, the nurse as advocate; and second, more formal but independent advocacy schemes. The first perspective concerns the efficacy of the nurse acting as advocate. This idea has been portrayed as particularly problematic by a number of commentators (Gates 1994, Teasdale 1994), and for some considerable period of time (Casteldine 1981, Smith 1980) and internationally (Abrams 1978, Evans 1992). The second perspective will explore whether advocacy schemes make a difference to the experience of, and/or outcome of, a mental ill-health episode. For a full analysis of nursing literature concerning this area the reader is advised to refer to two comprehensive reviews of the literature on advocacy (Evans 1992, Mallik 1997). It should be said that there has been an exponential explosion of literature related to advocacy in the field of mental health in the last 15 years. This has clearly necessitated, on the part of the author, a need to exclude a range of papers that may have been of interest to the reader. This does not imply that papers excluded are of little interest or importance, rather that constraints on word limit for this chapter have necessitated brief treatment of some of the literature, and it is for this reason that key texts for further reading are also provided for the reader at the end of the chapter.

Before exploring advocacy in mental health it would seem wise to commence this chapter by defining advocacy and then outline the various types of advocacy that can be found both in the literature and in practice.

ADVOCACY – ITS MEANING AND MANIFESTATIONS

The word advocate derives from the Latin 'advocactus' and is concerned with one who is summoned to give evidence. This point is interesting because advocacy has a long association with the legal profession and the word advocate in some countries, for example Scotland and South Africa, is still used to refer to a barrister. The *Webster Universal Dictionary* (1975) has defined advocacy as:

> the act of pleading in support of; intercession.
>
> *Webster Universal Dictionary* 1975:37

and an advocate is defined as:

> One called in to aid another, in legal cause, an advocate … to call to one's aid … one who pleads the cause of another … legal representative of the case for opposing canonisation . . one who supports, defends and recommends verbally, a cause, proposal, line of action.
>
> *Webster Universal Dictionary* 1975:37

This brings us briefly to consider the way in which the words 'advocate' and 'advocacy' are used in nursing. There are number of commentators who would argue that the nature of nursing and advocacy are practically and theoretically very different entities. Indeed, Gates (1994, 1995) has argued that nurses and advocates may essentially be, in any meaningful sense of either word, two mutually exclusive concepts. However, it is clear from the United Kingdom Central Council for Nursing, Midwifery and Health Visiting (UKCC) *Guidelines for Professional Practice* (1996) that there is a continuing expectation that nurses will act as a patient's advocate. Of particular interest are the latest guidelines for mental health and learning disability nurses from the UKCC (1998). Here it is stated that:

> When caring for your clients, you must

endeavour to promote and safeguard their interests. You must not practise in a way which assumes that only you know what is best for the client. This creates dependency and can interfere with the client's right to choose.

UKCC 1998:7

The UKCC in this document does endeavour to provide some realistic attempts at assisting practitioners to explore issues of practice that they are likely to encounter. For example, for the first time the UKCC suggests that nurses are clear about their role as advocate, especially in relation to the issue of conflict of interest:

You need to be clear about your role in advocating for clients. There is a potential for conflict when attempting to assume the role of an advocate for clients under the relevant mental health act. Your professional relationship with a client may mean that you cannot be objective about your input and may therefore be unable to identify and support the individual needs of the client. You must distinguish between your professional responsibility to advocate on behalf of your clients and the role of the professional advocate. In some instances an independent advocate can provide better objective support to clients.

UKCC 1998:7

It does seem to me that within this single paragraph lies the kernel of contradiction that myself and other commentators have raised on numerous occasions. This is that the nurse cannot act as an independent advocate, and the statutory body for the UK accepts this. This being the case, why does this body continue to promote something that practitioners cannot do? Would it not make more sense to dispose of the word 'advocate', that alludes to something that lies beyond the role of the nurse? Instead, adopt a word that more realistically describes what nurses are able and therefore should be expected to do. Despite the considerable energy and resource that the UKCC seems able to sustain in the deliverance of advice and guidance as to the nature of nursing

practice, there is little or no evidence that any of these guidelines are of any use whatsoever to practitioners in the very many different contexts in which they work. Therefore, despite these proclamations from the UKCC, it is not at all clear whether nurses are really able to assume an advocacy role with any authenticity or legitimacy. This is because of problems related, for example, to conflicts of loyalty, inadequate education and hegemonic power. This has led a number of commentators to conclude that nurses can *not* always be seen as an appropriate advocate (Allmark & Klarzynski 1992, Morrison 1991, Willard 1996).

The interface between role demands of nurse and advocate is clearly fraught with conflicts of loyalties and incumbent tensions (Gates 1994). In the field of mental health nursing, this has been demonstrated on numerous occasions, but of particular importance, in the folklore of mental health nursing, was the case of Walsh (1985). Walsh, a Senior Nursing Officer at Wrexham Hospital in Berkshire, was accused of managerial incompetence and gross misconduct warranting dismissal. Clearly such serious accusations must have been the result of some dreadful action on his part. Actually, Walsh challenged medical staff about their intrusion in attempting to determine the nature of nursing care. He made a series of counter accusations to that of managerial incompetence, including acting unlawfully within the Mental Health Act 1983, and requesting that nursing staff act forcibly against patients, almost in a punitive way. Walsh was eventually suspended because of his refusal to instruct staff to restrain a patient while they were administering a psychotropic drug. Walsh ostensibly challenged bad practice, and in a sense he might well have been acting as advocate. However, it is clear that in so doing he experienced the inevitable outcome of attempting to reconcile two mutually exclusive roles: those of nurse and advocate.

These tensions and potentially mutually exclusive role attributes of nurse and advocate are depicted in schematic form in Figure 19.1.

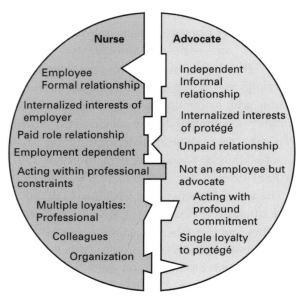

Figure 19.1 The interface between the role demands of advocate and nurse demonstrating the mutually exclusive nature of the two concepts (reproduced from Gates B 1994 Advocacy: A nurses' guide. Scutari Press, Middlesex).

It is the case that guidelines concerning advocates issued by the Citizen Advocacy Information and Training Scheme (CAIT 1994) have outlined very clearly the nature of the role of advocate:

> advocates owe those they represent a duty of loyalty, confidentiality, and a commitment to be zealous in the promotion of their [patients] cause.
>
> CAIT 1994

CAIT further identified that advocates must be unpaid, independent volunteers who represent only one individual at any given time. Clearly, these attributes are much more in keeping with the role attributes ascribed to advocates as opposed to nurses (see Fig. 19.1). This has led

Willard (1996), amongst others, to conclude that advocacy is an imposition to nursing rather than an obligation.

DIFFERENT TYPES OF ADVOCACY

Having briefly identified the role of advocate, it might be worth moving on at this point to briefly explore the different types of advocacy that are practised. It is anticipated that this portrayal will assist the reader in developing greater critical appreciation of a supposed role of nursing that has been polarised in much of the nursing literature.

Legal advocacy

This is a very specialised form of advocacy that Butler et al (1988) have described as:

> A process in which legally trained persons pursue and represent the rights and interests of people within existing legislative frameworks, or they seek to extend the parameters of legislation to protect and/or promote the rights of an individual.
>
> Butler et al 1988:2

This type of advocacy is frequently used in the specialism of mental health nursing. This is because the rights and integrity of people with mental health problems are so very easily compromised by human delivery services. A number of examples can be found in the literature that give details concerning the use of this very specialised form of advocacy. Diesfeld (1994) has reported on the importance of this type of representation and she provides refreshing evidence of the legal profession's commitment to the education of law students. She acknowledges the reciprocity of relationships of practitioners of law and those who are in need of representation.

Clearly the advocate occupies an extremely complex role and operates within an even more complex arena of practice, and that is why this type of advocacy is often only undertaken by legally trained persons.

Self-advocacy

In this type of advocacy, the advocate or facilitator attempts to shift the focus of control from himself or herself to the people with whom he or she is working. Williams & Schoultz (1982) have defined self-advocacy as:

> Individual people or groups speaking or acting on behalf of the people on issues which affect them in the same way as themselves.
>
> Williams & Schoultz 1982:87–89

In self-advocacy, people are encouraged to speak up for themselves, thus establishing an element of self-empowerment, rather than having an advocate speak for them. There is a strong ideological belief that self-advocacy enables people to grow and develop from the experience of speaking up for themselves. Probably the most widely known text concerning self-advocacy is that of Williams & Schoultz (1982). In their book they outline the life of Raymond Loomis who developed a self-advocacy group in Nebraska in North America. This group, known as the People First movement, gained national and international recognition. It demonstrated that people with learning disabilities were able to articulate their fears, aspirations and needs, and that human service delivery systems needed to learn how they might respond to such pressure. The idea that 'the user' of a service had an ability to articulate their ideas was, and it has to be said still is, a significant challenge to the attitudes and prejudices of some personnel and organisations. This movement undoubtedly inspired others to follow suit and one can find examples of numerous self-advocacy schemes that have been set up by people who have experience of mental health services and wish to see such services improve.

Campbell (1989) has described the emergence of the 'grass roots self advocacy' movement in the field of mental health. It is interesting to note that he has asserted that this movement has acknowledged that mental health workers are relatively powerless within the systems in which they are located. He has suggested that this was an important factor in the development of the self-advocacy movement. A fascinating account of the power of users to express opinion concerning their experiences of mental health episodes has been provided by the United Kingdom Advocacy Network (UKAN) (1995). In a national survey, questionnaires were distributed to elicit what people thought about their experiences of electroconvulsive therapy (ECT). Such opinions and experiences from the 'grass roots' have enormous potential to safeguard the rights, interests and integrity of people with mental health problems. Survivors Speak Out is probably the best known self-advocacy group in the field of mental health and has provided a focus for users, past and present, of mental health services to articulate ways in which services for people with mental health problems may be improved.

Peer advocacy

Conlan (1994) has pointed out that the first 'peer advocate' to be formally recorded was that of John Percival in the mid-nineteenth century, who was reported to have travelled to a psychiatric hospital in Northampton to seek the release of a poet, John Clare. It is suggested that the group he represented, The Alleged Lunatics Society, was the forerunner of the peer advocacy movement. Despite this gem of historical interest, it is fair to say that the term peer advocacy is still relatively new in the literature, but it has been described by Brandon (1994) as:

individual support by recovering or recovered users in helping other service users to express and fulfil their individual wishes.

Brandon 1994:218

Citizen advocacy

Probably the most widely known form of advocacy is that of citizen advocacy. It is likely that this form of advocacy developed in the USA some time during the 1960s and that conceptually the notion of citizen advocate was shaped by the writings of Wolfensberger (1972) and Sang & O'Brien (1984). Wolfensberger has defined a citizen advocate as:

> A mature, competent citizen volunteer representing, as if they were his own, the interests of another citizen who is impaired in his instrumental competency, or who has major expressive needs which are unmet and which are likely to remain unmet without special intervention.

Wolfensberger 1972

It is important to explore briefly the notion of instrumental competency and expressive need.

Instrumental competency refers to those behaviours that enable us to respond to and successfully interact with our environments, for example, earning a living, managing our financial affairs, painting and decorating, gardening, getting dressed – in other words, collections of fairly sophisticated daily living skills. These daily living skills become more extensive and refined as we develop and reach a relatively stable plateau during adult life. In some mental health experiences the ability to undertake these 'everyday' activities becomes severely impeded.

Expressive need refers to the emotional component of psychological being. Maslow (1954) in his model of human need described these as psychological needs. During our childhood these are met by deep meaningful relationships with our parents and significant others within our lives. Examples of such needs are a feeling of security, a need for love and understanding, friendship and the promotion of self-worth and self-esteem. Clearly we develop into better, more stable and well-adapted individuals, if these needs are successfully met during our formative years. As a child grows, these needs are met by an increasingly wide network of valued significant others. During our adult years we meet these expressive needs through the development of relationships with friends, partner and / or children.

Once again the experience of some users of mental health services, either during or after an episode of ill-health, may significantly affect the ability of an individual to meet such needs. McFadyen (1989), for example, has stated that a range of issues that might broadly be grouped under instrumental competency are important to people with mental health problems. These include:

> tenure and tenancy issues, employment relations, personal and family relations and welfare and state benefit rights are all areas where advocacy needs can be identified.

McFadyen 1989:46

Evidently these two concepts are very important to understanding the role of the citizen advocate in the field of mental health work. Finally, pivotal to the role of the citizen advocate are the *needs* of the protégé rather than the protégé having to conform to the provisions of particular caring agencies or professional groupings, such as nursing.

Class or collective advocacy

This type of advocacy is also referred to in some

literature as corporate advocacy. In essence, it is a type of advocacy that, through large organisations, pursues the rights and interests of a complete category of people. Perhaps the most widely known of these, in the field of mental health, is MIND, but there are other groups who also serve equally important sub-groups of people with mental heath problems.[1] Clearly these organisations have an enormous resource at their disposal and therefore they often appoint full-time officers as well as relying upon the use of volunteers. Much of the work of such organisations is concerned with the promotion of a more positive image of mental health disorders. But, in addition to this, many of these organisations attempt to pursue the rights of people experiencing mental health problems and/or their carers. More recently, a new term seems to have evolved to describe this type of advocacy provision. This is sometimes referred to as *formal advocacy* in some recent literature and this refers to individuals who are paid, and the organisation is said to adopt an 'expert' model. Essentially, formal or professional advocacy is the same as collective or class advocacy.

Having briefly outlined the various types of advocacy, and how they are used, the next section will consider a range of literature and explore some of the evidence surrounding advocacy in mental health nursing.

ADVOCACY IN MENTAL HEALTH NURSING – THE LITERATURE AND RESEARCH

There is considerable literature concerning issues of advocacy in the field of mental health nursing, but surprisingly little research to report on. Surprising because much of the literature puts forward passionate argument for the need for advocacy schemes in this field, and yet little attention has been paid to the important issue of whether they actually achieve the claims that are made about them. As far back as 1985, the issue of advocacy in mental health nursing was beginning to emerge as a consistent theme in nursing literature. Walsh (1985), during the week of the Mental Health Congress, questioned the appropriateness of nurses taking on the role of advocate. In the same issue of the nursing journal as the Walsh (1985) article, Brown (1985) produced a checklist of factors for nurses to ask themselves to direct any advocacy role that they might assume; the assumption presumably was that nurses should take on the role of advocate. These checklist factors were:

- quality of care as a response to patient needs
- Access to care appropriate to patient needs
- information being provided in a manner that a patient would understand
- alternative provision of care that might more adequately meet patient needs.

What is clear is the emergence of an almost polarised view 'for or against' nurses acting as advocates, and this may be found as a consistent theme from commentators of this subject in much nursing literature. McFadyen (1989), for example, has argued that the Mental Health Act 1983, in some senses, represented a major shift in issues concerning the protection of patients rights. However, by way of contrast, he acknowledged that never before had there been such a need for effective advocates. He also argued that nurses were not necessarily best placed to undertake this role. This article provides a valuable summary of advocacy schemes within the USA and McFadyen constructed arguments for 'properly empowered and organised advocacy ser-

---

[1]A list of useful addresses of such organisations is provided at the end of the chapter (p. 388).

vices', that he stated were not available in the UK.

> In fighting for resources and monitoring the rights of mentally ill people, such advocacy might help produce not only services that uphold the rights of the mentally ill, but services which are right for them.
>
> McFadyen 1989:48

Clarke (1995) has similarly argued the need to promote the rights of people with mental ill-health. He has asserted that there is considerable argument for rejecting the use of ECT and that nurses should advise their patients of alternatives. However, he constructs a convincing argument that nurses engage in an avoidance of the advocacy issues, and this avoidance is for many reasons. One of those reasons was:

> What little evidence there is suggests that nurses will still be construed as rogue elements[2] and sanctioned accordingly.
>
> Clarke 1995:330

It has already been said that there is little research concerning the effectiveness of advocacy in the mental health field.

> There is clearly a need for research in this area. Few empirical studies exist examining the effectiveness of patient advocacy programmes or comparing the effectiveness of different programmes.
>
> Olley & Ogloff 1995:374

Given that it has been suggested that advocacy services in England alone are estimated to cost somewhere in the region of £28 million (Tannahill & Lawson 1993), it does not seem unreasonable to seek out whether there is any evidence that suggests them to be of benefit to those in receipt of such a service. Those studies reported here represent small sample surveys that have used questionnaires and other more qualitative measures. Before moving on to consider the research basis for the use of advocacy schemes, it does seem appropriate to raise the problematic nature of what constitutes evidence. My own view is that evidence obtained through personal accounts, either autobiographical or biographical or in the form of poetry, are both legitimate and authentic sources and therefore may be considered in every sense of the word as 'evidence', in just the same ways as carefully controlled trials. There are, however, clear issues concerning both reliability and validity of such sources of evidence. Kitson (1997) has recently explored the notion of using 'evidence' to demonstrate the contribution of nursing and its effectiveness. She holds as problematic the use of the term evidence and makes a distinction between 'knowledge based upon opinion and practice as opposed to scientific evidence'. Sackett et al (1996) has defined evidence-based medicine as:

> Conscientious, explicit and judicious use of current evidence about the care of individual patients.
>
> Sackett et al 1996:71–72

The use of the term 'evidence' in nursing, and perhaps in medicine, seems to be adopting its own special meaning. It is the case that many contemporary definitions of the word 'evidence' talk of the establishment of fact and also of giving reason for believing something. In law, for example, evidence is used to mean proof of something, or to support a case. It does seem that if one uses the term 'evidence' in the sense that others use it, nursing does have at its disposal considerable evidence of both the utility and necessity for advocacy in mental health care. Perhaps what nursing does not have is a range of the so-called gold standard of evidence – the

---

[2] Here Clarke is making reference to the Pink case: Pink G 1993 Whistle down the drain. Nursing Standard 7(17):47.

apparently more sophisticated randomised controlled trials – to prove such an assertion.

Therefore, given the evidence provided in this chapter (i.e. using evidence in the special way that nursing and medicine perhaps use the term), it might be argued that there exists the necessary but not sufficient evidence upon which to validly and reliably base our practice. Perhaps, advocacy might one day occupy a place on the agenda in mental health of sufficient magnitude to be considered worthy of carefully controlled studies that would also combine qualitative elements, thus enhancing claims of generalisability. This section of the chapter will conclude with two extracts of personal accounts that perhaps might be seen as a different kind of evidence that supports advocacy in the field of mental health.

Tannahill & Lawson (1993) have reported on a survey of senior psychiatrists in Wales. The overwhelming view of these psychiatrists was one of support for advocacy in mental health, although it is interesting to note that the authors of the paper conclude that further and more extensive research is required in this area before resources are diverted to support such schemes. The paper reports on the long-fought adversarial relationship of advocacy with the medical profession. A questionnaire was distributed to 133 psychiatrists that sought to examine their knowledge of advocacy in general, advocacy locally, experience of advocacy in clinical work and attitudes and beliefs held by the psychiatrists toward advocacy.

Of the psychiatrists responding (86%), a large proportion (76%) thought that they had little general knowledge on advocacy, and 73% of the sample admitted to having little or no knowledge of advocacy services locally. Concerning clinical involvement, 62% stated that they had no patients involved with advocacy services. Interestingly, 87% of those surveyed felt that advocacy would not affect their professional status,

which apparently contradicts the experience of psychiatrists in the USA (Applebaum 1979). However, the response from the psychiatrists in Wales might have been predicted, as so few had any experiences of advocacy. It was clear from the survey that psychiatrists thought that patients would benefit from advocacy, especially in the areas of housing, finance and benefits, social and job skills along with health and therapeutic issues. This study concluded that advocacy clearly had the potential to be of benefit to a wide range of people with mental health problems, but that which people it could most help was not known; this led the authors to conclude that there was a need for further studies in this area.

The Evaluation and Development and Review Unit of the Tavistock Institute has produced a number of evaluative reports on the impact of a range of advocacy schemes (Holly & Webb 1992, Webb 1992). Of particular importance is the scheme reported from Whitby, to be discussed more fully later, under the auspices of the Advocacy Alliance. It is clear from the evaluation study undertaken, which used self-evaluation material, interviews conducted with members of management advisory groups and interviews with project co-ordinators, that a number of achievements may be illustrative of the success of this scheme.

Sellin (1995) reported on a qualitative study of advocacy in an institutional setting. In this study, a convenience sample comprising 27 clinical nurses, six nurse managers, four clinical nurse specialists and three nurse administrators was recruited from five clinical settings in two, large, urban, teaching hospitals. The researcher used formal, semi-structured interviews as the primary means of generating data. These interviews explored with participants definitions of advocacy, situations in which they acted as advocates, factors influencing their decisions to act as advocates and, finally, their willingness to take risks associated with advocacy. Participants also completed a decision-making inventory to further understand how participants gathered and processed information leading to a decision as whether to take a risk and act as advocate. Data from the interviews were analysed through the constant comparative approach that enabled the coding and categorisation of data.

The findings of the study point to the definitions of advocacy used by the participants being consistent with nursing ethics literature. Interestingly, participants saw information-gathering as the primary, preliminary activity of nurse advocacy. The further developed theoretical properties of nursing advocacy were concerned with protection from harm, supporting patients in their decisions, educating patients, explaining treatments and guiding patients 'through the system'. It was clear that situations that led nurses to experience ethical discomfort were strongly related to action as advocate. In other words, acting as advocate was highly subjective and idiosyncratic and perhaps had a lot to do with the degree of tension between internally held value bases and external lived experience. The greater the challenge or affront to an individual nurse's ethical value base, it would seem the more likely it is for a nurse to see his or her role as patient advocate. Clearly, this was a limited study: first, methodologically the sample size is small and unrepresentative and second, the study relates to another culture and another specialism within nursing. However, such studies are interesting, and it is worth noting that perhaps other specialisms in nursing should be undertaking research in order for us to construct evidence of the usefulness of advocacy.

Let me conclude this section with two accounts of a different kind of evidence that are concerned with the need for advocacy in the field of mental health. First, Jimmy Laing, a man who has experienced mental health problems, writes powerfully at the end of his book:

> I am angry, though, that there was no power of redress in the old days. There was no way that you could argue your case to try to prove that you shouldn't be in the system. Today there are various groups interested in the welfare of mental patients which keep their plight to the forefront and that is a great step forward. Mental patients need their support particularly when they're at the lowest ebb. When you're down at rock bottom, to know that someone is interested in you gives you the necessary to continue living.

> Laing & McQuarrie 1989:187

Next consider a poem by Ford (1995):

A case for self-advocacy *Post Mortem*

Although Sylvia herself is dead
she's made again, over and over.
They take her and make her over, over
again and again. In their heads they shape
and fashion her and have printed out,
more black than black on white, on paper.
It's always men, almost always, who mop up
where others have bled and make out
of being, doing; who make up a case
for themselves as mentor, progenitor. . .

She isn't Sylvia's Sylvia any longer,
she isn't herself now, she can't be.
Not so much as a shred of breath remains
unswept up from the flat in Fitzroy Road:
the nurse's bare. In her garden, grown
over with brambles, mist hangs dankly round
the yew tree. It's all empty. Dull. From the earth
brown bed where her wounds lie, her words lie,
they keep on bleeding, we keep on reading
all the doing of her undoing.

> Ford 1995:30

ADVOCACY SCHEMES IN MENTAL HEALTH

Clientbond

Glasman (1991a) has reported how the rights of people in receipt of psychiatric services in hospitals in the Netherlands could be safeguarded by the introduction of advocates into hospital services. Early in the 1970s, stories of ill-treatment and the abuse of human rights were emerging from the large psychiatric hospitals in the Netherlands. From the appalling stories emerged a new group to protect the rights and integrity of such people, known as 'Clientbond'. Originally the group evolved from a group of disaffected parents who were concerned at the sacking of a psychiatrist from a children's psychiatric unit. The 'Clientbond' developed into a radical user group who located their work in many of the psychiatric hospitals. By the late 1970s they began to flourish and to form patients' councils in hospitals throughout the Netherlands. In 1981, the National Association of Patients Councils was formed to provide professional support to each of the councils. The advocate's independence is supposedly assured by the funding mechanism, which was administered through central government rather than the local hospitals. Each hospital pays the equivalent of the advocate's wage to the patients' council which pays the advocate, thus ensuring that the advocate is an independent employee and not reliant upon the hospital for financial security. This scheme, however, is not without its critics who have complained that such schemes only truly extend their influence to the decor of buildings and the type of food on offer. This said, it is interesting to note that mental health legislation requires all psychiatric hospitals in the Netherlands to have a patients' council. The Patients Council Foundation continues to be funded by the Netherlands government, and the Foundation assists in the development and support of the local, hospital-based councils.

Nottingham Advocacy Group

Mullender (1991) has reported on the work of the Nottingham Advocacy Group (NAG). This scheme brought together three distinct types of advocacy. A number of self-advocacy groups were set up in hospitals surrounding Nottingham. This was augmented by patient advocacy, similar to that described by Glasman above. Lastly, the scheme used citizen advocacy as another approach in ensuring that this comprehensive advocacy scheme met the various and unique needs of the people concerned. Mullender (1991) concluded that:

> [The work of NAG] has already had a dramatic effect on the self esteem and confidence of a significant number of users and ex-users of the psychiatric services.
>
> Mullender 1991:11

The three types of advocacy used comprised:

- *Self-advocacy*. Here something approaching 20 different locations were involved in ensuring that user views were made known through user-only meetings. These meetings were held in hospital wards as well as community settings. Volunteers, those who had previously used mental health services, were charged with the responsibility of making representation of user views during the planning of service provision.
- *Citizen advocacy*. The Mental Health Foundation and Nottinghamshire Social Services Department provided the necessary funding for the appointment of a citizen advocacy co-ordinator. This person was charged with the responsibility of establishing a register of volunteers (citizen advocates) who were to be matched with users of mental health services in the area. In the first year, approximately 20 pairings were made between advocates and protégés. All advocates were prepared for their long-term relationship with their partners and were

chosen on the basis of their commitment to the project's philosophy of advocating on behalf of their partner as strongly as they would for one of their own relatives.

- *Patient advocacy*. The final type of advocacy reported from this scheme was described as patient advocacy. This type of advocacy was based upon a study undertaken by the Nottingham group of advocacy systems used in the Netherlands. It was envisaged that an individual would be appointed who would liaise with patients' councils and other community groups to explore the wider issues associated with representation.

These three types of advocacy represented an impressive 'front line' that was successfully used in the pursuit of rights for, and representation of, people with mental health problems

Whitby Advocacy Project

As mentioned earlier, the Evaluation Development and Review Unit of the Tavistock Institute has reported on four projects concerning advocacy. Of particular interest to this chapter is a scheme that was established and evaluated in Whitby (Holly & Webb 1992, Webb 1992). The Whitby Advocacy Project dealt exclusively with people, aged between 18 and 65, with mental health and/or emotional problems. Those people who required or requested advocates because of their mental health and/or emotional problems were known as partners. Partners may have been detained under the Mental Health Act 1983, but most partners lived in the community. The purpose of the intervention by the advocate was to assist in recovery from the mental ill-health episode and promote independence. This scheme encountered a number of difficulties that included: the co-ordinator working considerably longer hours than she was being paid for and advocates experiencing

difficulties regarding expenses (namely paying for travelling expenses for their partners without being reimbursed). In addition, enormous stress was experienced by some advocates because of some partners' attempts at self-harm or reported suicidal tendencies. This last difficulty required specific training and support group work. However, most problems encountered by advocates were responded to by the construction of an advocates' self-help support group. This group assisted with the sharing of experience to dissipate some of the difficulties that advocates encountered.

The evaluation reported that a number of achievements were realised by the advocacy project, including:

- *Public awareness*. It was clear that the activities of this advocacy group did much to raise public awareness about mental health and this was generally thought to be both constructive and helpful.
- *Support group*. A 'by-product' of the establishment of this advocacy group was the development of a support group. While this was seen by the evaluation group as an achievement, it should be noted that support groups and advocacy groups are both theoretically and practically very different things. Some might argue that if the advocacy group were to develop exclusively into a support group then this would compromise the central function of the group.
- *Cohesive group*. It was clear from the evaluation that the group developed into a strong and cohesive group. There was clear evidence of people working closely together – this type of cohesion is extremely useful to the productivity of a group.
- *Foundations for future development*. An important feature of such innovations is constructing a base that is sufficiently robust

to last. The evaluation team believed that the Whitby project achieved this. Making short-lived changes is relatively easy to achieve, but sustaining a service is much more difficult. Indeed professionals, rightly or wrongly, often criticise such groups because of their 'short-lived' nature.

- *Partnerships formed*. At the time of writing the report, 10 partnerships had been formed and two further partnerships were being established. Although these numbers may be seen as modest, each partnership has the potential to represent a unique opportunity to ensure adequate and proper representation of people experiencing mental ill-health, in order to protect their rights and interests.

Barnsley Hospital Advocacy Service

Another most interesting scheme, here in the UK, is that of the Barnsley Hospital Advocacy Service. This scheme was established by MIND in 1994 and is now in its 5th year of operation. It provides a hospital advocacy service for people who are experiencing mental health problems and who feel that they are not being listened to. The scheme provides an annual report of its activities that includes statistical data along with more qualitative accounts of the kinds of advocacy service provided. Examples in the 1996 annual report included:

> A patient is admitted onto the ward as a voluntary patient. The patient is told by the consultant that if he discharges himself/he will be sectioned under the Mental Health Act 1983.
>
> MIND 1996:2

The advocacy service's response to this individual included explanation of rights as a voluntary patient and liaison with a range of qualified practitioners. Lastly, if the patient wished to complain, the advocate would help write a letter of complaint to the Chief Executive Officer of the Trust. The advocacy service maintains data on the types of issues that are raised by patients, complaints, referrals to other agencies and the take-up of services by ward and date. These types of activities may at a superficial level seem rather ineffectual, but the evidence from MIND in Barnsley is that such advocacy schemes do make a difference in protecting the rights and integrity of people experiencing mental health distress and/or illness.

CONCLUSIONS

This chapter has attempted to demonstrate the importance of advocacy in mental health nursing. Mental health nurses are central and crucial in the treatment and prevention of mental health problems. They are ideally placed to act as a bridge and enable people with mental health problems to access truly independent advocacy services. Such a nursing intervention has the ability to empower this group of people. It has also been illustrated that there exists little empirical evidence that supports advocacy as a known contributor to effective treatment of mental health problems. However, in a sense, the traditions of advocacy do not claim to be able to do this. Rather, the various movements of advocacy do claim that they assist in the representation of the rights and integrity of disadvantaged and devalued people. They also claim to empower people to lead more valued lifestyles and this is borne out through the literature and life history accounts. A number of advocacy schemes have been reported in this chapter that have had a positive impact upon those who have experienced mental health problems. Mental health nurses have the power to empower and this should be at the heart of nursing interventions, even if this means seeking the assistance of others who are better placed to assist people to achieve this. All providers of care for people with mental ill-health should have constructed a charter for users of mental health services. A framework for such a charter is outlined in the NHS Executive's Mental Health Task Force User Group 'Guidelines for a local charter for users of mental health services' (1994). These guidelines outline a number of areas that should be addressed:

- *Personal dignity and respect*. This criterion requires the provider to make specific statements about being treated with dignity and respect, also to ensure that privacy and physical safety are guaranteed and, lastly, that an individual is to be protected against discrimination.
- *Information*. This requires information to be provided in a clear and objective way that is easily accessible. Information should also be provided concerning the diagnosis made and an individual's rights.
- *Accessibility*. People who use mental health services have a right to appropriate services and this includes local community services even when living in residential care.
- *Participation*. All people have a right to be fully involved in the planning of their own care. The framework is designed to promote this right along with the person with a mental illness being involved in the assessment process and any subsequent planning.
- *Choice*. Once again all people, within limits, have the right to choose. This does not just refer to a choice between treatment or non-treatment. Rather, individuals should be made aware of the range of treatments that are available to them. They should also have a choice in stating who they would prefer to be their key-worker.
- *Advocacy*. People with mental health problems have a right to someone of their own choice being present with them at any meeting which

is being attended by a professional worker. They also have the right to have access to an independent advocacy service.
- *Confidentiality and records*. The framework makes explicit the right to have access to records that are being held on an individual, to challenge the content of those records and yet simultaneously expect that those records will be maintained confidentially.
- *Complaints*. It seems almost unnecessary, but nonetheless it is important, to state that people in receipt of mental health services should have a right to have any complaint investigated, and that this should be done in a fair and methodical way. Individuals should also be provided with details about complaints procedures and, lastly, should not be victimised because of a complaint.
- *Treatment*. Mental health care has a long history and because of this treatments go back many centuries. Some of these treatments haunt the imaginations of people requiring care. Therefore, this area is one that needs to be dealt with in an honest and sensitive way. The framework requires that people receive the least-restrictive treatment. They must also be informed of any potentially harmful effects and alternative forms of treatment. They should be treated and/or cared for by a trained, supervised and competent individual and treatment should be compatible with an individual's belief system.
- *Mental Health Act 1983*. Finally, any person who is detained under this Act has fundamental rights that must once again be made available to them.

If nurses working in the specialism of mental health were to ensure that such a charter existed in any area where they should practise, and to ensure that all people in receipt of mental health services had access to an independent advocate,

Case study 19.1 Michael – a man without friends

Michael is a man with long-standing mental health problems. He has, until recently, spent the last decade in a large psychiatric hospital on the outskirts of an industrial city in the North-East of England. As a result of the closure of this hospital, 3 years ago, Michael was transferred to a new, purpose-built mental health unit in the grounds of a large, district general hospital. When Michael was first admitted to the old psychiatric hospital, he presented with an acute psychotic episode. He was homeless, experiencing frank delusions, hallucinations and in poor physical health. He also exhibited outward aggression on occasions to those around him, and for no apparent reason. Despite considerable efforts to treat Michael's problems, insufficient progress was made to consider Michael moving to a community-based form of care provision, hence his transfer to the psychiatric unit.

Staff at the new unit are committed to continuing working with Michael. Everyone's aim is that he leaves the unit and lives much more independently. Staff are concerned that Michael should have much more say in his lifestyle and planning for the future, but he finds it difficult speaking up for himself. Clearly a friend or relative might be in an ideal position to support him. However, because of the long period of time that Michael has been in receipt of care, he has lost contact with those people he knew before his admission, and therefore there is a general consensus amongst the multidisciplinary team that someone, or some organisation, should be approached to represent Michael's best interests. Michael is aware of these discussions and has agreed that he would like to be involved in some form of independent scheme that could identify someone to represent his interests.

Case study 19.2 Mr Kamal – a distressed man

Mr Kamal, an immigrant to England in the 1970s, lives in the Midlands. He is a married man with four children and what is described as a very happy marriage. He runs a series of small but successful businesses in the clothing trade. Approximately 6 months ago, he began to demonstrate signs of increasing anxiety. He visited his GP who suggested that Mr Kamal may have had a mild depression and prescribed him an antidepressant drug. Mr Kamal took this drug for 6 days and then stopped suddenly because of a number of side-effects that he said were interfering with his work. He felt disinclined to go back to his GP as he did not wish to 'take any more pills'. Over a short period of time, his condition worsened; he woke early in the morning and was fearful of the day ahead. He frequently experienced long periods of anxiety during the day but he was not sure why he was anxious. He found eating difficult as he frequently felt nauseous. His family noted that he became increasingly agitated and became irritated with him because he would frequently interfere with things without finishing off anything. He also, at this time, became increasingly suspicious of some of the managers who worked for him in some of his retail outlets.

Most recently, Mr Kamul completely 'broke down'. He was becoming increasingly distressed and was found weeping in the garage of his home, threatening to 'take his life' as he was worthless. His wife and family, not surprisingly, were themselves very distressed to see him so unwell. They called the local GP who managed to arrange an immediate informal admission to a local psychiatric unit. Following admission to the unit, Mr Kamal settled down a little and then demanded to leave. His wife, nursing staff and the duty psychiatrist felt that his condition warranted compulsory detention. Mr Kamal demanded to be released asking his wife what he had done to cause her to hate him so much.

should they wish, then this would do much to achieve a more realistic application of advocacy than is currently being recommended by some.

Exercise

Activity 1
Spend some time reading Case Studies 19.1 and 19.2 (p 387). Having read about the different types of advocacy which, if any, do you consider to be the most appropriate in meeting the needs of the people described? Identify your rationale for the decisions that you have reached.

Activity 2
Consider the two extracts provided on page 382. Do you think that these two accounts provide evidence of the importance of advocacy in the field of mental health? Do you think that these accounts have any reliability and or validity? Discuss your thoughts with a colleague.

USEFUL ADDRESSES

- Advocacy Alliance, 16 Chenies Street, London WC1E 7ET
- Citizen Advocacy Information and Training, 164 Lee Valley Technopark, Ashley Road, London N17 9LN
- Dutch Patients Council Foundation (LPR), 48 Meerkerthoef, Utrecht, Netherlands, 3582-DA
- Milton Keynes Advocacy Group, Campbell Centre, Milton Keynes General Hospital Campus, Milton Keynes, Buckinghamshire
- National Citizens Advocacy Resource and Advisory Centre, 2 St Pauls Road, London N1 2QR
- Nottingham Patients Council Support Group, Nottingham Advocacy Group, 9a Forest Road East, Nottingham NG1 4HJ
- Stanley Royds Patients Council, Stanley Royds Hospital, Aberford Road, Wakefield, Yorks
- Survivors Speak Out, 354 Osnaburgh Street, London NW1 3ND
- UKAN (United Kingdom Advocacy Network), Suite 417, Premier House, 14 Cross Street, Sheffield S1 2HG

KEY TEXTS FOR FURTHER READING

Gates B 1994 Advocacy: A nurses' guide. Scutari Press, Middlesex. *This book, especially written for nurses, serves as a useful introduction for the student to develop a conceptual framework as to what advocacy is, and its impact upon nursing.*
Teasdale K 1998 Advocacy in health care. Blackwell Science, London. *This excellent text is compulsory reading for those who wish to access an authoritative account of advocacy that attempts to provide balanced argument and discussion for health care practitioners on a very complex subject.*

Hunt G 1995 Whistleblowing in the health service: accountability, law and professional practice. Edward Arnold. London. *This is a most interesting book which explores an area that has become closely linked to issues of advocacy. Readers with an interest in legal implications of confidentiality and 'gagging' will find this book has much to offer. The book has been contributed to by a number of academics and this lends it an air of authority.*

REFERENCES

Abrams N 1978 A contrary view of the nurse as patient advocate. Nursing Forum XVII(3):259–267
Allmark P, Klarzynski R 1992 The case against nurse advocacy. British Journal of Nursing 2(1):33–36
Appelbaum P S 1979 Rotting with their rights on – constitutional theory and clinical reality in drug refusal by psychiatric patients. Bulletin of American Psychiatry Law 7:308–317
Brandon D 1994 Peer advocacy. Care in Place 1(3):218–224
Brown P 1985 Matter of commitment. Nursing Times

81(18):26–27
Butler K, Carr S, Sullivan F 1988 Citizen advocacy a powerful partnership. National Citizen Advocacy, London
Campbell P 1989 Speaking for themselves. Community Care 30 March: 22–23
Casteldine G 1981 The nurse as the patients advocate: pros and cons. Nursing Mirror 15(20):38–40
Citizen Advocacy Information and Training 1994 Advocacy: a code of practice. NHS Mental Health Task Force User Group. HMSO, London

REFERENCES (*contd*)

Clarke L 1995 Psychiatric nursing and electroconvulsive therapy. Nursing Ethics 2(4):321–331

Conlan E 1994 Peer advocacy. In Mental Health Task Force User Group Advocacy: A code of practice. HMSO, London, p 10

Diesfeld L 1994 Mental health law: innovations in education and representation. Disability and Society 9(3):337–354

Evans M 1992 Advocacy a role for nurses? In: Gray G, Pratt R (eds) Issues in Australian nursing 3. Churchill Livingstone, Edinburgh

Ford J (1995) A case for self-advocacy Post Mortem. In: Under the asylum tree: Survivors' poetry. Illustrated anthology. Survivors Press, London

Freddolono P, Moxley D 1992 Refining an advocacy model for homeless people coping with psychiatric disabilities. Community Mental Health Journal 28(4):337–354

Gates B 1994 Advocacy : A nurses' guide. Scutari Press, Middlesex

Gates B 1995 Advocacy. Whose best interest? Nursing Times 91(4):31–32

Glasman D 1991a The challenge of patient power. The Health Service Journal 101(5 September):16–17

Glasman D 1991b Divided opinions. The Health Service Journal 101(12 September):20

Holly L, Webb B 1992 The four projects in the advocacy alliance: Some commonalties and differences. The Tavistock Institute Evaluation and Development and Review Unit, London

Kitson A 1997 Using evidence to demonstate the value of nursing. Nursing Standard 2(11):34–39

Laing J, McQuarrie D 1989 Fifty years in the system. Mainstream, Edinburgh

Mallik M 1997 Advocacy in nursing – review of the literature. Journal of Advanced Nursing 25:130–138

Maslow 1954 Motivation and personality. Harper and Row. New York

McFadyen J A 1989 Who will speak for me? Nursing Times 85:45–48

MIND 1996 Barnsley Hospital Advocacy Service. Annual report. MIND, Barnsley

Morrison A 1991 The nurse's role in relation to advocacy. Nursing Standard 5(41):37–40

Mullender A 1991 Nottingham Advocacy Group: giving voice to the users of mental health services. Practice 5(1):5–12

Olley M C, Ogloff J R P 1995 Patients' rights and advocacy: implications for programme design and implementation. Journal of Mental Health Administration 22(4):368–376

Sackett D L, Rosenburg W M C, Gray J A M, Haynes R D, Richardson W S 1996 Evidence based medicine: what it is and what it isn't. British Medical Journal 31(2):71–72

Sang B, O'Brien J 1984 Advocacy: The UK and American experiences. Project paper No. 51. King Edward's Hospital Fund, London

Sellin S 1995 Out on a limb: a qualitative study of patient advocacy in institutional nursing. Nursing Ethics 2(1):19–29

Smith C 1980 Outrageous or outraged: a nurse advocate story. Nursing Outlook 28:624–625

Tannahill M, Lawson C 1993 Patient advocacy: psychiatrists perspectives. Health Trends 25(2):57–59

Teasdale K 1994 Advocacy and the nurse manager. Journal of Nursing Management 2:93–97

United Kingdom Advocacy Network 1995 A Code of practice. NHS Executive Mental Health Task Force User Group, Wetherby

United Kingdom Central Council for Nursing, Midwifery and Health Visiting 1996 Guidelines for professional practice. UKCC, London

United Kingdom Central Council for Nursing, Midwifery and Health Visiting 1998 Draft guidelines for mental health and learning disabilities nursing – a guide to working with vulnerable clients. UKCC, London

Walsh P 1985 Speaking up for the patient. Nursing Times 81(18):24–26

Webb B 1992 Views from inside and out: The management of the Advocacy Alliance. Advocacy in its wider setting. The Tavistock Institute Evaluation and Development and Review Unit, London

Webster Universal Dictionary 1975 Harvard Educational Services, New York

Willard C (1996) The nurses role as patient advocate: obligation or imposition. Journal of Advanced Nursing 24:60–66

Williams P, Schoultz B 1982 We can speak for ourselves. Souvenir Press, London

Wolfensberger W 1972 Citizen advocacy for the handicapped, impaired and disadvantaged: an overview. The President's Committee on Mental Retardation, Washington DC

CHAPTER CONTENTS

Key points 391

Introduction 392

Self-help – history and background 392
Terminology 392
Origins 393

Self-help today 393
Use 393
Self-help in the UK 393
UK self-help organisations 394

How helpful is self-help? 396
Efficacy and clinical effectiveness 396
Professional and paraprofessional treatments 397
Self-help treatments 398
No Panic study 399
What seems to be helpful in self-help? 401

Collaboration between professionals and self-help organisations 402

Exercise 403

Key text for further reading 404

References 404

20

Self-help initiatives

Bhavna Tanna   Kevin Gournay

KEY POINTS

- Interest in self-help is increasing not only from professionals but also from researchers and the general public.

- Self-help groups in the West date roughly from the 1930s and are now making a significant impact in health care services around the world.

- In the UK, members of self-help groups vary in age, background and in the length of time they have lived with their difficulties.

- Self-help organisations offer a range of services, including telephone help-lines, individual and group help, local meetings, information, support, advice and education to statutory and voluntary organisations and schools, and involvement in research.

- While there are some methodological difficulties with the research, it appears that paraprofessional and self-help interventions are very often as useful as professional interventions.

- The success of projects such as No Panic suggests that clinicians need to become more educated about and more involved in self-help initiatives, and that there is a need for self-help organisations and professionals to work together.

INTRODUCTION

10 years ago it would have been difficult to imagine that a chapter dealing with self-help initiatives would have been seen as an important contribution to the knowledge of health care professionals. Interest in self-help is increasing not only from professionals but also from researchers and the general public. One reason for this is the pressure on health care resources, with the consequence that there are more individuals presenting to health care services and there is an insufficient supply of resources to meet this increasing demand. This mismatch between demand and supply leads to pressure on professionals and the public to seek non-statutory forms of help, and self-help is one. Further, a recent catalyst has been the increased coverage by the media of self-help groups in daytime television talk shows, some of which frequently promote existing self-help groups at the end or involve members from specific groups speaking about their organisation and the help they provide. This coverage is further supported by exposure on the radio and in magazines and newspaper articles. These sources of public information are more than likely to have a large effect on the public awareness of self-help as a source of help which they may not have considered before.

It is becoming more apparent that self-help initiatives form an increasingly large and important aspect of helping services for those with mental health difficulties. They are making a significant impact in health care services around the world; this is particularly so in the USA (Jacobs & Goodman 1989) and it is likely that they will play an increasingly important role in the UK's health care services.

Given that surveys of prevalence indicate that the 1-year prevalence rate for all forms of psychiatric illness is around 25% (Department of Health 1993), it is clear that organisations other than statutory organisations need to be involved in providing services and it is increasingly realised that self-help groups can provide a very powerful alternative to professional services. The development of the self-help movement has also been linked to disillusionment with, and the limited access to, professional services and supportive institutions (Hatch & Kickbusch 1983).

Self-help organisations can be defined as:

> member governed voluntary associations of persons who share a common problem or who rely on experiential knowledge at least partly to solve or cope with their common concerns; emotional help is one kind of help given.
>
> Borkman 1990a:323

Such organisations can be seen to involve themselves in all aspects of social and individual concerns and psychological and behavioural difficulties are one aspect of this.

This chapter will first discuss some historical and background information about self-help, followed by a description of some of the UK self-help initiatives for those with mental health needs. This is then followed by a review of the research to date on the effectiveness of self-help and concludes with a description of a recent study of effectiveness in one typical UK organisation.

SELF-HELP – HISTORY AND BACKGROUND

Terminology

The literature on self-help is fraught with difficulties in terminology and definitions. The American literature speaks of 'mutual aid groups' and research in the USA seems to have advanced beyond testing the efficacy of self-help into exploring the ways in which mainstream health care services can develop positive relationships with these groups (Borkman 1990a).

The terms 'mutual aid' and 'self-help' are often used interchangeably in the literature. Borkman (1990a) attempts to differentiate these terms. She suggests that mutual aid groups have a membership of people who have come together to share a common interest or problem, housing co-operatives being an example. Such groups generally have a history amongst those who are politically and economically disadvantaged and these early groups were concerned with resource exchange and political activism. By contrast, self-help groups have their beginnings in health and human services; they rely on the sharing of experiential knowledge and emotional support. Members are responsible not only for obtaining from the group the support and help needed for their own welfare, but also for providing help to others. They are governed by their members rather than by professionals. Self-help is the term that will be used throughout this chapter with the intention of conveying that each member both receives and provides aid.

Origins

Self-help groups in the West date roughly from the 1930s. Alcoholics Anonymous (AA) is probably the most well known and now the largest self-help organisation. It was started in Akron, Ohio in 1935 by a surgeon and a banker who had received, to no avail, treatment for their alcoholism and who were deemed to be 'hopeless drunks'. In an act of despair, they attempted to help each other, finally became sober and started the setting-up of groups which are now worldwide. Membership of AA is now more than 1 million. The setting up of AA was quickly followed by groups for the parents of sick children, then by groups for those who were stigmatised in society, those with lifelong medical conditions such as diabetes and those who had undergone medical procedures such as heart surgery. Self-help groups for those coping with life transitions such as bereavement and for those dealing with psychological difficulties began in the 1950s and continue to proliferate today.

SELF-HELP TODAY

Use

Despite its increasing importance, relatively little research regarding the self-help movement in the UK has been published. There is an absence of good epidemiological data on 'who' and 'how many people' participate in self-help groups, not only in the UK but also in other countries. Differing estimates have been made regarding the numbers of people utilising self-help organisations. Jacobs & Goodman (1989) estimated that 6.25 million people in the USA use self-help groups each year, a figure that is equivalent to the number of people receiving psychotherapy from professionals (Borkman 1990a).

The National Institute of Mental Health has investigated the use of self-help groups as part of its research into the mental health service system in the USA. Lieberman & Snowden (1994) have attempted to calculate the prevalence of people using self-help organisations. They estimate that 2.8% of those with mental health needs had used self-help groups at some time in their lives. This compares with 15.7% who had sought professional mental health services. Of those individuals who had sought self-help, 71% had used both self-help groups and professional mental health services at some time in their lives. These data illustrate the important role that self-help plays as either the sole, or an additional service, for those with mental health needs.

Self-help in the UK

In the UK, the charting of the extent and use of self-help groups remains to be carried out.

However, an informative study regarding the nature of self-help organisations in the UK was carried out some time ago at the Policy Studies Institute by Richardson & Goodman (1983). They outline the nature and functions of self-help groups and make some broad-brush observations which are still applicable today:

- Members of self-help groups vary in age, background and in the length of time they have lived with their difficulties. This leads to varied demands on the group.
- Such groups are essentially small organisations and, as organisations, they have the usual structures in place such as chairs, committees and secretaries.
- Most groups tend to have a few key members who carry out most of the work, not only in terms of practical running of the group but also in terms of providing most of the help members gain from it.
- Self-help groups provide direct help to members in order to help them cope with the problem in question. They also act as pressure groups to obtain more resources and to educate the general public about their particular concerns.
- They have one advantage clearly not present in statutory services: the opportunity for members to gain from, and provide help to, other people with difficulties similar to their own.

UK self-help organisations

The picture of self-help in the UK is similar to the USA, although the literature indicates that organisations here have a lesser political role. In the UK, there are self-help groups for most types of psychological difficulties with groups focusing on addictions, eating disorders, depression, psychosis and bereavement. These organisations range from small, locally based organisations with membership funding to large, international organisations which have achieved charitable status and receive some local government and lottery funding. Some groups are formed around general problems, some are aimed at individuals who have very specific psychological difficulties and some are formed to provide help for those often overlooked by statutory services, the people who are carers for those with difficulties, such as families and partners. For example, ADFAM National offers support, advice and courses for carers of those with drug dependency, but does not offer help to those who are dependent on drugs themselves.

Self-help groups differ not only in terms of their structure and funding but also in ideology (Levine 1988). Antze (1976) drew attention to the importance of ideology as being the essence of the groups' teachings to its members. The most well-known organisation, Alcoholics Anonymous, and the more recent Overeaters Anonymous (OA), urge addicts to give themselves up to a 'higher power', while organisations such as No Panic (for those with anxiety problems) urge their members to realise that their symptoms are psychological and can be overcome through 'will power'. These sorts of differences in ideology are seen by Antze as reflecting the core problem of each difficulty – in AA, the alcoholic's main problem is seen as the mistaken belief of control over the drinking so the idea of appealing to a 'higher power' opposes this mistaken belief.

The ideology of these groups affects their language and practices. The AA and OA (both international groups) are examples of relatively tightly structured organisations. They both use the '12-step' approach to recovery, and the '12 traditions' which are aimed at guiding the group. One of the central aims of '12-step' type groups (which include other problem areas such as

Narcotics Anonymous for drug users) is that the groups should remain forever non-professional. Each step of the programme provides the member with a spiritual principle which is seen as central to 'recovery'. Meetings are held regularly and often focus on one of the 12 steps of the programme. A member will read out the relevant step and discuss this in the light of his or her experience. This is similar in many ways to study in religious or spiritual settings. One of the characteristics of some groups, particularly AA and OA, is that they provide an opportunity for individuals to 'confess' the ways in which they have 'slipped' from abstinence and the ways in which their difficulty has resulted in them hurting those around them. This can be a cathartic experience, enabling members to feel that they can begin each day as a new opportunity to succeed in their aim of abstinence.

Another aspect of the varying ideological elements of self-help organisations is their understanding of causation; some groups insist that members should not attempt to understand the cause of their difficulties, while, at the other extreme, some groups feel that it is very important that members and professional agencies accept their understanding of causation. There is a tendency in some self-help organisations to encourage the understanding of their members in biological or genetic models, rather than in psychological or social terms. The organisation Schizophrenia a National Emergency (SANE) is an example of this. It not only provides the usual help services to members, but it is also active in working with researchers in exploring the physiological and genetic links of the aetiology of schizophrenia.

Being able to both give and receive help is another valuable aspect of the groups. Self-help groups can offer members an opportunity to develop social roles and have access to role models. Maton (1988) has found that self-help group

members who both gave and received support had lower levels of depression, higher self-esteem and reported higher levels of satisfaction and more benefits than those who were either providers or receivers alone. This research focused on OA, Compassionate Friends (for the bereaved) and Multiple Sclerosis.

Usually, self-help organisations offer a range of services to their members and non-members, such as:

- Telephone help-lines which provide counselling and information daily between certain hours.
- Help programmes for members, which may take the form of either individual help or in groups, face to face, or over the telephone. The format for this help can range from very structured, specific help to more general assistance and information.
- Local self-help group meetings for members. Some of these meetings may be 'open meetings' at which non-members may attend – these may include professionals, carers and other interested individuals.
- Information, support, advice and education courses to statutory and voluntary services – these can include education in schools, provision of information for the media and courses for professionals.
- Research involvement – this can range from incorporating requests for participants into their regular literature to taking a major role in the design and recruitment of participants for research initiatives.

These services are usually provided by trained volunteers who are likely to have at some time experienced, or continue to experience, the difficulties addressed by the organisation. Volunteers are usually trained in counselling skills and are supervised by other members or professionals. Further training may include 'shadowing' more experienced volunteers. In some organisations, those having more of a helper role learn from others in the organisation by 'shadowing' a more experienced member. Some of the organisations offer help that is informed by professionals, may be supervised by professionals and so can be thought of as 'para-professional' rather than self-help alone.

HOW HELPFUL IS SELF-HELP?

As previously noted, the self-help movement is a growing service provider, but is it effective? The literature on self-help spans both diverse research designs and forms of self-help. This diversity ranges from studies which have randomised controlled trial designs in which the self-help is in the form of written, taped or computer-assisted treatment programmes, to studies which compare therapist-assisted and paraprofessionally assisted treatment, through to naturalistic designs carried out by researchers in close collaboration with self-help organisations themselves. The literature reviewed here presents this range, but prior to a discussion of the research, it is worth giving some thought to the types of designs that can be used in this area of outcome research.

Efficacy and clinical effectiveness

Roth & Fonagy (1996) make a clear distinction between the efficacy of a therapy and its clinical effectiveness. The former is a statement about the results a therapy achieves in a research trial, while the latter is an indicator of the results that the therapy achieves in routine clinical practice. These writers explore some of the difficulties encountered by those interested in carrying out research in the field of treatment outcomes. Design issues can confound the conclusions drawn from outcome research. Table 20.1 sum-

marises the different types of design along with the strengths and weaknesses of each.

Table 20.1 Overview of study designs

Design	Strengths	Weaknesses
Single case	Useful in looking at treatment innovations. Can provide rich data. Quick and convenient to carry out in clinical practice	Patients may not be representative as they are often highly selected. The lack of a control condition means interpretation of specific and non-specific factors in treatment are hard to differentiate
Randomised controlled trials	Allow differentiation of the effects of treatments and controls for extraneous variables	Time consuming and expensive. They are more difficult for longer-term therapies to utilise. Generalising may be difficult as the rigour in patient selection and those providing the treatment is not an accurate reflection of what occurs in clinical practice
Open trials	Allow naturalistic protocols relevant to clinical practice	Lack of control group makes it difficult to differentiate specific and non-specific factors in treatment

In addition to study design, further considerations include the types and breadth of measures used by researchers to assess the usefulness of a therapy. Roth & Fonagy suggest that studies should aim to incorporate measures from differing perspectives (e.g. patient and therapist) and that they consider different symptom domains (affect, cognition and behaviour) and differing domains of functioning, such as work and social functioning. They also suggest that studies incorporate one or several follow-up periods in order to provide some indication of the possibly longer-term effects of therapy and the maintenance of any treatment gains.

Professional and paraprofessional treatments

Individuals with psychological difficulties who receive professional treatment show better outcomes than those who receive no treatment at all. Since some self-help organisations can be said to be offering paraprofessional help, it is interesting to see if treatment offered by paraprofessionals achieves outcomes similar to those of professionals.

In 1979, Durlak carried out a review of 42 studies which compared professional and paraprofessional therapists for cases involving specific target problems such as insomnia, obesity and enuresis.

Professionals comprised experienced psychologists, psychiatrists and social workers. Paraprofessionals were defined as adults with professional backgrounds who had not completed a clinical training in mental health. Examples were medical students or community volunteers. Most of the studies reviewed found no difference between the two types of helpers in terms of effectiveness on measurable outcomes. Durlak concluded that 'paraprofessionals achieve clinical outcomes equal to or significantly better than those obtained by professionals' (Durlak 1979:80). Two further reviews and meta-analyses have been conducted, both of which have shown that either there are no differences between professionals and paraprofessionals or that the results favour paraprofessionals as more effective helpers (Hattie et al 1984, Nietzel & Fisher 1981). However, these outcomes were achieved by paraprofessionals who had either received close supervision from a professional or those who were treating less severe difficulties such as mild behaviour problems in college students.

Berman & Norton (1985) carried out a further review, which included the studies reviewed by Durlak. They note the difficulties encountered by previous researchers in ascribing 'professional' or 'paraprofessional' labels to helpers. In their review, they included as 'professional' only those helpers who had completed their training and excluded those 'paraprofessionals' who had had either extensive preparation or prior experience with the therapy task and those who had received close supervision from a professional. They looked at interventions for phobias, psychosis, obesity and social adjustment, using five common forms of treatment: behavioural, cognitive–behavioural, humanistic, crisis intervention and counselling. Outcomes were measured from four different sources: patient, therapist, independent observer and behavioural indicator.

Berman & Norton found that people achieved comparable levels of improvement across five different outcome measures (symptom distress, global adjustment, social adjustment, work–school adjustment and personality traits). whether treated by professionals or paraprofessionals. They were also interested in which conditions indicated which type of help as the treatment of choice. They found that when treatment was brief, professionals achieved better outcomes, while paraprofessionals appeared to be more effective with treatments of longer duration. They also found that professionals were more effective with patients who were older. One explanation given for this difference is the fact that the therapists were older than the paraprofessionals – therapists are more effective with patients closer to their own age.

Christensen & Jacobson (1994) point out some of the difficulties with studies comparing the effectiveness of professional and paraprofessional help. First, there is the issue of how one defines professionals and paraprofessionals and what is assumed about their potential to help. There is a also a lack of clarity in the literature about the definition of 'paraprofessional' – this makes comparison between studies at best difficult and at worst invalid. It seems that paraprofessionals can be seen as individuals who offer professionally based help without the qualifications or training of a professional. However, the skills overlap between paraprofessional and professional helpers may be higher than assumed in some studies. It is hard to identify what is being compared in such studies. Is it the skills of the helper, the benefits of the helper's training or the model of treatment being offered? Some of these difficulties are avoided in studies which have compared professional help with self-help and this body of work will now be discussed.

Self-help treatments

Research into the processes and outcomes of self-help carries with it many contradictions. There is a view that the self-help organisation is significantly different from statutory health services and therefore needs to be studied through a different methodology (Powell 1994). One of the difficulties is that those who choose to contact and take part in self-help groups may be more motivated for change than those who do not seek help or seek professional help. Further, those who continue their involvement are more likely to be those who find the self-help process helpful, while at the same time there is a paucity of information about those individuals who do not continue with them. Groups tend to provide a great deal of information about their history, ideology and services in the literature which they send to everyone who makes an initial contact. Given this, it follows that individuals who are attracted by the information they receive join, while those who are not, do not proceed with membership and are therefore not included. Research which examines the characteristics of those who seek, and take part in self-help, compared with those who seek but do not take part and those who do not seek self-help at all, would provide valuable

information about factors contributing to process and outcome. However, there is pressure from within self-help organisations and from the professional health care community for empirical evidence supporting the effectiveness of the assistance offered through self-help. This has led to some fruitful alliances between self-help organisations and researchers which are mutually beneficial. When outcome research shows self-help as successful, it can obviously provide the self-help organisation with the case for recruiting much needed resources.

Early accounts in the literature viewed self-help as merely an informal and less sophisticated form of traditional treatments offered by professionals. More recently, however, the focus has shifted towards viewing self-help as more of a social movement concerned with the broader links between individual, interpersonal and social change. Along with this shift, there has followed a change in the ways in which the self-help organisation is researched. There has been a movement away from treatment-efficacy-type studies towards an ecological framework; that is, an increasing amount of literature now exists on how self-help groups shape the social networks of their members and there is a growing interest in how self-help groups exist in a complex system of community support (Borkman 1984).

Researchers are also becoming increasingly aware of the need to understand the experiences of self-help members as the principal means of understanding the self-help phenomenon. This has meant the use of a narrative (or storytelling) approach to the investigation of the self-help process (Cain 1991). This body of research is perhaps less relevant for professionals, and as it is relatively poorly developed, it will not be discussed here.

Recent reviews of self-administered treatments, such as self-help books and audio tapes with or without minimal therapist contact, indicate outcomes comparable to those achieved with therapist help. Scogin et al (1990) carried out a meta-analysis of studies which compared such self-administered treatments with a no-treatment control condition or therapist-administered treatment. The problems treated fell into four broad categories of 'habit problems', such as smoking; 'emotional problems', such as depression, anxiety and phobias; 'skills' training, such as difficulties with parenting; and 'others', such as sleep problems. The researchers found that self-administered treatments were more effective than no treatment and as effective as therapist-administered treatments. However, they note that all of these difficulties are relatively circumscribed and that self-administered treatment may not be as effective with more global, less clearly identified difficulties.

In 1993, Gould & Clum published a meta-analysis of self-help treatment approaches: that of media-based treatment approaches such as manuals, audio-tapes and video tapes, which are used by individuals independently of a helping professional. Some of the studies did involve contact with a professional, but only at assessment or for ongoing monitoring. Only those studies incorporating randomised groups of self-help treatments with no-treatment, wait-list or placebo controls were included. A total of 40 studies were analysed.

The authors concluded that self-help treatments were more effective with skill deficits and specific psychological problems such as phobias and depression than with habit problems such as smoking. They found that self-help showed a similar drop-out rate to psychotherapy and control subjects. The results support the effectiveness of self-help approaches for the kinds of problems they target (i.e. those that use a behavioural approach). Furthermore, when the authors analysed the effectiveness of self-help in comparison with therapist-assisted intervention, the

results indicated similar effectiveness. They also found that these subjects generally maintained their treatment gains at follow-up. However, since few of the studies independently confirmed the diagnosis of conditions, it is impossible to say if the participants were equivalent to clinical populations seen by professionals.

Tyrer et al (1993) carried out a 2-year study comparing the effectiveness of drug treatment, cognitive–behaviour therapy and self-help with psychiatric out-patients suffering from anxiety disorders. Patients were randomly assigned to groups and given treatment for 6 weeks; contact was then reduced over another 4-week period. There were no overall differences in compliance rate or efficacy between the three modes of treatment, self-help being as effective as the other two interventions. The researchers were also interested in the effects of personality status on treatment. They found that those with personality disorders as defined by the Personality Assessment Schedule (PAS, Tyrer & Alexander, 1979) fared less well with self-help and cogitive–behaviour therapies, particularly between weeks 32 and 52 of the study.

No Panic study

The research indicates that self-help can be an effective form of treatment. There is a lack of published research examining the effectiveness of a self-help organisation currently offering structured treatment for its members. One study conducted by the first author has attempted to examine the effectiveness of the UK self-help organisation No Panic. This study was concerned with self-help treatment for those with panic and agoraphobia. It set out to examine any changes in the reported severity of symptoms for people taking part in a 12-week, telephone, self-help recovery programme offered by No Panic. Additionally, it set out to investigate whether any changes in symptoms were related to participants' pre-treatment histories, expectations of treatment or facilitator effects. 25 members of the self-help organisation completed the study.

Each participant was asked to complete questionnaires regarding the severity of panic over the last 7 days. The symptoms included:

- the severity of the physiological sensations of panic
- the severity of the accompanying catastrophic thoughts
- the frequency of panic attacks
- how often situations such as travelling on trains were avoided when alone and when accompanied
- the severity of feelings of anxiety and depression
- the degree to which the symptoms interfered with daily life.

These symptoms of panic were assessed at three points: before the programme began (pre), halfway through the programme (mid) and at the end (post). 14 participants were assessed further at 3-month follow-up. In addition to symptom questionnaires, participants were asked to complete satisfaction questionnaires at the end of treatment and at 3-month follow-up. Participants were also interviewed regarding their treatment histories and their expectations of the recovery programme.

The analysis of results comparing symptom severity at the beginning of the recovery programme and symptom severity at the end indicated a significant reduction in all of the symptoms measured, except for avoidance behaviour when alone. This finding, when contrasted with a significant reduction in avoidance behaviour when accompanied, indicated that participants avoid fearful situations less as the recovery programme progresses, but this only applies to situations in which they are accompanied.

Professional opinion would say this is a disappointing outcome since this is the core difficulty for those with agoraphobia. However, this measure did not correlate with participants' own degree of satisfaction with the recovery programme. One explanation for this finding is that during the recovery programme, participants are encouraged to set their own exposure goals. Group facilitators and group members encourage each other, but participants are asked to take responsibility in setting goals and are left to decide if they want to share this with the group. Given this, it is not surprising that individuals show least improvement on what, for many, is the most difficult aspect of the recovery programme. It is also understandable that they do not see this lack of improvement as being a reflection on the usefulness of the recovery programme.

It is likely that participants experience difficulties in carrying out exposure work for reasons not related to the content of the recovery programme, but more to the lack of individual contact with the facilitator. In the study by Hand et al (1974) which involved group exposure for agoraphobics, the participants commented that 'I didn't want to let the others down' or 'I didn't want to let the doctor down'. This study found that many of the participants would not engage in exposure tasks unless taught and accompanied by the therapist; they wanted the therapist to be with them during early exposure sessions. Hand et al explained their results in terms of low self-esteem in participants. A more recent study of housebound agoraphobics by McNamee et al (1989) suggested that while therapists do not need to accompany patients, therapist contact might be an important aspect of treatment effectiveness. It may be that this aspect of recovery is the most difficult to facilitate through the minimal support of a telephone self-help group.

It is interesting to note that virtually all participants in the study achieved a significant change in catastrophic thoughts during a panic attack. From participants' comments, this seemed attributable, in part at least, to increased knowledge about the symptoms of panic gained through taking part in the programme. As Clark (1986) and others note, people who experience panic attacks have a tendency to misinterpret the sensations of panic as indicative of an immediately impending physical or mental disaster. One of the aspects of the recovery programme offered by No Panic was that it provided an opportunity for all group members, including the facilitator, to talk about their experience of physiological sensations of panic and the fearful thoughts that accompany them. The group members then examine the reality of these catastrophic thoughts to see if they are a 'false alarm' rather than based on real threat. It may be that this aspect of the programme contributed to the change in cognitions which was detected at the end of treatment and at follow-up.

In terms of significant clinical change, nearly three-quarters of participants had improved on three or more symptom measures. All except one person had shown a significant reduction in the severity of the catastrophic cognitions associated with panic. However, only one-third of the participants were 'panic free' at the end of the recovery programme.

Satisfaction at the end of the recovery programme was correlated with the severity of fearful body sensations. Participants who reported a reduction in the severity of fearful body sensations also reported being more satisfied with the recovery programme. There were no significant relationships between symptom reduction and duration of illness, age of participant, group facilitator, helpfulness of the GP, and whether participants were taking medication.

A comparison of symptom severity at the end of recovery and at 3-month follow-up revealed a significant reduction in severity of fearful body sensations, catastrophic cognitions, anxiety and depression. However, there was no difference from the end of treatment to follow-up on how participants' daily lives were affected by the symptoms of panic. At follow-up, participants reported a reduction in the somatic and cognitive aspects of panic and agoraphobia, but they did not report a significant change in their agoraphobic avoidance behaviour, alone or accompanied.

Satisfaction at follow-up was related to a reduction in the severity of catastrophic cognitions; those reporting a decrease in severity of catastrophic thinking also reported being more satisfied with the recovery programme at follow-up. Interview data suggested that one of the satisfying aspects of the self-help recovery programme was the experience of being in a group with people who had similar difficulties.

This study lends support to the potential usefulness of self-help in the treatment of panic and agoraphobia. As this study did not include a control group, inferences regarding the causation of the significant reduction in symptom severity cannot be made with confidence. However, when seen in the context of other self-help research, which reports positive findings, it is likely that the experience of being part of the recovery programme made some contribution to positive outcome. Given this, it is clear that clinicians need to become more educated about and more involved in self-help initiatives such as the one offered by No Panic as they can potentially offer an effective alternative or addition to professionally assisted interventions.

What seems to be helpful in self-help?

Reissman (1990) suggests a number of benefits to being part of a self-help group, in both a help receiver and a help provider:

- being a helper leads to positive feelings about having something to give
- it is an active role rather than a passive role as may occur when receiving help alone
- helping is socially useful and may lead to feelings of increased status
- it encourages helpers to be open to learning, so that they can both help effectively and learn how to receive help.

It may be that being in the helper role assists people in making the most of their experience when they are in the role of helpee. This has important implications for professionally assisted therapies; active involvement of the client is likely to be more successful in creating change. Borkman (1990b) used the term 'experiential knowledge' to refer to the knowledge people acquire when they live through and resolve a problem. It has been assumed by self-help organisations and professionals that experiential knowledge is the essential ingredient that distinguishes self-help from other types of help and it is highly valued by members of self-help groups (Hasenfield & Gidron 1993). However, it is a challenge to researchers to operationalise the concept of experiential knowledge in investigating the nature of self-help.

Powell & Cameron (1991) highlight a number of issues relevant to how researchers can take a role in self-help initiatives. They note that policy makers and researchers often prefer quantitative research methods and findings as they lend themselves to policy initiatives based on sound reliable and valid data, which can be generalised across populations. Powell & Cameron suggest that research using a qualitative approach should be sponsored by research organisations since this is not only likely to be more acceptable to self-help leaders, but also because this method is more suited to the complexity of the self-help process. They also suggest that research moves

on from studies of effectiveness to studies about participation in self-help. However, the authors describe the issue of researchers being involved in observing self-help groups and the probable disruptive effect this can have on the group process. Powell & Cameron recommend collaborative working between professionals and self-help groups, as this can be useful to the self-help organisation in clarifying priorities and reflecting on current practice.

COLLABORATION BETWEEN PROFESSIONALS AND SELF-HELP ORGANISATIONS

The essential difference between self-help organisations and professional help is that the former comprise members who are both receiving and providing help to others. Professional help involves individuals who are either in the role of helper or helpee. The self-help approach enables many more people to offer help, thus expanding resources. This expansion through helpee also being helpers, provides an opportunity for professional resources to be used more efficiently. Professionals may therefore alter the focus of their work to educating lay members of the public in the skills and knowledge they have acquired. They may also concentrate their energies in providing help for those people who would benefit most from it or who actively choose that professional help.

At first glance, this new paradigm makes sense in a society in which professionals find themselves under ever-increasing pressure with limited resources. However, Reissman (1990) points to the resistance offered by some professionals about this change of paradigm. He states how, in Western society, there is a view that help is a commodity that is bought, sold, promoted and marketed. This context is often not talked about explicitly, but it often inevitably affects the ways in which professionals are trained and the attitudes that are fostered. It can set up an asymmetrical relationship in which professionals have a vested interest in not sharing their knowledge or their help-giving role. The process of years of training and specialising in a field of help-giving reflects the view that people can benefit only from receiving help from those trained to provide it.

The types of interaction that can be engendered by the view that professionals have a privileged access to skills and knowledge are that they can be seen by help-seekers as uninvolved. Those with many years of formal training (such as psychiatrists) may be especially at risk of being seen in this way. It is clear that self-help initiatives have a great deal of current success and future potential in the treatment of psychological distress. When seen in the context of the effectiveness research, which reports positive findings, it is clear that clinicians of all disciplines need to become more educated about, and more involved in, the self-help movement. This involvement is important for a number of reasons:

- some clients may find self-help more beneficial than professional help; clinicians need to bear this in mind when suggesting treatment options
- some clients may benefit from a combined treatment package of self-help and professional help, perhaps at different stages in recovery or these modes provided in parallel
- self-help organisations may value and benefit from collaboration with professionals. Collaborative work is possible at all levels, including clinical, research and training/supervision projects

- professionals can benefit from the experiential knowledge of self-help members. The accessibility of professional help and the ways in which treatment packages are implemented are of particular concern to people who are housebound through agoraphobia.
- professionals may benefit from collaborative work, as this may be a better use of their skills. It may enable them to spend more time working with individuals who require their specific skills and training.

Given the fact that resources are limited and that the demand for mental health care is increasing, it is likely that clinicians will have little choice but to become more involved with self-help organisations. Future collaborative work has the potential to produce some creative and valuable treatment innovations for a range of psychological difficulties, and the opportunities for increasing our knowledge and resources as professionals are clear if we can see self-help as an ally rather than a threat.

Exercise

Consider a member of your family, a friend or a colleague who suffers with a particular difficulty. How would self-help be relevant to such a person? How would you go about establishing a group which would address his or her needs? What issues would be different if you were acting as a professional facilitating the formation of such a group for clients with whom you were in contact?

KEY TEXT FOR FURTHER READING

Marks I 1987 Living with fear. McGraw Hill, London. *This is one of the best self-help texts available, and the material from this book has now been developed for use as a computer program.*

REFERENCES

Antze P 1976 The role of ideologies in peer psychotherapy organisations: some theoretical considerations and the three case studies. Journal of Applied Behavioural Science 12:323–346

Berman J S, Norton N C 1985 Does professional training make a therapist more effective? Psychological Bulletin 98:401–406

Borkman T S 1984 Mutual self-help groups: strengthening the selectively unsupportive personal and community networks of their members. In: Gartner A, Reissman F (eds) The self-help revolution. Human Sciences Press, New York

Borkman T 1990a Self-help groups at the turning point: emerging egalitarian alliances with the formal health care system? American Journal of Community Psychology 18(2):321–332

Borkman T 1990b Experiential, professional and lay frames of reference. In: Powell T J (ed) Working with self-help. NASW Press, Silver Spring, MD

Cain C 1991 Personal stories: identity acquisition and self-understanding in Alcoholics Anonymous. Ethos 19:210–251

Christensen A, Jacobson N S 1994 Who (or what) can do psychotherapy: the status and challenge of non-professional therapies. Psychological Science 5:8–14

Clark D 1986 A cognitive approach to panic. Behaviour Research and Therapy 24:461–470

Department of Health 1993 The health of the nation key area handbook. HMSO, London

Durlak J A 1979 Comparative effectiveness of paraprofessional and professional helpers. Psychological Bulletin 86:80–92

Gould R A, Clum G A 1993 A meta-analysis of self-help treatment approaches. Clinical Psychology Review 13:169–186

Hand I, Lamontagne Y, Marks I M 1974 Group exposure (flooding) in vivo for agoraphobics. British Journal of Psychiatry 124:588–602

Hasenfield Y, Gidron B 1993 Self-help groups and human service organisations: an interorganisational perspective. Social Service Review 2:217–235

Hatch S, Kickbusch I 1983 Self-help and health in Europe. World Health Organization, Copenhagen

Hattie J A, Sharpley C F, Rogers H J 1984 Comparative effectiveness of professional and paraprofessional helpers. Psychological Bulletin, 95:534–541

Jacobs M K, Goodman G 1989 Psychology and self-help groups: predictions on a partnership. American Psychologist 44:536–545

Levine M 1988 An analysis of mutual assistance. American Journal of Community Psychology 16:167–187

Lieberman A, Snowden R 1994 Problems in assessing prevalence and membership characteristics of self-help group participants. In: Powell T J (ed) Understanding the self-help organisation. Sage, Thousand Oaks, CA, p 32–50

Maton K I 1988 Social support, organizational characteristics, psychological well-being, and group appraisal in three self-help group populations. American Journal of Community Psychology 16(1):53–77

McNamee G, O'Sullivan G, Lelliot P, Marks I M 1989 Telephone guided treatment for housebound agoraphobics with panic disorder: exposure vs relaxation. Behaviour Therapy 20:491–497

Nietzel M, Fisher S G 1981 Effectiveness of professional and paraprofessional helpers: a comment on Durlak. Psychological Bulletin 89:555–565

Powell T J 1994 Self-help research and policy issues. In: Powell T J (ed) Understanding the self-help organisation. Sage, Thousand Oaks, CA, p 1–19

Powell T J, Cameron M J 1991 Self-help research and the public mental health system. American Journal of Community Psychology 19:797–805

Reissman F 1990 Restructuring help: a human service's paradigm for the 1990s. American Journal of Community Psychology 18:221–230

Richardson A, Goodman M 1983 Self-help and social care. Policy Studies Institute, London

Roth A, Fonagy P 1996 What works for whom? A critical review of psychotherapy research. Guilford Press, New York

Scogin F, Bynum J, Stephens G, Calhoon S 1990 Efficacy of self-administered treatment programs: meta-analytic review. Professional Psychology: Research and Practice 21:42–47

Tyrer P, Alexander J 1979 Classification of personality disorder. British Journal of Psychiatry 135:163–167

Tyrer P, Seivewright N, Ferguson B, Murphy S, Johnson A L 1993 The Nottingham study of neurotic disorder: effect of personality status on response to drug treatment, cognitive therapy and self-help over two years. British Journal of Psychiatry 162:219–226

CHAPTER CONTENTS

Key points 405

Introduction 406

**Alternative residential treatment for acutely ill
    patients 408**
    Cedar House, Colorado 408
    Venture, Vancouver 409
    Crossing Place, Washington DC 409
    Services in the Netherlands 409
    Comment 410

**Residential alternatives for severe mental illness
    410**
    Northwest Evaluation Center 410

**Innovative and non-traditional (less conventional)
    services for acutely ill patients 410**
    Soteria 410
    Soteria Berne 411
    Comment 411

**Community approaches for acutely ill patients
    411**
    Santa Clara County Clustered Apartment Project
    411
    Stockport Arts on Prescription 412
    Comment 413

**Community approaches for people with enduring
    and severe mental illness 413**
    Gwydir Project, Cambridge 413
    Critical time intervention, New York City 414

Critical components 415
    Selection criteria 415
    Service elements 415
    Medication 415
    Comparable patients 416
    Continuity of care 416
    Programme content 416
    Personnel 416
    Evidence 417

Conclusion 417

Exercise 417

Key texts for further reading 418

References 418

21

Alternatives to traditional mental health treatments

Peter Huxley

KEY POINTS

- By traditional treatments we mean those that are delivered from an institution in the form of in-patient or out-patient care; alternative provision can be divided into institutional and community-based models.

- Unfortunately, the evidence for the success of these programmes is more often asserted than demonstrated. As Warner (1995) points out most of the alternative in-patient treatment programmes have not been subject to rigorous controlled trials.

- While it is possible to treat most patients in alternative community settings, there are patients who, in certain settings and under certain circumstances, require more traditional in-patient care.

- Successful alternative treatment programmes have common characteristics – they tend to target people with severe mental illness; they are linked in with other community resources and services; they attempt to provide the full range of functions formerly provided in institutional care; they adopt individually tailored care planning; they are culturally relevant; they have specifically trained staff; they make liaison arrangements with

---

KEY POINTS (*contd*)

existing institutions providing in-patient care; and they subject themselves to some form of internal evaluation, often self-monitoring.

- In assessing the effectiveness of alternative models one has to be careful to examine whether it is more effective medication administration and prescribing practice that is creating an advantage for the alternative system of care.

- If alternative programmes have such narrow inclusion criteria as to exclude most patients, they are bound to have a therapeutic advantage that traditional all-encompassing service systems do not have. Comparing like with like patients cannot be achieved simply by ensuring that crude demographics and diagnosis are similar. Factors that make treatment more difficult need to be taken into account, such as non-compliance, social problems, previous treatment history and the presence of suicidality or assaultive behaviours.

- Another important aspect of the success of such programmes is the quality of the personnel involved and their knowledge, experience and supervision. It is no coincidence that successful programmes use more psychiatrist time, or use the time available to better purpose.

- Providing a single institutional or community solution is clearly going to be wrong in a lot of cases because it will be appropriate and successful for some patients and not others. A range of approaches is needed, and getting the right patients into the right setting is then the challenge.

INTRODUCTION

The title of this chapter contains the assumption that it is easy to identify traditional models of care, whereas in reality patterns and modes of care are continually developing, so that a common treatment approach of the day is frequently, if not inevitably, replaced by a more up-to-date model of care. This progression is most easily observed in respect of pharmacological treatment, but is also true of the way that 24-hour care is delivered. At one time, 24-hour care was provided exclusively by mental hospitals, then by units in general hospitals, and more recently in smaller, more community-based settings.

In this chapter, I assume that by traditional treatments we mean those that are delivered from an institution in the form of in-patient or out-patient care. In some services, day-hospital programmes are well-established and in others various forms of partial hospitalisation occur. 'Partial hospitalisation' subsumes a vast array of programmes and services including day hospitals, day care centres and day treatment. Unfortunately, attention has been focused on partial hospitalisation programmes and residential alternatives as substitutes for the hospital 'rather than as a treatment in its own right or as the most appropriate intervention for certain patients or clinical conditions' (Hoge et al 1992:346).

The penetration of partial hospitalisation programmes varies from place to place, and it is probably true to say that they are not yet commonly regarded as 'traditional' approaches. So, in some settings, a day hospital might be regarded as a radical alternative while in others a day hospital has operated for many years and is no longer regarded as either radical or alternative.

The concept of a 'traditional' treatment is, of course, culture-bound, and one has to recognise that the 'traditional' system in Western culture is very different from that in non-Western cultures. One can therefore introduce a different approach to treatment from one culture where it is regarded as traditional into another culture where it is regarded as a radical alternative. The introduction of psychopharmacological treatments in developing countries, or the use of acupuncture in the West are two examples. Given the limited space available here, I will be concentrating on the traditional Western mental health care systems. Appropriate care, and alternatives to hospital treatment, vary depending upon context, and culture is one of the main contextual factors that influences appropriate care and its delivery.

There are also limitations imposed upon what can be included in the present chapter by the need to provide evidence that the approaches to treatment can and do work. As Warner (1995) points out, most of the alternative in-patient treatment programmes have not been subjected to rigorous controlled trials (e.g. family sponsor homes in southwest Denver – Polak et al 1995), even though some have been replicated (e.g. the Windhorse programme in Boulder – Fortuna 1995 was replicated in Halifax, Nova Scotia and Northampton, Massachusetts). By contrast, the original alternative community programmes, such as assertive community treatment (ACT), have been systematically evaluated. Indeed, some people might argue that assertive community models of care are rapidly becoming the 'traditional' model for many patients. However, Marshall doubts whether the application of ACT in practice has actually followed the ACT model consistently, and he provides compelling evidence to support this view (Marshall & Lockwood 1997). We can therefore consider ACT as one of the genuine alternative community treatments that has been the subject of adequate empirical testing in North America, but not in the UK.

There is good clinical evidence, and even some theoretical evidence dating back many years, upon which to base a judgement about alternative forms of treatment and care. Warner (1995) argues that non-institutional residential settings produce different results because:

> people are called on to use their own inner resources. They must exercise a degree of self-control and accept responsibility for their actions and for the preservation of their living environment. Consequently, patients retain more of their self-respect, their skills and their sense of mastery. The domestic and noncoercive nature … makes human contact with the person in crisis easier than it is in hospitals.
>
> Warner 1995:xvi

It is perhaps worth commenting on this statement, because one could argue that the key elements in effective community treatment programmes are very similar, and furthermore, comparable elements are present in most successful rehabilitation programmes for people with severe and enduring mental illness.

A final word on the evidence-based approach before moving on. While double-blind controlled trials enable a greater degree of certainty about the efficacy of the proposed treatment, external factors, such as the culture or the service system, are treated as non-problematic because they are the same for the treated and control patients. However, unless the trial is undertaken within several cultures simultaneously, or different service systems are involved, we cannot be confident that treatment efficacy will generalise to other settings. Even multicentre trials can suffer from this problem. Thompson & Lyons (1996) have pointed out that service managers are not really in a position to say how their particular setting will affect treatment results. The same can be said about experimental alternatives to traditional treatments. At the end of the day we cannot be sure how well one approach will be suited to a setting in which it was not developed.

Almost two decades ago, Leona Bachrach (1980) examined the reasons why model programmes, often with substantial additional funding, did not translate well into standard services. She pointed out that 'questions concerning the "how" of programming for chronic mental patients must be determined largely by such extra-program considerations as timing, available resources, and other local conditions' (Bachrach 1980:1028). The context in which a whole mental health service system operates is different in important respects from the situation that applies to model programmes: systems have to serve all people in need, not just those who can be selected for a clinical trial; systems have to serve people who are hard to treat, among whom are those whose prospects of recovery or rehabilitation are very limited; systems have to provide for competing patient groups, such as acute and long-term groups; finally, systems are accountable to changing political and economic masters, whereas the testing of model programmes and treatments is subject to a predetermined methodological and funding protocol.

Bachrach suggested that model programmes (and the same suggestion applies in my view to all alternative treatment programmes) should be thought of as a way of testing an hypothesis; that is, as a test of a series of assumptions about the best way to care for psychiatric patients. Successful alternative treatment programmes have common characteristics – they tend to target people with severe mental illness; they are linked in with other community resources and services; they attempt to provide the full range of functions formerly provided in institutional care; they adopt individually tailored care planning; they are culturally relevant; they have specifically trained staff; they make liaison arrangements with existing institutions providing in-patient care; and they subject themselves to some form of internal evaluation, often self-monitoring.

In a literature review on user-involvement (Huxley 1996), I classified approaches to user-involvement in psychiatric services into information-sharing only, participation and opposition. In practice, alternative forms of care can sometimes be absorbed into mainstream services and come to constitute an integral part of the system; or they can remain external and complementary to mainstream services and are, in Warner's term, 'assertively unconventional'. For the most part this chapter will refer to the former rather than the latter, less conventional approaches.

An interesting unresolved question concerns the extent to which alternative modes of treatment inevitably become part of the system of provision, and which models adapt in this way and which ones do not. There may be no consistency across cultures in the extent to which this happens or in the pace of change involved.

ALTERNATIVE RESIDENTIAL TREATMENT FOR ACUTELY ILL PATIENTS

A small number of reasonably well-known, alternative programmes are briefly summarised below. My intention here is to point out some of the key features of these treatment models, rather than to describe them in detail. For readers who are interested in the more detailed descriptions, these can be obtained in Warner (1995).

Cedar House, Colorado

Cedar House is a 15-bed, 24-hour, residential home in a house in the community (Warner & Wollesen 1995). It aims to function as an alternative to psychiatric hospital for acutely ill patients. Staff and patients share household duties, and come and go freely. Fewer than 10% of residents are transferred to hospital, and the only people excluded from Cedar House are those who are a very serious suicide risk, confused, very violent, agitated and non-compliant, or have access to guns. The length of stay is brief, about 1 or 2 weeks. Patients are discharged to suitable living conditions in the community. Two staff members are always on duty, and there is a psychiatric presence for 3 hours every day. The weekly costs of provision are much lower than a hospital bed. There is high morale among the staff group, and the programme has been replicated in the north of Colorado state.

Venture, Vancouver

This is another 24-hour, residential, community treatment facility with 10 beds to provide short-term crisis resolution (expanded to 20 beds in 1990). Care is described as intermediate between community case management and hospitalisation (Sladen-Drew et al 1995). Like Cedar House, there is an informal, homelike atmosphere with intensive staffing. The patient's case manager and usual clinician retain clinical responsibility for the patient and this strong continuity link is said to facilitate earlier discharge, as does the maintenance of links with support networks in the community. Patients go to Venture on a trial basis, and 20% transfer to hospital after admission. Only 17% of the patients who are admitted have psychotic symptoms. Patients are excluded if they are a high suicide risk or require close supervision owing to disorganisation, or meet the criteria for involuntary treatment. Those who have been violent within the last 24 to 48 hours are not automatically excluded, but are carefully screened. The mean length of stay is 8 days. Patients benefit from respite and medication monitoring and engaging in daily chores. Psychiatric care is only available on 3 half-days a week. The daily costs are said to be about half of that of a hospital bed.

Crossing Place, Washington DC

Crossing Place was established in 1978 and adopts a psychosocial approach that reflects the significance of ethnic identity of staff and patients, the environmental realities of their lives, and the political and economic climate (Bourgeois 1995). The service aims to resolve crises in supportive milieu operating as a temporary family. (For a useful classification of types of crisis requiring different service responses, see Huxley & Kerfoot 1995.) Clients served are over 18, of voluntary status, have no serious, complicating, medical problem requiring hospital care, and have a primary problem other than substance abuse. Suicidal and assaultive patients are not excluded. One-to-one, intensive, interpersonal support is provided by specially trained staff, in a homelike environment, where residents learn to cope with their life crisis in a real-life setting. Individual treatment plans are drawn up with the residents and the length of stay varies from a few days to several months. A psychiatric evaluation is made within 24 hours of admission. About 60% of clients are schizophrenia sufferers. Costs are said to be $156 per day compared to the costs in Medicaid eligible hospitals in Washington of $900 a day. In common with other similar facilities referred to above, about 10% of patients have to be transferred to hospital for treatment.

Services in the Netherlands

The Groningen University Hospital Crisis Clinic has 10 beds for a population of 170 000 (Schudel 1995). There are 14 nurses and two psychiatric residents, and a social worker on the staff and there are always at least two nurses on duty day and night. Seriously psychotic and dangerous patients are not admitted. Admissions are accepted over 24 hours, but for safety reasons the doors are locked at night. Each patient receives a counselling plan before being returned to the care of their family doctor or psychiatric out-patient service. Team meetings are held twice a day. The service is operated like a normal home with patients undertaking chores and being encouraged to return home for brief visits or to collect belongings. The average length of stay is about 9 days, and about 25% of those admitted have a psychosis. 60% of the patients are discharged to their home. The costs are $300 per day.

Comment

All of these programmes can accept the most difficult patients, but all of them have exclusion criteria, and most transfer between 10 and 20% of patients to a hospital setting for treatment. Comparisons between these alternative services and standard services need to include all the patients they intended to treat, or attempt to match carefully the patients who are accepted for care. If this is not done, the alternative services may appear to be more successful because they exclude the most difficult (and costly) patients, such as those with the greatest history of admission or those with comorbid physical illnesses.

None of the services provides detailed cost data. Even traditional services have difficulty in providing comprehensive costs. In both traditional and alternative services there is frequently no attempt to include the costs incurred in other constituencies, such as the justice system. In the examples given above, the cost-savings, or opportunity costs of using patient labour for household chores may or may not have been included.

RESIDENTIAL ALTERNATIVES FOR SEVERE MENTAL ILLNESS

Northwest Evaluation Center

An example of an alternative service for some of the most difficult patients is the Northwest Evaluation Center (NEC) in Seattle (Ferguson & Dowd 1995). Involuntary detained patients are held in a locked residential treatment facility for up to 72 hours in the first instance and then for a further 90 or 180 days. Excluded are those people who are under 18, those who are non-ambulatory, have a medical condition requiring hospital treatment, are a felon requiring 24-hour armed guard, or have an organic brain syndrome. The average length of stay is 2 weeks. Pharmacology and reality orientation, recreational art and movement therapies are offered. There are four psychiatrists who work in 24-hour segments. Even though this is a secure facility, it is important to note that it also transfers 10% of its patients for treatment in the State Mental Hospital. The daily rate of $230 is said to be one-third of the hospital cost.

INNOVATIVE AND NON-TRADITIONAL (LESS CONVENTIONAL) SERVICES FOR ACUTELY ILL PATIENTS

Soteria

Perhaps the best known unconventional treatment service is the Soteria model developed by Mosher (1995). The original Soteria house had six bedrooms for patients and two for staff, and focused on growth, development and learning, not treatment. It was instigated with the intention of finding an informed and reliable alternative to drug treatment. There is part-time psychiatrist supervision of staff. Two cohorts of patients from Soteria were studied and compared with local community mental health centre patients. Matthews et al (1979) reported on the 1971–1976 cohort of 28 index and 11 control patients. They were similar on demographic and symptom measures at inception. At 6 weeks, both groups improved even though Soteria patients had received no neuroleptics. After

2 years, the Soteria group were working at a higher level, more often living independently or with peers, and had fewer re-admissions. 57% had not been treated with neuroleptic medication. Mosher et al (1990) reported on the 1976–1982 cohort. After 2 years, there were no significant differences in symptomatic outcome. More of the Soteria patients were living independently. The outcome was predominantly positive for 200 people on no or low-dose neuroleptics, but there were no significant differences in relapse rates. The Soteria cases had better social adjustment and lower treatment costs.

Soteria Berne

Soteria Berne is based on the integration of psychosocial and biological factors under medical supervision. It was opened in 1984 in a 12-room house in Berne for people aged 17 to 35 with a recent onset of schizophrenia or schizophreniform psychosis and two of six specific symptoms in the past 4 weeks (Ciompi et al 1995). People who are totally non-compliant and drug- or alcohol-dependent are excluded. The most acutely disturbed patients may bypass the system altogether by going from the emergency room directly to a hospital bed. System bypasses such as this could be regarded as another form of exclusion. There are two staff continually on duty and a part-time medical director, five psychiatric nurses and four paraprofessionals. The average stay is between 1 and 4 months.

Soteria Berne uses an educational approach, focuses on long-term after-care and relapse prevention, and generates positive expectations by providing everyone involved in care with up-to-date information. This also ensures better continuity of care. Low-dose, targeted medication is provided.

On the basis of a simple global evaluation of outcome, 65% had a good outcome. 14 matched patients were evaluated at 2 years and 71% relapsed in both groups. Patients on no medication or a low dose achieved better results, but the evaluation was based on small numbers. Patients and relatives found it less stigmatising than the control service and less upsetting. Similar results have been shown for intensive case management, so perhaps a less hospital-type environment should be the choice for first episodes if they are not extremely severe.

Comment

In spite of the caveats expressed earlier, these studies raise some interesting questions about the effects of non-institutional care. Institutions appear to foster an inability to live more independently. We do not know whether this happens more often in a group of vulnerable individuals, or what characteristics make them vulnerable, or whether there is a critical window of time after which the effect is irremediable. If we did know what these vulnerability characteristics were, we could perhaps take steps to avoid the problem by using non-institutional alternatives as a first course of treatment.

COMMUNITY APPROACHES FOR ACUTELY ILL PATIENTS

Santa Clara County Clustered Apartment Project (SCCCAP)

This programme was not established as an alternative to hospitalisation (Mandiberg 1995). The creators of the programme argue that to regard the patient sub-culture as a negative phenomenon is not appropriate, and this programme regards it as potentially positive and as a means of providing the permanent social supports that the wider culture and community seemed unwilling or unable to sustain. The model was based on the simple concept that if a patient community was given the resources and the assistance to form itself on a positive, mutually supportive basis, it could act as a permanent support system. The model used the clustering of patients' homes as one vehicle for fostering a community. In an ideal model, a patient could walk to any other patient's house within 5 minutes. Community organisers rather than clinicians would assist the clients in establishing a mutually supportive and interdependent community. The programme providers view independence as a false goal and substitute interdependence as the major objective. However, they aim to provide a substitute for treatment services in the long run.

Stockport Arts on Prescription

Creative activity has been shown to increase self-esteem, provide a sense of purpose, give structure to an otherwise shapeless day, help people engage in social relationships and friendships, enhance social skills and community integration and improve individual quality of life. Following the successful introduction of an Exercise on Prescription scheme, it was recognised that a wider range of activities might be of benefit to people in Stockport who were enduring stress-related illnesses. The Arts on Prescription scheme was offered to people with mild to moderate depression. A steering group was formed, consisting of people involved in mental health, the Arts in Health and the leisure services division of the local authority. The aim of Arts on Prescription is 'to increase the level of mental well-being of participants using a wide range of creative processes.' One objective was to 'raise self-esteem and self-confidence through involvement and achievement in creative activities.' Positive and negative self-concept were the same at evaluation times 1 and 2. There were some

positive changes in the social functioning items in the questionnaire, but these did not reach significance. However, the General Health Questionnaire (GHQ) showed a reduction in overall score from a mean of 14 items at time 1 to nine items at time 2, and this was almost a significant reduction (F = 3.89; $p = 0.058$). According to the GHQ results (using the 10/11 cut off), 65% of participants had a recognisable mental health problem at time 1, and only 35% by time 2.

Another objective was to 'encourage participants to take up further arts/leisure activities after the project and identify a range of possible future opportunities.' People increased their social activities, especially participative activities between times 1 and 2. At time 1, the mean number of social activities was between three and four, but by time 2, it was between six and seven activities per person. This difference is statistically significant (F = 7.12; $p = 0.012$).

Although the number of people assessed by questionnaire was not large (n = 33), the questionnaire results and subjective responses were remarkably consistent and suggest that the project may well have had the desired impact. People who remain in the project report a better self-concept, their mental health definitely does not appear to deteriorate, and for many it improves. They appear to be using fewer resources and participating more in social and leisure activity than the total group of referred patients, and more than they were when they joined the project. In four of the six specific objectives, the project was a success. Two quotations from participants in the creative writing group give a flavour of the personal magnitude of the impact of participation on their lives: 'A light in the darkness of depression, both socially and expressively' and 'the possibility in life that there is always writing, the adventure of writing, is quite exciting.'

Comment

Neither of these community-based services was acting as an alternative to hospitalisation; each of them offered something different as a key component of care. Both were, in Bachrach's terminology, testing hypotheses about the value of an alternative approach to aspects of care in the community. In both cases, there appeared to be benefit to clients, but without a controlled trial one could never be sure whether the observed improvements would have happened in time anyway. Also, without longitudinal studies of this type of programme, one cannot be sure whether the effects are lasting, or whether effects occur in the longer term which are undetectable in the short term.

COMMUNITY APPROACHES FOR PEOPLE WITH ENDURING AND SEVERE MENTAL ILLNESS

Gwydir Project, Cambridge

The Gwydir Project is a collaborative, supervised, discharge project between Turning Point, Cambridgeshire County Council Social Services Department, the Cambridgeshire Probation Service and the Cambridge and Huntingdon Health Commission. It was established as a multi-agency response to the need to provide intensive health and social care in the community for high-risk groups of people who have severe mental health problems and complex needs. A small group of workers, led by an experienced team leader, work intensively to engage clients who have been hard to help in the past, and who have severe mental illness and a history of contact with psychiatric services and the criminal justice system. They provide practical and emotional help aimed at maintaining clients in the community and improving their quality of life.

The criteria which were agreed for referral to the project were severe mental illness; vulnerability with a risk of harm to self and others; a history of non-engagement or non-co-operation with services; a need for intensive support to prevent breakdown of existing functioning, return to hospital or re-offending; subject to the Care Programme Approach and referred to the social services department for care management.

More men than women were referred to the project (24/17). They were predominantly young (52% were aged under 40), and white (92%). The majority (58%) were single and lived alone (60%). Many (38%) were at serious risk of going into institutional care. The referring agents emphasised the need for support, particularly at weekends when the statutory services are not available, and in an attempt to avoid a crisis. Many of the people referred had quite a history of being 'difficult to engage' with statutory services and it was felt that the intensive help that the project was offering, and its independence from the statutory services, might succeed in getting them engaged.

Four-fifths (80%) had a psychotic illness. The most common was schizophrenia (40%). Gwydir cases conform to published definitions of severe mental illness. They also have, on average, higher severity scores than comparable cases which have been assessed using the same techniques (Huxley et al 1997b).

One of the project's original features was that the service was contracted out to an independent sector provider, Turning Point, who employ and supervise the operational staff. The project successfully engaged a number of clients, a number of whom had difficulty engaging with statutory services. The outcome results are all consistent in showing that, over 3 months, the project had a significant impact on the quality of life of the service recipients, compared to their previous experience. The interview results show that all the cases had suffered abuse at some point in their lives and there were fewer admissions to hospital after referral to the project. The change in GHQ scores from time 1 to time 2 just failed to reach significance ($t = -2.14$, df 9, $p = 0.06$). However, two of the sub-scale changes *were* significant: social dysfunction improved significantly ($t = -2.38$, df 9, $p < 0.05$), as did the depression score ($t = 3.21$, df 9, $p = 0.01$).

In three of the quality of life domains, there was substantial improvement from below the norm to above the norm, but the changes were not significant. Global health improved from 4.1 to 4.6; social relations improved from 4.5 to 4.8; and safety also improved from 4.5 (below the norm) to 5.0 (above the norm). Leisure improved from 4 to 4.3, both below the norm. Work/education improved significantly from 4.0 (the norm) to 4.9 ($t = 2.95$, df 9, $p < 0.05$). None of the individual social functioning (SFS) items showed a significant difference, but the total score was improved significantly ($t = -2.34$, df 9, $p < 0.05$). The difference in the total Camberwell Assessment of Need (CAN) score between time 1 and time 2 was significant ($t = 3.27$, df 9, $p < 0.01$). The Service User Questionnaire covered such areas as satisfaction with times and places of appointments, with the amount of time available for talking about problems, with sensitivity for cultural/religious practices, with information provided and with treatment decision-making. The overall mean total score for the group was 22.7 initially but it was down to 14.7 at the final interview, a 35% decrease (towards better satisfaction) which was significant ($t = -4.55$, df 9, $p < 0.001$).

An analysis of the costs incurred by people using the service was compared with the costs of service in the period before coming to the project. The cost comparisons were not comprehensive, but like was compared with like, and showed that the project led to a reduction in average costs. Gwydir Project unit costs appeared to be similar to those of an occupational therapy visit. The project met its objectives to engage some of the most difficult, mentally ill client group, and had some considerable success in improving their quality of life and satisfaction with services. It would appear that, when targeted upon people who use large amounts of expensive hospital services, this type of intensive community service might well lead to a reduction in overall costs.

Critical Time Intervention, New York City

Susser et al (1997) describe the results of a study of critical time intervention (CTI) with 96 men with severe mental illness entering community housing from a shelter. The men were randomised to receive standard services or standard services plus CTI. Over the 18-month, follow-up period, the average number of homeless nights for the intervention group was 30 compared to 91 for the standard group. CTI has two components: the first is to strengthen the individual's long-term ties to services, family and friends; the second is to provide emotional and practical support during the critical time of transition. Although the programme was designed to reduce homelessness, this is obviously a central component in the acquisition and retention of community tenure for persons with severe mental illness. The same principles could be applied to discharged patients who do not have a history of homelessness but whose community tenure is insecure. Discontinuity, which occurs when hospitalisation takes place, makes re-integration hazardous, and as we have seen, continuity of care is vital to reduce future episodes of institutional care.

CTI involves workers in assisting patients to access their existing networks of care by attending appointments with them, assisting in the development of relationships with other agency workers, and tailoring individual supports. In the standard service, the connections between the different agencies involved in patient care were described as 'generally weak and unsystematised', a description that will be very familiar to anyone working in mental health services in most parts of the UK. By making existing networks function more appropriately, rather than creating yet another service for the client to depend upon, CTI offers the possibility of enhancing continuity of care, improving the efficiency of some existing services, and making better use of community resources in individual programmes of care.

CRITICAL COMPONENTS

What appear to be the critical components that lead to successful alternative treatment models? Are there aspects of alternative models that look promising and, consequently, suggest avenues for further research?

Selection criteria

While it is true, as Warner (1995) points out, that programmes that are integrated with or contract with a broader community treatment programme clearly do not exclude patients who are violent or on criminal charges, who actively resist treatment, who have AIDS or other medical problems, who prefer to live on the streets and who combine substance misuse with mental illness, most of the programmes mentioned in this chapter, individually, do have such exclusion criteria. So while it is possible to treat most of these patients in alternative community settings, there are patients who, in certain settings and under certain circumstances, require more traditional in-patient care. Even the NEC programme transferred 10% of its patients to hospital care. Most

commonly about 10 to 20% of patients served by the alternative facilities have to be treated at some stage in hospital. The question is which patients and under what circumstances? Broadly speaking, the exclusion criteria themselves give us the best clue to the type of patient where hospital care in a more restricted environment might be required: these are satisfying the legislative criteria for involuntary care, such as threat to the life of the patient or others, and co-existing medical conditions that do require care or investigation in an in-patient rather than an out-patient facility. Other than these, Warner is quite right that severity itself, self-harm or suicidality per se, intoxication, and lack of co-operation with treatment do not automatically mean treatment should be in a closed hospital environment.

Service elements

What we need urgently is a way of assessing how the different elements in the mental health service system interact. Even where services are less conventional, they are treating people in need. The patients they treat must *either* be being diverted from the other conventional treatment facilities or they must be those who would never have reached treatment otherwise. In terms of the cost-effectiveness of the whole service system, it is vital to know the answer to this question.

Medication

A critical element in many of the alternative services is the reduced dosage of medication required, and the use of oral medications and monitoring. On a recent visit to Sweden I was told that the UK practice of long-acting phenothiazine injections given in special 'depot' clinics is regarded in Sweden as bad clinical practice. Similarly, there is a marked contrast between the achievement of successful pharmacological treatment on both sides of the Atlantic; the North Americans are more prepared to use reduced doses and to achieve continuity either through more regular contact and monitoring of patients on oral medication, or (for those very small number of patients who are totally unco-operative) compulsory medication in the community. Monitored oral medication has at least two advantages: the first is the monitoring of side-effects on a regular basis, and the adjustment of medication to reduce these; and the second is that the monitoring demands face-to-face contact which may also be acting to enhance continuity of care.

In assessing the effectiveness of alternative models then, one has to be careful to examine whether it is more effective medication administration and prescribing practice that is creating an advantage for the alternative system of care.

Comparable patients

Another key issue is the comparability of the patient groups being studied. Clearly, as Bachrach suggested, if alternative programmes have such narrow inclusion criteria as to exclude most patients, they are bound to have a therapeutic advantage over traditional all-encompassing service systems. Comparing like with like patients cannot be achieved simply by ensuring that crude demographics and diagnosis are similar. Factors that make treatment more difficult need to be taken into account, such as non-compliance, social problems, previous treatment history and the presence of suicidality or assaultive behaviours (see Huxley et al 1997a).

Also, within a whole service system, it may be most appropriate for certain groups of patients to experience non-hospital settings as the preferred treatment option when they experience their first episode.

Continuity of care

Continuity of care emerges as a key variable in successful treatment. Several programmes feature ways of ensuring that the agency staff and community networks do not experience regular and dramatic changes in personnel. Warner argues that discharge planning as an integral part of the residential experience can help to ensure continuity of care after treatment.

Programme content

There appear to be benefits that derive from the nature of the residential programmes themselves. Characteristics summarised by Warner (1995) are:

- retain autonomy
- maintain community links
- carry less stigma
- maintain social skills
- provide more support = lower medications
- permit scarce hospital resources to be used for those who need them most
- improve access to care
- enhance continuity of care
- have lower costs.

Personnel

Another important aspect of the success of such programmes is the quality of the personnel involved and their knowledge, experience and supervision. It is no coincidence, I think, that successful programmes use more psychiatrist time, or use the time available to better purpose. This clearly emerges in Warner's book, but being a psychiatrist himself, he is perhaps wary of drawing attention to this, or perhaps he would not agree that it is evident. It is certainly not a popular assertion on either side of the Atlantic at the time of writing.

Evidence

Unfortunately, the evidence for the success of these programmes is more often asserted than demonstrated. The costing methodologies are unsophisticated at best; for example, not taking account of the contribution of patients to the care of the residential unit in opportunity cost terms, or counting the costs to other systems operating in the community such as the justice system.

CTI has been successfully used with homeless, severely mentally ill people and may well benefit other types of patients. ACT certainly benefits people with severe and enduring problems. Many residential alternatives seem to be as successful as day hospitals and can cope with all but the most difficult patients. In-patient care seems always to be required for a small number of patients.

Lack of scientific evidence for effectiveness or efficiency does not prevent programmes being replicated. Many of the ones described above have been replicated. The 'clubhouse' model, not considered in any detail here, has spread, successfully it would seem, throughout the world. The limited evidence that is available does confirm a beneficial impact on some patients and under certain circumstances (Huxley et al 1999).

CONCLUSION

There is a need to be more sophisticated in our approach; providing a single solution, whether this is the district general hospital unit model or the Soteria model, is clearly going to be wrong in a lot of cases because it will be appropriate and successful for some patients and not others. A range of approaches is needed, and getting the right patients into the right setting is then the challenge. This involves getting the patient the 'right' treatment, but also getting treatment in the most cost-effective setting. Success in both aspects of care can only be achieved by studying whole service systems in different cultures; only then will we begin to understand how to solve the problem of providing appropriate treatment at the same time as containing costs.

We need a methodology to study the interaction of elements within the mental health service system and also between the mental health services system and other systems such as housing and the justice system. It is no use simply following fashions either in residential services or in drug treatments. We need a more comprehensive approach to our understanding of the workings of the mental health service system and the part to be played in it by non-statutory mental health provision, alternative treatments and less conventional forms of care.

Exercise

Either (a) consider the most recent mental health service development in your area. To what extent could it be described as an alternative service? Look at its aims and objectives in relation to the other services available, and assess in what terms you think it is able to, or could, demonstrate the achievement of its aims and objectives. Or (b) examine the case for an alternative service in your area. How would it fit in with existing services, what would its aims be, and how could the achievement of its aims be demonstrated?

KEY TEXTS FOR FURTHER READING

Bachrach L L 1980 Overview: model programs for chronic mental patients. American Journal of Psychiatry 137:1023–1031

Bagley H, Hatfield B, Huxley P J 1996 Learning materials on mental health: An introduction. The University of Manchester and the Department of Health. Available from The School of Psychiatry and Behavioural Sciences, The University of Manchester, Oxford Road, Manchester M13 9PL

Stein L, Test M (eds) 1975 Alternatives to mental hospital treatment. Plenum Press, New York

Tansella M (ed) 1997 Making rational mental health services. II Piensero Scientifico Editore, Rome

Warner R (ed) 1995 Alternatives to the hospital for acute psychiatric treatment. Clinical Practice #32. American Psychiatric Press, Washington DC

REFERENCES

Bachrach L L 1980 Overview: model programs for chronic mental patients. American Journal of Psychiatry 137:1023–1031

Bourgeois P 1995 Crossing Place, Washington DC. In: Warner R (ed) Alternatives to the hospital for acute psychiatric treatment. Clinical Practice #32. American Psychiatric Press, Washington DC

Ciompi L, Dauwalder H, Maier C et al 1995 The pilot project 'Soteria Berne': clinical experiences and results. In: Warner R (ed) Alternatives to the hospital for acute psychiatric treatment. Clinical Practice #32. American Psychiatric Press, Washington DC

Ferguson W D, Dowd D 1995 Northwest Evaluation and Treatment Center, Seattle: alternative to hospitalization for involuntary detained patients. In: Warner R (ed) Alternatives to the hospital for acute psychiatric treatment. Clinical Practice #32. American Psychiatric Press, Washington DC

Fortuna J M 1995 The Windhorse Programme for Recovery. In: Warner R (ed) Alternatives to the hospital for acute psychiatric treatment. Clinical Practice #32. American Psychiatric Press, Washington DC

Hoge M A, Davidson L, Hill L W et al 1992 The promise of partial hospitalisation: a re-assessment. Hospital and Community Psychiatry 43:345–354

Huxley P 1996 Whose health is it anyway? Literature review on the involvement of users and carers in mental health services. Health Advisory Service, London (This was subsequently published in 1997 by the HAS as: Voices in Partnership: Involving Service Users in Commissioning and Delivering Mental Health Services, Firth M & Kerfoot M (eds))

Huxley P J, Kerfoot M 1995 Letter from Manchester: a typology of crisis services for mental health. Journal of Mental Health 4:431–435

Huxley P J, Reilly S, Butler T, Harrison J 1997a Information breakdown. Health Service Journal 5 June: 28–29

Huxley P J, Reilly S, Harrison J, Mohamad H 1997b Severe mental illness: the work of CPNs and social services staff compared. Mental Health Nursing 18:14–17

Huxley P J, Warner R, Berg T 1999 A case-control study of Clubhouse membership and quality of life. International Journal of Social Psychiatry (in press)

Mandiberg J 1995 Can interdependent mutual support function as an alternative to hospitalization? The Santa Clara County Clustered Apartment Project. In: Warner R

(ed) Alternatives to the hospital for acute psychiatric treatment. Clinical Practice #32. American Psychiatric Press, Washington DC

Marshall M, Lockwood A 1997 Systematic review of the effectiveness of case management and assertive community treatment for people with severe mental disorders. University of Manchester, School of Psychiatry and Behavioural Sciences, Royal Preston Hospital, Preston, UK

Matthews S M, Roper M T, Mosher L R et al 1979 A non-neuroleptic treatment for schizophrenia: analysis of the two-year post-discharge risk of relapse. Schizophrenia Bulletin 5:322–333

Mosher L R 1995 The Soteria Project: the first-generation American alternatives to psychiatric hospitalization. In: Warner R (ed) Alternatives to the hospital for acute psychiatric treatment. Clinical Practice #32. American Psychiatric Press, Washington DC

Mosher L, Vallone R, Menn A Z 1990 The treatment of acute psychosis without neuroleptics: new data from the Soteria Project. Paper presented at the annual meeting of the American Psychiatric Association, New York, May 1990

Polak P R, Kirby M W, Deitchman W S 1995 Treating acutely psychotic patients in private homes. In: Warner R (ed) Alternatives to the hospital for acute psychiatric treatment. Clinical Practice #32. American Psychiatric Press, Washington DC

Schudel W J 1995 Acute hospital alternatives in the Netherlands: crisis intervention centres. In: Warner R (ed) Alternatives to the hospital for acute psychiatric treatment. Clinical Practice #32. American Psychiatric Press, Washington DC

Sladen-Drew N, Young A, Parfitt H, Hamilton R 1995 Venture: The Vancouver experience. In: Warner R (ed) Alternatives to the hospital for acute psychiatric treatment. Clinical Practice #32. American Psychiatric Press, Washington DC

Susser E, Valencia E, Conover S, Felix A, Tsai W-Y, Wyatt R J 1997 Preventing recurrent homelessness among mentally ill men: a 'critical time' intervention after discharge from a shelter. American Journal of Public Health 87(2):256–262

Thompson B J, Lyons J S 1996 Lessons from the front: implementing outcomes projects. Behavioural Healthcare Tomorrow October: 85–87

Warner R 1995 From patient management to risk management. In: Warner R (ed) Alternatives to the hospital

REFERENCES (*contd*)

for acute psychiatric treatment. Clinical Practice #32. American Psychiatric Press, Washington DC

Warner R, Wollesen C 1995 Cedar House: a noncoercive hospital alternative in Boulder, Colorado. In: Warner R (ed) Alternatives to the hospital for acute psychiatric treatment. Clinical Practice #32. American Psychiatric Press, Washington DC

Index

A

ABC analysis of behaviour, 108, 211
Abdominal pain, recurrent, 328
Aberdeen Royal Mental Asylum, 33–34
Abnormal doctor behaviour, 231
Abnormal illness behaviour, 226, 230–231
Absconded patients, 67
Accessibility, mental health services, 386
Activity scheduling, in chronic fatigue syndrome, 237
ADFAM National, 394
Adherence, *see* Compliance
Adolescents
    anxiety disorders, 315–316, 330
    behavioural problems, 318–319
    dementia, 355
    depression, 317–318, 325, 330, 334
    mental health problems, *see* Child/adolescent mental health problems
    schizophrenia, 334
Adult, appropriate, 63
Adversity, chronic, 326
Advice, giving, 81–82
Advocacy, 13–14, 16–17, 373–388
    case studies, 387
    citizen, 378, 383
    class or collective (corporate), 378–379
    definition, 374
    formal, 379
    independent, 16–17
    legal, 376–377
    literature and research, 379–382
    meaning and manifestations, 374–376
    by nurses, 374–376, 379–380, 382
    patient, 384
    peer, 377–378
    rights, 386
    schemes, 382–385
    self-, 17, 377, 383
    useful addresses, 388
Advocacy Alliance, 381, 388
Affective disorders *see* Mood disorders
Age
    child mental health disorders and, 315
    suicide risk and, 192
Agenda setting, 86
Aggression
    in children and adolescents, 330
    definition, 272
    hostile/angry, 272
    instrumental/incentive, 272
    in intermittent explosive disorder, 268
    Novaco's model, 267–268
    prevention, 273–286
    self-directed, 272
    see also Anger; Violence

Agoraphobia, 216
    nurse therapists, 222
    in older people, 347, 348
    treatment, 216, 399–401
Aides, case management, 21, 154
AIDS (acquired immune deficiency syndrome), 193
AIDS dementia complex, 355
Aims, of consultations, 84
Albumin, serum, in anorexia nervosa, 256
Alcohol abuse
    in bi-polar disorder, 169
    in bulimia nervosa, 257
    in older people, 351–354
        assessment, 352–353
        characteristics and prevalence, 351–352
        interventions, 353–354
    in schizophrenia, 158–159
    suicide risk, 170, 191, 198
Alcoholics Anonymous (AA), 393, 394–395
Alcohol-related dementia, 355
Alienation, suicidal patients, 199, 200
Alienists, 28
The Alleged Lunatics Society, 377
Allen, Catherine, 31
Alternative treatments, 407–419
    community
        for acutely ill patients, 413–415
        for enduring and severe mental illness, 415–417
    comparable patients, 418
    continuity of care, 418
    critical components, 417–419
    evidence, 419
    medication, 417–418
    personnel, 418
    programme content, 418
    residential
        for acutely ill patients, 410–412
        for severe mental illness, 412
    selection criteria, 417
    service elements, 417
    unconventional, for acutely ill patients, 412–413
Alzheimer's disease (AD), 343, 354, 355
    anorexia nervosa and, 250
    early onset, 357
    personal experience of, 362
    treatment, 356
Alzheimer's Disease Society, 356–357, 358, 360, 361
Amenorrhoea, 248
Anchoring of effects, 267
Anger, 265–286
    in children and adolescents, 330
    dysfunctional, 266
    management, 273–286
        assessment, 275–276
        case study, 279–286
        cognitive preparation and assessment, 276

    evaluation, 278–279
    sessional structure, 278–279
    skill acquisition and rehearsal, 277
    skill application, 277–278
    stress inoculation therapy, 274–275
    mental health effects, 270–271
    Novaco's model, 266–268
    physical health effects, 269–270
    in PTSD, 308
    self-injury and, 271–272
    suppression, 270
    violence and, 272–273
    see also Aggression; Violence
Anger Expression Scale, 269
Anorexia nervosa, 244–256, 260
    aetiology, 245–247
    behavioural assessment, 248–249
    binge–purge sub-type, 244, 245
    clinical features, 247–248
    comorbidity, 245
    diagnosis and classification, 244–245
    measurement, 256
    medical complications, 249–252
    mental state assessment, 249
    prognosis, 255–256
    restricting sub-type, 244, 245
    treatment, 252–255
        current models, 254–255
        environment of care, 252–254
Antidepressants, 177
    in bulimia nervosa, 259
    in children and adolescents, 317, 334
    in obsessive–compulsive disorder, 219, 333
    in older people, 345–346
    in PTSD, 303
Anti-psychiatry, 42
Antipsychotic drugs, 151
    atypical, 151–152, 160
    in children and adolescents, 333–334
    depot injections, 152, 351, 417–418
    side effects, 151
Antisocial behaviour, 319
Anxiety
    and depressive disorder, mixed, 167
    management, 301, 348–349
    separation, 316–317, 323
    see also Somatic symptoms
Anxiety disorders, 209
    in children and adolescents, 315–316, 330
    in older people, 346–349
        assessment, 348
        characteristics and prevalence, 346–348
        interventions, 348–349
    self-help, 399
    see also Obsessive–compulsive disorder; Panic disorder; Phobias
Arousal
    cognitive, 266
    physiological
        in anger, 266, 277, 279–281
        in phobias, 215

Arousal (*contd*)
  symptoms, in PTSD, 292
Art therapies, creative, 331
Asperger's syndrome, 320
Assault
  nurses, 68
  serious, definition, 273
  victims, 306–307
  see also Sexual assault; Violence
Assertive community treatment
    (ACT), 153, 160, 409, 419
Assessment, 103–118
  aims, 86–87
  computers in, 77
  emergency, 57–58
  extended, 57, 58–59
  instruments, 114–115, 138
  interviewing skills, 86–89, 113–114
  joint, 106
  mental state, 107
  needs, 105, 138
  nursing, 106–109
    behavioural approach, 108
    content, 106
    definition, 106
    home visiting guidelines, 116–118
    initial referral, 112–113
    nursing models and, 107
    primary information, 113–115
    process, 112–117
    psychosocial approach, 107–108
    risk *see* Risk, assessment
    secondary information, 115–116
    versus medical assessment, 107
  problem, 108
Assessment order, 57, 58
Assistants, nursing, 140
Asylums, 12, 32–35
  break-up, 15, 43–44
  early history, 29–32
  military, 37–38
  reflections from within, 35–37
  see also Psychiatric hospitals
Atherosclerosis, 269
Attachment, 323
  avoidant, 323
  insecure, 253, 323
Attendants
  in nineteenth-century asylums, 34,
    35
  in military mental hospitals, 37, 38
Attentional cueing, 267
Attention-deficit–hyperactivity
    disorders, 319–320
  treatment, 330–331, 334
Attention deficits, in schizophrenia,
    150
Attributional error, 267
Attributions, illness, 233
Audit, 123, 124, 138
  see also Evaluation
Autism, 320, 325
Avoidance
  in anorexia nervosa, 244–245, 247,
    252–253

in panic disorder, 212
in PTSD, 292, 304, 306
in social phobia, 214–215
in somatic syndromes, 232–233

B

Bail Information Service, 64
Barbiturates, 39–40
Barnsley hospital advocacy service,
    385
Barry, John, 40
Battle fatigue, 292
Beck Anxiety Inventory, 211, 348
Beck Depression Inventory (BDI), 115,
    211, 298, 345
Beck Hopelessness Scale, 196
Beers, Clifford, 35–36
Behavioural assessment, 108
  in anorexia nervosa, 248–249
Behavioural (functional) analysis,
    87–88, 108
  anger, 274
  panic disorder, 211
  in somatic syndromes, 235
Behavioural model, PTSD, 293–294
Behavioural modification, in children
    and adolescents, 319–320,
    330–331
Behavioural problems, 318–319
Behaviour therapy
  children and adolescents, 317,
    328–329
  nurse therapists *see* Nurse
    therapists
  in obsessive–compulsive disorder
    (OCD), 217–218
  older people, 353
  training, 132, 221–222
Benzodiazepines, 348
Bereavement, suicide risk, 193
Binge-eating
  in anorexia nervosa, 244, 245, 249
  in bulimia nervosa, 256–257
Binge-eating disorder, 256, 257
Biological factors
  in child mental health problems,
    324–325
  in eating disorders, 246, 257–258
  in mood disorders, 171
Biological models, PTSD, 295–296
Bi-polar disorder
  aetiological theories, 171–172
  epidemiology, 168–169
  nursing roles, 179–182
  presenting symptoms, 168–169
  prognosis and outcome, 169
  relapse, early signs, 180
  self-management, 178–179
  social and occupational effects,
    172–176
  sub-types, 168
  suicide and parasuicide, 169–170
  treatment, 176–178

see also Depression
Blood chemistry, in anorexia nervosa,
    252
Body image disorder, 222, 249
Bolam test, 54
Bonding, 323
Bone marrow dysfunction, in anorexia
    nervosa, 251–252
Bowlby, J., 323
Brain abnormalities
  in anorexia nervosa, 250–251
  in schizophrenia, 150
Brief Psychiatric Rating Scale (BPRS),
    115
British Association of Behavioural and
    Cognitive Psychotherapy, 222
Browne, W.A.F., 34
Bulimia Investigatory Test, Edinburgh
    (BITE), 256
Bulimia nervosa, 244, 256–259, 260
  aetiology, 257–258
  clinical features, 256–257
  comorbidity, 257
  diagnosis and classification, 256, 257
  medical complications, 259
  prognosis, 259
  sociocultural factors, 258–259
  treatment, 259

C

Camberwell Assessment of Need
    (CAN), 115
Cameron, Dr K., 38
Campaign Against Psychiatric
    Oppression, 17–18
CANVAS (Clinical Assessment of
    Need: Violence Appraisal
    System), 108–109
Capacity (mental), 52–54
  to consent, 55–56, 59
  diminished, 50
  to manage financial affairs, 69
  test, 53
  testamentary, 69
Carbamazepine, 177
Cardiovascular disorders, in anorexia
    nervosa, 251
Cardiovascular reactivity, in anger,
    270
Care plan
  child/adolescent mental health
    problems, 323
  in relapse of schizophrenia, 156
  at-risk patients, 109
Care Programme Approach (CPA), 61,
    62, 105
  benefits to patients, 14, 17
  recent developments, 74
Carers
  formal, 113
    information from, 115
    see also Nurses; Staff
  informal (family), 113

Carers (*contd*)
  in dementia, 358, 359–361
  information from, 115–116,
    321–322
  see also Family
Carotid atherosclerosis, 269
Case law, 51
Case management, 105, 153–154
  aides, 21, 154
Casenotes, 115
Cedar House, Colorado, 410–411
Censorship, mail, 67
Central nervous system, in anorexia
    nervosa, 250–251
Centre for Reviews and Dissemination,
    4
Change management, 123
Charters, patients', 14, 385–386
Chest pain, non-cardiac, 229, 232, 239
Chilblains, in anorexia nervosa, 248,
    251
Child abuse, 273, 327–328
  in bulimia nervosa, 258–259
Child/adolescent mental health
    problems, 313–338
  aetiology/theoretical models,
    323–328
  assessment and detection, 320–323
  characteristic disorders, 316–320
  comorbidity, 315
  disorders, problems and difficulties,
    314
  epidemiology, 315–316
  formulation, 322–323
  future, 334–338
  historical background, 314–315
  treatment interventions, 328–334
    biological treatment, 333–334
    psychological therapies, 328–333
    residential settings, 333
Child/adolescent mental health
    services, 334–337
  four-tier model, 335–336
  future development, 76, 77, 337
  nursing skills and roles, 336–337
Children
  anxiety disorders, 315–316, 330
  behavioural problems, 318–319
  dementia, 355
  depression *see* Depression, in
    children and adolescents
  schizophrenia, 334
Chlorpromazine, 151
Choice, by mental patients, 18, 386
Chronic fatigue syndrome (CFS), 226,
    229, 230
  aetiology and model, 232–233
  cognitive–behaviour therapy (CBT),
    234–239
  evidence-based practice, 239
  illness attributions, 233
  interventions, 237–238
  nurse therapy, 222
Cicero, Marcus Tullius, 29
Circling swing, 30

Circulatory problems, in anorexia
    nervosa, 248, 251
Citizen Advocacy Information and
    Training (CAIT), 376, 388
Clientbond, Netherlands, 382–383
Clients *see* Patients, mental
Clinical effectiveness, 2, 3–5, 396
  lack of evidence for, 2–3
Clinical experience, 4–5
Clinical governance, 2
Clinical practice guidelines, 3, 124
Clinical significance, 125, 134–135
Clinical Standards Advisory Groups
    (CSAG), 74
Clinician-administered PTSD scale
    (CAPS), 298
Clomipramine, 219, 333
Clothier Inquiry Report (1994), 21–22
Clozapine, 151–152
Clubhouse model, 419
Clunis, Christopher, 23–24, 62, 108
Cocaine, crack, 158
Cochrane Collaboration, 4
Codes of Practice, 50–51
Cod-liver oil, 33
Cognitive–behavioural approach
  anger management, 275–286
  interviewing, 80–100
Cognitive–behaviour therapy (CBT),
    81–82, 324
  in anorexia nervosa, 255
  in children and adolescents,
    329–331
  medication compliance and, 177
  in mood disorders, 178
  nurse therapists *see* Nurse
    therapists
  in older people, 346, 349
  in panic disorder, 212
  in PTSD, 299–302, 304
  in schizophrenia, 154–155
  in somatic syndromes, 233–239
  in suicide prevention, 202, 203
  three systems model (Lang), 87–88,
    233–234, 239–240
  training, 221–222, 240
  see also Behaviour therapy;
    Cognitive therapy
Cognitive development, Piaget's
    theory, 323
Cognitive impairment
  in anorexia nervosa, 250–251
  in schizophrenia, 150
Cognitive processing models, PTSD,
    294–295
Cognitive processing therapy (CPT), in
    PTSD, 301–302
Cognitive restructuring
  in PTSD, 300, 301, 302
  in somatic syndromes, 237–238
Cognitive theory, depression and
    mania, 171
Cognitive therapy
  in PTSD, 306–307
  PTSD, 301–302, 303

Combat veterans, PTSD, 293, 299–300,
    302
Commission for Health Improvement
    (CHIMP), 73
Communication skills, 89–91
  in anorexia nervosa, 254
Community care, 13, 23–24
  alternatives to traditional, 409,
    413–417
    acutely ill patients, 413–415
    in enduring and severe mental
      illness, 415–417
  in dementia, 357, 358–359
  failures, 23–24
  government policies, 75, 76–77
  implications for nurses, 24–25
  legal provisions, 57, 61–63
  legislation, 105
  in mood disorders, 176
  suicidal patients, 198, 200–201
  transition to, 43–44
Community mental health teams
    (CMHT), 105–106
Community psychiatric nurses
    (CPNs), 44
  in child mental health care, 335, 336,
    337
  developing role, 76, 104, 105
  evaluation of training, 133
  forensic, 109
  historical background, 104
  in mood disorders, 176
  multidisciplinary working, 105–106
  nursing assessment, 106–118
  older people, 351
  primary care team attachment, 45
  problems, 44
Community tenure, 416
Compassionate Friends, 395
Compensation, 68–69
Competency, instrumental, 378
Complaints, 386
Complementary approaches, 2–3
Compliance
  interviewing skills and, 81
  in mood disorders, 169, 177
  promoting, 98–99, 153
  rape victims, 307
Compulsion, in mental health care, 18
Compulsions, 217
Computerised tomography, 150
Computers, in assessment and
    treatment, 77
Conditioning, 323–324
  classical, 293
  instrumental, 293
  operant, 98, 329
Conduct disorders, 318–319
Confessions of an Asylum Doctor
    (Montagu Lomax), 35, 36
Confidence, in depression and mania,
    174–175
Confidentiality, 69–70, 386
Conflict, interpersonal, 326–327
Connolly, Dr John, 32

Consent
    capacity to give, 55–56, 59
    informed, 55
    to searching a room, 66
    to treatment, 53–54, 59–61
Consultation (interviewing), 79–100
    aims and objectives, 84
    alliance-building and treatment
        orientation, 89–94
    approaching the client, 82–84
    for assessment, 86–89, 113–114
    children and adolescents, 321, 322
    engagement, 85–86
    goal-setting and planning, 94–99
    informal versus formal, 114
    non-directive approach, 80–81
    opening, 84–86
    planning, 84–85
    problems, 80–81
    process, 80
    questioning and advice-giving,
        81–82
    settings, 85
    timing, 84
Consumerism, 15, 16
Consumers of mental health care, 12
    mental patients as, 13, 16–17, 25
        beyond the concept, 19–20
        implications for nurses, 24–25
        limitations of concept, 17–19
    see also Patients, mental
Continuity of care, 418
Contracts
    drug, 16
    employment, 51
    suicidal patients, 201
Control, loss of sense of, 175
Control and restraint (C & R), 67
Control group, 131
Conversion disorder, 228
Coping
    rewarding client attempts, 92
    suicide risk and, 198
Cornelia de Lange syndrome, 272
Coronary atherosclerosis, 269
Coronary heart disease (CHD), anger
        and, 269–270
Coroners' verdicts, suicide, 189
Correlational analysis, 139
Cortisol, in anorexia nervosa, 250, 251
Cost-effectiveness, 3
Co-therapists, in obsessive–
        compulsive disorder, 218
Cotton, Nathaniel, 30
Counselling, in general practice, 2
Counter-transference, 254
Court, 63–66
    detention for report to, 57
    diversion, 64
    expert reports, 63
    fitness to plead, 64
    insanity and diminished
        responsibility, 64–65
    mandated restrictions, 57, 58, 65–66
    sentencing, 65–66

Court of Protection, 69
Cowper, William, 30
CPNs see Community psychiatric
        nurses
Creative art therapies, 331
Creutzfeldt–Jakob disease, 355
Criminal Injuries Compensation
        Board, 68–69
Criminal Law Act (1967), 67
Criminal offenders, anger
        management, 277, 279
Criminal Procedure (Insanity and
        Unfitness to Plead) Act (1991),
        58
Criminal proceedings, 63–66
    arrest and prosecution, 63
    court, 63–66
    remand for assessment, 57, 59
    remand for treatment, 57
Crisis
    assessment in, 114
    cards, 156
    services, 18, 112–113
        alternative residential settings,
            410–412
        unconventional services, 412–413
Critical time intervention (CTI), New
        York, 416–417, 419
Crossing Place, Washington DC, 411
Crown Prosecution Service, 63
Cueing, attentional, 267
Cues, following, 90
Cultural differences, 408–409
Cynical Distrust Scale, 269

D

Dangerous patients, 267–268
Dawson, Peter, 40
Day care centres, 408
Day hospitals, 408
Day treatment, 408
Day units, children and adolescents,
        333, 335–336
Deliberate self-harm (DSH), 187–204
    anger and, 271–272
    in bulimia nervosa, 257
    in children and adolescents, 318
    interventions, 199–203
    learning difficulty and, 272
    mental illness and, 272
    previous, 193–194
    psychosocial interventions, 199,
        201–203
    reasons given by patients for,
        194–195
    risk assessment, 197–199
    risk factors, 190–195
    suicide risk after, 194–195
    see also Parasuicide; Suicide
Delinquency, 318–319
Delusions
    in depression, 169
    therapeutic approaches, 155, 178

Dementia, 343, 354–364
    care nursing, 363–364
    causes, 355–356
    definition, 355
    early-onset, 355, 363
    family care/supportive
        interventions, 361
    financial affairs, 69
    historical and contemporary context,
        354–356
    impact on families, 359–361
    late-onset, 355
    personal experience of, 361–363
    policy and practice considerations,
        357–359
    presenile, 354
    prevalence, 356–357
    vascular, 355
Denial, in PTSD, 296
Dental changes, in anorexia nervosa,
        250
Department of Social Security (DSS)
        benefit regulations, 173–174
Dependent variables, 131, 134
Depot injections, 152, 417–418
    in paraphrenia, 351
Depression, 165–182
    aetiological theories, 171–172
    anger and, 271
    in bulimia nervosa, 257
    in children and adolescents, 317–318
        causation, 325
        treatment, 318, 330, 334
    clinical standards, 74
    nursing roles, 179–182
    in older people, 342–346, 348
        assessment, 344–345
        characteristics and prevalence,
            342–344
        interventions, 345–346
    parental, 326
    presenting features/epidemiology,
        169
    prognosis and outcome, 169
    in PTSD, 293, 307–308
    relapse, early signs, 180–181
    self-management, 178–179, 181, 399
    social and occupational effects,
        172–176
    in social phobia, 214–215
    spectrum of disorder, 167
    suicide and parasuicide, 170–171
    suicide prevention, 181–182, 203
    treatment approaches, 176–178, 203
Descartes, Rene, 227
Descriptive studies, 139
Desensitisation, 329
Detachment, emotional, in PTSD, 308
Detained patients, 66–68
    after-care of discharged, 61–63
    assault of nurses, 68
    mail censorship, 67
    residential alternatives, 412
    restricting visitors' access
    retaking absconded, 67

Detained patients (*contd*)
  searching a room, 66
  seclusion, 68
  therapeutic relationship, 179
  treatment
    not requiring consent, 60–61
    requiring consent or second
      opinion, 60
    requiring consent and second
      opinion, 61
    urgent, 60–61
  use of force, 67
Detention
  compulsory, 18, 55–59
  in anorexia nervosa, 255
  right of appeal against, 61
  without authority, 54, 55–56
Development
  childhood, history, 321
  psychological theories, 323–324
Developmental disorders, pervasive,
    320
Developmental model, supervision,
    129
Dexamphetamine, 334
Diagnostic and Statistical Manual
    (DSM), 148
Diaries, 211, 281
Dietary restriction, in anorexia
    nervosa, 244, 245, 249
Dignity, personal, 386
Diminished responsibility, 50, 64–65
Diploma in Psychological Medicine, 35
Direct therapeutic exposure, 299
Disability
  child mental health problems and,
    328
  in PTSD, 308–309
Disability Discrimination Act (1995),
    24
Disabled people, 13, 16, 24
Disabled Persons (Services,
    Consultation and
    Representation) Act (1986), 13
Disease, 227
Disinhibition, in aggression, 267
Dissemination, 3–4
Divorce, 326–327
Dizziness, unexplained, 229
Doctors
  in compulsory detention, 56
  in compulsory treatment, 60
  holding power, 57–58
  seclusion of patients, 68
  second opinion appointed (SOAD),
    60
Documentation *see* Records
Donepezil hydrochloride, 3556
Dopamine, 151
Drama therapy, 331
Drug misuse
  in bulimia nervosa, 257
  in schizophrenia, 158–159
  suicide risk, 191, 198
Drug overdose, 194, 201–202

  in children and adolescents, 318
Drug treatment *see* Medication
Dual diagnosis, 158–159
  suicide risk, 191
Dualism, mind–body, 226, 227, 239
Durkheim, E., 188
Dutch Patients Council Foundation
    (LPR), 383, 388
Duty of care, 54–55

E

Eating attitudes test (EAT), 256
Eating Disorder Examination, 256
Eating Disorder Inventory, 256
Eating disorders, 243–260
  see also Anorexia nervosa; Bulimia
    nervosa
Ecological analysis, 135–136
ECT *see* Electroconvulsive therapy
Education
  in autism, 320
  psychological *see* Psycho-education
  see also School
Educative groups, 331–332
Efficacy, 396
Efficiency, 125, 136–137
  nurse training, 136–137
Elderly *see* Older people
Electroconvulsive therapy (ECT), 40,
    177, 380
  consent to, 60
  in older people, 346
Embeddedness, of anger, 268
Emergency admission, 57, 58
Emergency assessment, 57–58
Emotional abuse, childhood, 327–328
Emotional disorders, in young life,
    316
Employment
  contracts, 51
  in mood disorders, 172–174
  suicide risk and, 192
Endocrine function
  in anorexia nervosa, 251
  antipsychotic drug effects, 151
Enduring and severe mental illness,
    148
  alternative community approaches,
    415–417
  see also Schizophrenia
Engagement, 85–86
  children and adolescents, 322
  in PTSD, 307
English National Board (ENB)
  course no. 603, 314, 337
  course no. 650, 77
Environmental factors, in
    schizophrenia, 149–150, 325
Environmental management
  in anger control, 276
  in children and adolescents, 333
Environmental theory, in nursing
    assessment, 107–108

Epilepsy, temporal lobe, 192–193
Equal opportunities, 16
Ethnic minority groups, 18
European Declaration of Human
    Rights, 51
Evaluation, 121–141
  historic background, 122–123
  service, 122–123, 137–140
  supervision, 129–130
  training, 124–137, 140–141
    discussion section, 141
    fundamental tasks, 137–140
    introduction section, 140
    issues, 125–130
    literature review, 130–137
    methods, 124–125, 140
    results, 141
  see also Audit; Research
Evidence, 380
  alternative treatments, 409, 419
  areas lacking, 2–3
  dissemination, 3–4
  levels, 4–5
  using, 4, 123
  see also Research
Evidence-based practice, 2, 3–5,
    123–124
  alternative treatments, 409, 419
  challenges to, 5–6
  definition, 124, 380
  need for, 5
  process, 4
  in somatic syndromes, 239
  stages, 3–4
Experience, clinical, 4–5
Experiential groups, 331
Experiential knowledge, 402
Experimental designs, 139–140
Expertise, professional, scepticism
    about, 15–16
Expert witnesses, 336
Explosive disorder, intermittent, 268
Exposure therapy
  in agoraphobia, 216, 400–401
  live, 306
  in obsessive–compulsive disorder,
    218
  in phobic disorders, 213, 214, 215
  in PTSD, 299–301, 303, 304–306
  see also Imaginal exposure
Expressed emotion, 157, 181
Expressive need, 378
External Reference Group (ERG), 73
Extrapyramidal side effects, 151
Eye contact, 215
Eye movement desensitisation and
    reprocessing (EMDR),
    302–303

F

Facial disfigurement, 91, 92
Facial pain, atypical, 229
False consensus, 267

Family
    adversity, chronic, 326
    in anorexia nervosa, 246–247,
        254–255
    in bulimia nervosa, 258
    carers see Carers, informal
    in dementia, 359–361
    interventions, in schizophrenia,
        135–136, 157–158
    older people, 345, 352
    in schizophrenia relapse prediction,
        156
    in somatic syndromes, 236–237
    in suicide prevention, 181
    support, 156, 320, 361
    violence, 273
Family history
    children and adolescents, 321–322
    suicide risk and, 193
Family therapists, 335
Family therapy, 332–333
Fatigue, chronic see Chronic fatigue
        syndrome
Fear Questionnaire, 211, 348
Feedback
    in consultations, 91, 96
    during therapy, 238
Ferriar, John, 31
Fertility, in anorexia nervosa, 251
Fibromyalgia, 229
Financial affairs, incapacitated
        patients, 69
Fitness to plead, 64
Flexibility, in consultations, 90
Flooding, 299
Force, 67
    unreasonable, 62
Formulation
    child mental health problems,
        322–323
    client's problems, 93
Fort Clarence Military Hospital,
        Chatham, 37
Fox, Edward, 31
Fractures, pathological, 250
Freud, Sigmund, 188, 324
Functional analysis see Behavioural
        (functional) analysis
Functional illness, 228–229
Functional overlay, 229

G

Gain
    primary, 228
    secondary, 228
Gangrene, in anorexia nervosa, 248,
        251
Gastrointestinal disorders, in anorexia
        nervosa, 251
Gender differences
    anorexia nervosa, 247
    child mental health problems, 315,
        318

    in mood disorders, 169, 173, 175
    PTSD, 293
    suicide risk, 192
Generalisation, 96, 306
Generalised anxiety disorder (GAD),
        in older people, 347, 348, 349
General practitioners (GPs), 77
    in child mental health care, 335
    contact with, before suicide, 193
    in dementia, 358
    in mood disorders, 176
    in paraphrenia, 351
    see also Primary care
Genetic factors
    in anorexia nervosa, 246
    in bulimia nervosa, 257–258
    in child mental health problems,
        325
    in mood disorders, 171, 325
    in schizophrenia, 149–150
George III, King, 30
Gestalt therapy, in children and
        adolescents, 331
Gilles de la Tourette syndrome (TS),
        220, 325, 333–334
Goals, 84
    assessment, 112
    effective, characteristics, 95–97
    interim, 87, 97–98
    promoting achievement, 98–99
    service, identifying, 137–138
    setting, 87, 94–99
    variety, 98
    working towards, 97
Government
    circulars, 50
    policy, 73–78
Greene, John, 38–39, 40
Greetings, in consultations, 85
Gronigen University Hospital crisis
        clinic, Netherlands, 411–412
Group Living Homes, 364
Groups
    interviewing in, 85
    self-help see Self-help groups
Group therapy
    in bulimia nervosa, 259
    children and adolescents, 331–332
    in obsessive–compulsive disorder,
        218
    in phobic disorders, 216
    in schizophrenia, 154, 155
Guardianship, 57, 63
Guardianship Order, 57
Guidelines
    clinical practice, 3, 124
    home visiting, 116–118
    'Guidelines for a Local Charter for
        Users of Mental Health
        Services' (1994), 14, 386
    Guidelines for Professional Practice
        (UKCC 1998), 374–375
Guilt, in PTSD, 308
Gwydir Project, Cambridge,
        415–416

H

Habit problems, 399
Habituation, 304, 306
Hair changes, in anorexia nervosa,
        249
Hallucinations, 155, 169
Handbook for the Instruction of the
        Attendants on the Insane, 35
Hawthorne effect, 133
Health education, 154
Health services
    contact with, before suicide, 193
    mental see Mental health services
Health visitors, 335
Helper Behaviour Rating Scale
        (HBRS), 132
Helpers, non-professional see
        Paraprofessional helpers
History of mental health care, 27–46
HIV infection, 193
Holding powers, nurse's, 57–58, 70
Home, visiting guidelines, 116–118
Home-based care, 153
Homelessness, 193, 416
Homicide Act (1957), 64
Hopelessness, 191, 197
Hopelessness Scale, 115
Hormone implants, 61
Hormone replacement therapy, 250
Hospital Direction Crime (Sentences)
        Act (1997), 58, 65
Hospital Direction Order, 58, 65
Hospitalisation, partial, 408
Hospital Order, 57, 65
    interim, 57, 65
Hospital Plan (1962), 42
Hospitals
    admissions
        compulsory, 55, 56–59
        emergency, 57, 58
        patients unable to consent, 55–56
        voluntary, 55
    compulsory retention, 57–58
    day, 408
    discharge, suicide risk, 200
    psychiatric see Psychiatric
        hospitals
    psychiatric units/wards, 43
    see also In-patient care; Residential
        care
Hospital ships, 38–39
House of Commons Social Services
        Select Committee Report on
        Community Care (1985), 13
Huntington's disease, 355
Hydrotherapy, 39
Hypertension, anger and, 269
Hyperventilation, 210
Hypochondriacal disorder, 229
Hypochondriasis, 226, 229–230
    illness attributions, 233
    perpetuating factors, 233
    treatment, 235, 236, 239
Hypomania, 168, 169

Hypothalamic–pituitary–adrenal
(HPA) axis, in anorexia nervosa,
246, 251
Hypothalamic–pituitary–gonadal axis,
in anorexia nervosa, 251
Hysteria, 228

I

Ideology, of self-help organisations,
394–395
Ignatieff, M., 42
Illness, 227
attributions, 233
Illness behaviour, 230–231
abnormal, 226, 230–231
normal, 230
Imaginal exposure
principles, 305–306
in PTSD, 304–306
rationale, 304–305
Impact of Events Scale (IES), 298
Implosive therapy, 299
Impulse control (disorder), 266, 268
treatment, 274
Incapacity *see* Capacity
Incontinence, phobia about, 213–214
Independent Reference Group (IRG),
73
Independent variables, 131
Index for Managing Memory Loss
(IMMEL), 362
Information
confidentiality, 69–70
for consent, 55
for family carers in dementia,
360–361
gathering, 86, 87–89
for mental patients, 16, 386
primary, 106, 113–115
rewarding client, 91–92
secondary, 106, 115–116
sources, 113
sufficient and necessary, 86–87
Information processing
in anger-prone individuals, 267
deficits, in schizophrenia, 150
models, PTSD, 295
In-patient care
alternatives to traditional, 409,
410–413
in anorexia nervosa, 255
children and adolescents, 333,
335–336
government policies, 76, 77–78
suicidal patients, 198–199, 200
see also Hospitals; Residential care
In-patients, suicide risk, 192, 200
Insanity, 64–65
Insight, 23
Instrumental competency, 378
Instruments
assessment, 114–115, 138
in evaluation, 134

Insulin growth factor, 250
Insulin therapy, 40
Intensive care, psychiatric, 78
Interactive staff training, 133
Interim hospital order, 57, 65
Intermittent explosive disorder, 268
International Classification of
Diseases, 148
International declarations, 51
Interpersonal psychotherapy, in
children and adolescents, 331
Inter-relatedness, of anger, 268
Interventions, therapeutic *see*
Treatment
Interviewing *see* Consultation
Intrusion, in PTSD, 296
Irritability, in PTSD, 308
Irritable bowel syndrome, 229
Isolation, in anorexia nervosa, 255

J

Jepson, George, 31

K

Keyworkers, 62, 157
Kilmainham, Royal Hospital, 37
Kindling, 296

L

Lanugo hair, 249
Law, 49–70
applying to mental health nurses, 51
case, 51
civil, affecting patients, 68–69
criminal, 63–66
arrest and prosecution, 63
court procedures, 63–66
legislation, 50–51, 105
mental health-related, 50–63
after-care/legal responsibilities,
61–63
compulsory detention/treatment,
55–61
enforcement, 52
principles and types of law, 50–51
status and rights of patients, 52–55
see also Mental Health Act (1983)
nursing detained patients, 66–68
preparing reports, 69–70
Law Commission (1995), 53
Laxative abuse, 244, 252
Learned helplessness, 171–172,
295–296
Learning disability, 52, 319
aetiology, 325
in autism, 320
self-injury and, 272
'Learning from each other' (English
National Board 1996), 14–15, 22

Learning Materials on Mental Health, 108
Learning theory, 323–324
Leave, hospital, suicide risk, 200
Legislation, 50–51, 105
Leptin, 246, 258
Lesch–Nyhan syndrome, 272
Lewis, Sir Aubrey, 39
Liability, vicarious, 55
Life events
anorexia nervosa and, 247
in mood disorders, 172
in somatic syndromes, 232
suicide risk, 193, 198
Lincoln Lunatic Asylum, 32–33
Lithium, 176–177, 178
Live exposure, 306
Liver dysfunction, in anorexia nervosa,
251
Liverpool University Neuroleptic Side
Effect Rating Scale (LUNSERS),
153
Living circumstances, suicide risk and,
193
Logs, anger, 275–276, 279
Lomax, Montagu, 35, 36
Loomis, Raymond, 377
Loss, in PTSD, 308–309
Lunatics Act (1845), 32

M

Madhouses, private, 29–31
Magnetic resonance imaging, 150
Mail censorship, 67
Management plan *see* Care plan
Manchester Rating Scale, 115
Mania, 165–182
clinical features, 168
treatment, 176–178
Manic–depression *see* Bi-polar
disorder
Manic Depression Fellowship, 170, 178
Measurement, in evaluation, 131–132,
134
Media, mass, 23–24
Medically unexplained symptoms,
226, 228
Medical Superintendents, 36, 40, 42–43
Medication
in alternative treatment services,
417–418
children and adolescents, 317,
319–320, 333–334
consent to, 60
in mood disorders, 176–177
nursing roles, 152–153
in obsessive–compulsive disorder,
219
in paraphrenia, 351
in schizophrenia, 150–153
self-, 178–179
Medico-Psychological Association
(MPA), 35
Memory deficits, in schizophrenia, 150

Menarche, early, in bulimia nervosa, 258
Mens rea, 64
Mental disorder
    criminal justice system, 63–66
    legal categories, 59
    parental, 326
    see also Mental illness
Mental guards, 38
Mental Health Act (1959), 56
Mental Health Act (1983), 56–61
    Codes of Practice, 50–51
    consent to treatment, 59–61
    formal admission procedures, 56–59
    protections for nurses, 52
    section 117, 62
    status and rights of patients, 13–14, 18, 52–54, 386
Mental Health Act Commission (MHAC), 56
Mental health care
    early forms, 29–32
    history, 27–46
    organisation, 73–78
Mental Health (Northern Ireland) Order (1986), 50
Mental health nurses
    changing status of mental patients and, 24–25
    children and adolescents, 336–337
    consent to treatment and, 60
    current problems, 45–46
    in early twentieth-century, 36–37
    law applying to, 51
    Mental Health Review Tribunals and, 61
    military, 38–39
    power over patients, 18
    primary care team attachment, 45
    recent history, 41, 43, 44
    reports for courts/statutory bodies, 69–70
    training *see* Training
    see also Community psychiatric nurses
Mental health nursing
    child and adolescent, 314–315
    evaluation, 122–141
    government policies, 76–78
    history, 27–46
    recent developments, 74–75
Mental Health (Patients in the Community) Act (1995), 18, 58, 62–63
Mental Health Review Tribunal (MHRT), 56, 61, 69
Mental Health (Scotland) Act (1984), 50
Mental health services
    children and adolescents, 334–337
    current difficulties, 44–46
    evaluation, 122–123, 137–140
    government policies for modernising, 75–78
    recent developments, 74–75
    in schizophrenia, 153–154

user involvement, 13–15, 19–20, 410
users *see* Patients, mental
    variability, 18
    see also Alternative treatments
Mental Health Task Force, 14
Mental hospitals *see* Psychiatric hospitals
Mental Hygiene movement, 35–36
Mental illness
    in anorexia nervosa, 245
    in nurses, 21–22
    patients as experts on, 22–23
    in PTSD, 293
    self-injury and, 272
    somatic syndromes, 232
    suicide risk, 190–192
    violence and, 273
    see also Mental disorder
Mental impairment, 59
Mental state
    in anorexia nervosa, 248
    assessment, 107
        in anorexia nervosa, 249
Meta-analyses, 5–6
Methylphenidate, 334
Military psychiatry, 37–39
Mills, Hannah, 31
Milton Keynes Advocacy Group, 388
Mind–body dualism, 226, 227, 239
MIND (National Association for Mental Health), 14, 154
    on advocacy, 379, 384
A Mind That Found Itself (Clifford Beers), 35
Modelling, 99, 218, 329
'Modernising Mental Health Services' (1998), 75–78
Monasteries, 29
Mood, self-monitoring, 179
Mood disorders, 165–182
    aetiological theories, 171–172
    concept, 166–167
    continuum, 167, 168
    epidemiology, 168–169
    nursing roles, 179–182
    presenting symptoms, 168–169
    prognosis and outcome, 169
    relapse, early signs, 179, 180–181
    social and occupational effects, 172–176
    suicide and parasuicide, 169–171, 190–191
    treatment approaches, 176–178
    see also Bi-polar disorder; Depression
Moral treatment movement, 31–32
'Muffling', 30
Multiple Sclerosis, 395
Musculoskeletal problems, in anorexia nervosa, 249–250
Mutual aid groups *see* Self-help groups
Mutuality concept, 360
Myalgic encephalitis (ME) *see* Chronic fatigue syndrome

N

Narcosis, continuous, 38, 39–40
Narcotics Anonymous, 395
National Boards, 74
National Citizens Advocacy Resource and Advisory Centre, 388
National Committee for Mental Hygiene, 35
National Health Service (NHS)
    early years, 40–41
    government policies, 75–77
National Health Service and Community Care Act (1990), 105, 358
National Hearing Voices Network, 22
National Institute for Clinical Excellence (NICE), 73
National Review of Mental Nursing (1924), 36–37
National Schizophrenia Fellowship, 154, 159
National Self-Harm Network, 22
National Service Framework (NSF), 73, 76, 77
Need
    assessment, 105, 138
    expressive, 378
Negative thoughts, 238
Neglect, childhood, 327–328
Negligence, law of, 54–55
Negotiation, 94
Netherlands
    Clientbond advocacy scheme, 382–383
    Gronigen University Hospital crisis clinic, 411–412
Netley Military Hospital, 37–38
Networking, by case managers, 154
Neurasthenia, 229
Neurodevelopmental factors, in child mental health problems, 325
Neuroleptic drugs *see* Antipsychotic drugs
Nightingale, Florence, 122
Non-accidental injury *see* Physical abuse, childhood
Non-compliance *see* Compliance
No Panic, 394, 399
Northwest Evaluation Center (NEC), Seattle, 412, 417
Nottingham Advocacy Group (NAG), 383–384
Nottingham Patients Council Support Group, 388
Novaco Anger Scale, 275
Numbing, emotional, in PTSD, 292, 308
Nurses
    in nineteenth-century asylums, 34–35
    as advocates, 374–376, 379–380, ?
    assault on, 68
    in criminal proceedings, 6?
    holding powers, 57–58, ?

Nurses (*contd*)
law of negligence, 54–55
mentally ill, 21–22
practice, 77
protections in law, 52
school, 335
seclusion of patients, 68
see also Community psychiatric
nurses; Mental health nurses
Nurses, Midwives and Health Visitors
Act (1997), 51
Nurse therapists, 77, 84, 221–222
efficacy, 222
in phobias and obsessive disorders,
208, 219, 222
training, 221–222
Nursing
assessment, 106–118
mental health *see* Mental health
nursing
models, 107
Nursing assistants, 140

O

Obesity, bulimia nervosa and, 258
Objectives, in consultations, 84
Observation
anger-prone individuals, 275
suicidal patients, 200
Obsessional personality, in anorexia
nervosa, 247, 248
Obsessions, 217
Obsessive–compulsive disorder
(OCD), 208, 217–220
in children and adolescents, 316,
325, 333–334
treatment, 217–219, 333–334
outcome measures, 220
ruminations versus rituals, 219
with/without tics, 220, 325
Obsessive rituals *see* Rituals, obsessive
Obsessive ruminations, 217
outcome of treatment, 219
treatment, 217–218, 219
Obsessive slowness, 219
Occupation
in mood disorders, 172–174
suicide risk and, 192
Occupational Stress Indicator, 138
Olanzapine, 152
Older people, 341–364
alcohol misuse, 351–354
anxiety disorders, 346–349
dementia, 354–364
depression, 342–346, 348
government policies, 76, 77
schizophrenia, paraphrenia and
paranoia, 349–351
suicide risk, 192, 344
Open-door policies, 41
Open trials, 396
Opinion, personal clinical, 4–5
Oppositional disorder, 318, 319

Orientation, treatment, 87, 89–94
Osteoporosis, 250
Outcomes
goal-setting and, 98
measuring
in evaluation, 134
in self-help studies, 396
treatment, 95
Overcrowding, in mental hospitals, 41
Overdose, drug *see* Drug overdose
Overeaters Anonymous (OA), 394–395

P

Padua Inventory, 348
Pain, chronic, 232–233, 235, 239
post-traumatic, 309
Panic attacks, 209–210
management, 210
in social phobia, 214–215
Panic Cognitions Inventory, 211
Panic disorder, 209–212
definition, 209
in older people, 349
treatment, 210–212
assessment, 210–211
evaluation, 212
interventions, 212
self-help, 399–401
Paradoxical intention, 215
Paranoia, in old age, 349–351
Paraphrenia, 349–351
late, 349, 350
Paraprofessional helpers, 396
training, 126–128
versus professionals, 397–398
Parasuicide, 169–171
perception of risk, 194
previous, 193–194, 197
in PTSD, 307–308
see also Deliberate self-harm; Suicide
Parenting characteristics, 327
Parents
adult child carers, 360
during child interviews, 321
early loss, 193, 326
history taking from, 321–322
mental disorder in, 326
Participation, 20, 386
Pathfinder Trust, 21
Patients, mental (service users, clients),
11–25
as advocates, 384
approaches to, in consultation, 82–84
in asylums, 33–34, 35–36
as care providers, 20–22, 154
as citizens, 23–24
civil law matters, 68–69
detained *see* Detained patients
as experts on madness, 22–23
individualism, 52–54
interviewing *see* Consultation
involvement in services, 13–15,
19–20, 410

self-advocacy, 377, 383
self-descriptions, 17
social problems, 45
status and rights, 12, 13–15, 25, 386
implications for nurses, 24–25
legal aspects, 13–14, 18, 52–55,
386
reasons for changes, 15–16
see also Consumers of mental health
care
Patients' Charter Mental Health
Services (1997), 18
Patients' charters, 14, 385–386
Pemoline, 334
Perceptual matching, 267
Percival, John, 377
Perfectionism, in anorexia nervosa,
247, 248, 253, 254
Personality, type A, 269–270
Personality disorder
in anorexia nervosa, 245
in bulimia nervosa, 257
self-help, 399
suicide risk, 191
Personal relationships, close, 172
Personhood, in dementia, 362
Personne *see* Staff
Pharmacotherapy *see* Medication
Phobias, 208, 209–216
in children and adolescents, 316
in older people, 347–348
panic disorder and, 209–212
school, 317
self-help treatments, 399
specific (simple), 212–214
in older people, 347
treatment, 213–214
see also Agoraphobia; Social phobia
Physical abuse, childhood, 273, 327
in bulimia nervosa, 258–259
Physical health
child mental health problems and,
328
effects of anger, 269–270
in schizophrenia, 77
suicide risk and, 192–193
Piaget, Jean, 323
Pick's disease, 354, 355
Place of Safety Order, 57
Planning
consultations, 84–85
treatment, 94–99
Play therapy, 324
Police, 63, 67
Police and Criminal Evidence Act
(1984), 63
Population statistics, 122
Positron emission tomography (PET),
150
Post-infectious fatigue syndrome *see*
Chronic fatigue syndrome
Post-traumatic disorders, 291–309
Post-traumatic stress disorder (PTSD),
222, 292–309
assessment, 297

Post-traumatic stress disorder (*contd*)
  bulimia nervosa, 257
  in children and adolescents, 325
  clinical features, 292
  clinical supervision, 309
  comorbidity, 293
  measurement, 298
  prevalence, 292–293
  theoretical models, 293–297
    behavioural model, 293–294
    biological models, 295–296
    cognitive/information processing
      models, 294–295
    psychodynamic models, 296
    psychosocial models, 296–297
  treatment, 298–304
    cognitive–behaviour therapy,
      299–302, 304, 305–307
    difficulties, 307–309
    exposure therapy, 299–301, 303,
      304–306
    eye movement desensitisation and
      reprocessing, 302–303
    medication, 303
    process, 304–309
    psycho-analytical therapy,
      298–299
    rationale, 304–305
    timing, 304
Post-traumatic stress disorder
    symptom scale (PSS), 298
Potassium iodide, 33
Powell, Enoch, 42
Practice nurses, 77
Prenatal factors, in schizophrenia,
    149–150, 325
Prestwick Asylum, 36
Primary care
  government policies, 76, 77–78
  somatic symptoms, 226–227
  team, 45, 77
  see also General practitioners
Prisoners, transfer of sentenced, 57, 61,
    65
Prison Transfer Order, 57, 65
Problem and targets rating, in PTSD,
    298
Problem assessment, 108
Problem-solving strategies, in suicide
    prevention, 201–203
Project 2000, 44, 45
Project Two, 377
Prolactin, 151
Prolonged exposure (PE), in PTSD,
    299–300
Proof, levels of, 52
Psychiatric disorders *see* Mental
    disorder; Mental illness
Psychiatric hospitals
  break-up, 15, 43–44
  history, 28, 36–37, 40–43
  military, 37–39
  see also Asylums
'Psychiatric Nursing Today and
    Tomorrow' (1968), 43

Psychiatric units/wards, 43
  substance misuse in, 158
Psychiatrists
  in alternative services, 418
  in case management, 153
  in child mental health care, 335
  in criminal proceedings, 65–66
  military, 38, 39, 40
  in mood disorders, 176
  support for advocacy, 381
Psychiatry
  history, 27–46
  military, 37–39
  post-war period, 39–41
  war-time, 38–39
Psycho-analytical therapy, PTSD,
    298–299
Psycho-analytic theory, depression and
    mania, 171
Psychodrama, 331
Psychodynamic theory
  child mental health problems, 324
  depression and mania, 171
  PTSD, 296
Psychodynamic therapy
  in children and adolescents, 331
  PTSD, 298–299
Psycho-education
  client, 97
    in mood disorders, 179, 181
  family
    in mood disorders, 181
    in schizophrenia, 157
    in suicide prevention, 181
Psychological factors, in anorexia
    nervosa, 247
Psychological theories of
    development, 323–324
Psychological treatments
  children and adolescents, 328–333
  in mood disorders, 178
  in schizophrenia, 154–155
Psychologists
  in criminal proceedings, 66
  educational, 335
  in mood disorders, 176
Psychopathic disorder, 59, 65
Psychosis
  in older people, 349–351
  symptom assessment, 114
  violence and, 273
Psychosocial assessment, 107–108
Psychosocial interventions
  in deliberate self-harm, 199,
    201–203
  in older people, 346, 351
  training, 133
Psychosocial models, PTSD, 296–297
Psychosomatic disorders, 227–228
Psychosurgery, 61
Psychotherapists
  child, 335
  in mood disorders, 176
Psychotherapy
  in anorexia nervosa, 255

  in bulimia nervosa, 259
  in children and adolescents, 317,
    331–332
  meta-analyses, 6
  in older people, 346
PTSD *see* Post-traumatic stress
    disorder
Pulling Together (Sainsbury Centre
    1997), 76, 104, 159
Punishment, 329

Q

Quality of life, in mood disorders, 172,
    176
Questions, 81–82
  closed, 89, 90
  general to specific, 89–90
  open, 90
  using statements as, 90
Quetiapine, 152

R

Random allocation, 131, 139
Randomised controlled trials (RCTs),
    3, 5, 396
Rape trauma syndrome, 292
Rape victims
  PTSD prevalence, 292–293
  PTSD treatment, 301, 307
  see also Sexual assault victims
Reassurance-seeking, in obsessive–
    compulsive disorder, 218
Re C (Adult: Refusal of Treatment)
    (1994), 53
Records
  access of patients to, 16
  in anger management, 275–276,
    279
  of consultations, 85
  legal aspects, 52, 68
  patients' rights, 386
  previous, 115
Redirecting clients, in consultations,
    90–91
Re-experiencing symptoms, in PTSD,
    292, 296
Referrals, 112–113
  children and adolescents, 321
  client awareness of, 113
  data provided in, 84–85
  risk assessment, 109
  urgency, 112–113
Rehearsal, in anger management, 277
Reinforcement, 80
  in children and adolescents, 329
  in consultations, 91–92, 98–99
  differential, 92, 329
  self-, 99
  in self-injury, 272
  in token economy systems, 154–155
  vicarious, 99

Relapse
early intervention, 156–157
early warning signs, 156, 179,
180–181
Relatives *see* Family
Relaxation techniques
in anger management, 277, 282
in anxious older people, 349
in children and adolescents, 329
Reliability, suicide rating scales, 196
Remand, 63–64
Remand Order, 57
Reports, for courts/statutory bodies,
63, 69–70
Representation, 20
Reproductive function, in anorexia
nervosa, 251
Research, 2
child mental health problems, 337
deficits in nursing, 6
explanatory, 123
pragmatic, 123
role of self-help groups, 395
study design *see* Study design
synopses of published, 6
versus service evaluation, 122–123
see also Evaluation; Evidence
Research and development
programme, 124, 125
Residential care
children and adolescents, 333,
335–336
in dementia, 357, 358, 364
government policies, 78
non-institutional alternatives, 409
acutely ill patients, 410–412
severe mental illness, 412
unconventional, 412–413
see also Hospitals; In-patient care
Resilience–protective factors, in
children, 328
Respect, personal, 386
Response-prevention, 217, 218
Responsibility, diminished, 50, 64–65
Responsible medical officer (RMO), 57,
60
Restraint, physical, 54, 67, 272
The Retreat, York, 31, 32
Risk
assessment, 108–109, 110–111
suicide *see* Suicide, risk
assessment
definition, 108
formulation, 198
Risk-taking behaviour, 170
Risperidone, 152
Rituals, obsessive, 217
in anorexia nervosa, 248
outcome of treatment, 219
treatment approaches, 217–218
Roberts, Sam, 30
Role play, 155, 277, 283
Room, searching, 66
Royal College of Nursing, 39
Royal Naval Hospital, Chatham, 38

Royal Naval Hospital, Great
Yarmouth, 37
*R. v. Bournewood Community and Mental
Health NHS Trust* (1997), 55–56

S

Safety
home visiting, 116–118
nursing detained patients, 66–68
Sainsbury Centre for Mental Health,
76, 104, 159, 160
Salivary gland hypertrophy, 251
Salmon Report (1966), 43
SANE, 24, 395
Santa Clara County clustered
apartment project (SCCCAP),
413–414
Scale for Predicting Subsequent
Suicidal Behaviour (SPSSB),
196, 197
Scene-setting, 85–86
Schemas, personal
in anger-prone individuals, 267
in anorexia nervosa, 253
in PTSD, 296
Schizophrenia, 147–161
causation, 149–150, 325
in children and adolescents, 334
clinical presentation and types,
148–149
clinical standards, 74
community approaches, 415–416
drug treatments, 150–153
dual diagnosis, 158–159
early intervention, 155–157
family-based interventions, 135–136,
157–158
late-onset, 349
models of service delivery, 153–154
in older people, 349–351
assessment and interventions,
350–351
characteristics and prevalence,
349–350
parental, 326
physical health, 77
psychological interventions, 154–155
relapse, 156–157, 180
self-injury, 272
suicide prevention, 203
suicide risk, 191
training, 133, 159–160
Schizophrenia a National Emergency
(SANE), 24, 395
School
in attention-deficit–hyperactivity
disorders, 319
history, 321
in in-patient units, 333
nurses, 335
phobia, 317
refusal, 317, 329
therapeutic community, 333

School medical officers, 335
Schwab–Gilleard Depression Scale, 345
Scott, Dr (military surgeon), 37
Searching, room, 66
Seclusion, 68
Second opinion, treatment requiring,
60, 61
Selective serotonin reuptake inhibitors
(SSRIs), 177, 219, 259, 333
Self, in anorexia nervosa, 253
Self-advocacy, 17, 377, 383
Self-esteem, 174–175, 270–271
Self-harm, deliberate *see* Deliberate
self-harm
Self-help, 391–403
in agoraphobia and panic, 216,
399–401
benefits, 401–402
efficacy and clinical effectiveness,
396
history and background, 392–393
literature review, 396–402
in mood disorders, 178–179, 181, 399
in PTSD, 300
in somatic syndromes, 239
terminology, 392–393
treatments, 398–399
trends, 15–16
versus professional treatments,
397–398
Self-help groups, 16, 19, 20–21, 239, 392
advocates, 384
collaboration with, 402–403
definition, 392
in dementia, 363
ideology, 394–395
numbers using, 393
origins, 393
range of services, 395–396
in UK, 393–396
Self-injury *see* Deliberate self-harm
Self-instructional training (SIT), in
anger management, 277, 282
Self-monitoring, anger, 275
Self-reinforcement, 99
Self-report questionnaires, 275, 315
Sensitivity, suicide rating scales,
196–197
Sentencing, mentally disordered
offenders, 65–66
Separation anxiety, 316–317, 323
Serotonin (5HT), in eating disorders,
246, 258
Services, mental health *see* Mental
health services
Service users *see* Patients, mental
Sex differences *see* Gender differences
Sexual abuse, childhood, 327, 328
in bulimia nervosa, 258–259
Sexual assault victims
exposure therapy, 300–301, 306
psycho-analytical therapy, 298–299
see also Rape victims
Shadowing, 396
Shaftesbury, Lord, 32

Shaping, 92, 329
Sheffield psychotherapy project, 132, 138
Short Risk Scale (SRS), 197
Significance
    clinical, 125, 134–135
    statistical, 134
Silcock, Ben, 23–24
Single photon emission tomography (SPET), 150
Single subject (n = 1) experiments, 94, 95, 139–140, 396
    ABAB (reversal) design, 139
    ABA (withdrawal) design, 139
    multiple baseline design, 139
    multiple phase design, 139
Skilled helping model (Egan), 81
Skin changes, in anorexia nervosa, 249
Sleep, routines, 237
Slowness, obsessive, 219
Social effects, depression, 172–176
Social factors
    in anorexia nervosa, 246
    in child mental health problems, 325–328
Social functioning
    children and adolescents, 322
    in depression and mania, 175–176
Social isolation, suicide risk, 193
Social learning theory, 98, 329
Social Network Scale (SNS), 115
Social phobia, 213, 214–216
    definition, 213
    in older people, 347
    three systems analysis, 88
    treatment, 215–216
Social services
    aftercare of discharged patients, 62, 63
    in dementia, 358–359
    government policies, 75–76
Social skills training
    in anger management, 277, 283
    in facial disfigurement, 91, 92
    in schizophrenia, 155
    in social phobia, 215–216
Social support
    older people, 349, 353
    somatic syndromes and, 232
Social workers
    in child mental health care, 335
    in compulsory detention, 56, 58
    in criminal proceedings, 66
Society of Registered Male Nurses, 39
Sociocultural factors, in bulimia nervosa, 258–259
Somatic symptoms (syndromes), 226
    aetiology and model, 231–233
    classification, 229
    cognitive–behaviour therapy (CBT), 233–239
    concepts and definitions, 227–231
    epidemiology, 226–227
    evidence-based practice, 239
    perpetuating factors, 231, 232–233

precipitating factors, 231, 232
predisposing factors, 231–232
Somatisation, 226, 227–228
    in children and adolescents, 328
    disorder, 229, 230
Somatoform disorders, 229–230
Sorbitol, 251
Soteria Berne, 413
Soteria Project, 412–413
Specificity, suicide rating scales, 196–197
Specifiers, 88–89
Speech therapists, 335
Speech therapy, 320
Spider phobia, 213
Spielberger State-Trait Anxiety Inventory, 348
Staff
    in nineteenth-century asylums, 34–35
    in alternative services, 418
    in anger management, 276
    assault against, 68
    mental hospitals in 1960s, 41, 43
    substance misuse by, 158
    violence towards, 273
    see also Doctors; Nurses
Standards
    of care, 74
    legal, 54–55
Standing Nursing Midwifery Advisory Committee (SNMAC), 78
Stanley Royds Patients Council, 388
State-Trait Anger Expression Inventory (STAXI), 271, 275
Stephenson, Dr G.V., 38
Stimulus–response theories, 329
Stockport Arts on Prescription, 414
Stress
    in child mental health problems, 325
    on family carers in dementia, 359–360
    in relapse of schizophrenia, 156–157
    staff, 44
    suicide risk, 198
    see also Life events
Stress inoculation training (SIT)
    in anger management, 274–275
    in PTSD, 299–300, 301, 303
Stress response syndrome, 296
Stress vulnerability model, 157
Structured Clinical Interview, 220
Study design, 139–140, 396
    nurse training evaluation, 134
Subjective units of discomfort (SUDS), 302
Substance abuse
    in PTSD, 293
    in schizophrenia, 158–159
    see also Alcohol abuse; Drug misuse
Sudden death, in anorexia nervosa, 251
Suicidal ideation (thoughts), 193, 197
Suicide, 187–204
    aetiology, 189–190

in bi-polar disorder, 169–170
in children and adolescents, 318
in dementia, 362–363
in depression, 169, 170–171, 190–191
interventions (prevention), 181–182, 199–203
in mood disorders, 169–171, 190–191
in older people, 192, 344
previous attempted, 193–194, 197
rating scales, 196–197
risk
    immediate, 200–201
    long-term, 199–200, 203
risk assessment, 197–199
    in clinical judgement, 198–199
    formulation, 198
    problems, 195–197
risk factors, 181, 190–195
    psychiatric, 190–192
    socioeconomic, 192–193
    in schizophrenia, 191
    theoretical explanations, 188–189
    see also Deliberate self-harm; Parasuicide
Superintendents, Medical, 36, 40, 42–43
Supervised Discharge Order (SDO), 58, 62, 105
Supervision, clinical, 128–130
    anorexia nervosa therapists, 254
    definition, 128
    evaluation, 129–130
    models, 128–129
    PTSD therapists, 309
Supervision Register, 62, 105
Support groups see Self-help groups
Survivors Speak Out, 377, 388
Swing, circling, 30
Symptoms
    medically unexplained, 226, 228
    somatic see Somatic symptoms

T

Teachers, 335
Teams
    community mental health (CMHT), 105–106
    primary health care, 45, 77
Temperament, 321, 324–325
Testamentary capacity, 69
Therapeutic alliance, 80
    in anger management, 276
    in anorexia nervosa, 253
    building, 89–94
    commencement, 87
    in mood disorders, 179–180
    in PTSD, 304
    in schizophrenia, 351
    in somatic syndromes, 234–235
Therapeutic community, 41
    schools, 333
Therapeutic milieu, 333
Therapeutic nihilism, 235

Therapists
non-professional *see*
Paraprofessional helpers
nurse *see* Nurse therapists
supervision *see* Supervision, clinical
training *see* Training
Thorn Programme, 104–105, 153,
159–160
Thought stopping, 277, 282
Three systems model (Lang), 87–88,
233–234, 239–240
Thunder and lightning phobia, 214
Tics, 220, 325
Time out, 329
Token economy systems, 154–155
Tourette's syndrome (TS), 220, 325,
333–334
Training
in nineteenth-century asylums,
34–35
in child and adolescent psychiatric
nursing, 314, 337
clinical significance, 134–135
cognitive–behaviour therapy (CBT),
221–222, 240
dependent variables, 134
effectiveness, 125–128
efficiency, 136–137
evaluation *see* Evaluation, training
external validity, 135–136
innovations, 104–105
internal validity, 130–134
in interviewing skills, 84
long-term effects, 160
non-professional helpers, 126–128
nurse therapists, 221–222
patient-centred, 136–137
Project 2000, 44, 45
recent history, 41, 44
in schizophrenia care, 159–160
Tranquillisers, minor, 348
Transformationality, of anger, 268
Traumatophobia, 292
Treatment
alternative *see* Alternative
treatments
compulsory, 18, 57, 60–61
computers in, 77
conditions for effective, 82
consent to, 53–54, 59–61
detained patients *see* Detained
patients, treatment

discharged patients, 62–63
forcible, 54
history, 30, 33, 39–40, 41, 43
information about, 16
orientation, 87, 89–94
patients' charter, 386
plan *see* Care plan
by professionals versus
paraprofessionals, 397–398
rationales, offering, 92–94
self-help, 398–399
traditional, 408–409
urgent, 60–61
Treatment Order, 57, 58, 59
Trespass law, 54
Tricyclic antidepressants, 177, 333
Truancy, 317
Tuke, William, 31, 32
Turning Point, 415–416
12-step approaches, 394–395
2000 year stare, 38
Type A personality, 269–270

U

Undernutrition, in anorexia nervosa,
248–249
Unipolar disorder, 166
United Kingdom Advocacy Network
(UKAN), 377, 388
United Kingdom Central Council for
Nursing, Midwifery and Health
Visiting (UKCC), 51, 74
Code of Professional Conduct, 51,
69–70
Guidelines for Professional Practice,
374–375
United Kingdom Council for
Psychotherapy, 222
Users, service *see* Patients, mental

V

Validity
external (ecological), 123, 125, 131,
135–136
internal, 123, 125, 130–132
in nurse training studies, 132–134
trade-off with external, 134
suicide rating scales, 196, 197

Validity of cognition (VOC) scale, 302
Venture Vancouver, 411
Violence, 266
anger and, 272–273
definition, 272
in dual diagnosis patients, 158
family (domestic), 273
prevention, 273–286
public perceptions, 24
risk assessment, 108–109
self-esteem and, 270–271
towards care staff, 273
see also Aggression; Anger
Visitors, detained patients, 67
Vita (hospital ship), 38–39
Volunteers, 395–396
see also Paraprofessional helpers
Vomiting, in anorexia nervosa, 250

W

Walsh, P., 375–376, 379
Ward Atmosphere Scale, 137
War neurosis, 292
War-time psychiatry, 38–39
War veterans, PTSD, 293, 299–300, 302
Watt, Christian, 33–34
Weight
in anorexia nervosa, 248–249, 256
control, in eating disorders, 245, 249,
257
Well-being, in dementia, 362
Whitby advocacy project, 384–385
Wills, making, 69
Women, service needs, 18
Worcester Pauper Lunatic Asylum, 33
Work *see* Employment
Work and Social Adjustment Scale, 298
'Working in Partnership. A
Collaborative Approach to
Care' (1994), 14, 74
Working through, 296
World War II, 38–39
Worry Scale, 348

Y

Yale Brown Obsessive Compulsive
Scale (YBOCS), 220
Young offenders, 277, 318–319